AF567081

Transcranial Magnetic Stimulation and Transcranial Direct Current Stimulation

Proceedings of the 2nd International TMS and tDCS Symposium

Transcranial Magnetic Stimulation and Transcranial Direct Current Stimulation

Proceedings of the 2nd International Transcranial Magnetic Stimulation (TMS) and Transcranial Direct Current Stimulation (tDCS) Symposium, Göttingen, Germany, 11–14 June, 2003

EDITED BY

W. PAULUS, F. TERGAU, M.A. NITSCHE

Department of Clinical Neurophysiology, University of Göttingen, Robert Koch Strasse 40, D-37075 Göttingen, Germany

J.G. ROTHWELL

Sobell Department of Neurophysiology, Institute of Neurology, Queen Square, London WC1N 3BG, UK

U. ZIEMANN

Clinic of Neurology, Johann Wolfgang Goethe-University Frankfurt, Schleusenweg 2–16, D-60528 Frankfurt am Main, Germany

M. HALLETT

National Institutes of Health, NINDS, NIH, Building 10, Room 5N226, 10 Center Drive, MSC 1428, Bethesda, MD 20892-1428, USA

SUPPLEMENTS TO CLINICAL NEUROPHYSIOLOGY
VOLUME 56
2003

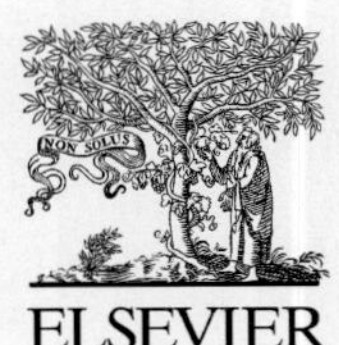

ELSEVIER

ELSEVIER SCIENCE B.V.
Sara Burgerhartstraat 25
P.O. Box 211, 1000 AE Amsterdam, The Netherlands

First edition 2003

Library of Congress Cataloging in Publication Data
A catalog record from the Library of Congress has been applied for.

British Library Cataloguing in Publication Data
A catalogue record from the British Library has been applied for.

ISBN: 0-444-51438-4 (this volume)
ISSN (series): 1567-424X

∞ The paper used in this publication meets the requirements of ANSI/NISO Z39.48-1992 (Permanence of Paper).
Printed in The Netherlands.

Welcome Address

Greetings from Lutz Stratmann, Minister of Science and Culture in Lower Saxony

2nd International TMS and tDCS Symposium, Göttingen, 11–14 June 2003

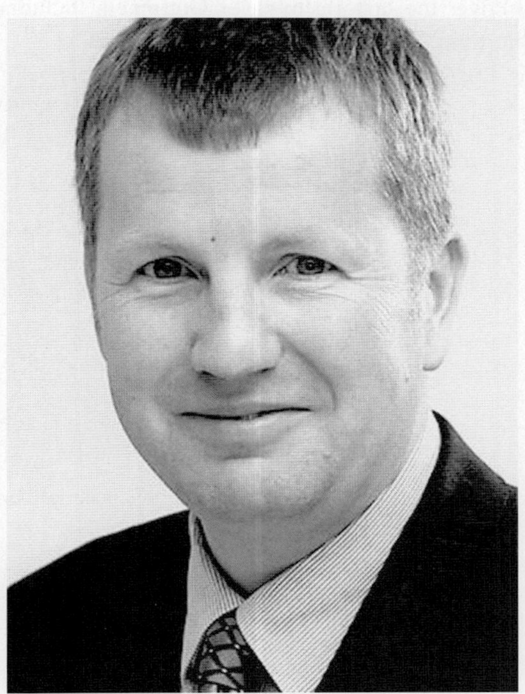

Dear Symposium Participants,

It is a great pleasure for me to welcome you all in Göttingen for the 2nd International Symposium on TMS and tDCS. The government of the *State* of Lower Saxony is particularly interested in the promotion of science. In Lower Saxony we have 26 Universities and Universities of Applied Sciences. The Georg August University, founded over 260 years ago in 1737, has the longest tradition. Since its foundation, this University has developed a worldwide reputation. Last year an exhibition presented all of the Nobel Prize winners who had ever lived or worked in Göttingen – an impressive total of over 40.

Göttingen also has a long-standing tradition in neuroscience dating back several decades. In recent years the first European Neuroscience Institute, a Centre of Molecular Physiology of the Brain (CMPB) and an MRI research group, as well as the research at the German Primate Centre, have seen Göttingen grow into an internationally recognized centre of neurosciences. The DFG European Graduiertenkolleg GRK 632 has just been funded for another 3 years. It strongly facilitates postgraduate training in an exchange between Göttingen and London; some of the project leaders are attending this symposium. As you may have noticed, this symposium is part of the long-established Göttingen Neurobiology Conference, which was founded by Otto Creutzfeldt some 30 years ago, and is now organized as a bi-annual meeting of the German Neuroscience Society by Norbert Elsner. I am delighted that the University is able to provide the conference facilities, thus facilitating the traditionally low conference fees. This in turn traditionally attracts a large number of young scientists and students.

I am quite sure that you will enjoy not only the scientific spirit of this meeting, but also be able to look beyond the bounds of transcranial magnetic and direct current stimulation into other areas of neuroscience. I would also encourage you to discover the historic town of Göttingen, including some of the university buildings, if this is possible within the time constraints of your conference.

Preface

TRANSCRANIAL MAGNETIC AND DIRECT CURRENT STIMULATION 2003: WHERE TO GO?

The 2nd International Conference on transcranial magnetic stimulation (TMS) and transcranial direct current stimulation (tDCS) brought together some 200 scientists from all over the world in order to discuss the most recent results on both techniques. Forty-four of the contributions are collected in this volume. TMS has the ability to examine the excitability of the brain and to explore cortical physiology. This has been investigated most extensively in the motor system, but other systems such as visual function and speech have also been studied.

A large variety of techniques are now available, and many of these were discussed at the conference. Here we summarize some recent developments in the field, due to space limitations only a small part of the book content can be referred to in this introductory chapter.

Motor cortex physiology

Single-pulse and paired-pulse TMS have now been developed as a sophisticated probe of motor cortex excitability. This is a relatively new field which has already enormously improved our understanding of motor cortex physiology and plasticity. Five major routes have contributed to progress of knowledge.

(1) Experiments in monkeys (laboratory of Roger Lemon, London, UK) focus on the nature of the direct or D-response to TMS and the more complex indirect or I-wave components. One important finding is that, in particular, the late I-waves (I2, I3 etc.) can be strongly facilitated by input from premotor areas. This research will enhance our understanding of cortico-cortical interactions. It is particularly relevant for understanding the effects of TMS and rTMS of premotor areas on the excitability of the primary motor cortex.

(2) Epidural recordings from the cervical spinal cord (laboratory of Vincenzo Di Lazzaro, Rome, Italy) explored systematically the conditions under which D- and I-waves are generated by TMS of the motor cortex in humans. D-waves originate from the cortico-spinal axon distal to the initial axon segment when either anodal transcranial electrical stimulation or a focal eight-shaped stimulating coil is used with the induced current in the brain directed from lateral to medial. This distal D-wave is resistant to changes of motor cortical excitability. A proximal D-wave is generated at the initial axon segment with a non-focal coil centered over the vertex, or when using a focal coil with the induced current in the brain directed from anterior to posterior. The first I-wave (I1) is preferentially activated by focal TMS with the induced current in the brain directed from posterior to anterior, while late I-waves (I2, I3, etc.) are preferentially activated with current in the reverse direction. The proximal D-wave and I-waves are sensitive to various extents to changes in motor cortical excitability. Inhibitory influences seem to affect late I-waves and leave the early I-waves unaffected. These experiments are extremely important because they open up avenues of how to

test effects of manipulation on the different parts of the cortico-spinal neuron and the network of motor cortical inter-neurons connected to it.

(3) Several different excitatory and inhibitory systems in the human motor cortex can be tested by TMS in conditioning–test protocols. These include short-interval intracortical inhibition (SICI), long-interval intracortical inhibition (LICI), intracortical facilitation (ICF), interhemispheric inhibition (IHI), short-latency afferent inhibition (SLAI) and long-latency afferent inhibition (LLAI). While considerable information has been known about most of these phenomena individually (see Proceedings to the International Symposium on TMS, Suppl. 51 to Electroencephalography and Clinical Neurophysiology, Elsevier 1999) recent studies started to explore the interactions between them (laboratory of Robert Chen, Toronto, Canada). Interactions are tested by looking at the changes of one excitability measure in the presence of another one. Clearly there are many types of inhibitory neurons in the brain, and these synapse on each other in addition to synapsing on excitatory neurons. TMS may well be able to work out some of the intracortical circuitry. Also the functional role of inhibition in normal and pathological movement is beginning to be explored. Important finding among many others are that different neuronal circuits mediate SICI and LICI and that LICI inhibits SICI. Very likely, SICI is regulated through the $GABA_A$ receptor, LICI through the $GABA_B$ receptor, and the inhibition of SICI by LICI is brought about by presynaptic $GABA_B$ receptor mediated auto-inhibition. This kind of experiments is extraordinarily important because they allow drawing models of interactions between different inhibitory and excitatory systems in human motor cortex. It is likely that this will be developed in the near future into a new way of studying the motor cortical pathophysiology of neurological and psychiatric disorders at the level of distinct inhibitory and excitatory circuits.

(4) While TMS studies have revealed many inhibitory mechanisms, the functional roles of inhibition still need to be worked out. Surround inhibition is the concept that motor activity not needed for a particular movement might be actively inhibited so that the selected movement might be more precise and motor performance would be enhanced. Mark Hallett described his group's work in this area that has demonstrated active inhibition of muscles in the contralateral extremity and within the same hand with movement of individual fingers. He also suggested that this process may well be deficient in dystonia and could be an explanation for overflow movement seen in this condition.

(5) Finally, knowledge of TMS motor cortex physiology has also advanced rapidly by studies of the effects of CNS active drugs on the various measures of motor cortical excitability (laboratory of Ulf Ziemann, Frankfurt, Germany). Acute pharmacological effects can distinguish between TMS measures which are mainly regulated by axon vs. synaptic excitability. Various neurotransmitter systems (GABA, glutamate) and neuromodulator systems (dopamine, norepinephrine, serotonin, acetylcholine) can be specifically tested. One important example is the distinction between several types of motor cortical inhibition regulated by the $GABA_A$ receptor (SICI), the muscarinic acetylcholine receptor (SLAI) and the $GABA_B$ receptor (cortical silent period). These experiments are extremely useful to delineate further the physiological properties of TMS excitability measures, and to understand better abnormalities of these measures in patients with neurological or psychiatric disorders.

Brain plasticity

TMS has been one of the central techniques for exploring human brain plasticity. A number of presenters showed how TMS could demonstrate plasticity in circumstances such as amputation and stroke. Leonardo Cohen et al. presented considerable material on the basic physiology of plasticity including its pharmacology and behavioral relevance. An exciting new development is that there is now clear evidence that TMS methods can actually be used to modulate plasticity and learning. The paired associate stimulation technique of Joseph

Classen seems particularly valuable in this regard. Pairing peripheral nerve stimulation with TMS to the motor cortex can give rise to robust changes in cortical excitability that may well be due to classical Hebbian learning principles.

Modification of interconnected areas has been the topic of a series of papers amongst others from the group of John Rothwell. These revealed clear after-effects of rTMS over either motor or premotor areas on the excitability of the motor cortex. These effects could be targeted towards intracortical circuitry (as tested in paired pulse paradigms) or to MEP excitability depending on the intensity and the frequency of stimulation. PET and fMRI studies confirm that rTMS to one site can have effects at distant connected sites at both cortical and subcortical levels, a feature that was also seen very clearly in the work of Paulus and colleagues. The tentative conclusion is that rTMS can be used to target specific neural circuits in the brain. An interesting feature of the data was that the effects in neurological patients may not be the same as those seen in healthy subjects. For example, a PET study showed that the effect of 1 Hz rTMS over premotor cortex appeared to be much more intense and widespread in patients with arm dystonia than in healthy subjects.

Finally, Nicolas Lang and Hartwig Siebner presented data on the interaction between DC and rTMS conditioning of the motor cortex. The unexpected finding was that preconditioning with anodal or cathodal DC stimulation could reverse the effects of 1 Hz rTMS, with anodal preconditioning leading to a depressive after-effect whilst cathodal preconditioning led to an excitatory after-effect. This was interpreted as a possible example of "homeostatic" plasticity that has been described in detail in several brain slice preparations, but never in the intact human cortex.

Modulation of cortical excitability by rTMS – therapeutic prospects

Repetitive transcranial magnetic stimulation (rTMS) – series of uniform stimulation of the same brain region with the similar stimulus characteristics at a given repetition rate – is capable of inducing long lasting modification of excitability of cortical neurons. The mechanisms underlying this phenomenon are fairly unclear but evidence is growing that rTMS-induced facilitation and inhibition of several minutes up to hours of duration may be explained by long-term potentiation (LTP) and long-term depression (LTD) like effects, respectively. Some time ago, it seemed well accepted that high frequencies above 1 Hz induce facilitation whereas frequencies below that produce inhibition. In the meantime it turned out that this does not hold true and numerous other parameters play important roles. Amongst others, Martin Sommer (Göttingen, Germany) presented evidence that the type of modification of cortical excitability also depends e.g. on pulse configuration and stimulus orientation, both for slow and fast frequency rTMS, with monophasic rTMS being more effective than biphasic rTMS concerning lasting corticospinal inhibition after 1 Hz rTMS and facilitation after 5 Hz rTMS. TMS – with very short pulses – and tDCS – with one very long "pulse" – may be seen as opposite ends of a continuous physical stimulation spectrum targeting different aspects of neuronal excitation.

Moreover, the after-effect induced in one brain region may be inverse in remote brain areas to which the stimulated neurons project. For therapeutic prospects it would appear necessary to explore what influence the underlying pathophysiology of a neurological disease may have on the effects of rTMS. Most experience exists regarding the treatment of depression and it is well accepted from controlled studies that some patients with major depression may improve, as reported by Mark George and Frank Padberg. It is not fully answered yet whether rTMS should be seen as an alternative to electroconvulsive therapy (ECT) and whether both principles share common mechanisms. Animal studies are performed to investigate whether rTMS can be used to induce more focally epileptic seizures that may be superior to ECT in its antidepressant efficacy as Sarah Lisanby had studied. Compared to other neurological diseases, the treatment of epilepsy by rTMS currently provides most promising results. After several open studies and case reports, evidence from two independent placebo-controlled studies exists that low-frequency rTMS may have antiepileptic efficacy of therapeutical usability. Nevertheless, the amount of seizure reduction with the current protocols is unsatisfactory and optimal stimulation conditions are still to be discovered.

Transcranial direct current stimulation (tDCS)

TMS has since its introduction in 1985 emerged as a tool mainly for inducing short electrical currents in the brain, which in turn most likely elicit spikes in dendrites or axons. A somewhat older technique, tDCS, was invented in the 1970s in the last century in man and even two decades earlier in the animal with direct intracranial stimulation. This method obviously targets at the membrane potentials of cortical neurons, as has been shown at that time in the animal experiment. Depolarizing currents increase, hyperpolarizing currents decrease the firing rate of cortical neurons. Early studies of direct current stimulation effects in humans had been performed by the group of N. Birbaumer. They found increased performance in forced choice reaction time tasks and polarity-specific shifts of the amplitude of cortical potentials due to direct current stimulation.

tDCS was reintroduced in the field in 2000 as a method for influencing neuroplasticity, when it was shown that at least a continuous stimulation of 3 min induced excitability changes outlasting the stimulation duration so far up to 1 h. This progress was achieved when the effects of tDCS were measured with TMS at the motor cortex. With these two methods it now seems to be possible to target preferentially the discharge of neurons directly by TMS or indirectly by altering membrane potentials by tDCS. The direction of the excitability shifts depends on stimulation polarity. They evolve intracortically and have a specific impact on intracortical inhibition and facilitation. Pharmacological studies show that the effects during stimulation are mediated by ion channels, which is in accordance with a primary polarity-specific hyper- or depolarizing effect of the stimulation, while the after-effects involve the modulation of the efficacy of NMDA receptors. Thus, tDCS may evolve as a powerful new tool to induce neuroplasticity in the human brain non-invasively and painlessly. The applicability of tDCS is not restricted to the motor cortex, it has been shown to be also effective in visual and prefrontal cortices. tDCS modulates visual evoked potentials, phosphene thresholds, contrast perception and may improve visuo-motor coordination. Due to existing safety criteria, limits and data presented at the conference, the tDCS protocols so far accomplished in the human have to be regarded as safe. However, the extension of these protocols is needed to give tDCS potential clinical relevance. Therefore, additional safety studies have to be performed to explore the limits of safe stimulation.

July 2003

Walter Paulus
Mark Hallett
Michael A. Nitsche
John C. Rothwell
Frithjof Tergau
Ulf Ziemann

List of Contributors

Amassian, V.E. Departments of Physiology and Pharmacology, and Neurology, State University of New York, Downstate Medical Center, 450 Clarkson Avenue, Box 31, Brooklyn, NY 11203, USA.

Angerer, B. Sensorimotor Integration Research Group, Klinikum Rechts der Isar ter TUM, Psychiatrische Klinik, Ismaningerstrasse 22, D-81675 Munich, Germany.

Antal, A. Department of Clinical Neurophysiology, Georg-August University, Robert-Koch-Strasse 40, D-37075 Göttingen, Germany.

Awiszus, F. Neuromuscular Research Group, Department of Orthopaedics, Otto-von-Guericke Universität, D-39120 Magdeburg, Germany.

Bajbouj, M. Clinic for Psychiatry and Psychotherapy, Medical School Benjamin Franklin, Free University of Berlin, Eschenallee 3, D-14050 Berlin, Germany.

Balestrieri, F. Unità Operativa di Neurologia, Azienda Sanitaria di Firenze, Ospedale S. Maria Nuova, Piazza S. Maria Nuova 1, 50122 Florence, Italy.

Baudewig, J. Biomedizinische NMR Forschungs GmbH, Max-Planck-Institut für Biophysikalische Chemie, D-37070 Göttingen, Germany.

Bäumer, T. Neurology Department, Hamburg University, Martinistrasse 52, D-20246 Hamburg, Germany.

Beck, S. Department of Neurobiology, Max Planck Institute for Biological Cybernetics, Tübingen, Germany.

Benvenuti, F. Ospedale INRCA 'I Fraticini', Florence, Italy.

Bestmann, S. Biomedizinische NMR Forschungs GmbH, Max-Planck-Institut für Biophysikalische Chemie, D-37070 Göttingen, Germany.

Birbaumer, N. Institute of Medical Psychology and Behavioral Neurobiology, University of Tübingen, Gartenstrasse 29, D-72072 Tübingen, Germany, and Center for Cognitive Neuroscience, University of Trento, Trento, Italy.

Bohning, D.E. Department of Radiology, Medical University of South Carolina, 169 Ashley Avenue, Charleston, SC 29425, USA.

Bohning, P.A. Department of Psychiatry, Medical University of South Carolina, 169 Ashley Avenue, Charleston, SC 29425, USA.

Borgheresi, A. Unità Operativa di Neurologia, Azienda Sanitaria di Firenze, Ospedale S. Maria Nuova, Piazza S. Maria Nuova 1, 50122 Florence, Italy.

Boroojerdi, B. Department of Neurology, University Hospital Aachen, Pauwelstrasse 30, D-52074 Aachen, Germany.

Braune, H.-J. Department of Neurology, Center of Nervous Diseases, Philipps-University of Marburg, Rudolf-Bultmann-Strasse 8, D-35033 Marburg, Germany.

Bütefisch, C.M. Neurological Therapeutic Center, Institute at the Heinrich-Heine University, Hohensandweg 37, D-40591 Düsseldorf, Germany.

Cappa, S.F. Centro di Neuroscienze Cognitive, Università Vita-Salute S. Raffaele, Milan, Italy.

Cincotta, M. Unità Operativa di Neurologia, Azienda Sanitaria di Firenze, Ospedale S. Maria Nuova, Piazza S. Maria Nuova 1, 50122 Florence, Italy.

Cohen, L. Human Cortical Physiology Section, NINDS, National Institutes of Health, Bethesda, MD 20892, USA.

Denslow, S. Department of Radiology, Medical University of South Carolina, 169 Ashley Avenue, Charleston, SC 29425, USA.

Dambeck, N. Department of Neurology, University Hospital Aachen, Pauwelstrasse 30, D-52074 Aachen, Germany.

Däuper, J. Department of Neurology and Clinical Neurophysiology, Medical School of Hannover, D-30623 Hannover, Germany.

Dengler, R. Department of Neurology and Clinical Neurophysiology, Medical School of Hannover, D-30623 Hannover, Germany.

Di Lazzaro, V. Department of Neurology, Università Cattolica, L.go A. Gemelli 8, 00168 Rome, Italy.

Dileone, M. Department of Neurology, Università Cattolica, L.go A. Gemelli 8, 00168 Rome, Italy.

Ellison, A. Cognitive Neuroscience Research Unit, Wolfson Research Institute, University of Durham Queen's Campus, University Boulevard, Stockton-on-Tees TS17 6BH, UK.

Fink, M. Department of Physical Medicine and Rehabilitation, Medical School of Hannover, D-30623 Hannover, Germany.

Feredoes, E.A. Neuropsychiatric Institute, Euroa Centre, Prince of Wales Hospital, Sydney, NSW 2031, Australia.

Foltys, H. Department of Neurology, University Hospital Aachen, Pauwelstrasse 30, D-52074 Aachen, Germany.

Frahm, J. Biomedizinische NMR Forschungs GmbH, Max-Planck-Institut für Biophysikalische Chemie, D-37070 Göttingen, Germany.

Gallinat, J. Clinic for Psychiatry and Psychotherapy, Medical School Benjamin Franklin, Free University of Berlin, Eschenallee 3, D-14050 Berlin, Germany, and Clinic for Psychiatry and Psychotherapy, University Clinic Charité, Berlin, Germany.

George, M.S. Department of Radiology, Medical University of South Carolina, 169 Ashley Avenue, Charleston, SC 29425, USA, and The Ralph H. Johnson Veterans Hospital, Charleston, SC, USA.

Gerloff, C. Department of Neurology, Cortical Physiology Research Group, Eberhard-Karls University Tübingen, Hoppe-Seyler-Strasse 3, D-72076 Tübingen, Germany.

Godde, B. Institute of Medical Psychology and Behavioral Neurobiology, University of Tübingen, Gartenstrasse 29, D-72072 Tübingen, Germany.

Goldstein-Müller, B. Department of Psychiatry, Ludwig-Maximilian University, Nussbaumstrasse 7, D-80336 Munich, Germany.

Haeske, H. Department of Neurology, Center of Nervous Diseases, Philipps-University of Marburg, Rudolf-Bultmann-Strasse 8, D-35033 Marburg, Germany.

Hallett, M. Human Motor Control Section, NINDS, NIH, Building 10, Room 5N226, 10 Center Drive, MSC 1428, Bethesda, MD 20892-1428, USA.

Hamdy, S. Clinical Sciences Building, Department of GI Sciences, Hope Hospital, Eccles Old Road, Salford M6 8HD, UK.

Havel, P. Sensorimotor Integration Research Group, Klinikum Rechts der Isar ter TUM, Psychiatrische Klinik, Ismaningerstrasse 22, D-81675 Munich, Germany.

Hayashi, T. Department of Investigative Radiology, National Cardio-Vascular Center, Research Institute, University of Tokyo, Tokyo, Japan.

Hinterberger, T. Institute of Medical Psychology and Behavioral Neurobiology, University of Tübingen, Gartenstrasse 29, D-72072 Tübingen, Germany.

Hummel, F. Department of Neurology, Cortical Physiology Research Group, Eberhard-Karls University Tübingen, Hoppe-Seyler-Strasse 3, D-72076 Tübingen, Germany.

Iida, H. Department of Investigative Radiology, National Cardio-Vascular Center, Research Institute, University of Tokyo, Tokyo, Japan.

Kammer, T. Department of Neurology, University Hospital of Tübingen, Hoppe-Seyler-Strasse 3, D-72076 Tübingen, Germany.

Karim, A.A. Institute of Medical Psychology and Behavioral Neurobiology, University of Tübingen, Gartenstrasse 29, D-72072 Tübingen, Germany.

Karst, M. Department of Anesthesiology, Pain Clinic, Medical School of Hannover, D-30623 Hannover, Germany.

Keck, M.E. Max Planck Institute of Psychiatry, Kraepelinstrasse 2–10, D-80804 Munich, Germany.

Kobayashi, M. Laboratory for Magnetic Brain Stimulation, Beth Israel Deaconess Medical Center, Harvard Medical School, 330 Brookline Avenue, Boston, MA 02215, USA.

Kossev, A. Department of Biophysics, Bulgarian Academy of Sciences, Sofia, Bulgaria.

Krause, P. Department of Neurology, University of Munich, Klinikum Grosshadern, Marchioninistrasse 15, D-81377 Munich, Germany.

Krings, T. Department of Neuroradiology, University Hospital Aachen, Pauwelstrasse 30, D-52074 Aachen, Germany.

Lang, N. Department of Clinical Neurophysiology, University of Göttingen, Robert-Koch-Strasse 40, D-37075 Göttingen, Germany, and Sobell Department of Motor Neuroscience and Movement Disorders, Institute of Neurology, University College London, Queen Square, London WC1N 3BG, UK.

Lang, U.E. Clinic for Psychiatry and Psychotherapy, Medical School Benjamin Franklin, Free University of Berlin, Eschenallee 3, D-14050 Berlin, Germany.

Lee, L. Wellcome Department of Imaging Neuroscience, Institute of Neurology, University College London, London WC1N 3BG, UK.

Liebetanz, D. Department of Clinical Neurophysiology, University of Göttingen, Robert-Koch-Strasse 40, D-37075 Göttingen, Germany.

Liepert, J. Department of Neurology, University Hospital Eppendorf, Martinistrasse 52, D-20246 Hamburg, Germany.

Lisanby, S.H. Magnetic Brain Stimulation Laboratory, Department of Biological Psychiatry, New York State Psychiatric Institute, 1051 Riverside Drive, Unit 126, New York, NY 10032, USA, and Department of Psychiatry, College of Physicians and Surgeons, Columbia University, New York, NY, USA.

Lomarev, M.P. Department of Radiology, Medical University of South Carolina, 169 Ashley Avenue, Charleston, SC 29425, USA.

Lotze, M. Institute of Medical Psychology and Behavioral Neurobiology, University of Tübingen, Gartenstrasse 29, D-72072 Tübingen, Germany.

Luber, B. Magnetic Brain Stimulation Laboratory, Department of Biological Psychiatry, New York State Psychiatric Institute, 1051 Riverside Drive, Unit 126, New York, NY 10032, USA.

Magistris, M.R. Unité d'Electroneuromyographie et des Affections Neuromusculaires, Clinique de Neurologie, Hôpitaux Universitaires de Genève, CH-1211 Geneva 14, Switzerland.

Maier, C. Department of Pain Treatment, BG-Kliniken Bergmannsheil, Ruhr-University, Buerkle-de-la-Camp-Platz 1, D-44789 Bochum, Germany.

Mansouri, S. Department of Neurology and Clinical Neurophysiology, Medical School of Hannover, D-30623 Hannover, Germany.

Matsuda, H. Department of Radiology, National Center Hospital of Mental, Nervous and Muscular Disorders, National Center of Neurology and Psychiatry, Tokyo, Japan.

Mazzone, P. Neurosurgery CTO, Via S. Nemesio 21, 00145 Rome, Italy.

Meister, I.G. Department of Neurology, University Hospital Aachen, Pauwelstrasse 30, D-52074 Aachen, Germany.

Meyer, B.-U.[†] Deceased 24 November 2001.

Miniussi, C. IRCCS "San Giovanni di Dio – FBF", Via Pilastroni 4, 25125 Brescia, Italy.

Möller, H.-J. Department of Psychiatry, Ludwig-Maximilian University, Nussbaumstrasse 7, D-80336 Munich, Germany.

Morales, O. Magnetic Brain Stimulation Laboratory, Department of Biological Psychiatry, New York State Psychiatric Institute, 1051 Riverside Drive, Unit 126, New York, NY 10032, USA, and Department of Psychiatry, College of Physicians and Surgeons, Columbia University, New York, NY, USA.

Mortensen, J. Brigham Young University, Provo, UT, USA.

Moscrip, T. Magnetic Brain Stimulation Laboratory, Department of Biological Psychiatry, New York State Psychiatric Institute, 1051 Riverside Drive, Unit 126, New York, NY 10032, USA.

Müller, H.-H. Institute for Medical Biometry and Epidemiology, Medical Center for Methodology and Health Research, Philipps-University of Marburg, D-35033 Marburg, Germany.

Münchau, A. Neurology Department, Hamburg University, Martinistrasse 52, D-20246 Hamburg, Germany.

Neumann, D. Epilepsy Center Kork, Kehl-Kork, Germany.

Niehaus, L. Department of Neurology, Charité, Campus Virchow-Klinikum, Humboldt-Universität, Augustenburger Platz 1, D-13353 Berlin, Germany.

Nitsche, M.A. Department of Clinical Neurophysiology, University of Göttingen, Robert-Koch-Strasse 40, D-37075 Göttingen, Germany.

Nonaka, Y. Neurology Division, Nihon Kohden Corporation, Tokyo, Japan.

Oertel, W.H. Department of Neurology, Center of Nervous Diseases, Philipps-University of Marburg, Rudolf-Bultmann-Strasse 8, D-35033 Marburg, Germany.

Ohnishi, T. Department of Radiology, National Center Hospital of Mental, Nervous and Muscular Disorders, National Center of Neurology and Psychiatry, Tokyo, Japan.

Okabe, S. Department of Neurology, Division of Neuroscience, Graduate School of Medicine, University of Tokyo, 7-3-1 Hongo, Bunkyo-ku, Tokyo 113-8655, Japan.

Oliviero, A. Department of Neurology, Università Cattolica, L.go A. Gemelli 8, 00168 Rome, Italy.

Padberg, F. Department of Psychiatry, Ludwig-Maximilian University, Nussbaumstrasse 7, D-80336 Munich, Germany.

Pascual-Leone, A. Department of Neurology, Beth Israel Deaconess Medical Center, 330 Brookline Avenue, KS-454, Boston, MA 02215, USA.

Paulus, W. Department of Clinical Neurophysiology, University of Göttingen, Robert-Koch-Strasse 40, D-37075 Göttingen, Germany.

Peller, M. Department of Neurology, Christian-Albrechts-University of Kiel, Niemannsweg 147, D-24105 Kiel, Germany.

Pilato, P. Department of Neurology, Università Cattolica, L.go A. Gemelli 8, 00168 Rome, Italy.

Puls, K. Department of Neurobiology, Max Planck Institute for Biological Cybernetics, Tübingen, Germany.

Ragazzoni, A. Unità Operativa di Neurologia, Azienda Sanitaria di Firenze, Ospedale S. Maria Nuova, Piazza S. Maria Nuova 1, 50122 Florence, Italy.

Roether, C. Department of Neurobiology, Max Planck Institute for Biological Cybernetics, Tübingen, Germany.

Rollnik, J.D. Department of Neurology and Clinical Neurophysiology, Medical School of Hannover, D-30623 Hannover, Germany.

Rosenow, F. Interdisciplinary Epilepsy Center, Department of Neurology, University of Marburg, Rudolf-Bultmann-Strasse 8, D-35033 Marburg, Germany.

Rossini, P.M. Neurologia, Università Campus Biomedico, Rome, Italy.

Rossi, S. Dipartimento di Neuroscienze, Sezione Neurologia, Università di Siena, Siena, Italy.

Rothwell, J.C. Sobell Department of Neurophysiology, Institute of Neurology, University College London, Queen Square, London WC1N 3BG, UK.

Ruohonen, J. Research and Development, Nexstim Ltd., Elimäenkatu 22B, FIN-00510 Helsinki, Finland.

Rushworth, M. Department of Experimental Psychology, University of Oxford, South Parks Road, Oxford OX1 3UD, UK.

Sachdev, P.S. School of Psychiatry, Faculty of Medicine, University of New South Wales, Sydney, Australia, and Neuropsychiatric Institute, Euroa Centre, Prince of Wales Hospital, Sydney, NSW 2031, Australia.

Sackeim, H.A. Magnetic Brain Stimulation Laboratory, Department of Biological Psychiatry, New York State Psychiatric Institute, 1051 Riverside Drive, Unit 126, New York, NY 10032, USA, and Department of Psychiatry, College of Physicians and Surgeons, Columbia University, New York, NY, USA.

Sandrini, M. IRCCS "San Giovanni di Dio – FBF", Via Pilastroni 4, 25125 Brescia, Italy.

Saturno, E. Department of Neurology, Università Cattolica, L.go A. Gemelli 8, 00168 Rome, Italy.

Schroeder, C. Nathan Kline Insitute, Orangeberg, NY, USA.

Schwenkreis, P. Department of Neurology, BG-Kliniken Bergmannsheil, Ruhr-University, Buerkle-de-la-Camp-Platz 1, D-44789 Bochum, Germany.

Siebner, H.R. Department of Neurology, Christian-Albrechts-University of Kiel, Niemannsweg 147, D-24105 Kiel, Germany.

Sommer, M. Department of Clinical Neurophysiology, Center for Neurological Medicine, University of Göttingen, Robert-Koch-Strasse 40, D-37075 Göttingen, Germany.

Sparing, R. Department of Neurology, University Hospital Aachen, Pauwelstrasse 30, D-52074 Aachen, Germany.

Steinhoff, B. Epilepsy Center Kork, Kehl-Kork, Germany.

Stewart, M. Department of Physiology and Pharmacology, State University of New York, Downstate Medical Center, 450 Clarkson Avenue, Box 31, Brooklyn, NY 11203, USA.

Stiasny-Kolster, K. Department of Neurology, Center of Nervous Diseases, Philipps-University of Marburg, Rudolf-Bultmann-Strasse 8, D-35033 Marburg, Germany.

Straube, A. Department of Neurology, University of Munich, Klinikum Grosshadern, Marchioninistrasse 15, D-81377 Munich, Germany.

Struppler, A. Sensorimotor Integration Research Group, Klinikum Rechts der Isar ter TUM, Psychiatrische Klinik, Ismaningerstrasse 22, D-81675 Munich, Germany.

K.M. Rösler Department of Neurology, University Hospital, Berne, Switzerland.

Tegenthoff, M. Department of Neurology, BG-Kliniken Bergmannsheil, Ruhr-University, Buerkle-de-la-Camp-Platz 1, D-44789 Bochum, Germany.

Teramoto, N. Department of Investigative Radiology, National Cardio-Vascular Center, Research Institute, University of Tokyo, Tokyo, Japan.

Tergau, F. Department of Clinical Neurophysiology, University of Göttingen, Robert-Koch-Strasse 40, D-37075 Göttingen, Germany.

Théoret, H. Laboratory for Magnetic Brain Stimulation, Beth Israel Deaconess Medical Center, Harvard Medical School, 330 Brookline Avenue, Boston, MA 02215, USA.

Thielscher, A. Department of Psychiatry III, University of Ulm, Ulm, Germany.

Thron, A. Department of Neuroradiology, University Hospital Aachen, Pauwelstrasse 30, D-52074 Aachen, Germany.

Tonali, P.A. Department of Neurology, Università Cattolica, L.go A. Gemelli 8, 00168 Rome, Italy.

Ueno, S. Bioimaging and Biomagnetics Laboratory, Department of Biomedical Engineering, Graduate School of Medicine, University of Tokyo, 7-3-1 Hongo, Bunkyo-ku, Tokyo 113-8655, Japan.

Ugawa, Y. Department of Neurology, Division of Neuroscience, Graduate School of Medicine, University of Tokyo, 7-3-1 Hongo, Bunkyo-ku, Tokyo 113-8655, Japan.

Urban, P.P. Department of Neurology, University of Mainz, Langenbeckstrasse 1, D-55101 Mainz, Germany.

Valero-Cabré, A. Laboratory for Magnetic Brain Stimulation, Beth Israel Deaconess Medical Center, Harvard Medical School, 330 Brookline Avenue, Boston, MA 02215, USA.

Van Boven, R.W. Laboratory of Brain and Cognition, National Institute of Neurological Disorders and Stroke, Bethesda, MD, USA.

Vanni, P. Unità Operativa di Neurologia, Azienda Sanitaria di Firenze, Ospedale S. Maria Nuova, Piazza S. Maria Nuova 1, 50122 Florence, Italy.

Walsh, V. Institute of Cognitive Neuroscience, University College London, Alexandra House, 17 Queen Square, London WC1N 3AR, UK.

Watabe, H. Department of Investigative Radiology, National Cardio-Vascular Center, Research Institute, University of Tokyo, Tokyo, Japan.

Weidemann, J. Department of Neuroradiology, University Hospital Aachen, Pauwelstrasse 30, D-52074 Aachen, Germany.

Wen, W. Neuropsychiatric Institute, Euroa Centre, Prince of Wales Hospital, Sydney, NSW 2031, Australia.

Werhahn, K.J. Department of Neurology, University of Mainz, Langenbeckstrasse 1, D-55131 Mainz, Germany.

Wessel, K. Department of Neurology, Municipal Hospital, and Cognitive Neurology, Institute at the Technical University, Salzdahlumer Strasse 90, D-38126 Braunschweig, Germany.

Wüstefeld, S. Department of Neurology and Clinical Neurophysiology, Medical School of Hannover, D-30623 Hannover, Germany.

Zaccara, G. Unità Operativa di Neurologia, Azienda Sanitaria di Firenze, Ospedale S. Maria Nuova, Piazza S. Maria Nuova 1, 50122 Florence, Italy.

Ziemann, U. Neurologische Klinik, Johann Wolfgang Goethe-University, Schleusenweg 2–16, D-60528 Frankfurt am Main, Germany.

Zwanzger, P. Department of Psychiatry, Ludwig-Maximilian University, Nussbaumstrasse 7, D-80336 Munich, Germany.

Contents

Section III. Motor Control

Section I

Methodology

Transcranial Magnetic Stimulation and Transcranial Direct Current Stimulation (Supplements to Clinical Neurophysiology, Vol. 56)
Editors: W. Paulus, F. Tergau, M.A. Nitsche, J.C. Rothwell, U. Ziemann, M. Hallett

Chapter 1

Background physics for magnetic stimulation

Jarmo Ruohonen

Nexstim Ltd., Elimäenkatu 22B, FIN-00510 Helsinki (Finland)

1. Introduction

With increasing use of magnetic stimulation in science and clinics, it is most important to consider and revisit the basic phenomena behind the technique. This chapter includes a simplified introduction to the basic physical principles. As examples, the chapter outlines how coil positioning affects where magnetic stimulation touches the brain. Moreover, advanced computation helps position the stimuli more accurately to desired spots. This chapter introduces starting points for engineering models that can be applied to further develop brain stimulation devices into advanced navigated brain stimulation (NBS) scanners that can produce important information complementary to fMRI, MEG and PET.

2. Basic principles

Electrical current can excite excitable cells (neurons, muscles). The tingling sensation when short-circuiting a low-power battery with fingers is a good demonstration of this. Even very strong electrical pulses can be beneficially applied in medicine, for instance, in cardiac defibrillators.

Magnetic stimulation can "mimic" direct stimulation with electrical current: it generates, or induces, an electrical current in the tissue. This has beneficial consequences. Unlike electrical stimulation, magnetic stimulation can reach the tissue without need for physical contact.

The mechanism of action is similar for both electrical and magnetic stimulation. In order to stimulate neuronal cells, an electric field $\mathbf{E}$ must be applied to the tissue; it forces coherent motion of free charges in intra- and extracellular spaces. In other words, the electric field drives an intracranial electrical current $\mathbf{J} = \sigma\mathbf{E}$, where σ is the electrical conductivity in the brain. Cell membranes that interrupt the current will depolarize or hyperpolarize. Eventually, the depolarization of the axon membrane will trigger a progressing depolarization front, or action potential. Figure 1 illustrates the chain of events in magnetic stimulation.

2.1. *Faraday's law of induction*

The physical phenomenon behind magnetic stimulation is electromagnetic induction, and is governed

* *Correspondence to*: Dr. Jarmo Ruohonen, Ph.D., Director, Research and Development, Nexstim Ltd., Elimäenkatu 22B, FIN-00510 Helsinki, Finland.
Tel: +358-9-2727 1711; Fax: +358-9-2727 1717;
E-mail: jarmo.ruohonen@nexstim.com
Internet: www.nexstim.com

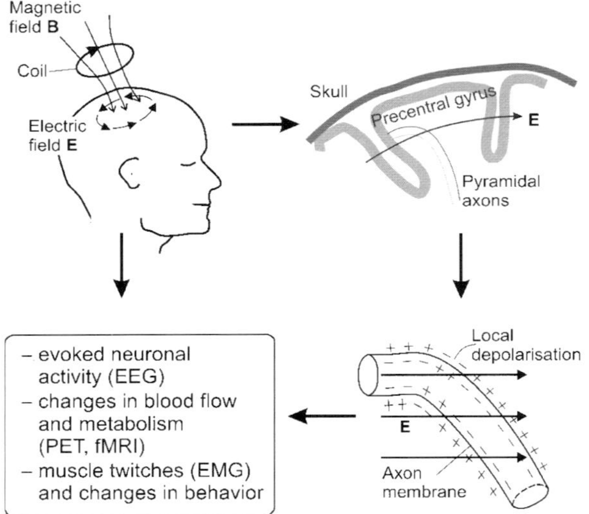

Fig. 1. Principles of TMS. Current pulse $I(t)$ in the coil generates a magnetic field **B** that induces an electric field **E**. The lines of **B** go through the coil; the lines of **E** follow the shape of the coil. The upper-right drawing illustrates two pyramidal axons, together with a typical orientation of the intracranial **E**. The E-field affects the transmembrane potential, which may lead to local membrane depolarization and firing of the neurons. Events following TMS include: (1) coherent activation of neurons; (2) metabolic and hemodynamic changes; and (3) behavioral changes. Reactions of the brain can be recorded with EEG (Ilmoniemi et al., 1997), or with fMRI (Bohning et al., 1998), PET (Paus et al., 1997) or NIRS (Oliviero et al., 1999). Macroscopic responses are seen also with surface EMG or as behavioral changes.

by a basic law of physics, namely, Faraday's law:

$$\nabla \times \mathbf{E} = -\, \partial \mathbf{B}/\partial t.$$

In practice, this relation states that an electric field **E**, and thereby electrical current **J**, is *induced* in tissue by the time-varying magnetic field **B** from the coil. Solution to the equation above gives an estimate of the induced **E** that ignores the effects of conductivity variations between and within the brain, skull and scalp.

Magnetic fields encountered in magnetic stimulation travel freely in air and can easily penetrate through tissue. Therefore, magnetic stimulation can readily reach brain cells even through the highly resistive skull.

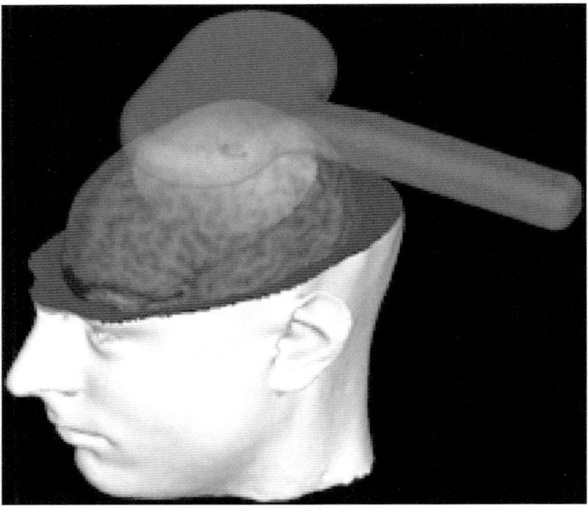

Fig. 2. Accurate localization of the stimulating coil and real-time calculation of the electric field induced in the brain offer interactive targeting and mapping. The image shows the electric field on 3-D MR images while navigation is used to guide the coil optimally for motor cortex stimulation. (Courtesy of Nexstim Ltd., Helsinki, Finland.)

Several references include detailed information on the physical formulas governing magnetic stimulation (Barker, 1991; Grandori and Ravazzani, 1991; Ilmoniemi et al., 1999; Ruohonen and Ilmoniemi, 2002).

3. "Hot spot" modeling

Modeling of magnetic stimulation can be divided into two main parts:

(1) computation of the macroscopic electric field **E** in the brain, and
(2) cellular mechanisms.

3.1. Hot spots of activation

Figure 2 illustrates results from straightforward modeling. The figure shows a 3-D reconstruction of the MR images of a subject's head together with the computed induced field **E** that touches the cortex.

The coil has been positioned optimally to obtain muscle twitches in the right hand fingers with help of eXimia NBS navigation system (Nexstim Ltd., Finland). The "hot spot" of the electric field coincides nicely with the location of the hand motor area, identified from structural MRIs in the precentral omega-shaped knob.

The calculation of the electric field **E** induced in the tissue has several benefits. Most importantly, together with accurate localization of the coil with respect to anatomical landmarks, the induced **E** can be used to determine the cortical areas influenced by stimulation. This can significantly help interpret the experimental findings and enables new paradigms, for instance, based on functional information acquired with other brain scanning modalities.

3.2. E-field computation

Generally, the electric field induced in the tissue depends on

(1) coil shape;
(2) coil location and orientation; and
(3) electrical conductivity structure of the head.

The computation of the electromagnetic fields induced in the brain is well understood. The total field is the sum of the directly induced field from Faraday's law and the secondary field arising from surfaces of different conductivity (Fig. 3) (Roth et al., 1991; Durand et al., 1992; Ruohonen and Ilmoniemi, 2002). Accurate calculation would require knowledge of the exact electrical conductivity and its preferential direction in the subject's head (Wang et al., 1994; Cerri et al., 1995; D'Inzeo et al., 1995). However, computational algorithms that can make use of such information are extremely complicated and time consuming, and hence cannot be used in practical investigations.

Although dedicated MR imaging sequences can be used to estimate the conductivity profile of the head, the actually achievable resolution is poor, and the values determined are questionable – at least until otherwise proven. And, the procedure should be repeated for every patient examined. For these reasons, conductivity profiles such as the spherical model have been developed that approximate the shape of the head and brain (Eaton, 1992; Heller and Van Hulsteyn, 1992). Such models are still complicated, but modern computers allow for fast and reproducible computation.

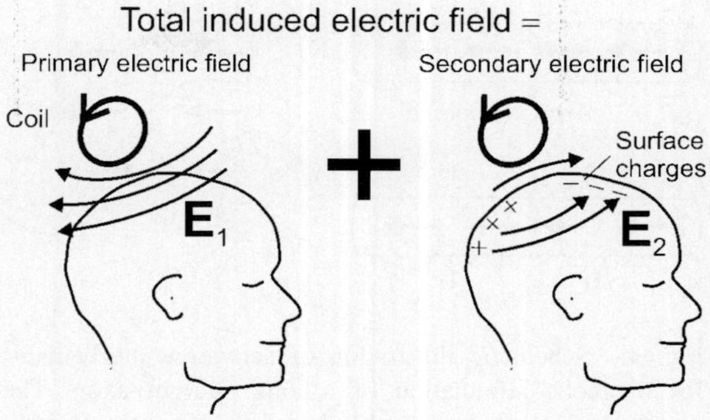

The spherical head model has relatively good accuracy for biomagnetic studies of the brain (Hämäläinen et al., 1993). There is little information regarding the spherical model's usefulness in special circumstances such as a stroke.

Fig. 3. The total induced electric field is the sum of primary and secondary fields: $\mathbf{E} = \mathbf{E}_1 + \mathbf{E}_2$. The primary field is induced by the coil according to Faraday's law (left). The secondary field arises from charges that accumulate on surfaces where conductivity changes (right).

4. Cellular mechanisms

There is considerable theoretical and physiological evidence that the cerebral cortex is activated predominantly at the location of the maximum of the induced electric field. Of course, the strength and focus of the magnetic field are irrelevant.

The complex shape of the neurons makes it difficult to predict precisely the effects of stimulation. Modeling studies suggest that TMS predominantly causes excitation at bends of corticocortical or of corticospinal fibers or at nerve endings near the surface of the cortex (Basser and Roth, 1990; Nagarajan et al., 1993; Abdeen and Stuchly, 1994). Experimental data seem to support these conclusions (Maccabee et al., 1993; Nagarajan et al., 1997;

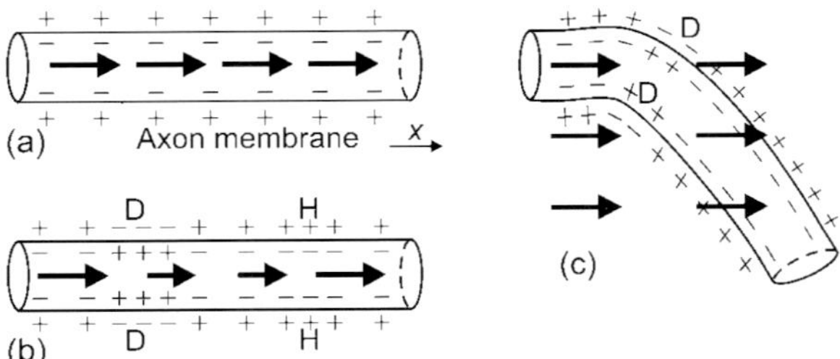

Fig. 4. Schematic illustration of activation mechanisms for magnetic stimulation of a long straight axon. The membrane polarization is sketched for different externally applied electric field patterns (arrows): (a) uniform **E** along the axon, no change from the resting state; (b) gradient activation, with $\partial E_x/\partial x \neq 0$; (c) gradient activation for a bent axon in uniform **E**. Regions of depolarization and hyperpolarization are indicated by D and H, respectively.

Amassian et al., 1998). The major implications from models are (see also Fig. 4):

(1) straight long axons are most easily stimulated where the gradient of the electric field along the axon is the strongest (dE_x/dx for axons along x axis);
(2) short axons are most easily stimulated at their ends; and
(3) curved axons are most easily stimulated at the bends, where the effective electric field gradient along the axon is the strongest.

In summary, TMS most likely stimulates short and curved cortical neurons near bends, and where the induced electric field is the strongest. The orientation of the electric field affects it as well. The practical strength to elicit hand muscle twitches is on the order of 100 mV/mm.

The basic mechanisms and effects of TMS have been recently reviewed by Terao and Ugawa (2002).

4.1. Transcranial electrical vs. magnetic stimulation

In their fundamental works, Day et al. (1989) and Amassian et al. (1989) reported that the CMAPs with TMS are about 2 ms longer than with transcranial electrical stimulation (TCES), which most likely stimulates pyramidal axons in the white matter. This means that TMS probably stimulates more superficial structures than TCES. The site of excitation in TMS is possibly in the grey matter and in TCES in the white matter. By appropriately orienting the TMS coil, the CMAPs match, leaving the possibility that TMS can activate the pyramidal axons also directly.

Distribution and orientation of the electric fields in TCES and TMS are significantly different. In TMS, the field is always in the direction along the scalp; there is no radial electric field. This probably explains the observed differences in the CMAP latencies. In TCES, there are both field directions: the relative strengths of the field components parallel and perpendicular to the scalp depend on the electrode configuration.

4.2. Comparison with fMRI, MEG and PET findings

Comparative results from localization of the somatosensory cortex indicate that the activation occurs near, or at the site of, the strongest externally applied **E**. Krings et al. (1997) compared stereotactic magnetic stimulation maps with direct cortical stimulation results, finding agreement to within less than 5–10 mm. The site of the strongest **E** has been found to agree with the localization results from MEG (Morioka et al., 1995a, b; Ruohonen et al., 1996), PET (Wassermann et al., 1996) and fMRI (Terao et al., 1998a; Herwig et al., 2002) to within 5–20 mm. Similarly, fMRI, PET and TMS have localized the frontal eye field to the precentral gyrus (Carter and Zee, 1997; Paus et al., 1997; Terao et al., 1998b).

5. TMS devices

A circuit containing a discharge capacitor connected in series with the coil by a thyristor, generates the current pulses in a TMS coil (Cadwell, 1990; Barker, 1991). With the capacitor first charged to 2–3 kV, the gating of the thyristor into the conducting state will cause the discharging of the capacitor through the coil. The

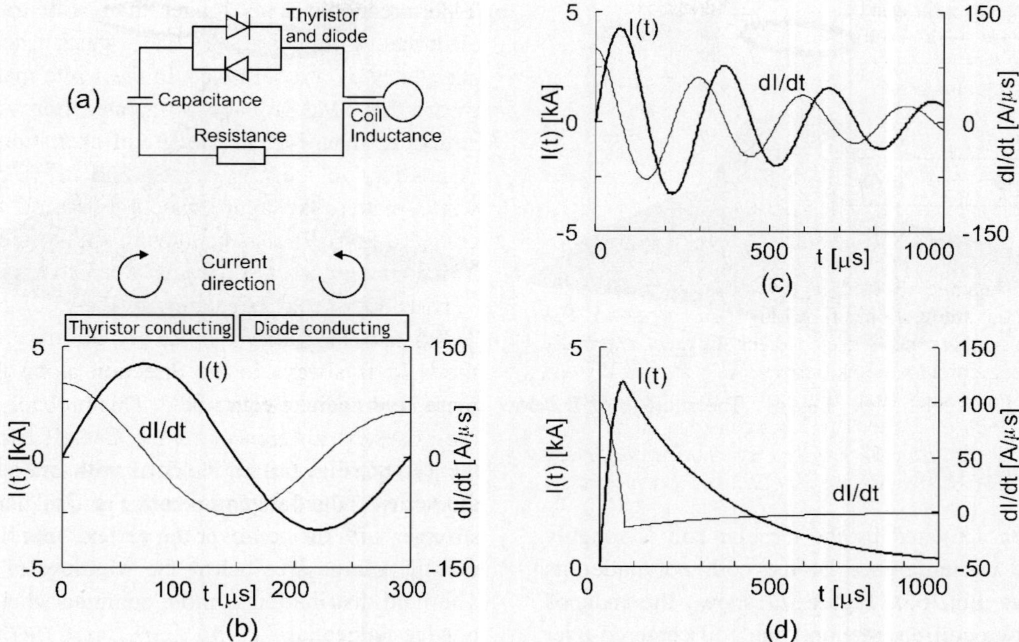

Fig. 5. (a) Schematic illustration of the stimulator circuit. The current *I(t)* and its rate of change *dI/dt* for (b) biphasic, (c) polyphasic, and (d) monophasic current pulses. Inserts to (b) depict the conducting periods of the thyristor T and diode D and the direction of the current in the coil. Parameters used: coil inductance $L = 15$ μH, capacitance 100 μF, resistance 50 mΩ, initial capacitor voltage 2,000 V.

resulting current waveform is typically a damped sinusoidal pulse that has a peak value of 5–10 kA. Typically, the power consumption is 2–3 kW at maximum stimulus intensity and 1-Hz repetition rate.

The current pulse properties vary among manufacturers. Three pulse waveforms are available (Fig. 5):

(1) monophasic, i.e. rapid rise from zero to peak and slower decrease to zero;
(2) biphasic, i.e. one damped cycle of sinusoid; and
(3) polyphasic, i.e. multiple-cycle damped sinusoid.

The duration of the pulse is typically 200–300 μs for biphasic and about 600 μs for monophasic pulses. Unlike in electrical stimulation, it is difficult to modify the pulse shape in magnetic stimulation.

rTMS devices operate at 10–60 Hz at 40–100% of the maximum intensity of single pulses. The duration of sustained operation is limited by coil heating to 100–1000 pulses at maximum power. With proper coil cooling, the duration of the stimulus train is not limited by heating.

6. Coils

The size of the stimulated area, and the direction of the induced current flow, depend greatly on the coil's shape. Successful targeting of stimulation requires that the field pattern from the coil is taken into account. Likewise, significant improvements in stimulator design can be achieved only through good understanding of the electromagnetic fields around the coil.

Effective coil design is challenged by the high amount of energy that must be driven through the coil in a very short time. In brain stimulation, this energy is about 500 J, which would suffice to throw a weight of 1 kg to a height of 50 m. This section describes some available coil types with their excitation fields.

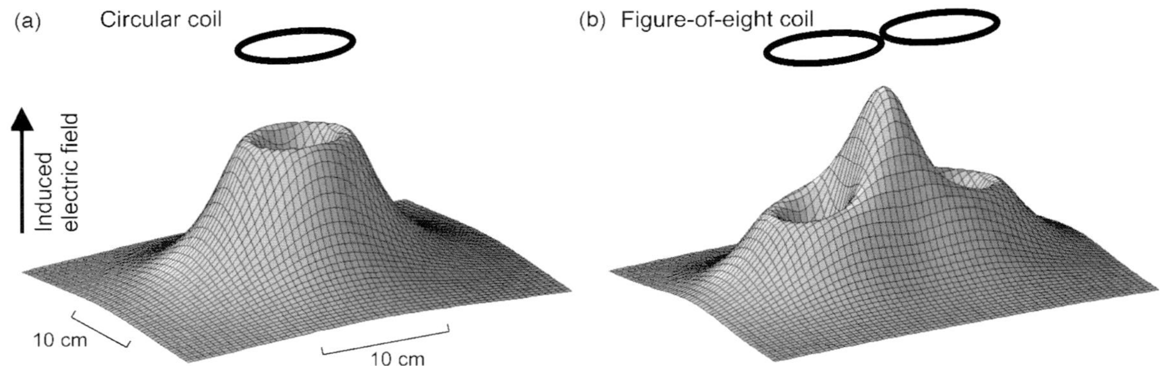

Fig. 6. The strength of **E** below circular and figure-of-eight coil.

6.1. Circular coil

The region activated by the circular coil is roughly under the circumference of the coil, not under its center (see Fig. 6a). Figure 7a shows the induced field for two coil orientations: the coil centered over the vertex (Fig. 6a) and shifted with one edge over the vertex (edge-tangential coil, Fig. 7b). The field is stronger with the coil over the vertex, but it is distributed in a large area below the windings of the coil. The field distribution is more confined when the coil is edge-tangential.

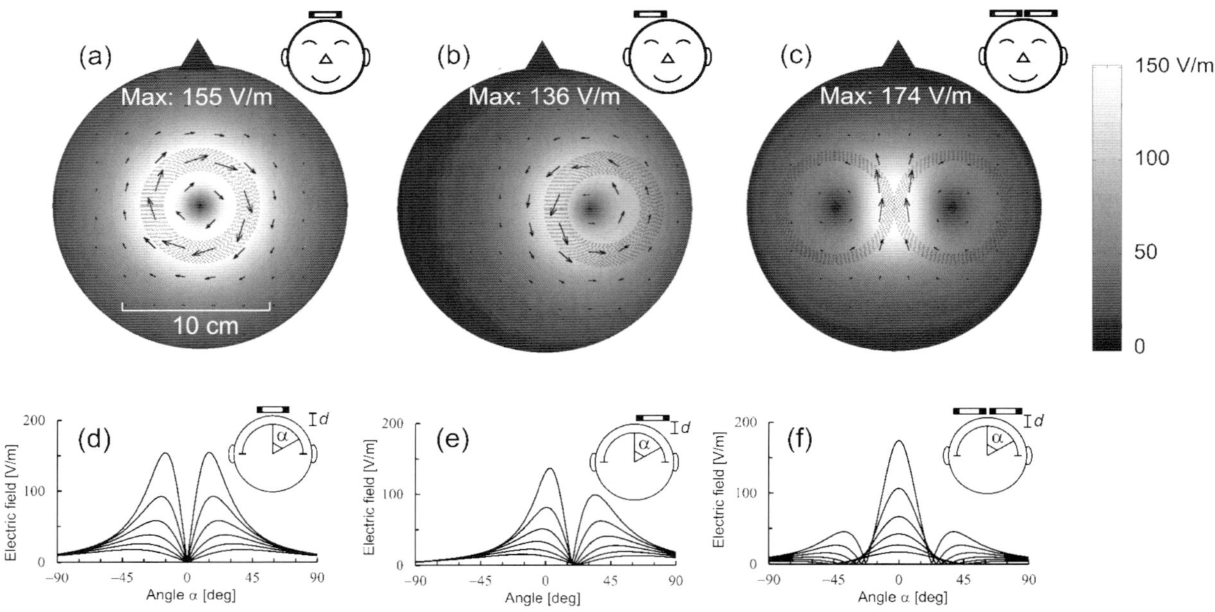

Fig. 7. Pattern of the electric field induced by: (a) circular coil over the vertex; (b) circular coil edge-tangential over the vertex; (c) figure-of-eight coil. The illustrations show the field strength on a spherical surface, 20 mm below the coils as gray level maps. The plots in (d, e, f) show the field in points of a circular arc going from the left ear to the right ear, when the arc is at different distances from the coil (d =, 20, 30, 40, 50, 60, 70 mm). The coils consisted of 16 concentric turns (2×8, 8-shaped coil) 60 mm in diameter and were driven with $dI/dt = 10^8$ A/s. The spherical head model was used.

Figures 7d and 7e show the field strengths for the vertex and edge-tangential coils along a semicircle at different depths below the coil (20 to 70 mm). The field strength decreases quickly with distance from the coil. Notably, the strength of the secondary peak at $\alpha \approx 35°$ produced by the edge-tangential coil orientation is 73% of the primary peak. This secondary peak should be taken into account when positioning the coil since it may stimulate undesired cortical areas.

6.2. *Figure-of-eight coil*

The region activated by the figure-of-eight coil is under its center (Fig. 6b). The total induced field is the sum of the fields from the two wings of the coil. The resulting field is much more focused than the field produced by a single coil of the same size. Also, the figure-of-eight coil produces a stronger field than single coils, provided that the coils are driven with the same energy. The field strength from the figure-of-eight coil decreases about as quickly with distance (Fig. 7f) as the field from the single coils. The field strength exceeds its half-maximum value over an arc of about 25°. The secondary peak strength from the figure-of-eight coil is about 25% of the primary peak.

6.3. *Cap-shaped and cone coils*

Cap-shaped or cone coils are constructed with a pair of circular windings at such an angle with respect to each other that they fit the curvature of the head. The cone coils are somewhat more effective than the normal planar coils, but at the cost of focality. The secondary peaks from the cone figure-of-eight coil are about 40% of the primary peaks. The primary peak is slightly wider for the cone coil than for the planar figure-of-eight coil.

6.4. *Sham/placebo coils*

Sham stimulation is required in many TMS studies to control any side-effects due to the coil click or somatosensory scalp stimulation. The aim of sham TMS is to apply pulses without stimulating the brain but still causing the perception of real TMS. Sham stimulation can be obtained, for instance, by tilting or lifting the coil so that the electric field induced in the brain will decrease. Generally the disadvantage of these solutions is that the auditory and/or somatosensory sensations may be significantly different from those in real TMS.

An advanced approach is to use a special figure-of-eight coil that is suitable for both real and sham TMS. This can be realized by switching the direction of the current in one of the wings of the coil (Ruohonen et al., 2000). As compared to the normal figure-of-eight coil, the sham coil induces no primary peak below the coil's center. This type of sham stimulation requires a two-channel computerized stimulator device and allows interleaved and randomized trains of real and sham stimuli.

7. Navigated brain stimulation systems

TMS responses are often highly variable. An important source of variability is the variation in the positioning of the coil. Shifts of a few millimeters or small angling of the coil may change the electromagnetic fields in the brain significantly, and thereby cause the response to change or even disappear. Accurate coil positioning, preferably frameless image guidance, is clearly needed (Ruohonen et al., 1996; Miranda et al., 1997; Paus and Wolforth, 1998; Ilmoniemi et al., 1999; Krings et al., 2001). Visualization of the electric field on individual MR images of the subject greatly enhances targeting to predefined cortical loci.

Navigated brain stimulation (NBS) systems have been developed that record automatically the location and orientation of the coil (Fig. 8). The motor response strengths, and other responses, can be linked with individual stimulation pulses to produce immediate colored maps of the stimulation effects. The data reviewing possibilities include browsing of the "hot spots" and comparison of the response maps with the realized strength and direction of the electric field at different locations of the brain. And when

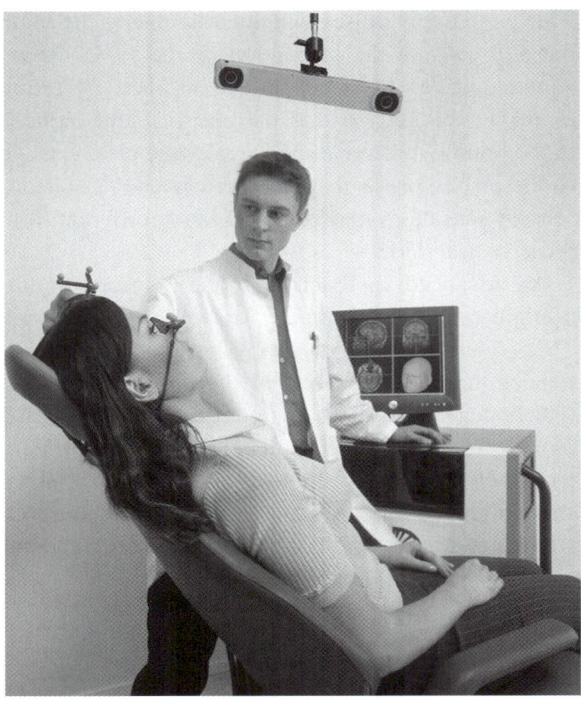

Fig. 8. Navigated brain stimulation (NBS) system. (Courtesy of Nexstim Ltd., Helsinki, Finland.)

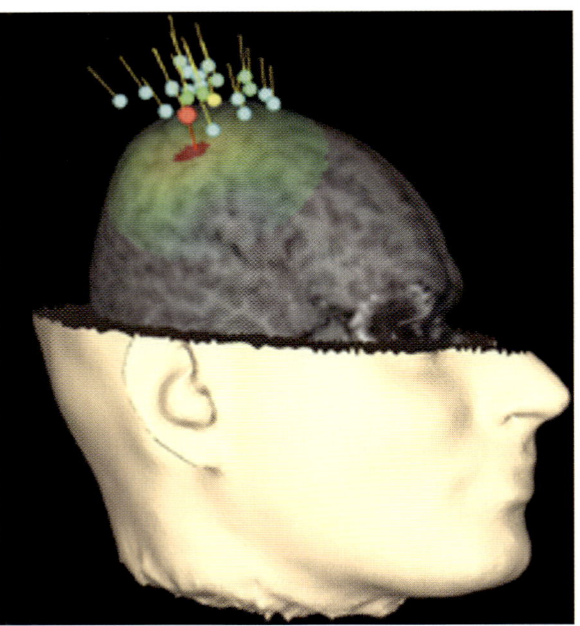

Fig. 9. Motor cortex localization experiment with navigated brain stimulation. The colored dots represent coil positioning; the color indicates the corresponding motor response strength. The induced electric field is shown in the 3-D MRIs is for the selected coil placement.

stimuli are delivered in sequence, navigation can produce "dose" distributions that are the cumulative sum of the electromagnetic exposure everywhere in the brain. Figure 9 shows an example from motor cortex mapping with Navigated Brain Stimulation (NBS).

8. Conclusions

Transcranial magnetic stimulation is based on the well-understood phenomenon of electromagnetic induction. The electric field induced in the neuronal tissue drives ionic currents, which charge the capacitances of neuronal membranes and thereby trigger the firing of neurons. The most likely location of neuronal stimulation in the cerebral cortex is the location of the strongest electric field induced by the stimulation coil.

Frameless stereotaxy combined with MR images is gradually becoming the preferred way of doing TMS. Such Navigated Brain Stimulation equipment, or NBS scanners, comprise a "hot spot" localization system with 3-D visualization of the stimulating field locations within the brain and automatic generation of reaction maps. This allows new clinical concepts such as reporting of the dose of stimulation for improved reliability of clinical examinations.

References

Abdeen, M.A. and Stuchly, M.A. Modeling of magnetic field stimulation of bent neurons. *IEEE Trans. Biomed. Eng.*, 1994, 41: 1092–1095.

Amassian, V.E., Cracco, R.Q. and Maccabee, P.J. Focal stimulation of human cerebral cortex with the magnetic coil: a comparison with electrical stimulation. *Electroenceph. Clin. Neurophysiol.*, 1989, 74: 401–416.

Amassian, V.E., Rothwell, J.C., Cracco, R.Q., Maccabee, P.J., Vergara, M., Hasan, N. and Eberle, L. What is excited by near-threshold twin magnetic stimuli over human cerebral cortex? *J. Physiol.*, 1998, 506: 122pp.

Barker, A.T. An introduction to the basic principles of magnetic nerve stimulation. *J. Clin. Neurophysiol.*, 1991, 8: 26–37.

Basser, P.J. and Roth, B.J. Stimulation of myelinated nerve axon by electromagnetic induction. *Med. Biol. Eng. Comput.*, 1991, 29: 261–268.

Bohning, D.E., Shastri, A., Nahas, Z., Lorberbaum, J.P., Andersen, S.W., Dannels, W.R., Haxthausen, E.U., Vincent, D.J. and George, M.S. Echoplanar BOLD fMRI of brain activation induced by concurrent transcranial magnetic stimulation. *Invest. Radiol.*, 1998, 33: 336–340.

Cadwell, J. Principles of magnetoelectric stimulation. In: S. Chokroverty (Ed.), *Magnetic Stimulation in Clinical Neurophysiology*. Butterworth, Boston, 1990: 13–32.

Carter, N. and Zee, D.S. The anatomical localization of saccades using functional imaging studies and transcranial magnetic stimulation. *Curr. Opin. Neurol.*, 1997, 10: 10–17.

Cerri, G., De Leo, R., Moglie, F. and Schiavoni, A. An accurate 3-D model for magnetic stimulation of the brain cortex. *J. Med. Eng. Technol.*, 1995, 19: 7–16.

Day, B., Dressler, D., de Noordhart, C., Marsden, C., Nakashima, K., Rothwell, J. and Thompson, P. Electrical and magnetic stimulation of the human motor cortex: surface EMG and single motor unit responses. *J Physiol.* (*Lond.*), 1989, 412: 449–473.

D'Inzeo, G., Esselle, K.P., Pisa, S. and Stuchly, M. A. Comparison of homogeneous and heterogeneous tissue models for coil optimization in neural stimulation. *Radio Sci.*, 1995, 30: 245–253.

Durand, D., Ferguson, S. and Dalbasti, T. Effect of surface boundary charge on neuronal magnetic stimulation. *IEEE Trans. Biomed. Eng.*, 1992, 39: 58–64.

Eaton, H. Electric field induced in a spherical volume conductor from arbitrary coils: application to magnetic stimulation and MEG. *Med. Biol. Eng. Comput.*, 1992, 30: 433–440.

Esselle, K.P. and Stuchly, M.A. Cylindrical tissue model for magnetic field stimulation of neurons: effects of coil geometry. *IEEE Trans. Biomed. Eng.*, 1995, 42: 934–941.

Grandori, F. and Ravazzani, P. Magnetic stimulation of the motor cortex – theoretical considerations. *IEEE Trans. Biomed. Eng.*, 1991, 38: 180–191.

Hämäläinen, M., Hari, R., Ilmoniemi, R.J., Knuutila, J. and Lounasmaa, O.V. Magnetoencephalography(theory, instrumentation, and applications to noninvasive studies of the working human brain. *Rev. Mod. Phys.*, 1993, 65: 413–497.

Heller, L. and Van Hulsteyn, D.B. Brain stimulation using electromagnetic sources: theoretical aspects. *Biophys. J.*, 1992, 63: 129–138.

Herwig, U., Kolbel, K., Wunderlich, A.P., Thielscher, A., Von Tiesenhausen, C., Spitzer, M. and Schonfeldt-Lecuona, C. Spatial congruence of neuronavigated transcranial magnetic stimulation and functional neuroimaging. *Clin. Neurophysiol.*, 2002, 113: 462–468.

Ilmoniemi, R.J., Virtanen, J., Ruohonen, J., Karhu, J., Aronen, H., Näätänen, R. and Katila, T. Neuronal responses to magnetic stimulation reveal cortical reactivity and connectivity. *NeuroReport*, 1997, 8: 3537–3540.

Ilmoniemi, R.J., Ruohonen, J., and Karhu, J. Transcranial magnetic stimulation – A new tool for functional imaging of the brain. *Crit. Rev. Biomed. Eng.*, 1999, 27: 241–284.

Krings, T., Buchbinder B.R., Butler W.E., Chiappa, K.H., Jiang, H.J., Rosen, B.R. and Cosgrove, G.R. Stereotactic transcranial magnetic stimulation: correlation with direct electrical cortical stimulation. *Neurosurgery*, 1997, 41: 1319–1325.

Krings, T., Reinges, M.H.T., Foltys, H., Cosgrove, G.R. and Thron, A. Multimodality neuroimaging: research and clinical applications. *Neurology and Clin. Neurophysiol.*, 2001, Number 1A, 1–12.

Maccabee, P.J., Amassian, V.E., Eberle, L. and Cracco, R.Q. Magnetic coil stimulation of straight and bent amphibian and mammalian peripheral nerves in vitro: locus of excitation. *J. Physiol.*, 1993, 460: 201–219.

Miranda, P.C., De Carvalho, M., Conceicao, I., Luis, M.L. and Ducla-Soares, E. A new method for reproducible coil positioning in transcranial magnetic stimulation mapping. *Electroencephalogr. Clin. Neurophysiol.*, 1997, 105: 116–123.

Morioka, T., Mizushima, A., Yamamoto, T., Tobimatsu, S., Matsumoto, S., Hasuo, K., Fujii, K. and Fukui, M. Functional mapping of the sensorimotor cortex: combined use of magnetoencephalography, functional MRI, and motor evoked potentials. *Neuroradiol.*, 1995a, 37: 526–530.

Morioka, T., Yamamoto, T., Mizushima, A., Tombimatsu, S., Shigeto, H., Hasuo, K., Fujiki, K. and Fukui, M. Comparison of magnetoencephalography, functional MRI, and motor evoked potentials in the localization of the sensory-motor cortex. *Neurol. Res.*, 1995b, 17: 361–367.

Nagarajan, S.S., Durand, D.M. and Warman, E.N. Effects of induced electric fields on finite neuronal structures: a simulation study. *IEEE Trans. Biomed. Eng.*, 1993, 40: 1175–1188.

Nagarajan, S.S., Durand, D.M. and Hsuing-Hsu, K. Mapping location of excitation during magnetic stimulation: effects of coil position. *Ann. Biomed. Eng.*, 1997, 25: 112–125.

Oliviero, A., Di Lazzaro, V., Piazza, O., Profice, P., Pennisi, M. A., Della Corte, F. and Tonali, P. Cerebral blood flow and metabolic changes by repetitive magnetic brain stimulation. *J. Neurol.*, 1999, 246: 1164–1168.

Paus, T., Jech, R., Thompson, C.J., Comeau, R., Peters, T. and Evans, A.C. Transcranial magnetic stimulation during positron emission tomography: a new method for studying connectivity of the human cerebral cortex. *J. Neurosci.*, 1997, 17: 3178–3184.

Paus, T. and Wolforth, M. Transcranial magnetic stimulation during PET: reaching and verifying the target site. *Human Brain Mapping*, 1998, 6: 399–402.

Roth, B.J., Saypol, J.M., Hallett, M. and Cohen, L.G. A theoretical calculation of the field induced in the cortex during magnetic stimulation. *Electroenceph. Clin. Neurophysiol.*, 1991, 81: 47–56.

Ruohonen, J., Ravazzani, P., Ilmoniemi, R.J., Galardi, G., Nilsson, J., Panizza, M., Amadio, S., Grandori, F. and Comi, G. Motor cortex mapping with combined MEG and magnetic stimulation. *Electroenceph. Clin. Neurophysiol., Suppl., 1996*, 46: 317–322.

Ruohonen, J., Ollikainen, M., Nikouline, V., Virtanen, J. and Ilmoniemi, R.J. Coil design for real and sham transcranial magnetic stimulation. *IEEE Trans. Biomed. Eng.*, 2000, 47: 145–148.

Ruohonen, J. and Ilmoniemi, R.J. Physical principles for TMS. In: A. Pascual-Leone, N.J. Davey, J.C. Rothwell, E.M. Wassermann and B.K. Puri (Eds.), *Handbook of Magnetic Stimulation*. Arnold Publishers, London, 2002: 18–29.

Terao, Y., Fukuda, H., Ugawa, Y., Hikosaka, O., Hanajima, R., Furubayashi, T., Sakai, K., Miyauchi, S., Sasaki, Y. and Kanazawa I. Visualization of the information flow through human oculomotor cortical regions by transcranial magnetic stimulation. *J. Neurophysiol.*, 1998a, 80: 936–946.

Terao, Y., Ugawa, Y., Sakai, K., Miyauchi, S., Fukuda, H., Sasaki, Y., Takino, R., Hanajima, R., Furubayashi, T., Pütz, B. and Kanazawa, I. Localizing the site of magnetic brain stimulation by functional MRI. *Exp. Brain Res.*, 1998b, 121: 145–152.

Terao, Y. and Ugawa, Y. Basic mechanisms of TMS. *J. Clin. Neurophysiol.*, 2002, 19: 322–343.

Wang, W. and Eisenberg, S.R.A Three-dimensional finite element method for computing magnetically induced currents in tissues. *IEEE Trans. Magn.*, 1994, 30: 5015–5023.

Wassermann, E.M., Wang, B., Zeffiro, T.A., Sadato, N., Pascual-Leone, A., Toro, C. and Hallett, M. Locating the motor cortex on the MRI with transcranial magnetic stimulation and PET. *Neuroimage*, 1996, 3: 1–9.

Transcranial Magnetic Stimulation and Transcranial Direct Current Stimulation (Supplements to Clinical Neurophysiology, Vol. 56)
Editors: W. Paulus, F. Tergau, M.A. Nitsche, J.C. Rothwell, U. Ziemann, M. Hallett

Chapter 2

TMS and threshold hunting

Friedemann Awiszus

Neuromuscular Research Group, Department of Orthopaedics, Otto-von-Guericke Universität, D-39120 Magdeburg (Germany)

1. Introduction

Threshold is a general concept that is often used to describe a basic property of stimulus-response experiments (Carley and Raymond, 1983). While for threshold definition it is essential that the stimulus is characterised by a continuous variable (stimulus strength), each response needs to be classified as either a success or a failure. For excitable membranes, the probability to observe a success increases monotonically with increasing stimulus strength in a sigmoidal fashion that may be described by a cumulative Gaussian (Rubinstein, 1995). The threshold value is then defined as the stimulus strength at which the response probability equals 0.5. Such a threshold concept is especially important for all fields of transcranial magnetic stimulation (TMS) research. Motor threshold is believed to reflect membrane excitability of corticospinal neurones and interneurones projecting on to these neurones in the motor cortex, as well as the excitability of motor neurones in the spinal cord, neuromuscular junctions and muscle (Chen, 2000; Abbruzzese and Trompetto, 2002; Curra et al., 2002; Kobayashi and Pascual-Leone, 2003) while the phosphene threshold is regarded as an excitability measure of the visual cortical areas (Stewart et al., 2001). Moreover, estimating a threshold value is important for stimulus standardisation in double-pulse TMS (Kujirai et al., 1993; Ilic et al., 2002) and good threshold estimates for other brain areas would be helpful in therapeutical applications of TMS (Lisanby et al., 2002).

Despite this fundamental importance of the threshold concept, only a few research efforts were directed towards an optimisation of the threshold estimation procedure for TMS experiments. Most researchers adopt a threshold estimation strategy that is based on the proposals of an IFCN committee (Rossini et al., 1994; Rothwell et al., 1999). These proposals define successes in motor cortex stimulation experiments as stimuli for which a motor evoked potential (MEP) is observed that exceeds some peak-to-peak amplitude (usually 50 μV). Threshold is then approximated by the stimulus strength at which 50% of successes are obtained in a *finite* number of trials (usually 10) which is motivated by the threshold definition given above (a success probability of 0.5 corresponds to 50% of successes in an *infinite* number of trials). However, neither the original version of the IFCN proposals (Rossini

* *Correspondence to*: Prof. Dr. Friedemann Awiszus, Orthopädische Universitätsklinik, Leipziger Straße 44, D-39120 Magdeburg, Germany.
Tel: +49 391 6714067; Fax: +49 391 6714006;
E-mail: friedemann.awiszus@medizin.uni-magdeburg.de

et al., 1994) nor the revised version (Rothwell et al., 1999) give a clear algorithm how to proceed after the stimulating coil has been placed. In particular, in the original version of the committee's proposals, it is assumed that the process is started with some subthreshold value, as the stimulus intensity should be increased in steps of 5% of maximal stimulator output until a stimulus strength is reached with "approximately" 50% successes in 10–20 consecutive stimuli (Rossini et al., 1994). The revised version of the proposals (Rothwell et al., 1999) state in contrast to the earlier version that the procedure should start with a suprathreshold value from which the strength is decreased in steps of 2% or 5% of maximal stimulator output, until a level is reached below which reliable responses disappear. The definition of a reliable response is based on the stimulus strength at which 50% of successes occur in 10–20 stimuli. Neither procedure describes in detail how the sub- or suprathreshold start strength to initialise the procedure should be obtained.

Considering the shortcomings of the IFCN procedure, an alternative way for threshold estimation was developed by Mills and Nithi (1997). In contrast to the IFCN procedures, the Mills–Nithi procedure is given as a completely defined algorithm. This procedure estimates the threshold as the arithmetic mean of the "lower" (largest stimulus strength with no success within 10 trials) and the "upper" threshold (smallest stimulus strength with 10 successes within 10 trials). Clinical applications of the Mills–Nithi procedure (Mills and Nithi, 1997a; Tremblay and Tremblay, 2002) propose that it may be more accurate than the IFCN procedures.

Recently, a third type of threshold-estimation procedure, "adaptive threshold-hunting", has been proposed for threshold estimation in TMS experiments (Awiszus et al., 1999; Fisher et al., 2002). These procedures estimate threshold continuously throughout the stimulus sequence, where the stimulus strength that is to be used for the next stimulus is calculated from the information obtained from the previous stimuli.

While it has been speculated that the adaptive procedures may be more sensitive for threshold estimation (Strens et al., 2002) a rigorous comparison of all three types of threshold estimation procedures has not been performed so far. The aim of the present study was to perform such a comparison. This was achieved by measuring the complete relationship between stimulus strength, and success probability, in experiments on some hand and leg muscles, and to use these measured properties to perform Monte-Carlo simulations that allow a valid comparison of the different TMS-threshold-estimation strategies.

2. Materials and methods

2.1. *Threshold property measurements*

Experiments were performed on four healthy male volunteers who had given their informed consent (all right handed; age range 31–44 years). Additionally, all experimental procedures were approved by the local Ethics Committee. All subjects were involved in previous long-duration TMS experiments performed in this laboratory (Awiszus and Feistner, 1999; Awiszus et al., 1999) and were experienced to maintain a constant active relaxation throughout prolonged periods of TMS. Subjects lay supine, and were instructed to close their eyes while relaxing as completely as possible. Conventional silver/silver chloride electrodes (3M Red Dot) were used to record the surface electromyographic (EMG) activity of seven different target muscles that were obtained in two sessions for each subject. During the hand session three muscles of the right hand (abductor policis brevis (APB); first dorsal interosseus (FDI); abductor digiti minimi (ADM)) were recorded, and during the leg session surface EMG activity of four muscles of the left leg (rectus femoris (RF); vastus medialis (VM); tibialis anterior (TA); extensor digitorum brevis (EDB)) was obtained. For each muscle the different electrode was mounted on the motor point of the particular muscle and the indifferent electrode was placed on a bony landmark close to the target muscle (proximal phalanx of thumb, index and little finger for ADB, FDI and ADM respectively; patella for RF and VM; tibia for TA; malleolus for EDB). The surface EMG signal was amplified by a conventional electromyograph (Counterpoint, Dantec, Skovlunde, Denmark) with a bandpass filter (20 Hz to 5 kHz). The amplified signal was digitised by a laboratory computer with an analog-digital (AD)-conversion card at a sampling rate of 25 kHz per channel.

Transcranial magnetic stimulation was applied with a Magstim 200 stimulator with remote-control interface (The Magstim Company, Dyfed, UK). For hand sessions a flat figure-of-eight coil with an outer wing diameter of 9.5 cm was used. This coil was centred 5 cm left of the vertex and the orientation was adjusted in such a way that the induced current flowed from posterior to anterior approximately perpendicular to the central sulcus. For leg sessions the double-coned coil (The Magstim Company, Dyfed, UK) was used, that was centred 1 cm right of the vertex with the induced current flowing from posterior to anterior. Coil movement during the recording sessions was minimised by mounting the coil to a tripod.

The interstimulus interval was chosen to be equally distributed between 3.5 s and 4.5 s to avoid stimulus anticipation and carry-over effects. Digitised EMG data from 25 ms before to 100 ms after each stimulus were stored on disk for further analysis. In particular the post-stimulus-peak-to-peak amplitude was determined immediately after each stimulus and the stimulus was classified as a success if the peak-to-peak amplitude exceeded 50 μV and as a failure if the amplitude was below that amplitude threshold. TMS strengths, TMS triggers, and data acquisition were controlled by a laboratory computer using purpose-written software.

Each stimulus session started by estimating the resting motor thresholds of all recorded muscles employing the maximum-likelihood threshold-hunting procedure (see below) with 20 stimuli. Then a range of stimulus strengths was chosen containing all thresholds and reaching at least 2% of maximal stimulator output above the highest threshold and 2% of maximal stimulator output below the lowest threshold. For the eight sessions performed during this study, the ranges thus obtained contained between 11 and 17 different stimulus strengths. After range determination the recording session was started during which each chosen stimulus strength was applied 50 times. The order of application of these 550 to 850 stimuli was randomised by the laboratory computer. For three of the eight sessions, the full number of stimuli could not be applied due to coil heating. In these cases the session was terminated prematurely leaving between 27 to 45 applications of each chosen stimulus strength. However, the data-analysis procedure appeared to be rather robust and the results obtained for these shortened sessions did not differ in any obvious way from those obtained during full-length experiments.

2.2. *Analysis of experimental data*

The probability p to obtain a success at a particular magnetic stimulus strength m was modelled by a cumulative Gaussian as

$$p(m,t,s) = \frac{1}{s\sqrt{2\pi}} \int_{-\infty}^{m} e^{\frac{(\tau-t)^2}{2s^2}} \, d\tau$$

parameters t (“threshold” corresponding to the stimulus strength for which $p = 0.5$) and s (“threshold spread” corresponding to the extra amount of stimulus strength that is necessary to increase p from 0.5 to 0.84).

The log-likelihood function L for an experiment during which n stimuli were applied that yielded j successes at magnetic stimulus strengths of $ms_1, \ldots, ms_j$ and k failures at stimulus strengths of $mf_1, \ldots, mf_k$ (where $j + k = n$) was defined as

$$L(t,s) = \sum_{i=1}^{j} \ln(1-p(ms_i, t, s)) + \sum_{i=1}^{k} \ln(p(mf_i, t, s))$$

where ln denotes the natural logarithm. The values of t and s that maximised L were defined as the maximum-likelihood threshold estimate and the maximum-likelihood threshold spread estimate respectively.

For each muscle recorded, estimates of threshold and threshold spread were obtained by minimising $-L$ with a Levenberg–Marquard algorithm.

Monte-Carlo simulations of threshold-estimation procedures

For a given value t of threshold and s of threshold spread, simulated responses at a TMS strength of m were obtained in the following way. A random number r was generated that was equally distributed in the interval from 0 to 1. If $p(m, t, s)$ was smaller than r the simulated response was classified as a success and if it was larger or equal to r it was regarded as a failure. With this procedure the simulated responses had identical statistical properties to responses obtained from a real muscle with these threshold properties.

Simulated responses were used to evaluate three different types of threshold-estimation procedures.

The IFCN procedure. This procedure tried to give an implementation of the threshold-determination procedures of an IFCN committee (Rossini et al., 1994). For all physically realisable stimulus strengths of the Magstim 200 stimulator (i.e. all 100 values from 1% to 100% of maximal stimulator output) 10 simulated responses were obtained yielding 1000 simulated stimuli for each threshold determination. The IFCN threshold estimate was calculated as the smallest stimulus strength with five successes or more.

The Mills–Nithi procedure. This procedure followed the algorithm given in the original publication (Mills and Nithi, 1997b). In particular, single simulated magnetic stimuli were given at intervals of 10% of maximal stimulator strength increasing from 10% until a success was obtained. Then the stimulus strength was reduced in steps of 1% until 10 stimuli applied at a particular strength were classified as failures. This strength was taken as the "lower threshold". Thereafter, the stimulus strength was increased again in steps of 1% of maximal stimulator output until the smallest strength with 10 successes within 10 stimuli was obtained representing the so-called "upper threshold". The procedure incorporated the bookkeeping strategy proposed (see Fig. 1 in Mills and Nithi, 1997b) that allowed to reject most stimulus strengths as candidates for upper or lower threshold even if less than 10 stimuli are applied at each particular strength. The Mills–Nithi threshold estimate was defined as the arithmetic mean of upper and lower threshold.

The maximum-likelihood threshold-hunting procedure. This procedure was implemented as a variant of the so-called "best parameter estimation by sequential testing" (best PEST) strategy (Pentland, 1980). After n stimuli were applied the $n + 1$ stimulus was given at the physically realisable strength m that maximised $L(m, 0.07m)$. If more than one stimulus strength qualified to be the next stimulus the physically realisable strength closest to the mid-point of the interval containing all candidates was chosen. Initially, the procedure was started with two "pseudo responses" (a failure at 0% and a success at 100% of maximal stimulator output) that identify the interval within which the threshold hunting procedure will search for the threshold value. Additionally, if a single candidate was available for the next strength, Brent's method was used to identify the maximum of $L(m, 0.07m)$ that is attained at a stimulus strength m that represents the best estimator of the underlying threshold considering the information gathered during all previous stimuli. This best threshold estimate is not necessarily physically realisable. Maximum-likelihood threshold hunting procedures employing from 10 to 50 stimuli were evaluated in the Monte-Carlo simulations.

For each value of the true threshold t and the threshold spread s, each of the threshold estimation procedures was repeated 10,000 times. For each estimated threshold value t_e the relative error e was calculated as $e = 100\,|\,t{-}t_e\,|\,/t$ giving the absolute distance of the estimate from the true threshold expressed as percentage of the true threshold. The (95%) error limit for each threshold estimation procedure was obtained as the 95%-percentile of the 10,000 error values for this procedure.

2.3. Statistical methods

Measured values are given as mean ± standard deviation. Assumptions about the normality of a distribution were tested with the one-sample Kolmogorov–Smirnov test. A significant correlation between variables was assumed, if the Pearson correlation coefficient differed significantly from zero. An unpaired *t*-test was used to compare experimental results obtained for different motor cortex areas.

For all tests statistical significance was assumed if $p < 0.05$. All statistical evaluations were performed with the software package SPSS version 10.07.

3. Results

3.1. Threshold-property measurements

All subjects were able to maintain an active relaxation of all recorded target muscle throughout the two recording sessions. Figure 1 shows typical results for two muscles of one subject (filled circles fitted with continuous line: FDI; open circles fitted with dashed line: TA). It can be seen that the success rate (i.e. the percentage of successes at each stimulus strength) increases with stimulus strength in a sigmoidal fashion that resembles a cumulative Gaussian. For all 28 muscles the maximum-likelihood estimator for

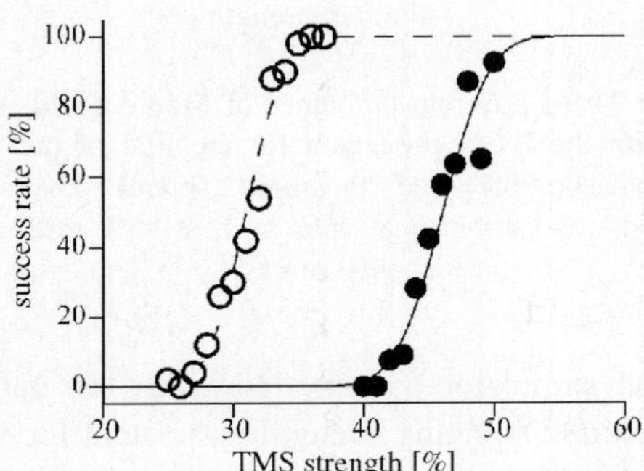

Fig. 1. Experimental results for two muscles of the author. The filled circles with the continuous line represent results obtained for the FDI during the hand session (550 stimuli) and the open circles fitted with the dashed line represent results for the TA obtained during the leg session. The curves were fitted with a maximum-likelihood procedure to the corresponding experimental data with parameters: FDI threshold 46.06%; FDI threshold spread 2.8%; TA threshold 31%; TA threshold spread 2.28%.

threshold and threshold spread gave a reasonable fit for the underlying success rates, thus validating the assumptions for the subsequent Monte-Carlo simulations.

The mean threshold for the leg muscles obtained with the double-coned coil ($46.58 \pm 9.54\%$ of maximal stimulator output) did not differ significantly from the mean threshold of the hand muscles ($47.45 \pm 2.79\%$ of maximal stimulator output; unpaired *t*-test $t = -0.346$, $p = 0.733$). Also the threshold spread parameter ($3.26 \pm 1.03\%$ of maximal stimulator output for leg muscles and $3.37 \pm 0.64\%$ of maximal stimulator output for hand muscles) did not differ between leg and hand muscles (unpaired *t*-test $t = -0.349$, $p = 0.73$).

There was, however, a significant positive correlation between threshold and threshold spread. The scatter diagram of Fig. 2a shows all 28 pairs of threshold and corresponding threshold spread obtained from four subjects where open symbols represent values obtained during the leg and filled symbols represent values obtained during the hand sessions. The correlation coefficient was 0.76 indicating that more than 50% of the variance of threshold spread could be explained by variations of the threshold. Moreover, the regression line almost passed through the origin of Fig. 2a which indicates that the relative threshold spread (threshold spread divided by threshold expressed as percentage of the underlying threshold) is rather constant. This is shown in Fig. 2b which gives the distribution of relative threshold spreads for leg (dashed line) and hand muscles (continuous line). Moreover, the relative threshold spread did not differ between hand ($6.93 \pm 1.31\%$ of threshold) and leg muscles ($7.08 \pm 1.22\%$ of threshold; unpaired *t*-test, $t = -0.31$, $p = 0.76$). For all 28 muscles the relative threshold spread was $7 \pm 1.25\%$ of the threshold and the assumption of a normal distribution of relative threshold spreads could not be rejected (Kolmogorov–Smirnov test, $p = 0.82$).

3.2. Monte-Carlo simulations

With the measured values of the threshold properties Monte-Carlo simulations of the threshold estimation

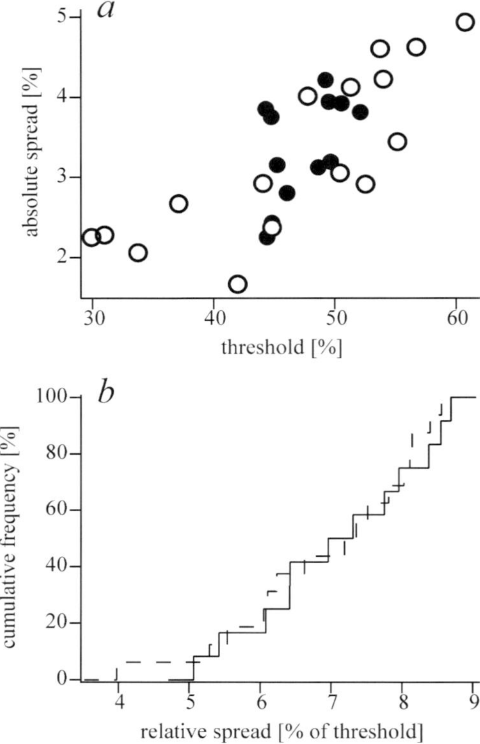

Fig. 2. Summary of the threshold properties for the 28 muscles investigated in this study. A scatter diagram of threshold and corresponding threshold spread is given in Fig. 2a. Filled symbols correspond to muscles recorded during hand sessions and open symbols correspond to muscles recorded during the leg sessions. Figure 2b shows the distributions of the relative threshold spread for all hand (continuous line) and all leg muscles (dashed line).

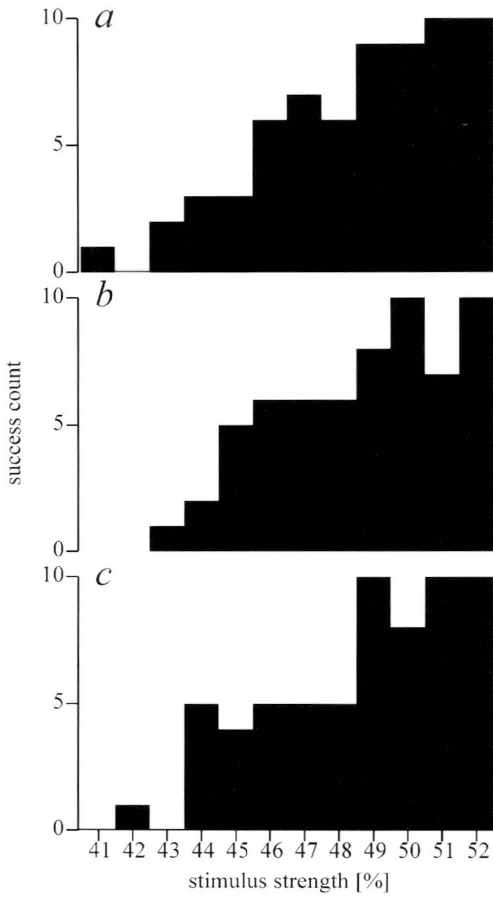

Fig. 3. Three different outcomes of Monte-Carlo simulations with the IFCN procedure for the FDI of the author (threshold 46.06% and threshold spread 2.8%). The threshold was estimated at 46% in *a*, at 45% in *b*, and at 44% in *c*.

procedures for all 28 muscles were performed. Results for three of the 10,000 threshold estimations for the right FDI of the author (threshold 46.06%, threshold spread 2.8% of maximal stimulator output) with the IFCN procedure are shown in Fig. 3. The original proposals of the IFCN procedure (Rossini et al., 1994) suggested that the threshold is assumed at the stimulus strength with 50% of successes. For the threshold estimation trial shown in Fig. 3b there is indeed a unique stimulus strength at which five successes were obtained for 10 stimuli (at 45% of maximal stimulator output). However, the outcome that a unique stimulus strength was found for which five successes within 10 stimuli were obtained was the exception rather than the rule. For more than half of the IFCN Monte-Carlo threshold estimations either no stimulus strength with five successes in 10 stimuli (as in Fig. 3a) or more than one stimulus strength fulfilling the 50% success condition (as in Fig. 3c) was observed. These results indicate that the IFCN estimation procedure requires a definition of the threshold estimate representing an extension of the original definitions in so far that the estimate is at the smallest stimulus strength at which 50% or more successes are observed.

The distribution of all 10,000 IFCN threshold estimates for the right FDI of the author is shown in Fig. 4a. It can be seen that the estimates are distributed fairly symmetrically around the true value of 46.06% of maximal stimulator output and the central 95% of the estimates were contained in the range from 44% to 48% of maximal stimulator output. Calculating the (95%) error limit for the results shown in Fig. 4a yields a value of 4.47% of the true threshold.

Threshold estimates obtained from the Mills–Nithi procedure for the same threshold properties are given in Fig. 4b. As the threshold estimate is defined as the arithmetic mean of two stimulus strength values, it can assume values that are not realisable physically. The central 95% of the Mills–Nithi estimates for this muscle were within the range from 44.5% to 47.5% of maximal stimulator output which yields a (95%) error limit of 3.39% of the true threshold. The number of stimuli required for the Mills–Nithi procedure to reach the results of Fig. 4b was 54 on average.

Threshold-estimation results for the maximum-likelihood threshold hunting procedure for the right FDI of the author are shown in Fig. 4c. The continuous line shows the distribution of estimates observed after 24 stimuli. The central 95% of these estimates ranged from 44.5% to 47.5% yielding an error limit identical to the Mills–Nithi procedure. One should note, however, that the Mills–Nithi procedure required, on average, more than twice the number of stimuli to reach this level of accuracy. When the maximum-likelihood threshold estimation procedure is performed with the number of stimuli required by the Mills–Nithi procedure for these values of the threshold properties (in this case 54), the threshold estimates obtained were much closer to the true value (dashed line in Fig. 4c). In this case the central 95% of the threshold estimates are within the range from 45.08% to 47.04% of maximal stimulator output and the error limit was 2.13% of the true threshold.

These results are summarised in Fig. 5a. The dashed line indicates the error level achievable with the IFCN procedure and the filled circle represents the results of the Mills–Nithi procedure. The continuous line represents error limits obtained for the maximum-likelihood threshold-hunting procedure. It can be seen that the maximum likelihood results cross the dashed line after 16 stimuli. On the other hand, the Mills–Nithi procedure yields a clear error reduction when compared to the IFCN procedure. However, when the Mills–Nithi procedure is compared to the maximum-likelihood procedure, it

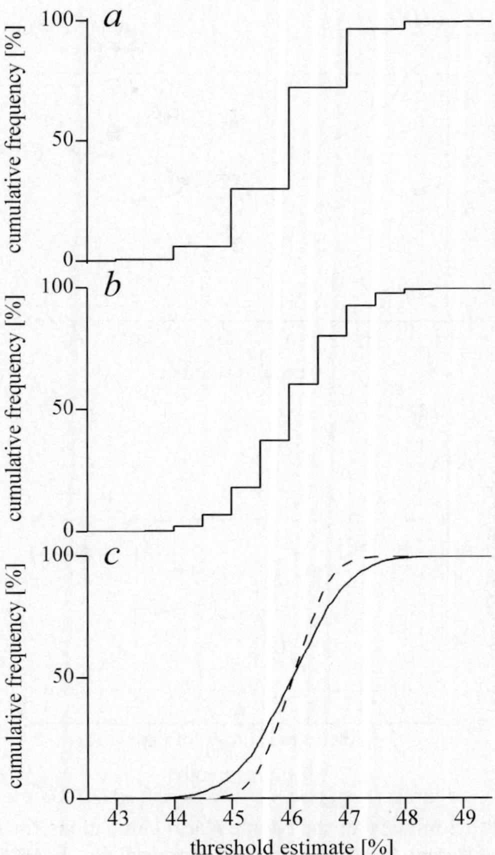

Fig. 4. Distribution of the threshold estimates for the right FDI of the author (true threshold 46.06%; threshold spread 2.8% of maximal stimulator output). Fig. 4a shows the estimates obtained with the IFCN procedure, Fig. 4b gives the estimates of the Mills–Nithi procedure, and Fig. 4c shows the distribution of threshold estimates obtained with the maximum-likelihood threshold-hunting procedure with 24 stimuli (continuous line) or 54 stimuli (dashed line).

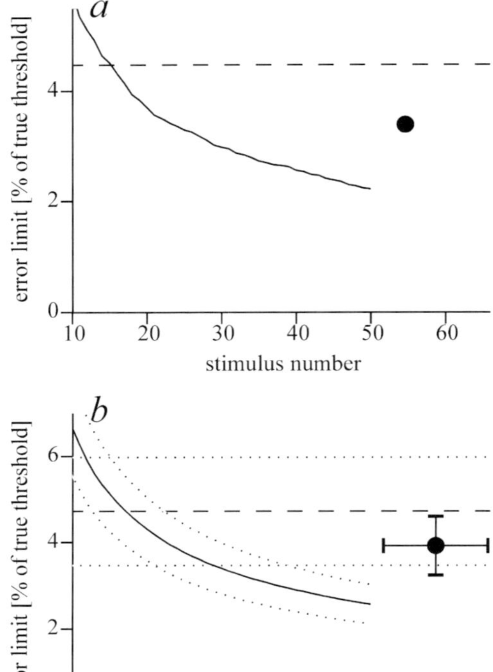

Fig. 5. Summary of the Monte-Carlo simulations for the three different threshold estimation procedures. Figure 5a shows the error limits obtained for a muscle with threshold properties of the FDI of the author and Fig. 5b the average procedure behaviour when the error limits for all 28 muscles were averaged. Dashed lines give the error limit of the IFCN procedure, the filled circle corresponds to the error limit with corresponding average number of stimuli achieved by the Mills–Nithi procedure and the continuous line represents the behaviour of the maximum-likelihood threshold-hunting procedure. Error bars and dotted lines around the dashed and the continuous line represent mean ± standard deviation.

is apparent that the Mills–Nithi procedure, requiring on average 54 stimuli for this particular muscle, gives an accuracy that is reached by just 24 stimuli of the maximum-likelihood procedure. Consequently, using the maximum-likelihood procedure, instead of the Mills–Nithi procedure saves 30 stimuli.

Similar results were obtained for all 28 muscles studied. This is shown in Fig. 5b, giving the averaged error limits for all procedures. The error bars and the dotted lines represent standard deviation. For all but two muscles the Mills–Nithi procedure was superior to the IFCN procedure. However, the maximum-likelihood procedure required less stimuli to reach an accuracy superior to the other procedures. In particular, the maximum-likelihood procedure yielded an error level superior to the IFCN procedure on average after 19 ± 6 stimuli, and an accuracy greater than the Mills–Nithi procedure after 24 ± 3.4 stimuli. Moreover, as the Mills–Nithi procedure required on average 58.7 ± 7 stimuli to reach a threshold estimate, selecting the maximum-likelihood procedure instead of the Mills–Nithi procedure allowed to save on average 34.5 ± 6 stimuli while maintaining the same accuracy.

4. Discussion

The experimental results of this study confirm that TMS threshold behaviour is similar to that of simple excitable membranes (Rubinstein, 1995). In particular, the success probability increases monotonically with increasing stimulus strength in a sigmoidal fashion that may well be described by a cumulative Gaussian. Thus, the complete threshold behaviour can be described by two parameters, the threshold and the threshold spread. The threshold spread parameter is believed to represent the number and the statistical properties of the sodium channels at the action potential initiating site (Rubinstein, 1995), although for TMS experiments it cannot be excluded that synaptic transmission parameters at the interneuronal stages of the action-potential transmission influence this parameter as well. The results of the present study show that the relative threshold spreads were rather constant for different areas of the motor cortex (approximately 7% of the threshold value). However, to what an extent such a threshold behaviour is also present for brain areas other than the motor cortex, for example, visual cortex, remains to be determined in future studies.

Performing the three different threshold estimation strategies on simulated muscles with the measured properties, revealed an important result, that the IFCN procedure yields only a relatively inaccurate estimate. This poor estimation behaviour is remarkable in so far as the IFCN simulations of the present study used 1% steps of maximal stimulator output while the original IFCN proposals suggest that stimulus strength is varied either in 2% or 5% of maximal stimulator output. A coarser stimulator will reduce the number of stimuli necessary to reach the threshold estimate. However, omitting stimulus strengths will decrease accuracy still further, and thus, the IFCN error limits given by the current Monte-Carlo simulations represent an upper limit for the accuracy that is achievable by such a procedure.

The reason for this poor behaviour resides in the fact that the IFCN procedure represents a variant of the so-called "method of constant stimuli" which is known for some time to be an inefficient procedure for threshold estimation in the field of psychophysics (Watson and Fitzhugh, 1990).

Considering the Mills–Nithi procedure as an alternative, it was found, for the 28 muscles investigated in this study, that the average number of stimuli to reach a threshold estimate with the Mills–Nithi procedure was 58.7 ± 7 stimuli which is rather similar to the number of stimuli, required in the original publication reporting a range from 25 to 85 stimuli with a median of 48 for experimental Mills–Nithi threshold estimation on 102 healthy hand muscles (Mills and Nithi, 1997b). The current Monte-Carlo results confirm the assumption of previous clinical applications of the Mills–Nithi procedure (Mills and Nithi, 1997a; Tremblay and Tremblay, 2002) that this procedure is more accurate than an IFCN procedure.

Despite the fact that the Mills–Nithi procedure represents a considerable improvement with respect to IFCN procedures, the current Monte-Carlo simulations clearly show that adaptive threshold-hunting procedures, like the maximum-likelihood threshold-hunting procedure investigated here, will outperform the Mills–Nithi procedure, in so far as either considerably higher accuracy can be reached with the same number of stimuli (see dashed line in Fig. 4c) or a considerable number of stimuli may be saved in order to reach the same level of accuracy.

Recently, adaptive threshold estimation strategies have become popular in peripheral nerve physiology (Bostock et al., 1998). Extensions of this peripheral nerve algorithms have been given for H-reflex thresholds (Chan et al., 2002; Lin et al., 2002) and TMS thresholds (Awiszus et al., 1999; Fisher et al., 2002). The adaptive threshold-hunting strategy proposed in these publications is similar to the maximum-likelihood strategy proposed here. However, the so-called proportional tracking strategy employed by the laboratories of Hugh Bostock and David Burke requires some knowledge of the underlying input-output curve (the relationship between stimulus strength and response amplitude) which may be difficult to measure reliably in the threshold region of motor cortex TMS experiments (Carroll et al., 2001). Moreover, for TMS effects like phosphenes (with a typical yes–no outcome), it is not possible to define a classical input–output curve, and thus, proportional tracking is not possible in this cases. The maximum-likelihood strategy on the other hand, does not require any knowledge of the underlying stimulus-strength-to-response-amplitude relation. For the application of this procedure, it is sufficient to have some idea how the probability of a success increases with increasing stimulus strength which was shown by the present experiments to be rather similar to that of simple excitable membranes (Rubinstein, 1995).

The main disadvantage of the maximum-likelihood threshold-hunting procedure is that considerable computations employing the outcome of all previous stimuli need to be performed to calculate the next stimulus strength. For current laboratory computers, however, the computational power is more than sufficient, to perform these calculations within a fraction of a second, and as the interstimulus interval between subsequent stimuli should be more than three seconds to avoid carryover effects (Rothwell et al., 1999), the computational burden does not represent an obstacle in using the maximum-likelihood procedure. An implementation of the maximum-likelihood threshold-hunting procedure is available from the author and may be downloaded from http://www.med.uni-magdeburg.de/fme/ortho/forsch.htm.

The superiority of adaptive threshold estimation strategies has been known for some time in psychophysics (Pentland, 1980; Emerson, 1984; Watson and Fitzhugh, 1990; Green, 1993) where applications of a single stimulus may be quite time consuming (Weiler and Awiszus, 1998) and thus, strategies that reduce the number of stimuli as far as possible are vital to manage a reasonable threshold estimate. For TMS threshold estimation, stimuli may be applied quite rapidly, and thus, IFCN and Mills–Nithi procedures may be performed within a reasonable amount of time. One should note, however, that all threshold estimation strategies require stationary threshold conditions (i.e. neither threshold nor threshold spread vary with time). For motor-cortex TMS such a stationarity is assumed to require a constant relaxation for resting motor threshold or a constant amount of preinnervation for active motor threshold (Rossini et al., 1994; Rothwell et al., 1999). While subjects with profound experience in TMS (as those investigated in the present study) may easily maintain stationary conditions for a considerable amount of time (e.g. one hour in the present study), the time window within which stationarity may be assumed for subjects or patients being exposed to TMS for the first time may be much more narrow. Consequently, reduction of the total time necessary for threshold estimation may be important to achieve reasonable threshold estimates not only for trained subjects giving further support to use the maximum-likelihood strategy.

Recently, Wassermann (2002) reached the disappointing conclusion that due to the considerable amount of within and across-subject variability, TMS motor threshold measurement is not useful as a clinical test for individual subjects or even for groups with minor differences. This paper employed an IFCN procedure to estimate the motor thresholds (Wassermann, 2002). The results of the present study indicate that such a procedure for threshold estimation has a large procedure-related error that can be avoided, if maximum-likelihood threshold-hunting is used instead. To what an extent, such a shift of threshold-estimation strategies towards adaptive threshold-hunting allows to establish an excitability test with at least some clinical usefulness remains to be determined in future studies.

References

Abbruzzese, G. and Trompetto, C. Clinical and research methods for evaluating cortical excitability. *J. Clin. Neurophysiol.*, 2002, 19: 307–321.

Awiszus, F. and Feistner, H. Recruitment order of single motor units of the anterior tibial muscle in man. *Electroencephalogr. Clin. Neurophysiol. Suppl.*, 1999, 51: 102–112.

Awiszus, F., Feistner, H., Urbach, D. and Bostock, H. Characterisation of paired-pulse transcranial magnetic stimulation conditions yielding intracortical inhibition or I-wave facilitation using a threshold-hunting paradigm. *Exp. Brain Res.*, 1999, 129: 317–324.

Bostock, H., Cikurel, K. and Burke, D. Threshold tracking techniques in the study of human peripheral nerve. *Muscle Nerve*, 1998, 21: 137–158.

Carley, L.R. and Raymond, S.A. Threshold measurement: applications to excitable membranes of nerve and muscle. *J. Neurosci. Methods*, 1983, 9: 309–333.

Carroll, T.J., Riek, S. and Carson, R.G. Reliability of the input-output properties of the cortico-spinal pathway obtained from transcranial magnetic and electrical stimulation. *J. Neurosci. Methods*, 2001, 112: 193–202.

Chan, J.H., Lin, C.S., Pierrot-Deseilligny, E. and Burke, D. Excitability changes in human peripheral nerve axons in a paradigm mimicking paired-pulse transcranial magnetic stimulation. *J. Physiol.*, 2002, 542: 951–961.

Chen, R. Studies of human motor physiology with transcranial magnetic stimulation. *Muscle Nerve*, 2000, 999: S26-S32.

Curra, A., Modugno, N., Inghilleri, M., Manfredi, M., Hallett, M. and Berardelli, A. Transcranial magnetic stimulation techniques in clinical investigation. *Neurology*, 2002, 59: 1851–1859.

Emerson, P.L. Observations on a maximum likelihood method of sequential threshold estimation and a simplified approximation. *Percept. Psychophys.*, 1984, 36: 199–203.

Fisher, J., Nakamura, Y., Bestmann, S., Rothwell, C. and Bostock, H. Two phases of intracortical inhibition revealed by transcranial magnetic threshold tracking. *Exp. Brain Res.*, 2002, 143: 240–248.

Green, D.M. A maximum-likelihood method for estimating thresholds in a yes-no task. *J. Acoust. Soc. Am.*, 1993, 93: 2096–2105.

Ilic, T.V., Meintzschel, F., Cleff, U., Ruge, D., Kessler, K.R. and Ziemann, U. Short-interval paired-pulse inhibition and facilitation of human motor cortex: the dimension of stimulus intensity. *J. Physiol.*, 2002, 545: 153–167.

Kobayashi, M. and Pascual-Leone, A. Transcranial magnetic stimulation in neurology. *Lancet Neurology*, 2003, 2: 145–156.

Kujirai, T., Caramia, M.D., Rothwell, J.C., Day, B.L., Thompson, P.D., Ferbert, A., Wroe, S., Asselman, P. and Marsden, C.D.

Corticocortical inhibition in human motor cortex. *J. Physiol.*, 1993, 471: 501–519.

Lin, C.S., Chan, J.H., Pierrot-Deseilligny, E. and Burke, D. Excitability of human muscle afferents studied using threshold tracking of the H reflex. *J. Physiol.*, 2002, 545: 661–669.

Lisanby, S.H., Kinnunen, L.H. and Crupain, M.J. Applications of TMS to therapy in psychiatry. *J. Clin. Neurophysiol.*, 2002, 19: 344–360.

Mills, K.R. and Nithi, K.A. Corticomotor threshold is reduced in early sporadic amyotrophic lateral sclerosis. *Muscle Nerve*, 1997a, 20: 1137–1141.

Mills, K.R. and Nithi, K.A. Corticomotor threshold to magnetic stimulation: normal values and repeatability. *Muscle Nerve,* 1997b, 20: 570–576.

Pentland, A. Maximum likelihood estimation: the best PEST. *Percept. Psychophys.*, 1980, 28: 377–379.

Rossini, P.M., Barker, A.T., Berardelli, A., Caramia, M.D., Caruso, G., Cracco, R.Q., Dimitrijevic, M.R., Hallett, M., Katayama, Y. and Lucking, C.H. Non-invasive electrical and magnetic stimulation of the brain, spinal cord and roots: basic principles and procedures for routine clinical application. Report of an IFCN committee. *Electroencephalogr. Clin. Neurophysiol.*, 1994, 91: 79–92.

Rothwell, J.C., Hallett, M., Berardelli, A., Eisen, A., Rossini, P. and Paulus, W. Magnetic stimulation: motor evoked potentials. The International Federation of Clinical Neurophysiology. *Electroencephalogr. Clin. Neurophysiol. Suppl.*, 1999, 52: 97–103.

Rubinstein, J.T. Threshold fluctuations in an N sodium channel model of the node of Ranvier. *Biophys. J.*, 1995, 68: 779–785.

Stewart, L.M., Walsh, V. and Rothwell, J.C. Motor and phosphene thresholds: a transcranial magnetic stimulation correlation study. *Neuropsychologia*, 2001, 39: 415–419.

Strens, L.H., Oliviero, A., Bloem, B.R., Gerschlager, W., Rothwell, J.C. and Brown, P. The effects of subthreshold 1 Hz repetitive TMS on cortico-cortical and interhemispheric coherence. *Clin. Neurophysiol.*, 2002, 113: 1279–1285.

Tremblay, F. and Tremblay, L.E. Cortico-motor excitability of the lower limb motor representation: a comparative study in Parkinson's disease and healthy controls. *Clin. Neurophysiol.*, 2002, 113: 2006–2012.

Wassermann, E.M. Variation in the response to transcranial magnetic brain stimulation in the general population. *Clin. Neurophysiol.*, 2002, 113: 1165–1171.

Watson, A.B. and Fitzhugh, A. The method of constant stimuli is inefficient. *Percept. Psychophys.*, 1990, 47: 87–91.

Weiler, H.T. and Awiszus, F. Characterization of human joint proprioception by means of a threshold hunting paradigm. *J. Neurosci. Methods,* 1998, 85: 73–80.

Transcranial Magnetic Stimulation and Transcranial Direct Current Stimulation (Supplements to Clinical Neurophysiology, Vol. 56)
Editors: W. Paulus, F. Tergau, M.A. Nitsche, J.C. Rothwell, U. Ziemann, M. Hallett

Chapter 3

The triple stimulation technique to study corticospinal conduction

M.R. Magistris[a,*] and K.M. Rösler[b]

Departments of Neurology, University Hospitals of [a]Geneva and [b]Berne (Switzerland)

1. Introduction

Motor evoked potentials (MEPs) are presently widely used to study the physiology of corticospinal conduction in healthy subjects and in patients with diseases of the central nervous system (cf. review in Mills, 2000). Main parameters studied by "conventional" MEPs are the *central motor conduction time* (CMCT) and the *size of the MEP* (amplitude, duration and area); other parameters of interest (such as stimulation thresholds, silent period, etc.) will not be considered in this chapter. Measurement of the *CMCT* is of interest since it can disclose slowings of central conduction that could otherwise remain subclinical (Beer et al., 1995). The evaluation of the *size of the MEP* should allow assessing deficits of corticospinal conduction causing the handicap of a patient, because theoretically the size of a MEP should be related to the number of conducting corticospinal motor neurons. However, this relation is obscured by some particular characteristics of MEPs, making the interpretation of MEP size measurements difficult. First, the size of a MEP is reduced (as compared to the peripheral response), and it varies from subject to subject and from one stimulus to the next (Hess et al., 1987). The magnitude of this reduction of amplitude, varies among subjects and is unpredictable (Magistris et al., 1998; Rösler et al., 2002). Second, the MEP is influenced by the excitability of the corticospinal pathway, which is variable and can be facilitated by a number of mechanisms (Hess et al., 1986; Andersen et al., 1999). In particular, voluntary "background" contraction of the target muscle facilitates the MEP, reducing its threshold, shortening its latency and – most notably – increasing its size. The relation between MEP size and background contraction force is not linear and differs between muscles (Hess et al., 1987; Kischka et al., 1993; Rösler et al., 2002). Finally, a MEP includes responses of spinal motor neurons discharging more than once in response to the transcranial stimulus. Probably, the number of such multiple spinal motor neuron discharges differs between subjects, may be facilitated by voluntary contraction, and may be affected by diseases (Naka and Mills, 2000), yet their contribution to the MEP size of a given subject or patient is not known. For these reasons, conventional MEPs do not allow for an accurate assessment of corticospinal deficits.

* *Correspondence to*: Prof. Michel R. Magistris, Unité d'Electroneuromyographie et des Affections Neuromusculaires, Clinique de Neurologie, Hôpitaux Universitaires de Genève, CH-1211 Geneva 14, Switzerland. Tel: (+4122) 37 28 348; Fax (+4122) 37 28 350; E-mail: michel.magistris@hcuge.ch

The triple stimulation technique (TST) was first developed to measure conduction blocks at the peripheral nerve level (Roth and Magistris, 1989). It has been adapted for the use with transcranial brain stimulation (Magistris et al., 1998). It resolves the above mentioned difficulties of conventional MEPs. We shall describe the technique and discuss its yield and limitations in the study of corticospinal conduction.

2. Methods

The TST has been described in detail in several publications (Magistris et al., 1998, 1999; Rösler et al., 1999, 2000; Bühler et al., 2001). In short, three sequential stimuli are given with appropriate delays (Fig. 1). Two collisions of the evoked action potentials can occur. The first stimulus is the transcranial brain stimulus. It is followed by two supramaximal stimuli of the nerve supplying the target muscle, distal then proximal. Two different TST protocols were developed, one for the study of a small hand muscle (abductor digiti minimi; ADM), and one for a foot muscle (abductor hallucis; AH). The peripheral stimuli in the TST-ADM procedure are applied over the ulnar nerve at the wrist, and over the brachial plexus (Magistris et al., 1998). Those for the TST-AH are given over the tibial nerve at the internal malleolus, and to the sciatic nerve at the gluteal fold (Bühler et al., 2001). For the latter, a monopolar needle electrode is used, which is brought into the nerve's proximity to reduce the current needed to reach supramaximal stimulation (Yap and Hirota, 1967). The descending action potentials evoked by the transcranial stimulus collide with the action

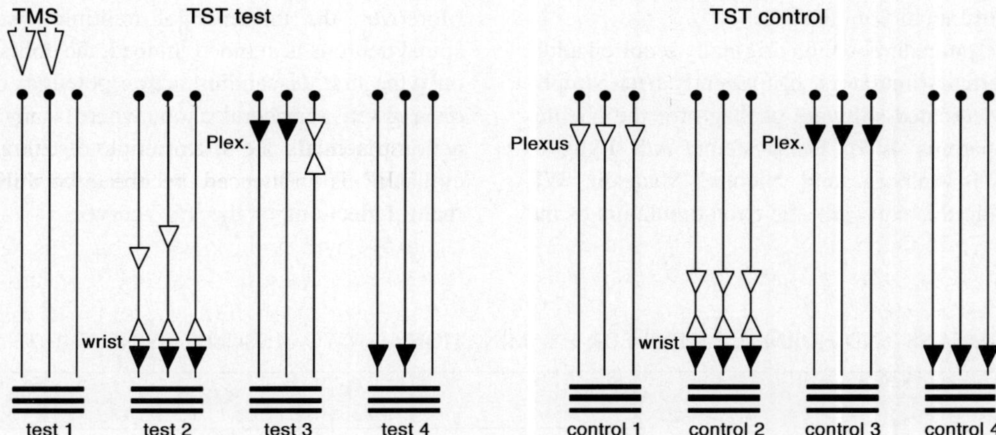

Fig. 1. Triple stimulation technique (TST) principle. The motor tract is simplified to three spinal motor neurons; horizontal lines represent the muscle fibres of the three motor units. Black arrows depict action potentials that cause a trace deflection, open arrows those that do not. (test 1) A submaximal transcranial stimulus excites two spinal motor neurons out of three (large open arrows). (test 2) On 2/3 neurons, TMS induced action potentials descend. Desynchronisation of the two action potentials has occurred (possibly at spinal cell level). After a delay, a maximal stimulus is applied to the peripheral nerve at the wrist. It gives rise to a first negative deflection of the recording trace. The antidromic action potentials collide with the descending action potentials on motor neurons 1 and 2. The action potential on neuron 3 continues to ascend. (test 3) after a second delay a maximal stimulus is applied at the brachial plexus (Plex.). On motor neuron 3, the descending action potential collides with the ascending action potential. (test 4) A synchronised response from the two motor neurons that were initially excited by the transcranial stimulus is recorded as the second deflection of the TST test trace. (control 1) A maximal stimulus is applied at Erb's point. (control 2) after a delay, a maximal stimulus applied at the wrist is recorded as the first deflection of the TST control trace. (control 3) after a delay a maximal stimulus is applied at Erb's point. (control 4) a synchronised response from the three motor neurons is recorded as the second deflection of the TST control trace. The test response is quantified as the ratio of TST test (test 4): TST control (control 4).

potentials evoked by the second, distal stimulus, which is given after a first delay (Fig. 1). After a second delay, the third stimulus, proximal, evokes the response that will be studied. This is the response of those motor units which were initially excited by the transcranial stimulus. However, whereas the descending activity evoked by the brain stimulus was desynchronised, the activity of the same motor units is now synchronised by the collisions, in the same manner as it would in response to a single proximal nerve stimulus (Fig. 1). The response is compared to that of a control curve, obtained by a triple stimulation procedure performed on the peripheral nerve (where the first transcranial stimulus is replaced by a stimulus applied at the proximal site, Fig. 1). The size ratio of the TST test and TST control curves was termed "TST amplitude ratio" or "TST area ratio"; it is an estimate of the proportion of the motor neuron pool of the target muscle that was driven to discharge by the transcranial stimulus.

The TST procedure, which originally required additional external stimulators, has recently been simplified by a dedicated software package for the Nicolet Viking apparatus (Judex Datasystemer A/S, Lyngvej 8, DK-9000 Aalborg, and Nicolet, Madison, WI, USA). Using this software, the two stimulators of the EMG machine are sequentially triggered at preselected intervals, to provide the stimulations needed during both TST test and TST control procedures. For transcranial stimulation, a standard magnetic stimulator is used, and choice of coils and coil placements are the same as for conventional MEPs. A high voltage electrical stimulator (Digitimer, Welwyn Garden City, UK) may replace the magnetic stimulator when direct stimulation of the pyramidal axon hillock is required. Table 2 details the TST procedures.

3. Results

3.1. Neurophysiological aspects

The three stimuli of the TST couple central and peripheral conductions through the two collisions (Fig. 1). This results in a "resynchronisation" of the action potentials evoked by the transcranial stimulus. Moreover, the influence of multiple discharges of spinal neurons is avoided. Indeed, the collision affects only the first descending action potential descending on a given peripheral axon, whereas any following action potentials (i.e. the multiple discharges) escape collision. The latter are recorded between the two main deflections of the TST curve.

TABLE 1

NORMAL MEANS AND NORMAL LIMITS FOR EXAMINATION OF TWO MUSCLES USING THE TST

	ADM *		AH **	
	Mean (SD)	Normal limit	Mean (SD)	Normal limit
TST amplitude ratio	99.1% (2.14)	≥ 93%	95.0% (4.06)	≥ 88%
TST area ratio	98.5% (2.48)	≥ 92%	96.1% (8.30)	≥ 84%
MEP amplitude ratio	66.1% (12.99)	≥ 33%	37.2% (9.72)	≥ 21%
MEP area ratio	96.8% (17.95)	≥ 52%	99.7% (38.45)	≥ 43%
Mean amplitude loss	34.3% ***		57.8% (9.12)	
Mean area loss	16.2% ***		58.9% (11.36)	
TST amplitude variability (CoV)	2.6% *			
MEP amplitude variability (CoV)	8.1% *			

* Magistris et al., 1998. ** Bühler et al., 2000. *** Rösler et al., 2002. CoV: Coefficient of Variation.

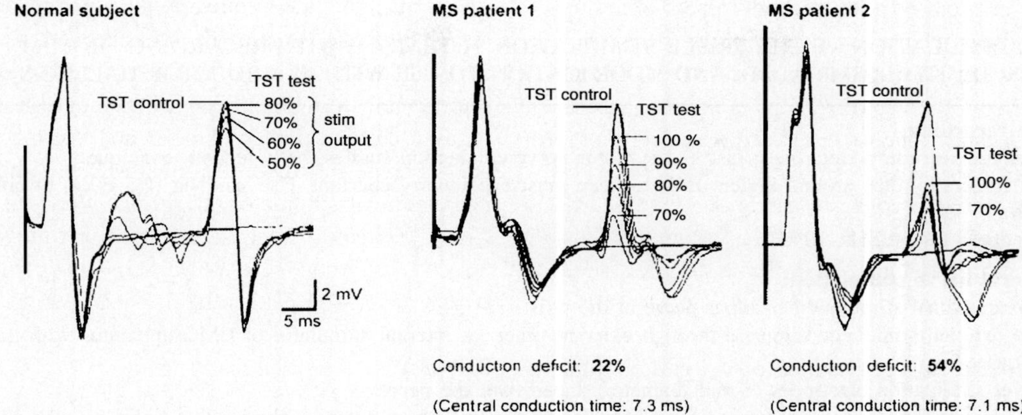

Fig. 2. Examples of TST recordings in a normal subject and in two patients with multiple sclerosis. Several recordings are superimposed: The TST control curve (which calibrates the TST test recordings), and TST test curves obtained with increasing stimulus intensity. Note that in the normal subjects, a superposition of the TST test and TST control curves is obtained (TST amplitude ratio = 100%), whereas in the two MS patients, the TST test curve does not reach the TST control curve even with 100% of stimulator output. Thus, the TST demonstrates a conduction deficit in both patients. The central motor conduction time is normal in both patients.

In both target muscles (ADM and AH) and in all healthy subjects studied, the TST amplitude and area ratios were close to 100%, indicating that nearly all target motor units were driven to discharge by the transcranial stimulus (an example is given in Fig. 2). Moreover, the variability of the TST amplitude and area ratios was markedly reduced compared to MEPs (Magistris et al., 1998). These observations demonstrate that size reduction and variability of MEPs are mainly caused by varying synchronisation of the descending action potentials evoked by the transcranial stimulus, and by the associated phase cancellation phenomena (Fig. 3). The mean values of the TST amplitude and area ratio in normal subjects are given along with the respective normal limits in Table 1.

Comparison of the TST results with those of the conventional MEPs allows an estimate of the degree of size reduction caused by the discharge desynchronisation. For ADM, four previous studies suggested a rather uniform average MEP amplitude loss in healthy subjects and patients, of about one third of the "true" size (Magistris et al., 1998, 1999; Rösler et al., 2000, 2002; Table 1). For AH, the average amplitude loss is greater (approximately 55%), due to the considerably greater degree of discharge desynchronisation (Bühler et al., 2001; Table 1). The size reducing effect of the discharge desynchronisation was not influenced by submaximal stimulation, but differed greatly (and unpredictably) between subjects (Rösler et al., 2002).

An important aspect of the TST is the fact that it does not only resynchronise the motor unit discharges, but that it also suppresses the effects of multiple spinal motor neuron discharges. This effect appeared particularly important for studies involving the AH (Bühler et al., 2001), where multiple spinal motor neuron discharges sometimes appeared to artificially amplify the MEP responses. One of the reasons for the proneness of AH-MEP to be contaminated by multiple discharges probably relates to the fact that the background contraction needed to obtain discharge of all motor units is higher than in ADM. Multiple spinal motor neuron discharges are markedly facilitated by voluntary background contraction (Naka and Mills, 2000; Magistris, Rösler et al., in preparation).

Summarised, the following conclusions can be drawn from the TST studies in healthy subjects:

TABLE 2

CLINICAL APPLICATION OF THE TRIPLE STIMULATION TECHNIQUE WITH RECORDING FROM M. ABDUCTOR DIGITI MINIMI (ADM); AND MODIFICATION TO USE WITH M. ABDUCTOR HALLUCIS (AH)

(1) Muscle recording:

(a) Standard recording electrodes, just as for motor nerve conduction studies, belly-tendon technique.
(b) Fix fingers by tape around fingers II–V to keep muscle geometry constant. Use sandbag (2.5–5 kg) to hold hand down.
(c) Bandpass filters 2 Hz–10 kHz.

(2) Peripheral nerve stimulation:

(a) Supramaximal stimulation of ulnar nerve at the wrist.
(b) Use external stimulator triggered through external timer, or internal stimulator of EMG apparatus with timer software.
(c) Silver stimulation electrodes (8 mm diameter), taped over the nerve.
(d) To account for volume conduction from brachial plexus by Erb stimulation, the median nerve may be stimulated simultaneously.
(e) Apply same facilitation manoeuvre during peripheral stimulation than during transcranial magnetic stimulation (e.g. slight voluntary contraction).

(3) Proximal nerve stimulation:

(a) Brachial plexus stimulation using monopolar cathode at Erb's point (surface 1 cm^2) and large remote anode (30 cm^2) taped over internal region of suprascapular fossa. Supramaximal stimulation often requires application of some external pressure on the stimulating cathode.
(b) Use external stimulator triggered through external timer, or internal stimulator of EMG apparatus with timer software.
(c) Supramaximal stimulation! (is always possible).
(d) Apply same facilitation manoeuvre during peripheral stimulation than during transcranial magnetic stimulation (e.g. slight voluntary contraction).

(4) Transcranial magnetic stimulation:

(a) Any magnetic stimulator can be used.
(b) Circular coil (or other coils depending on purpose of study, e.g. mapping with figure-of-eight coil).
(c) Coil placement as for conventional motor evoked potentials.

(5) Procedure:

(a) Patient lays supine. Fingers fixed by tape and hand fixed by sandbag.
(b) Supramaximal ulnar nerve stimulation at wrist, during slight voluntary contraction.
(c) Supramaximal stimulation at Erb's point, during slight voluntary contraction.
(d) Conventional TMS, several stimuli using increasing stimulation intensity and slight voluntary contraction to facilitate the responses. Measurement of shortest latency and largest amplitude of the motor evoked potential (MEP).
(e) Calculation of delay I = latency of MEP - latency of CMAP wrist (rounded down to nearest ms).
(f) Calculation of delay II = latency of CMAP Erb – latency of CMAP wrist (rounded down to nearest ms).
(g) TST control curve: 3 stimuli are given: Erb – wrist – Erb. Interval between stimuli = delay II.
(h) TST test curve: 3 stimuli are given: TMS – wrist – Erb. Interval between stimuli = delay I (TMS – wrist) and delay II (wrist – Erb).
(i) Several TST test curves are obtained by increasing stimulation intensity of TMS, and applying facilitation manoeuvres, until TST test response size does not increase further.
(j) Repeat TST control curve, perform wrist stimulation alone to insure that no change has occurred during the procedure.
(k) Evoke F-waves by wrist stimulation, for calculation of central motor conduction time.

6) Measurement:

(a) Compare size of TST test curve with that of TST control curve (see Fig. 2). TST amplitude ratio = TST test: TST control; in normal subjects always near 100%; may be reduced in patients in case of conduction failure. Normal limit for ADM > 93% (Table 1).

TABLE 2

CONTINUED

((7) Modifications for leg examination:
(a) Recording from m. abductor hallucis (AH)
(b) Distal nerve stimulation: tibial nerve at ankle.
(c) Proximal nerve stimulation: sciatic nerve at gluteal fold, using "near nerve" needle cathode electrode with large surface anode (30 cm^2) over ventral thigh.
(d) Patient prone; assistant (technician) needed to hold leg.
(e) Double cone coil.
(f) To facilitate responses: flexion and abduction of big toe.

- the transcranial stimulus (whether magnetic or electrical) can excite virtually all axons innervating the target muscle (Magistris et al., 1998; Bühler et al., 2001);
- the reduction in size of the MEP (as compared to the peripheral response) is mainly caused by the desynchronisation of the motor unit potentials that compose the MEP (Fig. 3), and this size reduction is unpredictable and differs between subjects (Magistris et al., 1998; Rösler et al., 2002);
- when all motor units are driven to discharge by the transcranial stimulus, the variability of the MEP size from one response to the next is largely caused by changing degrees of discharge synchronicity (Magistris et al., 1998);
- Multiple discharges of spinal motor neurons may importantly influence the size of a MEP (Magistris et al., 1998; Bühler et al., 2001).

3.2. Clinical application of the TST

Because of the methodological advantages described above, the TST allows detection of corticospinal conduction deficits in patients with central nervous system disorders (for examples see Fig. 2). In many of these patients, the conventional MEP recordings are normal. Thus, the sensitivity of the TST to detect a conduction disorder is considerably greater than that of conventional MEPs. In a large study of 271 patients with various disorders of corticospinal

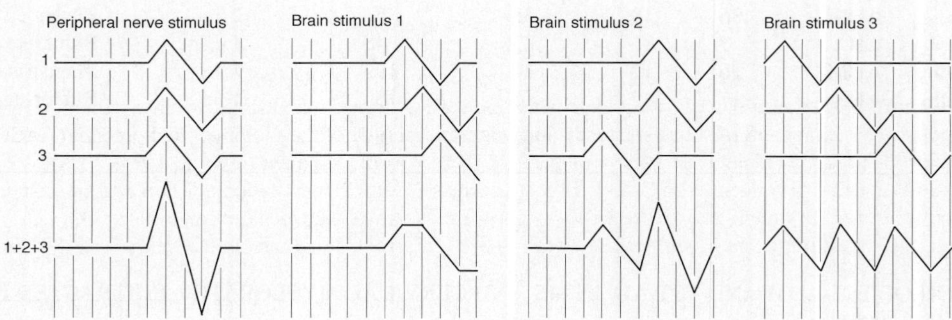

Fig. 3. Phase cancellation. Three identical action potentials (1, 2, and 3) are summated, and the sum potential is shown (1 + 2 + 3). The sum potential varies greatly in shape and size, which is caused by the varying degree of synchronicity of the 3 action potentials. The situation in the left panel is comparable to peripheral nerve stimulation, where action potentials are well aligned; here the amplitude of the sum potential is indicative of the number of action potentials of which it is composed. The situation in the three panels to the right is comparable to transcranial magnetic brain stimulation, where the synchronicity of the potentials varies from one stimulus to the next. The resulting sum varies from stimulus to stimulus, and the size of the resulting potential does not reflect the number of action potentials that composes it.

conduction, the TST disclosed conduction deficits in 212 of 489 arms, while conventional MEPs found abnormalities in 116 sides only (Magistris et al., 1999). Combining MEP and TST results led to an overall increase of diagnostic sensitivity of 1.9-fold. In all but one of the diseases studied, conduction deficits were more common than conduction slowing (Table 3). The only exception to this concerned patients with spondylotic cervical myelopathies, in which prolongations of the CMCT was found more often than deficits of conduction. Still, combining the results of the conventional MEPs with those of the TST increased the sensitivity to detect abnormalities in these patients also (Magistris et al., 1999). Favourable results were also reported in a large series of patients with amyotrophic lateral sclerosis (ALS; Rösler et al., 2000). In ALS, the challenge for the clinician and the electrophysiologist is to detect upper motor neuron dysfunction occurring along with (and masked by) lower motor neuron dysfunction. In our study, the TST-ADM disclosed central conduction deficits attributable to upper motor neuron loss in 15 of 42 sides without any clinical signs of pyramidal tract involvement (Rösler et al., 2000).

Recordings from the AH muscle corroborated the results obtained from ADM, in that the sensitivity increase compared to the conventional MEPs was in a similar range (Bühler et al., 2001; Table 3). Combining the TST-ADM and the TST-AH further increased the diagnostic yield of the method (Table 4).

The TST not only increases the sensitivity of transcranial stimulation to detect conduction deficits, but it also offers a way to quantify the deficit. The measured conduction deficit correlates to the

TABLE 3

NUMBER OF ABNORMAL SIDES IN PATIENTS WITH MS, ALS, OR CERVICAL MYELOPATHIES

Disease	Recording muscle	Sides *n*	Abnormal MEPs Sides *n*	Abnormal TST Sides *n*	Abnormal MEP and TST Sides *n*	Increase in sensitivity	Reference
MS	ADM	221	60	106	113	1.9×	Magistris et al., 1999
MS	AH	27	9	15	17	1.9×	Bühler et al., 2000
ALS	ADM	28	6	13	13	2.2×	Magistris et al., 1999
ALS	ADM	86	18	38	38	2.1×	Rösler et al., 2000
ALS	AH	7	3	3	4	1.3×	Bühler et al., 2000
Cerv. myelopathy	ADM	26	17	14	19	1.1×	Magistris et al., 1999
Cerv. myelopathy	AH	17	12	15	15	1.3×	Bühler et al., 2000
Total		412	125	204	219	1.8×	

TABLE 4

COMBINATION OF TST-ADM AND TST-AH, IN MS AND CERVICAL MYELOPATHY (EXTRACTED FROM BÜHLER ET AL., 2000)

Disease	Sides *n*	Abnormal TST-ADM	Abnormal TST-AH	Both abnormal	Additional gain by TST-AH
MS	25	12	12	17	1.4×
ALS	7	4	2	5	1.3×
Cervical myelopathy	6	2	4	4	2.0×

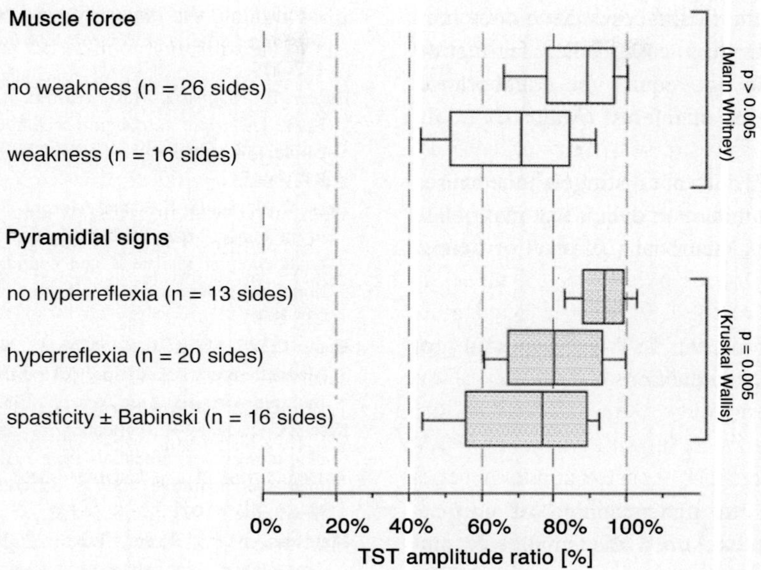

Fig. 4. Relation between motor deficit and TST amplitude ratio in patients with MS, ALS, and cervical myelopathies (extracted from Bühler et al., 2001). Boxes and whiskers give the 5th, 25th, 50th, 75th, and 95th percentiles.

clinical motor deficit suffered by the patients. An example of such a relation is given in Fig. 4. Thus, TST recordings assess the effect of lesions that are relevant in causing the patients deficit. It may be inferred that the TST could serve as a tool to follow the disease progression, e.g. in treatment trials.

Pathophysiologically a reduction of the TST amplitude ratio in a patient can relate to different pathologies. Loss of axons, central conduction block, or increased stimulation threshold will equally affect the response. Considering the result of TST together with the CMCT and with the clinical deficit, helps to distinguish these abnormalities.

3.3. Limitations of the TST

The TST faces several limitations:

- The proximal nerve stimulus (third stimulus) is uncomfortable for the subject. In the TST-ADM, the discomfort of Erb's point stimulus is reduced by use of "monopolar" stimulation (Roth and Magistris, 1987). For the TST-AH, proximal stimulation may be delivered in different ways. Percutaneous transabdominal stimulation, as described by Troni et al. (1996) is very unpleasant, so that one may prefer use of needle stimulation performed at the gluteal fold (Yap and Hirota, 1967).
- The TST cannot use recording from a proximal muscle since this does not allow for a sufficient interval between second and third stimuli.
- An accurate quantification of a corticospinal conduction deficit is sometimes difficult and may require several trials using transcranial stimuli of increasing intensities and different facilitation manoeuvres (Fig. 2). Indeed, whereas the TST easily demonstrates the absence of a corticospinal conduction deficit (when superimposition of test and control curves has been obtained), it is more difficult to determine the precise value of a deficit when the "ceiling effect" given by a control value is no longer available. One has to ascertain that the transcranial stimulus is supramaximal; this is more difficult to achieve than at the peripheral nerve level, due to the larger number of factors that influence corticospinal excitability.
- On some occasions, such as coma, general anaesthesia, hysteria, malingering, absent cooperation of

the subject during the facilitation manoeuvres may be a limitation. In this case, other facilitation manoeuvres that do not require the collaboration of the subject may be of interest (Magistris et al., in preparation).

- Eventually, the TST does not distinguish the causes of a corticospinal conduction deficit that may relate to conduction block, neuronal (cellular) or axonal lesion.

Despite these limitations, the TST is a powerful tool to study corticospinal conduction.

4. Conclusions

The TST improved our understanding of corticospinal conduction. It explained the small size and variable configuration of the conventional MEPs and demonstrated that transcranial stimuli were able to depolarize virtually all motor units of the target muscle. The TST markedly improves the study of corticospinal conduction. It allows better detection and quantification of corticospinal conduction deficits. It offers interesting perspectives for studies that conventional MEPs do not allow. In particular, it may be used as an objective method of assessment of the effects of treatments. Eventually, it will play a role in the further understanding of the physiology of the corticospinal conduction.

Acknowledgements

This work was supported by the Swiss National Foundation for Research (Grants 31-43454.95 and 31-53748.98).

References

Andersen, B., Rösler, K.M. and Lauritzen, M. Non-specific facilitation of responses to transcranial magnetic stimulation. *Muscle Nerve*, 1999, 22: 857–863.

Beer, S., Rösler, K.M. and Hess, C.W. Diagnostic value of paraclinical tests in multiple sclerosis. Relative sensitivities and specificities for reclassification according to the Poser committee criteria. *J. Neurol. Neurosurg. Psychiatry*, 1995, 59: 152–159.

Bühler, R., Magistris, M.R., Truffert, A., Hess, C.W. and Rösler, K.M. The triple stimulation technique to study central motor conduction to the lower limbs. *Clin. Neurophysiol.*, 2001, 112: 938–949.

Hess, C.W., Mills, K.R. and Murray, N.M. Magnetic stimulation of the human brain: facilitation of motor responses by voluntary contraction of ipsilateral and contralateral muscles with additional observations on an amputee. *Neurosci. Lett.*, 1986, 71: 235–240.

Hess, C.W., Mills, K.R., Murray, N.M. and Schriefer, T.N. Magnetic brain stimulation: central motor conduction studies in multiple sclerosis. *Ann. Neurol.*, 1987, 22: 744–752.

Kischka, U., Fajfr, R., Fellenberg, T. and Hess, C.W. Facilitation of motor evoked potentials from magnetic brain stimulation in man: a comparative study of different target muscles. *J. Clin. Neurophys.*, 1993, 10: 505–512.

Magistris, M.R., Rösler, K.M., Truffert, A. and Myers, P. Transcranial stimulation excites virtually all motor neurons supplying the target muscle: A demonstration and a method improving the study of motor evoked potentials. *Brain*, 1998, 121: 437–450.

Magistris, M.R., Rösler, K.M., Truffert, A., Landis, T. and Hess, C.W. A clinical study of motor evoked potentials using a triple stimulation technique. *Brain*, 1999, 122: 265–279.

Mills, K.R. (Ed.). *Magnetic Stimulation of the Human Nervous System*. Oxford University Press, Oxford, 2000.

Naka, D. and Mills, K.R. Further evidence for corticomotor hyperexcitability in amyotrophic lateral sclerosis. *Muscle Nerve*, 2000, 23: 1044–1150.

Rösler, K.M., Etter, C., Truffert, A., Hess, C.W. and Magistris, M.R. Cortical motor output map changes assessed by the triple stimulation technique. *NeuroReport*, 1999, 10: 579–583.

Rösler, K.M., Truffert, A., Hess, C.W. and Magistris, M.R. Quantification of upper motor neuron loss in amyotrophic lateral sclerosis. *Clin. Neurophysiol.*, 2000, 111: 2208–2218.

Rösler, K.M., Petrow, E., Mathis, J., Arányi Z., Hess, C.W. and Magistris, M.R. Effect of discharge desynchronisation on the size of motor evoked potentials: an analysis. *Clin. Neurophysiol.*, 2002, 113: 1680–1687.

Roth, G. and Magistris, M.R. Detection of conduction block by monopolar percutaneous stimulation of the brachial plexus. *Electromyogr. Clin. Neurophysiol.*, 1987, 27: 45–53.

Roth, G. and Magistris, M.R. Identification of motor conduction block despite desynchronisation. A method. *Electromyogr. Clin. Neurophysiol.*, 1989, 29: 305–313.

Yap, C.B. and Hirota, T. Sciatic nerve motor conduction velocity study. *J. Neurol. Neurosurg. Psychiatry*, 1967, 30: 233–239.

Transcranial Magnetic Stimulation and Transcranial Direct Current Stimulation (Supplements to Clinical Neurophysiology, Vol. 56)
Editors: W. Paulus, F. Tergau, M.A. Nitsche, J.C. Rothwell, U. Ziemann, M. Hallett

Chapter 4

Pulse configuration and rTMS efficacy: a review of clinical studies

Martin Sommer* and Walter Paulus

Department of Clinical Neurophysiology, Center for Neurological Medicine, University of Göttingen, Robert-Koch-Str. 40, D-37075 Göttingen (Germany)

1. Introduction

The potential of repetitive transcranial magnetic stimulation (rTMS) to modify the excitability of human cerebral neurons in a non-invasive and lasting manner has incited much interest and hopes in its potential clinical usefulness. However, the results of clinical trials in a variety of neuro-psychiatric disorders have yielded an unexpectedly wide range of responses, from clear clinical benefit to no change or even deleterious effects. Therefore, a recent review concludes that overall evidence for a therapeutic application is lacking so far (Wassermann and Lisanby, 2001).

It is not clear why the results are so inconsistent. We have recently discovered that the configuration of the magnetic pulse exerts a pivotal influence on the outcome of slow-frequency rTMS on the corticospinal excitability in healthy humans (Sommer et al., 2002b). This extends earlier data that demonstrated an influence of stimulus configuration and current direction on the effect of single-pulse TMS, such as motor threshold (Corthout et al., 2001; Kammer et al., 2001). On the basis of these findings we speculated that biphasic pulses may be more suitable to discharge neuronal action potentials, and that monophasic pulses may be more appropriate to induce lasting changes of membrane excitability. We therefore wondered whether pulse configuration and current direction were optimally chosen in published clinical rTMS trials, and whether these factors could have contributed to the wide range of results. Another motivation to go into the detail of potential mechanisms, was the development of transcranial direct current stimulation (Nitsche and Paulus, 2000). This is a different technique to influence human cortical excitability in a lasting fashion (Nitsche and Paulus, 2001), potentially by tissue polarization as seen in animal experiments (Girvin, 1978).

Thus, we reviewed key publications on rTMS trials in depression, Parkinson's disease, writer's cramp and epilepsy, with particular respect to stimulator set-up, stimulus configuration, and current direction. The aforementioned disorders are the ones most intensively studied with rTMS. In addition, we reviewed studies on corticospinal excitability after 1 Hz rTMS in healthy subjects.

2. Studies on 1 Hz rTMS in healthy subjects

With rTMS applied over the primary motor cortex at a frequency of about 1 Hz, Wassermann et al. (1996) and Chen et al. (1997) were the first to report a lasting inhibition of the corticospinal tract as indicated by a

* *Correspondence to*: E-mail msommer@gwdg.de

reduced motor evoked potential (MEP) amplitude after the end of rTMS. Later on, various authors have used comparable paradigms with similar (Wassermann et al., 1998; Maeda et al., 2000; Muellbacher et al., 2000) or dissimilar (Siebner et al., 1999b; Gerschlager et al., 2001; Sommer et al., 2002a; Sommer et al., 2003) results (see Table 1). What can explain these divergent results?

Concerning pulse configuration, a post-rTMS inhibition of the corticospinal tract has been observed with Dantec MagPro (Dantec S.A., Skovlunde, Denmark) (Wassermann et al., 1996), with the Cadwell high-speed stimulator (Cadwell Laboratories Inc, Kennewick, WA, USA) (Chen et al., 1997; Muellbacher et al., 2000), and with the Magstim Rapid stimulator (The Magstim Company, Spring Gardens, Wales, UK) (Maeda et al., 2000). Negative findings exist for the Dantec MagPro (Siebner et al., 1999b) and the Magstim Rapid (Sommer et al., 2002a; Sommer et al., 2003). We are not aware of a negative finding with the Cadwell high-speed stimulator. All of these stimulators have been used with biphasic pulse configurations, except for one study (Sommer et al., 2002b). Unfortunately, a detailed comparison of pulse configurations of these stimulators is not possible, since the exact pulse configuration of the Cadwell high-speed stimulator is not known (the published data refer to another Cadwell single-pulse stimulator (Brasil-Neto et al., 1992)). Experimental data indicate that even slight differences in rise time and zero crossing of the current waveform may profoundly change the induced current (Maccabee et al., 1998). Our data obtained in humans (Sommer et al., 2002b) suggest that monophasic pulses may be more efficacious in inducing a lasting corticospinal inhibition.

The direction of current flow is another factor of importance, especially for the motor threshold, which is the lowest, with the current flowing from posterior to anterior in the brain (i.e. anterior to posterior in the coil (Barker, 1996)), in a direction perpendicular to the central sulcus (Ziemann et al., 1996). Gerschlager and colleagues demonstrated the absence of any post-rTMS inhibition with the coil rotated by 90°, i.e. the current flowing parallel to the central sulcus, while the post-rTMS inhibition was about equally strong with the anterior-posterior and posterior-anterior directions of current flow (Gerschlager et al., 2001). Unfortunately, most studies do not clearly indicate the current direction used, and if it is indicated, it is not always clear whether it refers to the coil or the brain. To further confuse this issue, the direction of current flow in an 8-shaped coil varies according to the manufacturer (e.g. a-p in the Magstim Rapid 8-shaped coil, p-a in the Dantec MC-B70 coil, according to the coil specifications).

So far the physical coil configuration does not seem to be important, however, further developments are currently being studied. Positive and negative findings have been reported with both flat (Maeda et al., 2000; Sommer et al., 2002a; Sommer et al., 2003) and slightly bent 8-shaped coils (Wassermann et al., 1996; Siebner et al., 1999b).

The occurrence of the MEP inhibition is clearly frequency-dependent, since it is absent with rTMS frequencies as low as 0.1 Hz (Chen et al., 1997). The only exception for this seems to be when cortical disinhibition induced at the same time by ischemic deafferentation (Ziemann et al., 1998). Also, with rTMS frequencies considerably faster than 1 Hz no inhibition was shown (Wassermann et al., 1996; Maeda et al., 2000). One explanation for the absence of inhibition with higher frequencies may be the breakdown of cortical inhibitory activity during 5 Hz rTMS, but not during 1 Hz and 2 Hz rTMS (Sommer et al., 2001).

Whether the post-rTMS MEP inhibition depends on the stimulation intensity is questionable. An inhibition was observed after stimulus intensities of 90% motor threshold (MT) (Maeda et al., 2000), 120% (Chen et al., 1997) or 125% MT (Wassermann et al., 1996). No inhibition was found after rTMS of 90% active motor threshold (AMT) (Gerschlager et al., 2001), 90% resting motor threshold (RMT) (Siebner et al., 1999b), or about 120% RMT (Sommer et al., 2002a; Sommer et al., 2003). Obviously, a wide range of stimulus intensities can be used to induce corticospinal inhibition after 1 Hz rTMS.

The site of stimulation is certainly of relevance, with a dorsolateral premotor site 2.5 cm anterior to

TABLE 1

OVERVIEW OVER TRIALS WITH RTMS IN HEALTHY SUBJECTS USING A FREQUENCY OF ABOUT 1 HZ

Author	Year	Nr	Design	Site	Intensity	Freq [Hz]	Duration [seconds]	Intertrain interval [seconds]	Trains per session	Number of sessions	Sum of pulses	Stimulator	Coil	Pulse	Current Direction in brain	% MEP inhibition
Wassermann et al.	1996	10	Open, crossover	M1 + 5 other	125% MT	1	204	NA	1	1 each site	204	Dantec MP	8/50 mm	bi, width 200µs	?	MEP inhibition in 3 of 4 subjects after M1 stim; Tapping faster after rTMS at either site
"	"	"	"	"	100% MT	20	2	58	10	1 each site	400	"	"	"	?	No consistent MEP change after M1 stim; Contralaeral tapping faster after rTMS at either site
Chen et al.	1997	9	Open, no sham	M1	115% MT	0.9	15 min	NA	NA	1	810	Cadwell HS	8/70 mm	bi ?	?	MEP amp signif reduced by 19.5%, no change in tapping rate
"	"	5	"	"	105% MT	0.1	60 min	NA	NA	1	360	"	"	"	?	No signif change in MEP amp
Wassermann et al	1998	11	Blind, crossover	M1	> MT	1	15 min	NA	NA	1	900	Cadwell HS	8/? mm	bi ?	p-a	Input-Output curves reduced bilaterally (tested with circular coil)
"	"	7	"	M1	"	"	"	"	"	"	"	"	"	"	"	No signif change of Input/output curves (tested with circular coil)
Siebner et al.	1999	7	Open, no sham	M1	90% RMT	1	30 min	NA	NA	1	1800	Dantec MP	8/50 mm	bi, width 200µs, rise time 50 µs	?	No signif change of ICE 20 min after rTMS
"	"	11	"	"	"	"	"	"	"	"	"	"	"		"	"No signif change of MT, I/O curve or SP immediately after rTMS
Maeda et al.	2000	20	Open, crossover	M1?	90% MT	1	240	NA	NA	2	480	Mag R	8/70 mm	polyphasic	post-lat ?	MEP amp reduced by 16.1% (day 1)/18.5% (day2), signif interaction site by time
"	"		"	"	"	10	8	72	3	2	480	"	"	"	(in coil?)	No signif change of MEP amp
"	"		"	"	"	20	2	38	6	2	480	"	"	"	"	MEP amp enlarged by 10.8%/24.6%
Muellbacher	2000	7	Open, no sham	M1	115% RMT	1	15 min	NA	NA	1	900	Cadwell HS	8/? mm	bi ?	?	RMT increased, I/O curve less steep; No change of finger force and acceleration
Gerschlager	2001	8	Open, crossover	M1	90% AMT	1	5 min	60	5	1	1500	Mag R	8/90 mm	bi	?	No signif change of MEP amp
"	"	8	"	prefrontal	"	"	"	"	"	"	"	"	"	"	"	No signif change of MEP amp
"	"	8	"	ant parietal	"	"	"	"	"	"	"	"	"	"	"	No signif change of MEP amp
"	"	8	"	premotor	"	"	"	"	"	"	"	"	"	"	"	MEP amp signif reduced by 54%
"	"	2	"	premotor	"	"	"	"	"	"	"	"	"	"	rot.180°	Similar MEP inhibition
"	"	2	"	premotor	"	"	"	"	"	"	"	"	"	"	rot. 90°	No signif MEP inhibition
Touge et al.	2001	13	Open, crossover	M1	95% RMT	1	5 min	60	5	1	1500	Mag R	8/90 mm	?	?	MEP amp signif reduced by 32% after 300 and by 49% after 1500 pulses
"	"	5	"	"	"	"	?	?	?	"	750	"	"	"	"	Less MEP inhibition than after 1500 pulses
"	"	5	"	"	"	"	?	?	?	"	150	"	"	"	"	"
Sommer et al.	2002	9	Blind, crossover	M1	~120% RMT	1	15 min	NA	1	3*	900	Mag R	8/? mm	bi, width ~300µs	p-a	No signif change of MEP amp, finger tapping worsened after real rTMS
"	"	"	"	sham 70∞	"	"	"	"	"	"	"	"	"	"	"	No signif change of MEP amp, finger tapping unchanged
Sommer et al.	2002	10	Blind, crossover	M1	90% RMT	1	15 min	NA	1	1	900	Dantec MP	8/50 mm	bi, width 200µs	a-p	No signif change of MEP amp
"	"	"	"	"	"	"	"	"	"	"	"	"	"	mono, width ~100µs	a-p	MEP amp signif reduced by 34.7%
Plewnia et al.	2003	8	Open, no sham	M1	115% MT	1	13,3 min	NA	NA	2	1600	Mag R	8/70 mm	?	?	MEP amp reduced by 19.5% in the hemisphere stimulated, ICI reduced contralaterally
Sommer et al.	#	8	Open, no sham	M1	~120% RMT	1	15 min	NA	1	2*	900	Mag R	8/? mm	bi, width ~300µs	p-a	No signif change of MEP amp or I/O curve; finger tapping and grip force worsened

Abbreviations: Nr = number of subjects studied, Freq = rTMS frequency, M1 = primary motor cortex, MT = motor threshold, RMT = resting MT, AMT = active MT, # = unpublished, Dantec MP = Dantec MagPro stimulator, Cadwell HS = Cadwell High-Speed stimulator, Mag R = Magstim Rapid stimulator, 0 = circular coil with a diameter of x mm, 8 = 8-shaped coil with a diameter of each wing in mm, usually the outer diameter is indicated, bi = biphasic, mono = monophasic, NA = not applicable, ? = not known, rot = coil rotated, * different types of real rTMS, p-a = posterior-anterior, a-p = anterior-posterior, MEP = motor evoked potential amplitude.

the hot spot for evoking MEPs in hand muscles being potentially more efficacious than the hot spot itself (Gerschlager et al., 2001).

The duration of rTMS and the number of stimuli applied at about 1 Hz is important, since the post-rTMS inhibition is more pronounced with long trains than with short trains of pulses (Touge et al., 2001).

In summary, decisive factors to induce a lasting corticospinal inhibition after 1 Hz rTMS include the site and duration of stimulation as well as the direction of current flow; the pulse configuration is likely to play a role.

3. Studies on movement disorders

Several studies exist on rTMS in Parkinson's disease. Since earlier studies on motor effects during rTMS were inconsistent (Pascual-Leone et al., 1994; Ghabra et al., 1998), we will focus on effects on bradykinesia outlasting rTMS (Table 2). Here, the site of stimulation may be relevant, since rTMS over the supplementary motor area (SMA) yielded a transient worsening (Boylan et al., 2001), while positive reports exist for rTMS over M1 (Siebner et al., 1998; Siebner et al., 1999a; Siebner et al., 2000; Sommer et al., 2002a) and over frontal cortices (Shimamoto et al., 1999; Shimamoto et al., 2001). In addition, the duration of rTMS seems relevant, since long-lasting clinical effects were only reported in trials with rTMS sessions repeated over several days or even weeks (Shimamoto et al., 1999; Shimamoto et al., 2001). However, these reports need to be reproduced with appropriate sham control conditions.

Improvements of motor function have been reported with a variety of stimulus intensities (20% MT to 120% RMT), frequencies (0.2–5 Hz), stimulators and coils. The pulse configuration and current direction were usually not specified (Table 2). In addition, the measures of motor performance varied widely, including overall clinical scales (Siebner et al., 2000; Shimamoto et al., 2001), subtests like finger tapping (Sommer et al., 2002a), and specific pointing movements (Siebner et al., 1999a). Because these measures are difficult to compare, and because only few negative reports have been published (Tergau et al., 1999b), it is very difficult to draw conclusions on how to optimize rTMS in order to maximize clinical effects.

We are aware of a single study on rTMS in writer's cramp (Siebner et al., 1999b), where a subgroup of patients showed improved writing performance and normalized intracortical excitability after 30 min of subthreshold contralateral M1 rTMS. Here, as well as in a study on Parkinson's disease (Sommer et al., 2002a), findings in patients with movement disorders were dissociated from the results in healthy control subjects obtained with the same rTMS protocols. Therefore, it seems that one cannot conclude from rTMS effects in control subjects on rTMS effects in patients. In fact, it may even be possible that effects are reverse between controls and patients and in treated and untreated conditions.

4. Studies on epilepsy

We are aware of two published trials on rTMS in refractory epilepsy, with divergent results (Table 2). They are difficult to compare since site, frequency and duration of stimulation as well as the stimulator set-up differ (Tergau et al., 1999a; Theodore et al., 2002). It seems noticeable, however, that the open study with positive effects (Tergau et al., 1999a) used the same stimulator in the monophasic mode we have used in the above-mentioned study comparing different pulse configurations (Sommer et al., 2002b).

5. Studies on major depression

The widest range of rTMS trials exists for major depressive disorders (Table 1). Positive results have been reported with high (Pascual-Leone et al., 1996) as well as low (Padberg et al., 1999) frequencies, with high (Klein et al., 1999) as well as low (Triggs et al., 1999) stimulus intensities, and with a variety of stimulators. In most trials, the site of stimulation was the left dorsolateral prefrontal cortex, known to be involved in this disorder (see Padberg et al., in this volume). In most studies, the stimulus configuration and current direction were not defined (Table 1). Hence, one cannot unequivocally decide

TABLE 2

OVERVIEW OVER TRIALS WITH rTMS IN PARKINSON'S DISEASE, WRITER'S CRAMP OR EPILEPSY

Author	Year	Nr	Design	Site	Intensity	Freq [Hz]	Duration [seconds]	Intertrain interval [seconds]	Trains per session	Number of sessions	Sum of pulses	Stimulator	Coil	Pulse	Current Direction in brain	Medication	Effects
Parkinson's disease, effects after rTMS																	
Tergau et al.	1999	7	Open, crossover	Vertex	90% MT	1	500	?	2	1	1000	Dantec MP	0/90 mm	bi	?	stable, add-on	No significant effect on UPDRS, RT, Walking speed, self-assessment
"	"	"	"	"	"	5	5	30	40	1	1000	"	"	"	"	"	"
"	"	"	"	"	"	10	2	20	50	1	1000	"	"	"	"	"	"
"	"	"	"	"	"	20	2	45	25	1	1000	"	"	"	"	"	"
Siebner et al.	1999	12	Blind, crossover	M1	90 % RMT	5	30	10	15	1	2250	Dantec MP	8/?	bi, width 200µs,	?	defined off	Movement times significantly more reduced than after sham
"	"	"	"	3cm ant 45° sham	"	"	"	"	"		"	"	"	rise time 50 µs	"		"
Shimamoto et al.	1999	8	Blind, parallel	Frontal	78% Max	0.2	30		2 per week**	9 months	?	Ni	0/152 mm	?	?	stable, add-on	Signif improvement of UPDRS, H/Y scores after 3, 6 and 9 months
"	"	7	"	sham (?)	"	"	"	"	"	"	"	"	"	"	"	"	No signif.change of UPDRS and H/Y scores
Shimamoto et al.	2001	9	Blind, parallel	Frontal	78% Max	0.2	30		2 per week**	2 months	?	Ni	0/152 mm	?	?	stable, add-on	Signif improvement of UPDRS after 1 and 2 months
"	"	9	"	sham (?)	"	"	"	"	"	"	"	"	"	"	"	"	No change of UPDRS
Boylan et al.	2001	10	Blind, crossover	SMA	<=110% MT	10	5	55	40	1	2000	Mag R	8/70 mm	bi, width ~250 µs	?	defined off	Worsening of spiral drawing; UPDRS, RT, threshold unchanged; 2 drop-outs
"	"	"	"	sham 90°	"	"	"	"	"	"	"	"	"	"	"	"	
Siebner et al.	2000	10	Blind, crossover	M1	90 % RMT	5	30	10	15	1	2250	Dantec MP	8/? mm	bi, width 200µs,	?	defined off	UPDRS improvement (rigidity, bradykinesia, tremor)
"	"	"	"	5cm ant 45° sham	"	"	"	"	"	"	"	"	"	rise time 50 µs	"	"	Less improvement than real rTMS
So mmer et al.	2002	11	Blind, crossover	M1	~120% RMT	1	15 min	NA	1	3*	900	Mag R	8/? mm	bi	p-a	stable, add-on	Finger tapping improved, tremor freq and amplitude unchanged
"	"	"	"	sham 70°	"	"	"	"	"	"	"	"	"	"	"	"	No signif change in finger tapping or t remor
Okabe et al	2003	~28	Blind, parallel	M1	110% AMT	0.2	~8 min	6 days	1	8	800	Ni or Mag 200	0, 140-180	?/mono	p-a and a-p	stable, add-on	Similar improvement in all 3 groups
"	"		"	occipital	"	"	"	"	"	"	"	"	"	"	"	"	"
"	"	"	"	sham	200% ST	"	"	"	"	"	"	Electrical	cup electr	?	?	"	"
Writer's cramp																	
Siebner et al.	1999	7	Open, no sham	M1	90% RMT	1	30 min	NA	NA	1	1800	Dantec MP	8/50 mm	bi, width 200µs,	?	none	Normalization of decreased ICI 20 min after rTMS
"	"	16	"	"	"	"	"	"	"	"	"	"	"	rise time 50 µs	"	none	Writing improvement in 8/16, SP prolonged; no change in MT or I/O curve
Epilepsy																	
Tergau et al.	1999	9	Open, no sham	Vertex	90% RMT	0.33	25 min	30	2	5	5000	Dantec MP	0/90 mm	mono	p-a and a-p	stable, add-on	Seizures per week reduced by 38.6
Theodore et al.	2002	24	Blind, parallel	ictal focus	120% MT	1	15 min	?	2	5	9000	Cadwell HS	8/70 mm	?	?	stable, add-on	Insignificant transient improvement of seizure frequency

Abbreviations as in Table 1, Max = maximum stimulator output, ** = one session for either hemisphere, Ni = Nihon Kohden SMN 1100 stimulator, Mag 200 = Magstim 200 stimulator, ST = sensory threshold.

TABLE 3

OVERVIEW OVER TRIALS WITH rTMS IN MAJOR DEPRESSIVE DISORDERS

Author	Year	Nr	Design	Site	Intensity	Freq [Hz]	Duration [seconds]	Interval [seconds]	Session	Sessions	Pulses	Stimulator	Coil	Pulse	Direction in brain	HDRS % increase	Notes
H˚flich et al.	1993	2	Open	Vertex	105-130 % ?	0.3	75	60	10	10	2500	Mag 200	0/140 mm	mono	?	21/0	1 improved by 21%, the other did not improve
George et al.	1995	6	Open	Left DLPFC	80 % MT	20	2	60	20	>= 5	>2000	?	8/? mm	?	?	26	
Grisaru et al.	1995	10	Open	Vertex	2 T	0.017	?	?	?	1	60	?	0/? mm	?	?	?	4 slight improvement, 1 worse, 5 no change
Kolbinger et al.	1995	5	Open	Vertex	MT + 0,3 T	0,25-0,5	?	?	?	5	1250	?	0/? mm	?	?	15	
"	"	5	Open	Vertex	MT - 0,3 T	0,25-0,5	?	?	?	5	1250	?	?	?	?	34	
Conca et al.	1996	12	Open	8 areas	100% Max	<0,17	?	?	?	10	400	Dantec16E05	?	mono, rise 163μs, decay 4 ms	?	58	add on to medication, better than medication alone
Pascual-Leone et al.	1996	17	Blind, crossover	Left DLPFC	90% MT	10	10	60	20	5	10000	Cadwell HS	8/? mm	?	?	45	Nimodipine co-medication
George et al.	1997	12	Blind, crossover	Left DLPFC	80% MT	20	2	>58	20	10	8000	Cadwell HS	8/? mm	?	?	17	superior to sham
Epstein et al.	1998	32	Open	Left DLPFC	110%	10	5	30	10	5	2500	Custom***	8/***	damped cosine	?	52	
Figiel et al.	1998	56	Open	Left DLPFC	110%	10	5	30	10	5	2500	Custom***	8/***	damped cosine	?	?	
Klein et al.	1999	70	Blind, parallel	Right DLPFC	110% MT	1	60	180	2	10	1200	Cadwell HS	0/90 mm	0,1 ms duration	?	50	significantly better than sham
Padberg et al.	1999	6	Blind, parallel	Left DLPFC	90%	10	5	?	5	5	1250	?	?	?	?	?	3/6 responders
"	"	6	Blind, parallel	Left DLPFC	90%	0.3	7	?	10	5	1250	?	?	?	?	?	5/6 responders
"	"	6	Blind, parallel	Left DLPFC	Sham	?	?	?	?	?	?	?	?	?	?	?	none
Triggs et al.	1999	10	Open	Left DLPFC	80% MT	20	2	28	50	10	20000	Mag R	8/~70 mm	?	?	41	9/10 responders
Loo et al.	1999	18	Blind, parallel	Left DLPFC	110% MT	10	5	30	30	>10 ?	>15000?	Mag?	8/70 mm	?	?	?	not better than sham
Kimbrell et al.	1999	9	Blind, crossover	Left DLPFC	80% MT	1	20 min?	NA	1	10	8000	Cadwell HS	8/? mm	?	?	?	trend for improvement, more pronounced with 1 Hz
"	"	13	Blind, crossover	Left DLPFC	"	20	2	60	20	10	8000	"	"	"	"	?	"
Grunhaus et al.	2000	20	Blind, parallel	Left DLPFC	90% MT	10	2 or 6	?	20	20	8000 or 24000	Mag R	8/100 mm	?	?	40	rTMS equal to ECT in non-psychotic depression
George et al.	2000	10	Blind, parallel	Left DLPFC	100% MT	5	8	28	40	10	16000	Cadwell MS	8/? mm	?	?	44	6/10 responders
"	"	10	Blind, parallel	Left DLPFC	100% MT	20	2	22	40	10	16000	Cadwell MS	8/? mm	?	?	28	3/10 responders
"	"	10	Blind, parallel	Left DLPFC	Sham 45∞	20	2	28/22	40	10	16000	Cadwell MS	8/? mm	?	?	24	none
Berman et al.	2000	10	Blind, parallel	Left DLPFC	80% MT	20	2	58	20	10	8000	Cadwell MS	8/? mm	?	?	?	1/10 full responder, 3/10 partial responders
"	"	10	Blind, parallel	Left DLPFC	Sham 45∞	20	2	58	20	10	8000	Cadwell MS	8/? mm	?	?	?	0/10 full or partial responders
Loo et al.	2001	18	Blind, parallel	Left DLPFC	110% MT	10	5	25	30	10	15000	Mag?	8/70 mm	?	?	?	no deterioration of neurophsych measures
Garcia-Toro	2001	20	Blind, parallel	Left DLPFC	90%MT	20	2	20-40	30	10	12000	Dantec MP	8/? mm	?	?	?	significantly better than placebo, 5/20 full responders
"	"	20	Blind, parallel	Left DLPFC	Sham 90°	20	2	20-40	30	10	12000	Dantec MP	8/? mm	?	?	?	1/20 full responders
Manes et al	2001	20	?	Left DLPFC	80% MT	20	2	?	20	5	4000	?	?	?	?	?	no difference real/sham

Abbreviations as in Table 1, *** = custom-built stimulator with iron-filled 8-shaped coil.

on optimal rTMS parameters to maximise effects in patients suffering from major depression.

6. Conclusion

The overview of the studies in healthy subjects using 1 Hz rTMS suggests a rather important role in the site and duration of stimulation, as well as the direction of current flow. Likely, the pulse configuration also determines the rTMS outcome.

The site and duration of stimulation have been taken into account in the existing rTMS trials on major depressive disorder and Parkinson's disease. Unfortunately, current flow and pulse configuration were poorly controlled in these trials. In addition, Parkinson's disease trials are further complicated by the huge range measures indicating clinical impairment and potential improvement.

Therefore, in future rTMS trials, it seems necessary to provide a minimum data set on stimulator and pulse configuration used and the current direction in the brain, and to standardize clinical outcome measures.

Acknowledgements

We used summaries on rTMS trials in depression by George et al. (1999) and on the web (http://www.ists.unibe.ch/TMSAvery.htm). M. S. was supported by the DFG (Deutsche Forschungsgemeinschaft) grant SO 429/2-1, W. P. by the DFG Graduiertenkolleg GRK 632.

References

Barker, A.T. Magnetic nerve stimulation. Basic principles and development. In: J. Nilsson, M. Panizza and F. Grandori (Eds.), *Advances in Magnetic Stimulation. Mathematical Modeling and Clinical Applications*, Vol 2. Pavia, Fondazione Salvatore Maugeri Edizioni, 1996: 1–11.

Berman, R.M., Narasimhan, M., Sanacora, G., Miano, A.P., Hoffman, R.E., Hu, X.S., Charney, D.S. and Boutros, N.N. A randomized clinical trial of repetitive transcranial magnetic stimulation in the treatment of major depression. *Biol. Psychiatry*, 2000, 47: 332–337.

Boylan, L.S., Pullmann, S.L., Lisanby, S.H., Spicknall, K.E. and Sackeim, H.A. Repetitive transcranial magnetic stimulation to SMA worsens complex movements in Parkinson's disease. *Clin. Neurophysiol*., 2001, 112: 259–264.

Brasil-Neto, J.P., Cohen, L.G., Panizza, M., Nilsson, J., Roth, B.J. and Hallett, M. Optimal focal transcranial magnetic activation of the human motor cortex: effects of coil orientation, shape of the induced current pulse, and stimulus intensity. *J. Clin. Neurophysiol.*, 1992, 9: 132–136.

Chen, R., Classen, J., Gerloff, C., Celnik, P., Wassermann, E.M., Hallett, M. and Cohen, L.G. Depression of motor cortex excitability by low-frequency transcranial magnetic stimulation. *Neurology*, 1997, 48: 1398–1403.

Corthout, E., Barker, A.T. and Cowey, A. Transcranial magnetic stimulation Which part of the current waveform causes the stimulation? *Exp. Brain Res.*, 2001, 141: 128–132..

Epstein, C., Figiel, G.S., McDonald, W.M., Amazon-Leece, J. and Figiel, L. Rapid rate transcranial magnetic stimulation in young and middle-aged refractory depressed patients. *Psychiatr. Ann.*, 1998, 28: 36–39.

Garcia-Toro, M., Mayol, A., Arnillas, H., Capllonch, I., Ibarra, O., Crespi, M., Mico, J. and Lafau, O.L.L. Modest adjunctive benefit with transcranial magnetic stimulation in medication-resistant depression. *J. Affect. Disord.*, 2001, 64: 271–275.

George, M.S., Wassermann, E.M., Williams, W.A., Callahan, A., Ketter, T.A., Basser, P., Hallett, M. and Post, R.M. Daily repetitive transcranial magnetic stimulation (rTMS) improves mood in depression. *NeuroReport*, 1995, 6: 1853–1856.

George, M.S., Wassermann, E.M., Kimbrell, T.A., Little, J.T., Williams, W.E., Danielson, A.L., Greenberg, B.D., Hallett, M. and Post, R.M. Mood improvement following daily left prefrontal repetitive transcranial magnetic stimulation in patients with depression: a placebo-controlled crossover trial. *Am. J. Psychiatry*, 1997, 154: 1752–1756.

George, M.S., Nahas, Z., Molloy, M., Speer, A.M., Oliver, N.C., Li, X.B., Arana, G.W., Risch, S.C. and Ballenger, J.C. A controlled trial of daily left prefrontal cortex TMS for treating depression. *Biol. Psychiatry*, 2000, 48: 962–970.

Gerschlager, W., Siebner, H.R. and Rothwell, J.C. Decreased corticospinal excitability after subthreshold 1 Hz rTMS over lateral premotor cortex. *Neurology*, 2001, 57: 449–455.

Ghabra, M., Hallett, M. and Wassermann, E.M. Lack of beneficial effect of repetitive transcranial magnetic stimulation (rTMS) on the Grooved Pegboard task in Parkinson's disease (PD). *Mov. Disord.*, 1998, 13: 288.

Girvin, J.P. A review of basic aspects concerning chronic cerebral stimulation. In: I.S. Cooper (Ed.), *Cerebellar Stimulation in Man*. New York. Raven Press, 1978: 1–12.

Grisaru, N., Yaroslavsky, Y., Abarbanel, J., Lamberg, T. and Belmaker, R.H. Transcranial magnetic stimulation in depression and schizophrenia. *Eur. Neuropsychopharmacol*., 1994, 4: 1608–1610.

Grunhaus, L., Dannon, P.N., Schreiber, S., Dolberg, O.H., Amiaz, R., Ziv, R. and Lefkifker, E. Repetitive transcranial magnetic stimulation is as effective as electroconvulsive therapy in the treatment of nondelusional major depressive disorder: an open study. *Biol. Psychiatry*, 2000, 47: 314–324.

Höflich, G., Kasper, S., Hufnagel, A., Ruhrmann, S. and Möller, H.J. Application of transcranial magnetic stimulation in treatment of drug- resistant major depression – a report of two cases. *Hum. Psychopharmacol.*, 1993, 8: 361–365.

Kammer, T., Beck, S., Thielscher, A., Laubis-Herrmann, U. and Topka, H. Motor threshold in humans: a transcranial magnetic stimulation study comparing different pulse waveforms, current directions and stimulator types. *Clin. Neurophysiol.*, 2001, 112: 250–258.

Kimbrell, T.A., Little, J.T., Dunn, R.T., Frye, M.A., Greenberg, B.D., Wassermann, E.M., Repella, J.D., Danielson, A.L., Willis, M.W., Benson, B.E., Speer, A.M., Osuch, E., George, M.S. and Post, R.M. Frequency dependence of antidepressant response to left prefrontal repetitive transcranial magnetic stimulation (rTMS) as a function of baseline cerebral glucose metabolism. *Biol. Psychiatry*, 1999, 46: 1603–1613..

Klein, E., Kreinin, I., Chistyakov, A., Koren, D., Mecz, L., Marmur, S., Ben-Shachar, D. and Feinsod, M. Therapeutic efficacy of right prefrontal slow repetitive transcranial magnetic stimulation in major depression. A double-blind controlled study. *Arch. Gen. Psychiatry*, 1999, 56: 315–320.

Kolbinger, H.M., Höflich, G., Hufnagel, A., Möller, H.J. and Kasper, S. Transcranial magnetic stimulation (TMS) in the treatment of major depression. *Hum. Psychopharmacol.*, 1995, 10: 305–310..

Loo, C., Mitchell, P., Sachdev, P., McDarmont, B., Parker, G. and Gandeviam S. Double-blind controlled investigation of transcranial magnetic stimulation for the treatment of resistant major depression. *Am. J. Psychiatry*, 1999, 156: 946–948.

Loo, C., Sachdev, P., Elsayed, H., McDarmont, B., Mitchell, P., Wilkinson, M., Parker, G. and Gandevia, S. Effects of a 2- to 4-week course of repetitive transcranial magnetic stimulation (rTMS) on neuropsychologic functioning, electroencephalogram, and auditory threshold in depressed patients. *Biol. Psychiatry*, 2001, 49: 615–623.

Maccabee, P.J., Nagaranjan, S.S., Amassian, V.E., Durand, D.M., Szabo, A.Z., Ahad, A.B., Cracco, R.Q., Lai, K.S. and Eberle, L.P. Influence of pulse sequence, polarity and amplitude on magnetic stimulation of human and porcine periheral nerve. *J. Physiol.*, 1998, 513: 571–585.

Maeda, F., Keenan, J.P., Tormos, J.M., Topka, H. and Pascual-Leone, A. Modulation of corticospinal excitability by repetitive transcranial magnetic stimulation. *Clin. Neurophysiol.*, 2000, 111: 800–905.

Manes, F., Jorge, R., Morcuende, M., Yamada, T., Paradiso, S. and Robinson, R.G. A controlled study of repetitive transcranial magnetic stimulation as a treatment of depression in the elderly. *Int. Psychogeriatr.*, 2001, 13: 225–231.

Muellbacher, W., Ziemann, U., Boroojerdi, B. and Hallett, M. Effects of low-frequency transcranial magnetic stimulation on motor excitability and basic motor behavior. *Clin. Neurophysiol.*, 2000, 111: 1002–1007.

Nitsche, M.A. and Paulus, W. Excitability changes induced in the human motor cortex by weak transcranial direct current stimulation. *J. Physiol.*, 2000, 527: 633–639.

Nitsche, M.A. and Paulus, W. Sustained excitability elevations induced by transcranial DC motor cortex stimulations in humans. *Neurology*, 2001, 57: 1899–1901.

Okabe, S, Ugawa, Y. and Kanazawa, I. 0.2-Hz repetitive transcranial magnetic stimulation has no add-on effects as compared to a realistic sham stimulation in Parkinson's disease. *Mov. Disord.*, 2003, 18: 382–388..

Padberg, F., Zwanzger, P., Thoma, H., Kathmann, N., Haag, C., Greenberg, B.D., Hampel, H. and Moller, H.J. Repetitive transcranial magnetic stimulation (rTMS) in pharmacotherapy-refractory major depression: comparative study of fast, slow and sham rTMS. *Psychiatry Res.*, 1999, 88: 163–171.

Pascual-Leone, A., Valls-Solé, J., Brasil-Neto, J.P., Cammarota, A., Grafman, J. and Hallett, M. Akinesia in Parkinson's disease. II. Effects of subthreshold repetitive transcranial motor cortex stimulation. *Neurology*, 1994, 44: 892–898.

Pascual-Leone, A., Rubio, B., Pallardo, F. and Catala, M.D. Rapid-rate transcranial magnetic stimulation of left dorsolateral prefrontal cortex in drug-resistant depression. *Lancet*, 1996, 348: 233–237.

Plewnia, C., Lotze, M. and Gerloff, C. Disinhibition of the contralateral motor cortex by low-frequency rTMS. *NeuroReport*, 2003, 14: 609–612.

Shimamoto, H., Morimitsu, H., Sugita, S., Nakahara, K. and Shigemori, M. Therapeutic effect of repetitive transcranial magnetic stimulation in Parkinson's disease. *Rinsho Shinkeigaku*, 1999, 39: 1264–1267.

Shimamoto, H., Takasaki, K., Shigemori, M., Imaizumi, T., Ayabe, M. and Shoji, H. Therapeutic effect and mechanism of repetitive transcranial magnetic stimulation in Parkinson's disease. *J. Neurol.*, 2001, 248(Suppl 3): III/48–III/52.

Siebner, H.R., Auer, C., Weindl, D., Mentschel, C. and Conrad, B. 5 Hz transcranial magnetic stimulation applied to the motor cortex has a beneficial effect on skilled drawing movements in Parkinson's disease. *J. Neurol.*, 1998, 245: 362.

Siebner, H.R., Mentschel, C., Auer, C. and Conrad, B. Repetitive transcranial magnetic stimulation has a beneficial effect on bradykinesia in Parkinson's disease. *NeuroReport*, 1999a, 10: 589–594.

Siebner, H.R., Tormos, J.M., Ceballos-Baumann, A.O., Auer, C., Catala, M.D., Conrad, B., Pascual-Leone, A. Low-frequency repetitive transcranial magnetic stimulation of the motor cortex in writer's cramp. *Neurology*, 1999b, 52: 529–537.

Siebner, H.R., Rossmeier, C., Mentschel, C., Peinemann, A. and Conrad B. Short-term motor improvement after sub-threshold 5-Hz repetitive transcranial magnetic stimulation of the primary motor hand area in Parkinson's disease. *J. Neurol. Sci.*, 2000, 178: 91–94.

Sommer, M., Tergau, F., Wischer, S. and Paulus, W. Paired-pulse repetitive transcranial magnetic stimulation of the human motor cortex. *Exp. Brain Res.*, 2001, 139: 465–472.

Sommer, M., Kamm, T., Tergau, F., Ulm, G. and Paulus, W. Repetitive paired-pulse transcranial magnetic stimulation affects corticospinal excitability and finger tapping in Parkinson's disease. *Clin. Neurophysiol.*, 2002a, 113: 944–950.

Sommer, M., Lang, N., Tergau, F. and Paulus, W. Neuronal tissue polarization induced by repetitive transcranial magnetic stimulation? *NeuroReport*, 2002b, 13: 809–811.

Sommer, M., Heise, A., Tings, T., Tergau, F. and Paulus, W. Transient motor lesion induced in healthy humans by biphasic repetitive transcranial magnetic stimulation. Poster presented at the international meeting on transcranial magnetic stimulation in movment disorders, Santa Margherita Ligure, Italy, March 14–15, 2003.

Tergau, F., Wassermann, E.M., Ziemann, U. and Paulus, W. Lack of clinical improvements in patients with Parkinson's disease after low and high frequency repetitive magnetic stimulation. *Electroencephalogr. Clin. Neurophysiol.*, 1999(Suppl.), 51: 281–288.

Touge, T., Gerschlager, W., Brown, P. and Rothwell, J. Are the after-effects of low-frequency rTMS on motor cortex excitability due to changes in the efficacy of cortical synapses? *Clin. Neurophysiol.*, 2001, 112: 2138–2145.

Triggs, W.J., McCoy, K.J.M., Greer, R., Rossi, F., Bowers, D., Kortenkamp, S., Nadeau, S.E., Heilman, K.M. and Goodman, W.K. Effects of left frontal transcranial magnetic stimulation on depressed mood, cognition, and corticomotor threshold. *Biol. Psychiatry*, 1999, 45: 1440–1446.

Wassermann, E.M. and Lisanby, S.H. Therapeutic application of repetitive transcranial magnetic stimulation: a review. *Clin. Neurophysiol.*, 2001, 112: 1367–1377.

Wassermann, E.M., Grafman, J., Berry, C., Hollnagel, C., Wild, K., Clark, K. and Hallett M. Use and safety of a new repetitive transcranial magnetic stimulator. *Electroencephalogr. Clin. Neurophysiol.*, 1996, 101: 412–417.

Wassermann, E.M., Wedegaertner, F.R., Ziemann, U., George, M.S. and Chen, R. Crossed reduction of human motor cortex excitability by 1-Hz transcranial magnetic stimulation. *Neurosci. Lett.*, 1998, 250: 141–144.

Ziemann, U., Rothwell, J.C. and Ridding, M.C. Interaction between intracortical inhibition and facilitation in human motor cortex. *J. Physiol.*, 1996, 496: 873–881.

Ziemann, U., Corwell, B. and Cohen, L.G. Modulation of plasticity in human motor cortex after forearm ischemic nerve block. *J. Neurosci.*, 1998, 18: 1115–1123.

Transcranial Magnetic Stimulation and Transcranial Direct Current Stimulation (Supplements to Clinical Neurophysiology, Vol. 56)
Editors: W. Paulus, F. Tergau, M.A. Nitsche, J.C. Rothwell, U. Ziemann, M. Hallett

Chapter 5

Interleaving fMRI and rTMS

D.E. Bohning[a,*], S. Denslow[a], P.A. Bohning[b], M.P. Lomarev[a] and M.S. George[a–d]

Center for Advanced Imaging Research, Departments of [a]Radiology, [b]Psychiatry, and [c]Neurology, Medical University of South Carolina, Charleston, SC 29425 (USA) and [d]The Ralph H. Johnson Veterans Hospital, Charleston, SC (USA)

1. Introduction

Transcranial magnetic stimulation (TMS) can be interleaved with fMRI to visualize regional brain activity in response to direct, non-invasive, TMS stimulation. We would like to think it is a promising tool for studying brain function. This chapter is a brief overview of the methodology, some of our recent work, and what we plan to do to try to convince ourselves that that is true.

1.1. Review of practical problems encountered in interleaving fMRI with rTMS

Issues involved in performing interleaved fMRI and rTMS include safety, the problems with static and dynamic artifacts, the problem of radiofrequency interference, and the requirements for minimizing the interaction between the TMS pulse and MR image acquisition.

* *Correspondence to*: Dr. Daryl E. Bohning, Radiology Department, Medical University of South Carolina, 169 Ashley Avenue, Charleston, SC 29425, USA.
Tel: (843) 792-6171; Fax: (843) 792-5067;
E-mail: bohninde@musc.edu

1.2. Where are we stimulating – MR-guided rTMS?

A major practical difficulty is the accurate positioning of the TMS coil within the MRI scanner for stimulating a particular area of an individual's brain cortical anatomy, especially when there is no overt response associated with that area. We have designed and built a self-contained hardware/software system for MR-guided TMS coil positioning in interleaved TMS/fMRI studies.

1.3. Repeatability of TMS interleaved with fMRI

In a study of 11 healthy adults, each scanned three times, we assessed both within-subject and between-subject variation of the BOLD response associated with 1 Hz TMS-induced thumb movement (TMS) and compared it with the response associated with a similar, volitionally-induced movement (VOL). BOLD Talairach normalized locations and intensities for TMS and VOL were not significantly different, dx = LR = 0.9 ± 7.1; dy = AP = 2.3 ± 6.0; dz = HF = 0.7 ± 4.3 and dI = 0.36 ± 1.3, respectively. Coil placement relative to BOLD location varied more than did BOLD location (dx = 17.3 ± 9.5, dy = 21.8 ± 8.7, dz = 11.0 ± 9.0) over repeated studies.

1.4. *Can temporal resolution be improved with paired-pulse rTMS?*

We have combined the TMS paired-pulse technique, a well-characterized physiological tool for testing intracortical inhibition and facilitation, with BOLD-fMRI neuroimaging. A Macintosh G3 laptop controlled the firing of two stimulators, synchronously interleaved with the fMRI acquisition, through a single TMS coil as a list of paired-pulse events with different interstimulus intervals (ISI). We hope to use this technique both for testing cortical sensitivity in areas other than motor cortex, and for using the BOLD response amplitude dependence on ISI to investigate brain communication at high time resolution.

1.5. *Does TMS directly induce a BOLD-fMRI response?*

The question of whether or not TMS directly induces a BOLD-fMRI response is central to its application as a tool for neuroscience; some pros and cons and future work.

2. Review of practical problems encountered in interleaving fMRI with rTMS

Shortly after Paus et al. (1997) and Fox et al. (1997) showed that TMS could be be interleaved with PET, we were able to demonstrate that TMS could be interleaved with fMRI (Bohning et al., 1998). Since the methodology has already been described (Bohning et al., 1998; Shastri et al., 1999), and others have since more thoroughly investigated the artifacts (Baudewig et al., 2000; Bestmann et al., 2003), we will refer the reader to those papers and here give only an overview.

The general arrangement for interleaving TMS with fMRI is shown in Fig. 1. To minimize interference with the scanner, the TMS stimulator is kept in the MR instrument room behind the scanner. The TMS coil cable is fed through a custom RF filter (Fig. 2) and the MR room penetration panel, and to the subject through the back of the magnet.

2.1. *Safety*

The first consideration is that of the safety of the subject and the research personnel. Initially, there was concern that the interaction of the TMS coil's magnetic field, roughly 1–2 Tesla, with that of the MR scanner's magnetic field, 1.5 Tesla, might cause the coil to move or break violently, causing injury. Using a flat figure-8 coil consisting of two wire loops with counter-rotating currents, the torques on the two loops are in opposite direction, so, in theory, they cancel in the MR scanner's uniform field, eliminating net motion. In practice, coils, even the same model from

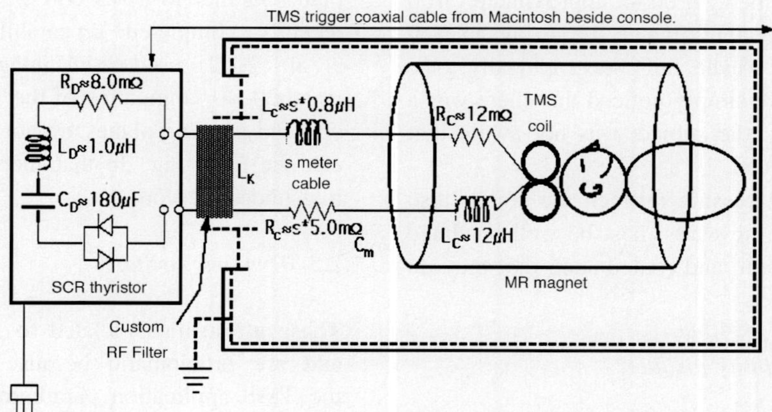

Fig. 1. General layout for TMS interleaved with fMRI.

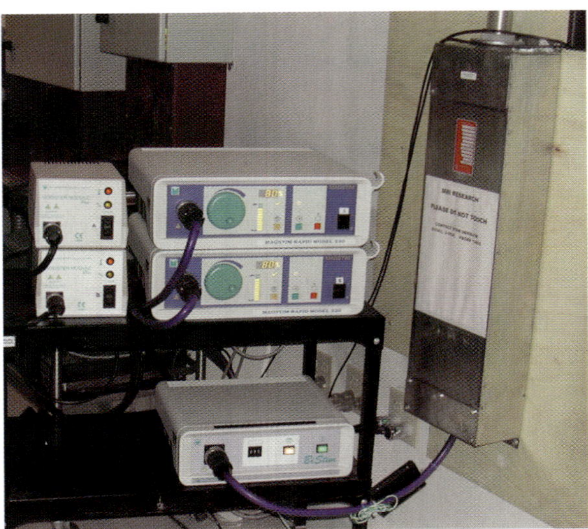

Fig. 2. TMS stimulator and custom RF filter.

the same manufacturer, vary in their symmetry, so they should be checked by holding them inside the scanner and firing them, first starting with a very low intensity and then gradually increasing the intensity, feeling carefully for any tendency to move or flex. The opposing torques on the two loops do try to fold the figure-8 coil, creating internal stresses which can crack or break the coil. Though the modified Dantec MC-B70 (Dantec Medical A/S, Skovlunde, Denmark) coil used in our laboratory for TMS interleaved with fMRI has proven to be quite strong, it did, eventually crack, but only after being used for approximately 100 studies consisting of approximately 150 firings in each study. It did not, however, fail catastrophically. One day after a study, we simply noticed that there was a crack in the casing; the subject was not aware that anything had happened.

The high current passing through the coil is also of concern, and all the wires must be well insulated and in good condition, and routed such that they do not touch the subject.

2.2. *Static susceptibility artifacts*

For interleaved TMS/fMRI, a pure copper coil embedded in some MR benign material to give it rigidity is best. Additional wires, switches, or sensors, usually cause artifacts. If they contain ferromagnetic materials, the artifacts can be so severe that the MR signal is completely destroyed in a large area around the coil. Even without such additional sources of artifact, the coil itself will cause noticeable artifact, which varies both with coil orientation with respect to the magnet field of the MR magnet (B_0) and the orientation of the imaging plane to the TMS coil (Bestmann, 2003). To include both motor and auditory bilaterally, our original studies used a coil tilted 20–40° from the axial plane with coronal imaging planes, roughly perpendicular to the plane of the figure-8. At the time, we also felt that the 2 mm pixel dimension in the direction of the coil, as opposed to the larger 5 mm slice thickness, would minimize the susceptibility artifact and would make it easier to see the area affected and how badly it was compromised. Phantom studies showed that, at the depth of the cerebral cortex, the reduction of signal was only 10–15%. Since the artifact is static and does not correlate with the fMRI paradigm, it did not seriously affected the ability to perform TMS interleaved with fMRI. Figure 3a shows an axial image of a phantom in which the susceptibility difference has been mapped for the TMS coil tilted about 30° from the coronal plane, long axis perpendicular to the image plane. The 0.006 Gauss contour intersects the white line at a depth of about 15 mm. Bestmann et al. (2003) have reported that an imaging plane parallel to TMS coil was preferable, and our recently completed repeatability study (Denslow et al., 2002) used axial imaging planes with the usual 20–40° angulation of the TMS coil. Though the coil and imaging planes are not far from parallel, one can see from Fig. 3b that there is still some signal loss under the coil.

2.3. *Dynamic artifacts*

These are artifacts related to the firing of the coil and are problematic because they correlate with the TMS application paradigm. There is the major interaction of the coil's short, strong pulsed magnetic field with the MR imaging process, and secondary

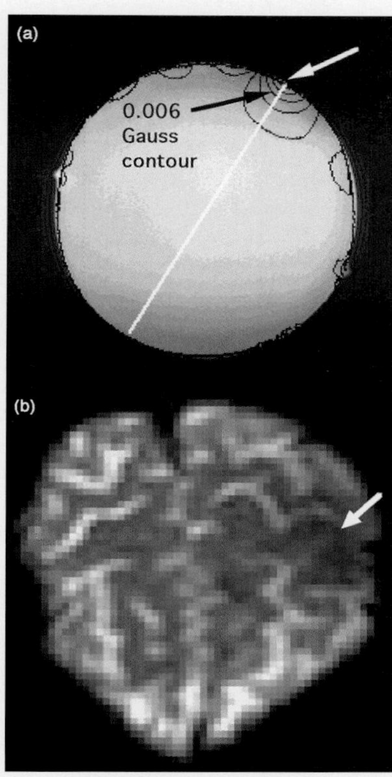

Fig. 3. TMS coil induced susceptibility artifacts: (a) phase shift map in phantom and (b) signal loss in axial fMRI image.

effects caused by movements and/or induced currents because the coil is not symmetric. The TMS pulse duration is quite short (250–350 μs), and can easily be interleaved with the MR image acquisition after the sampling of the MR signal and before the next excitation using a personal computer to synchronize the firing of the TMS coil with a timing pulse from the MR scanner (Bohning et al., 1998; Shastri et al., 1999) as shown in Fig. 4.

Our group uses a Macintosh G4 with a general purpose I/O board and Labview software (National Instruments, Inc, Austin, TX). However, depending on the TMS intensity, the effects of the TMS pulse can last considerably longer. In Fig. 5, the relative timing and amplitudes of the TMS and MR acquisition induced signals can be seen in a combined plot of the signal induced in a pickup coil placed near the TMS coil and the signal induced in the open leads of the TMS coil during an fMRI image acquisition; here, the effects of the TMS pulse last 40–50 ms. There were two voltage pulses induced in the TMS coil leads during the RF fat saturation of up to approximately ± 3 and ± 12 V, respectively, and the RF excitation gave a large, short pulse in the TMS coil of up to ± 30 V. Though the RF-induced pulses had no apparent affect on the stimulator, serious interference with the imaging process was observed if the

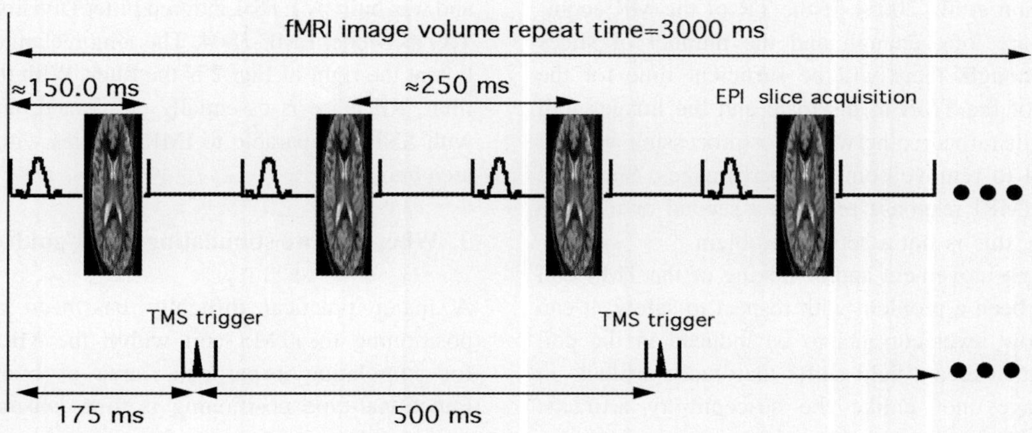

Fig. 4. Typical timimg of TMS interleaved with block design fMRI paradigm.

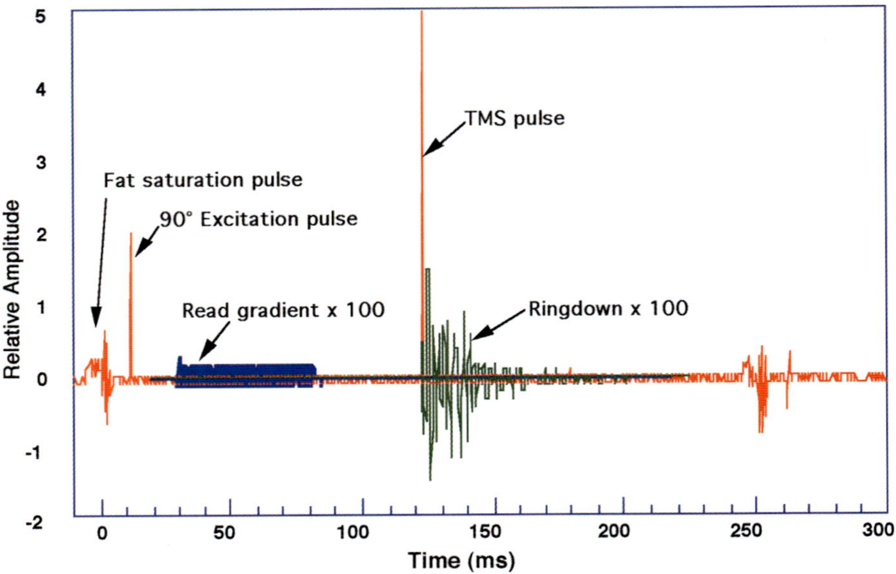

Fig. 5. Combined plot of the signal induced in a pickup coil placed near the TMS coil and the signal induced in the open leads of the TMS coil during an fMRI image acquisition.

delay between the TMS and the following RF excitation was shorter than 50 ms. Pulses from the switched gradients were two orders of magnitude.

In addition, the period during the applications of the RF pulses should be strictly avoided since this can create effects that are even longer lasting (Bestmann et al., 2003). If the TR of the MR acquisitions are long enough and the number of slices small enough, there will be sufficient time for the effects of the TMS to dissipate and the images will not be disturbed; otherwise, postprocessing will be required to remove compromised images. Since the BOLD-fMRI response requires a second or more to develop, this is not a serious problem.

Though movement and/or flexing of the TMS coil has not been a problem with respect to safety, it can cause low level currents to be induced in the coil which then create field shifts that cause artifacts in the images not unlike the susceptibilty artifacts. Unfortunately, they are dynamic and change in correlation with the TMS paradigm, so can confound the analysis of the fMRI data; they are best avoided, if possible with a rigid, well-balanced TMS coil.

2.4. RF noise and SNR

A custom RF filter was designed in collaboration with and was built by ETS-Lindgren Filter Division (Austin, TX) as Model LMF-3804. The long rectangular metal box at the right of Fig. 2 is the filter. With the custom filter, RF noise is essentially eliminated, and images with SNR comparable to fMRI studies without TMS are obtained.

3. Where are we stimulating – MR-guided rTMS?

A major practical difficulty has been accurately positioning the TMS coil within the MRI scanner for stimulating a particular area of brain cortex. Functional-type positioning is time-consuming, and operator dependent, and only works for areas of the brain, e.g. motor cortex, for which TMS induces an

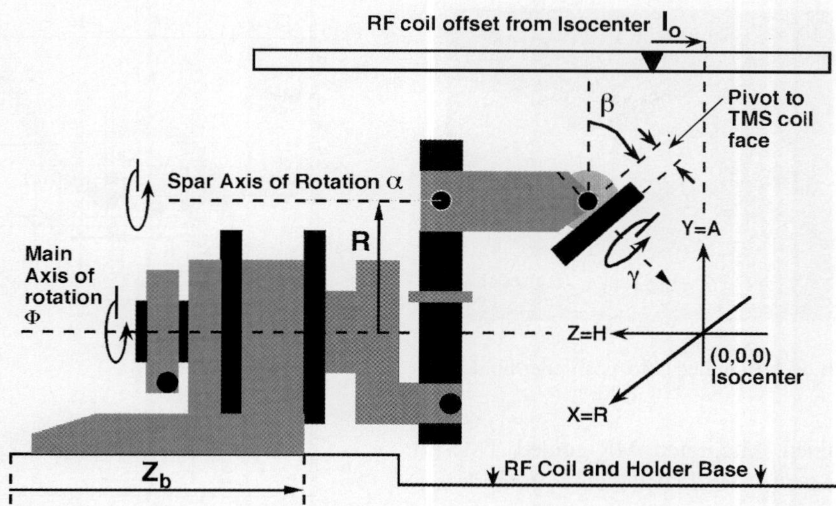

Fig. 6. Schematic of MRGuidedTMS positioner holder illustrating degrees of freedom.

overt response. Neuro-navigation system are very expensive and, since they cannot be used near the MR scanner, they require a complicated series of operations. A set of MR images is first acquired of the subject's brain, then loaded into the neuro-navigational workstation and displayed. Then, a locating pointer at the end of a moveable arm, of some sort, is moved over the subject's scalp while a marker, displayed on the MR images, tracks the position of the pointer relative to the cortical anatomy displayed in the MR images. Once the anatomical location to be selected as the target for the TMS stimulation is chosen, the pointer's position on the subject's scalp over which the TMS coil is to be placed for stimulating a desired target area is marked. The subject can then be returned to the MR scanner, the TMS coil positioned over the mark that has been made on the subject's scalp, and, finally, the coil rigidly fixed for the study by some other apparatus.

Feeling that the neuro-navigation apparatus and the TMS coil fixation apparatus could be combined, we have designed and built a self-contained hardware/software system for MR-guided TMS coil positioning/holding in interleaved TMS/fMRI studies. It allows us to accurately position the TMS coil for stimulation of a point in the subject's brain selected on an anatomical MR image acquired at the beginning of the study, then lock the coil into position for the study without moving the subject from the scanner bed. This self-contained hardware/software system consists of an articulated TMS coil positioner/holder with six calibrated degrees of freedom, sufficiently compact for use inside a cylindrical RF head coil, along with a software package for transforming between MR image coordinates, MR scanner space coordinates, and positioner/holder settings. Figure 6 shows a schematic illustrating the six degrees of freedom that allow it to be moved to a point on the subject's scalp and oriented so as to stimulate the desired target point.

Figure 7 shows a photograph of the actual device.

Phantom calibration studies indicate that the device gives an accuracy for positioning within setups of dx = LR = ± 1.9 mm, dy = AP = ± 1.4 mm, dz = FH = ± 0.8 mm and a precision for multiple setups of dx = LR = ± 0.8 mm, dy = AP = ± 0.1 mm, dz = FH = ± 0.1 mm. Preliminary results from the first study to use this system – targeting "motor knob" – have shown 100% success in achieving motor movement with the settings provided by the MR-guidance software; only rotation about its axis was required to point the B-field relative to the central sulcus.

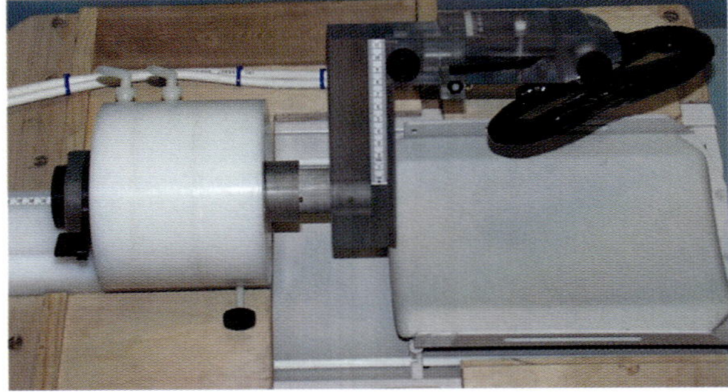

Fig. 7. Photograph of MRGuidedTMS positioner/holder.

This self-contained, integrated MR-guided TMS system for interleaved TMS/fMRI studies provides fast, accurate location of motor cortex stimulation sites traditionally located functionally, and a means of consistent, anatomy-based TMS coil positioning for stimulation of brain areas without overt response.

4. Repeatability of TMS interleaved with fMRI

In a study similar to earlier work (Bohning et al., 2000), but with 11 subjects and measurements repeated three times (Denslow et al., 2002), we sought to assess the magnitude of both within-subject and between-subject variations of the BOLD response associated with TMS-induced movement compared with that for similar volitionally-induced movement (VOL), as well as their respective anatomical locations. As in the earlier study, interleaved with fMRI, 1 Hz TMS was applied over motor cortex for thumb movement in 21-pulse trains in alternation with VOL every 126 s. Data were analyzed within each subject using anatomically defined regions of interest.

Activation locations: Locations of centers of gravity (COGs) of primary motor BOLD clusters relative to anatomic reference points on the central sulcus are shown in Fig. 8a. In agreement with the Penfield homunculus, the locations tend toward the lateral aspect of the hand knob, and there is considerable overlap between TMS-induced and volitionally induced cluster locations. Figure 8b shows these locations of TMS clusters relative to their paired volitional locations mapped to the origin. This presentation shows no obvious tendency for a consistent direction of displacement of one type of activation (TMS, VOL) relative to the other.

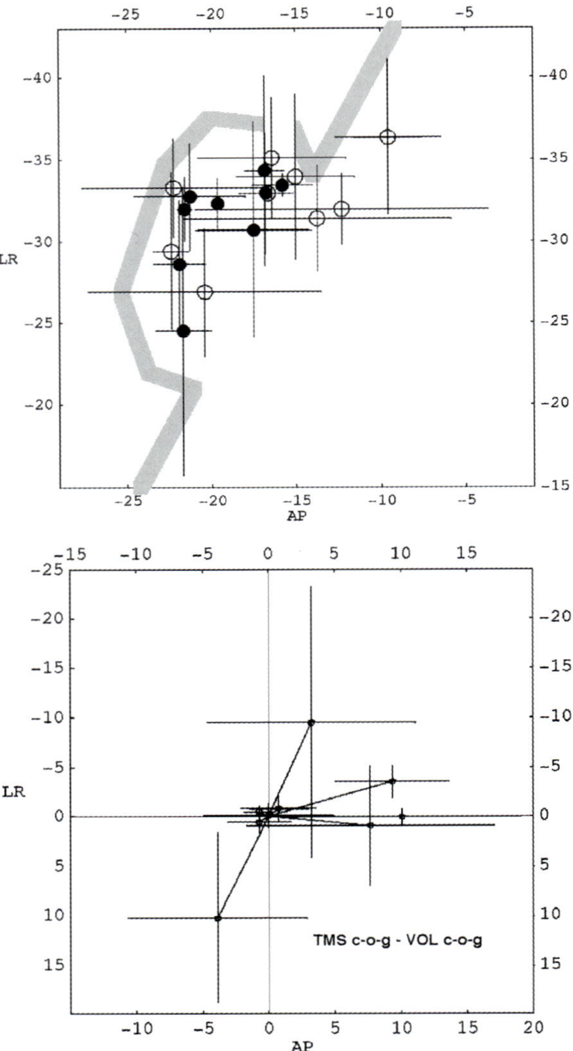

Fig. 8. (a) Centers of gravity (c-o-g) of BOLD-fMRI activity after TMS (filled circles) and volitional movement (VOL) (open circles) relative to motor knob and (b) relative displacement of TMS and VOL centers of gravity.

Pooling data across all subjects and all visits revealed that TMS and VOL BOLD locations were not significantly different statistically (dx = LR = 0.9 ± 7.1 mm; dy = AP = 2.3 ± 6.0 mm; dz = HF = 0.7 ± 4.3 mm) nor were BOLD intensities (dI = 0.36 ± 1.3%).

The observed intra-subject standard deviations in the principle directions ranged between 3 and 6 mm or approximately two to three pixels. Both LR and AP variations were greater between subjects as would be expected due to inter-subject variations in sulcal anatomy. The small head-foot inter-subject variation may reflect the lower variability of anatomy with respect to depth from the cortex. In the AP and LR directions, the presently determined locations of the TMS and VOL COGs are within a few millimeters of the locations reported previously (Lotze et al., 1999; Herwig et al., 2001). The mean HF coordinate found in the present study was about 5 mm lower than those found by others. Based on the location of the cortex in the Talairach atlas and the HF variance in location, this mean location is about 10 ± 2 mm below the cortical surface.

In general, there was no detectable difference in Talairach COG location between TMS-induced and volitionally induced activations. There were, however, clearly detectable inter-subject differences in location as would be expected based on the large inter-subject variation in the Talairach location of the precentral gyrus (Talairach and Tournoux, 1988). Interestingly, an ANOVA detected a significant difference across runs within subjects for the AP direction. The mean locations of both TMS- and VOL-induced activations in the final scans was 7 mm anterior to the mean location in the initial scans. The highly variable time-spans between scans for different subjects (1 week to 7 months) makes interpretation of this detected difference problematic.

BOLD magnitude and time courses: The average values of the Z-statistic within TMS and VOL clusters were similar and no significant difference was detected by ANOVA. When TMS and VOL clusters are analyzed independently, time courses from the hand knob region show peaks in both task epochs with the greater intensity peak occurring in the epoch on which the t-test was based. However,

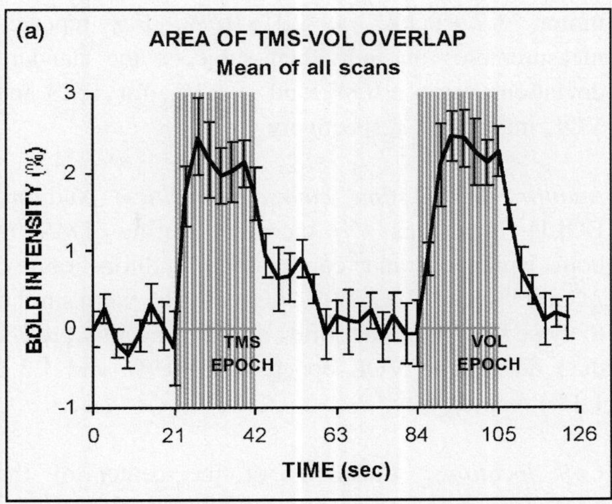

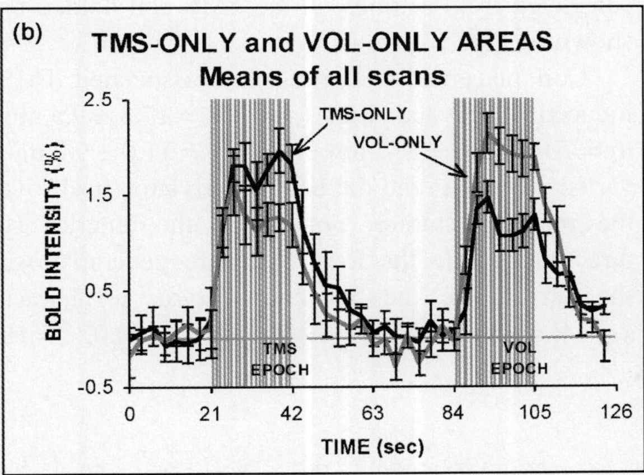

Fig. 9. BOLD-fMRI time curves from, (a) voxels common to both TMS and VOL activations and (b) voxels in TMS only and VOL-only activations.

when cluster voxels are segregated according to inclusion in one or both of the detected clusters, those voxels included in both types of clusters (overlap area) show equal peaks in the two epochs (Fig. 9a) and a higher intensity than those voxels included in only one or the other of the clusters (Fig. 9b). This again is the pattern observed previously (Bohning et al., 2000).

Primary motor BOLD time course intensities: There was not a significant difference between TMS and VOL intensities (% increase) observed in primary motor, 1.7 ± 0.7% vs. 2.1 ± 0.7%. For repeated measurements on individual subjects, the standard deviations were ± 0.8% and ± 1.1%, for TMS and VOL intensities, respectively.

Auditory BOLD time course intensities: Auditory BOLD intensities (% increase) during TMS in both ispilateral and contralateral auditory cortex, 2.3 ± 0.9% and 1.9 ± 1.0%, respectively, were similar to those seen in motor cortex and significantly greater than during the VOL epoch, 1.4 ± 0.7% and 1.3 ± 1.1%, respectively.

Coil locations: Locations of the center of the TMS coil and its HF projection to the cortex, calculated from settings on the TMS coil holder, are shown in Fig. 10.

Coil placement relative to its associated TMS-induced BOLD activation (dx = LR = 17.3 ± 9.5 mm, dy = AP = 21.8 ± 8.7 mm, dz = HF = 11.0 ± 9.0 mm) varied more than did the BOLD activation itself over the repeated studies, notably in the anterior (y) direction. While the locations were generally over the crown of the precentral gyrus (Talairach: x = LR = −35.4 ± 6.1, y = AP = −21.7 ± 10.0, z = HF = 53.4 ± 1.1), they clearly tend to be anterior to the location of the majority of Brodman's area 4 on the posterior bank of the central sulcus (Wassermann et al., 1996; Classen et al., 1998; Hervig et al., 2002). The observed range of location was greater than the dimensions of the hand knob along the precentral gyrus from medial to lateral and superior to inferior. This variation in location of the coil was also greater than the variation observed for the cortical activations induced by the coil.

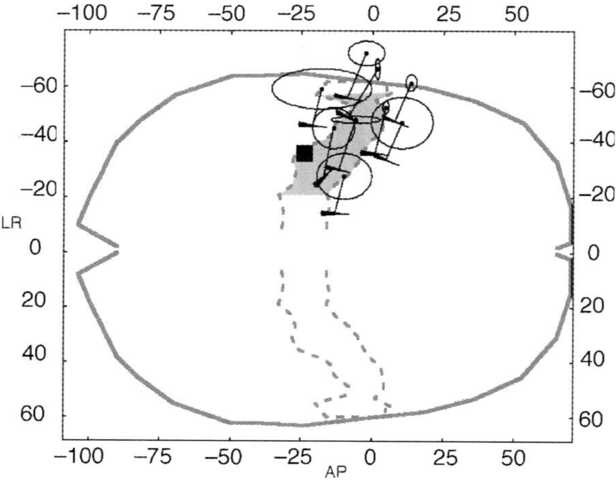

Fig. 10. Locations of the center of the TMS coil and its projection to the cortex calculated from settings of the TMS positioner/holder.

5. Can temporal resolution be improved with paired-pulse rTMS?

In the TMS paired-pulse technique for demonstrating intracortical inhibition (ICI) (Kujirai, 1993), two TMS pulses, separated by a variable interstimulus interval (ISI) are applied to motor cortex while electromyographic (EMG) recordings are made of the motor evoked potentials (MEPs) induced. It is a well characterized physiological tool for testing intracortical inhibition and facilitation, in health and disease, as well as the influence of CNS-active drugs (Ziemann et al., 1996). We have combined the TMS paired-pulse technique in its long-interval intracortical inhibition (LICI) form (Sanger, 2001) with BOLD-fMRI neuroimaging both to try to use it to test cortical sensitivity in areas other than motor cortex, and to try to use the BOLD response amplitude dependence on TMS ISI to investigate brain communication at high time resolution.

After obtaining informed consent, interleaved paired-pulse TMS/fMRI was performed on five healthy volunteers (to-date) in a whole body 1.5 T MR system (Philips Intera, Rel.8.1.1, Philips Medical Systems, Best, The Netherlands) using a 20 cm diameter circular phased array coil pair and a single shot gradient-echo EPI pulse sequence (TR = 1500 ms, TE = 40 ms a = 80°, matrix 64 × 64, FOV 256 mm, 11 slices, slice thickness 4 mm, gap 1 mm). A Macintosh G3 laptop with NI DAQCard-AI-16E-4 general purpose I/O board and custom Labview software controlled the firing of two Magstim 220 Stimulators through a BiStim Multiplexer synchronously interleaved with the fMRI acquisition. Using

Mathematica, a list of paired-pulse events with ISI of 50, 100, 150, 200, 250, 300, and 1000 ms, pseudo-randomly ordered and spaced, was generated so that the TMS pulses would minimally affect the MR pulse sequence RF pulses. The same event list was later used both to remove TMS compromised images and as the paradigm event list for data analysis with SPM to find areas of BOLD activation.

One data set was discarded due to excess movement. Analysis of the other four data sets revealed clusters of pixels with locally high *t*-values in motor and auditory cortex. Time curves of BOLD response were extracted from the clusters, cycle-averaged and, finally, averaged across subjects. In Fig. 11a and 11b, the cycle-averaged paired-pulse data have been rearranged in order of increasing ISI and plotted for ipsi-lateral motor cortex and contra-lateral auditory cortex activations, respectively. A mathematical model made up of a hemodynamice response function multiplied by an exponential recovery function (Bohning et al., 2003) with independent amplitude scaling factors (relative to the ISI = 1000 amplitude a1000, set to 1.0) for the different ISI has been fit to the data and superimposed on the plots as a thick red line. In Fig. 11c and 11d, the amplitude scaling factors for the fits (normalized to the coefficient a1000 = 1.0) have been plotted against ISI for motor and auditory cortex activations, respectively. Because these were determined from a single fit to the subject-averaged data, we were not able to give errors for the amplitude scaling factors.

The data analyzed to-date demonstrate the feasibility of combining paired-pulse TMS with fMRI. The auditory data (Fig. 10d) show a clearly reduced response for ISI = 250 ms, similar to that seen for visual stimuli (Chen et al., 2000); the lack of clear modulation of

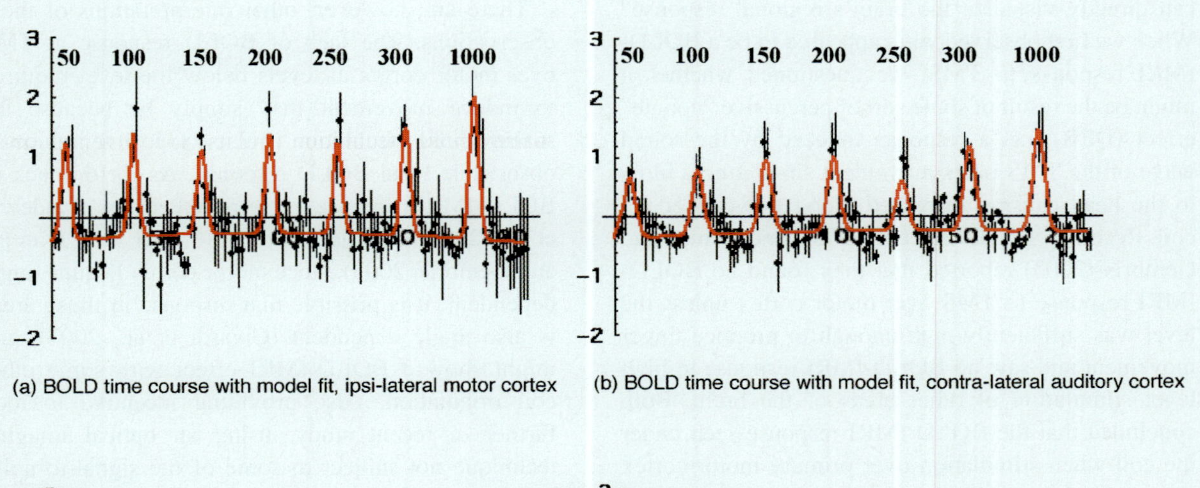

(a) BOLD time course with model fit, ipsi-lateral motor cortex

(b) BOLD time course with model fit, contra-lateral auditory cortex

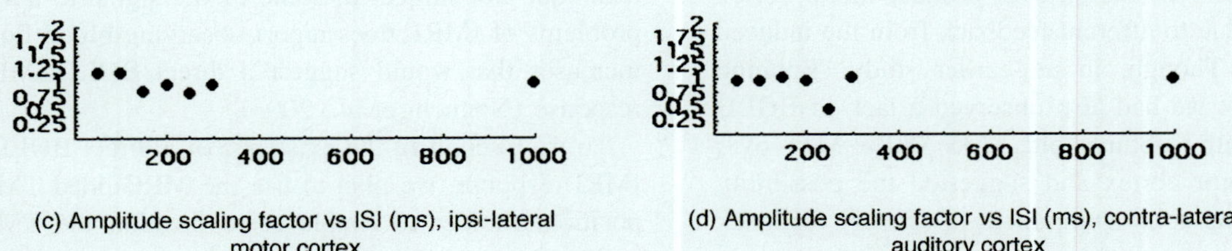

(c) Amplitude scaling factor vs ISI (ms), ipsi-lateral motor cortex

(d) Amplitude scaling factor vs ISI (ms), contra-lateral auditory cortex

Fig. 11. (a) BOLD time course with model fit, ipsi-lateral motor cortex; (b) BOLD time course with model fit, contra-lateral auditory cortex; (c) amplitude scaling factor vs ISI (ms), ipsi-lateral motor cortex; and (d) amplitude scaling factor vs ISI (ms), contra-lateral auditory cortex

response in motor cortex is likely because ISI = 50 used for these first studies is longer than the 1–20 ms where motor inhibition and facilitation are usually observed (Ogawa et al., 2000). Despite that, the data demonstrate that it might be possible to use the modulation of the BOLD response amplitude as a function of the ISI between pairs of TMS pulses to test intracortical inhibition and facilitation over the entire brain cortex in health and disease (Ziemann, 1996), as well as to investigate brain communication at time resolutions an order of magnitude greater than that of the hemodynamic response itself (Chen et al., 2000; Ogawa et al., 2000).

6. Does TMS directly induce a BOLD-fMRI response?

Transcranial magnetic stimulation (TMS) can be interleaved with fMRI, and one can perform direct, non-invasive, TMS stimulation, but is it clear that one can directly visualize the brain's regional response? When we first observed what appeared to be a BOLD-fMRI response to TMS, we questioned whether it might be the result of some sort of percussive "noogie" effect (DEB), i.e. a response induced by the sound wave of the TMS or its movement simulating a blow to the head causing increased blood flow under the coil. Recently, Baudewig et al. (2001) and Kemna and Gembris (2003) reported that they found no BOLD-fMRI response to TMS over motor cortex unless the level was sufficiently high enough to produce finger movement and saw no BOLD-fMRI response to high level stimulation of other areas of the brain. Both concluded that the BOLD-fMRI response seen under the coil when stimulation over primary motor cortex is actually due to afferent feedback from the induced movement. Though, in an earlier study (Bohning et al., 1999), we had also observed a lack of BOLD response with subthreshold TMS (80% MT) over primary motor cortex and suggested the possibility of there being some component of sensory feedback in the response, at the time, we did not seriously question that there was, at least, some direct response. However, the only study from our group reporting BOLD-fMRI response under the coil when stimulating over a non-motor area (DLPFC), is questionable, since the volume acquired was too thin for effective renormalization and response localization. Looking back over our own work and the TMS/fMRI and TMS/PET literature, our impression is that the data, generally because of poor localization and/or inconsistency, do not refute the interpretation of Baudewig et al. (2001) and Kemna and Gembris (2003).

This might also be in line with the observations of Logothetis et al. (2001). They suggested that BOLD activation reflects the neural activity related to the input and local processing in any given area, rather than the spiking activity associated with the output of the area. In that case, the TMS might depolarize spiking pyramidal cell which synapse elsewhere to induce movement, and that is where they are re-energized (causing increased bloodflow and BOLD), rather than under the coil. This also bring to mind the different signal pathways described by Amassian et al. (1987) and Ilic et al. (2001).

There are, however, other interpretations of these observations. The lack of BOLD response at TMS over motor cortex at levels below the level required to induce movement may simply be because the subthreshold stimulation is also too low to induce an observable local BOLD response. As for the lack of BOLD-fMRI response in prefrontal cortex (Baudewig et al., 2001) or adjacent to the motor area (Kemna and Gembris, 2003), since motor cortex is quite angle dependent, it is possible that response in those areas is also angle dependent (Civardi et al., 2001), and might show a BOLD-fMRI effect with some other coil orientation. Also providing incentive to look further, a recent study, using an optical imaging technique not subject to some of the signal-to-noise problems of fMRI, does report observing blood flow increases that would suggest a direct BOLD-fMRI response (Noguchi et al., 2003).

To try to confirm the existence of a direct BOLD-fMRI response, we plan to use the MRGuided TMS positioner/holder to enable us to position the TMS coil to target the same specific cortical structure with the same field direction. We will then use the more flexible single-event hardware/software developed for our work testing the feasibility of paired-pulse TMS interleaved with fMRI to investigate the conditions, if any, under which BOLD response appears to try to gain a better understanding of TMS action.

Acknowledgements

This work was supported by funding from the Dana Foundation, NINDS (RO1 RR14080-02), the Defense Advanced Research Projects Agency, and the South Carolina Commission on Higher Education.

References

Amassian, V.E., Stewart, M., Quirk, G.J. and Rosenthal J.L. Physiological basis of motor effects of a transient stimulation to cerebral stimulus. *Neurosurgery*, 1987, 20: 74–93.

Baudewig, J., Paulus, W. and Frahm, J. Artifacts caused by transcranial magnetic stimulation coils and EEG electrodes in T_2*-weighted echo-planar imaging. *Magn. Reson. Imag.*, 2000, 18: 479–484.

Baudewig, J., Siebner, H.R., Bestmann, S., Tergau, F., Tings, T., Paulus, W. and Frahm, J. Functional MRI of cortical activations induced by transcranial magnetic stimulation (TMS). *NeuroReport*, 2001, 12: 3543–3548.

Bestmann, S., Baudewig, J. and Frahm, J. On the synchronization of transcranial magnetic stimulation and functional echo-planar imaging. *J. Magn. Reson. Imag.*, 2003, 17: 309–316.

Bohning, D.E., Shastri, A., Nahas, Z., Lorberbaum, J.P., Anderson, S.W., Dannels, W., Vincent, D.J. and George, M.S. Echoplanar BOLD fMRI of Brain Activation Induced by Concurrent Transcranial Magnetic Stimulation (TMS). *Invest. Radiol.*, 1998, 33: 336–340.

Bohning, D.E., Shastri, A., McConnell, K.A., Nahas, Z., Lorberbaum, J.P., Roberts, D.R., Teneback, C., Vincent, D.J. and George, M.S. A combined TMS/fMRI study of intensity-dependent TMS over motor cortex. *Biol. Psych.*, 1999, 45: 385–394.

Bohning, D.E., Shastri, A., McGavin, L., McConnell, K.A., Nahas, Z., Lorberbaum, J.P., Roberts, D.R. and George, M.S. Motor cortex brain activity induced by 1-Hz transcranial magnetic stimulation is similar in location and level to that for volitional movement. *Invest. Radiol.*, 2000, 35: 676–83.

Bohning, D.E., Shastri, A., Lomarev, M.P., Lorberbaum, J.P., Nahas, Z. and George, M.S. BOLD-fMRI response vs transcranial magnetic stimulation (TMS) pulse-train length: testing for linearity. *J. Magn. Reson. Imag.*, 2003, 17: 279–290.

Chen, W., Zhu, X.-H., Ogawa, S. and Ugurbil, K. Probing fast neuronal events and neuronal interaction in human visual cortex during short visual stimulation based on fMRI BOLD response. *Proc. Intl. Soc. Mag Reson. Med.*, 2000, 8: 501.

Civardi, C., Cangtello, R., Asselman, P. and Rothwell, J.C. Transcranial magnetic stimulation can be used to test connections to primary motor areas from frontal and medial cortex in humans. *NeuroImage*, 2001, 14: 1444–1453.

Classen, J., Knorr, U., Werhahn, K.J., Schlaug, G., Kunesch, E., Cohen, L.G., Seitz, R.J. and Benecke, R. Multimodal output mapping of human central motor representation on different spatial scales. *J Physiol.* (Lond), 1998, 512(Part 1): 163–179.

Denslow, S., Bohning, D.E., Lomarev, M.P. and George, M.S. (2002). BOLD activation of motor cortex induced by transcranial magnetic stimulation and volitional movement: repeatability and comparison of location assessed by interleaved TMS/fMRI. *Proc. Intl. Soc. Mag. Reson. Med.*, 2002, Abs # 1479.

Fox, P., Ingham, R., George, M.S., Mayberg, H.S., Ingham, J., Roby, J., Martin, C. and Jerabek, P. Imaging Human Intra-Cerebral Connectivity by PET During TMS. *NeuroReport*, 1997, 8: 2787–2791.

Herwig, U., Kolbel, K., Wunderlich, A.P., Thielscher, A., Von Tiesenhausen, C. and Schonfeldt-Lecuona, C. Spatial congruence of neuronavigated transcranial magnetic stimulation and functional neuroimaging. *Clin. Neurophysiol.*, 2002, 113: 462–468.

Ilic, T.V., Meintzschel, F., Cleff, U., Ruge, D., Kessler, K.R. and Ziemann, U. Short-interval paired-pulse inhibition and facilitation of human cortex: the dimension of stimulus intensity. *J. Physiol.*, 2002, 545: 153–167.

Kemna, L.J. and Gembris, D. Repetitive transcranial magnetic stimulation induces different responses in different cortical areas: a functional magnetic resonance study in humans. *Neuroscience Letters*, 2003, 336: 85–88.

Kujiai, J., Caramis, M.D., Rothwell, J.C., Day, B.L., Thompson, P.D., Ferbert, A., Wroes, S., Asselman, P. and Marsden, C.D. Corticocortical inhibition in motor cortex. *J. Physiol.* (London), 1993, 471: 501–519.

Logothetis, N.K., Pauls, J., Augath, M., Trinath, T. and Oeltermann, A. Neurophysiological investigation of the basis of the fMRI signal. *Nature*, 2001, 412: 150–157.

Nahas, Z., Lomarev, M., Roberts, D.R., Shastri, A., Lorberbaum, J.P., Teneback, C.T., McConnell, K., Vincent, D.J., Li, X., George, M.S. and Bohning, D.E. Unilateral Left Prefrontal Transcranial Magnetic Stimulation (TMS) Produces Intensity-Dependent Bilateral Effects as Measured by Interleaved BOLD fMRI. *Biol. Psych.*, 2001, 50(9): 712–720.

Noguchi, Y., Watanabe, E. and Sakai, K.L. An event-related optical topography study of cortical activation induced by single-pulse transcranial magnetic stimulation, *NeuroImage*, 2003, in press.

Ogawa, S., Lee, T.-M., Stepnoski, R. and Chen, W. Probing neural events by fMRI at the neural time scale of milliseconds. *Proc. Natl. Acad. Sci.*, 2000, 97: 11026–11031.

Paus, T., Jech, R., Thompson, C.J., Comeau, R., Peters, T. and Evans, A.C. Transcranial Magnetic Stimulation during Positron Emission Tomography: A new method for studying connectivity of the human cerebral cortex. *J. Neuroscience*, 1997, 17: 3178–3184.

Sanger, T.D., Garg, R.R. and Chen, R. Interactions between two different inhibitory systems in the human motor cortex. *J. Physiol.*, 2001, 530(Pt. 2): 307–317.

Shastri, A., George, M.S. and Bohning, D.E. Performance of a system for Interleaving Transcranial Magnetic Stimulation with Steady State Functional Magnetic Resonance Imaging. In: W. Paulus, M. Hallett, P.M. Rossini and J.C. Rothwell (Eds.), *Transcranial Magnetic Stimulation, Electroencephalogr. Clin. Neurophysiol.*, 1999(Suppl.), 51: 55–64.

Talairach, J. and Tournoux, P. *Co-planar Stereotaxic Atlas of the Human Brain: an approach to medical cerebral imaging*. New York, *Thieme Medical*, 1988: 122.

Wassermann, E.M., Wang, B., Zeffiro, T.A., Sadato, N., Pascual-Leone, A., Toro, C. and Hallett, M. Locating the motor cortex on the MRI with transcranial magnetic stimulation and PET. *NeuroImage*, 1996, 3: 1–9.

Ziemann, U., Lonnecker, S., Steinhoff, B.J. and Paulus, W. Effects of antiepileptic drugs on motor cortex excitability in humans: a transcranial magnetic stimulation study. *Ann Neurol*, 1996, 40: 367–378.

Transcranial Magnetic Stimulation and Transcranial Direct Current Stimulation (Supplements to Clinical Neurophysiology, Vol. 56)
Editors: W. Paulus, F. Tergau, M.A. Nitsche, J.C. Rothwell, U. Ziemann, M. Hallett

Chapter 6

Is functional magnetic resonance imaging capable of mapping transcranial magnetic cortex stimulation?

Sven Bestmann[a,b,*], Jürgen Baudewig[a], Hartwig R. Siebner[c], John C. Rothwell[b] and Jens Frahm[a]

[a]*Biomedizinische NMR Forschungs GmbH, Max-Planck-Institut für Biophysikalische Chemie, D-37077 Göttingen (Germany)*
[b]*Sobell Department of Motor Neuroscience and Movement Disorders, Institute of Neurology, University College of London, London (UK)*
[c]*Institute of Neurology, University of Kiel, Kiel (Germany)*

1. Introduction

Over the past decade, transcranial magnetic stimulation (TMS) has become a prime tool for non-invasive stimulation of the human cortex. A rapidly increasing number of studies have employed TMS to investigate the physiology of the primary motor cortex (Chen, 2000; Ziemann and Rothwell, 2001), cortical plasticity (Siebner and Rothwell, 2003), as well as cognitive neuroscience (Walsh and Cowey, 2000).

Despite its widespread use, the exact mechanisms by which TMS exerts its effects on cortical circuits are yet to be fully understood. In this regard, neuroimaging techniques, such as electroencephalography (EEG) (Ilmoniemi et al., 1997), positron emission tomography (PET) (Siebner et al., 2000; Strafella and Paus, 2001; Siebner et al., this volume), single-photon emission computed tomography (SPECT) (Nahas et al., 2001a), and functional magnetic resonance imaging (fMRI) (Bohning et al., 1998; Baudewig et al., 2001) provide important tools to clarify how TMS interacts with both the stimulated cortex and remote connected brain regions.

In comparison with PET, the main advantages of fMRI based on blood-oxygenation-level-dependent (BOLD) contrast are the absence of limitations for the number of investigations in a single subject, as well as access to a superior temporal and spatial resolution. The MRI approach to functional brain mapping takes advantage of the fact that neuronal activation is accompanied by an increased blood flow which then leads to a washout of deoxyhemoglobin in venous compartments. Because deoxyhemoglobin is paramagnetic, it attenuates the signal intensity of gradient-echo MR images. Consequently, a decreased

* *Correspondence to*: Dr. Sven Bestmann, Biomedizinische NMR Forschungs GmbH, Max-Planck-Institut für Biophysikalische Chemie, D-37070 Göttingen, Germany.
Tel: +49-551-201-1720; Fax: +49-551-201-1307;
E-mail: sbestma@gwdg.de

intravascular concentration results in an increased MRI signal. This may be regarded as an indirect reflection of cortical activity and has been shown to be spatially tightly coupled to the site of neuronal activation (Logothetis et al., 2001). Moreover, it provides a means for directly visualising changes in regional hemodynamics following stimulation of the cortex.

As noted previously (Shastri et al., 1999), the combination of TMS and fMRI is technically challenging. For example, the introduction of local field inhomogeneities by the mere presence of the TMS coil can result in severe image distortions (Baudewig et al., 2000) that avert any predications about possible changes in cortical hemodynamics. Bohning et al. (1997) were the first to demonstrate the technical feasibility of TMS during MRI using low-frequency (1 Hz) repetitive TMS (rTMS) over primary motor cortex (M1) (Bohning et al., 1999, 2000, 2003).

In this chapter, we briefly discuss technical solutions for fMRI-TMS combinations and the resulting limitations affecting experimental protocols, imaging parameters, and data quality. Furthermore, we provide new data contributing to the ongoing debate whether cortical stimulation induced by TMS can be visualised using BOLD-sensitive fMRI and present the first TMS-fMRI results at 3.0 T.

2. fMRI strategies for mapping TMS-induced cortical hemodynamics

Combining TMS and fMRI can give rise to static and dynamic image distortions. Static image distortions result from susceptibility artefacts introduced by the interaction of the TMS coil with the imaging gradients and can lead to signal dropouts of up to 2 cm underneath the coil (Baudewig et al., 2000; Bestmann et al., 2003). In human studies, these problems can be largely avoided as the distance between the TMS coil which is placed tangentially to the scalp and the cortical target area usually exceeds 2 cm (Baudewig et al., 2000).

Dynamic image distortions reflect the interference of TMS pulses with MRI signal excitation and detection during BOLD-sensitive echo-planar imaging (EPI). Using EPI, coverage of the entire brain is accomplished within a repetition time (TR) of typically 2–4 s. To avoid confounding effects of TMS on image quality, it is necessary to prevent the application of TMS pulses during imaging. For example, TMS pulses during data acquisition operate as effective spoiling gradients and thus destroy all relevant signals of the affected image section (Shastri et al., 1999; Bestmann et al., 2003). An even more serious pitfall emerges when TMS pulses are applied during slice-selective RF excitation. The resulting effects on the longitudinal magnetization can last for up to several seconds and are likely to exceed signal changes induced by physiologic processes. As demonstrated in Fig. 1, this can result in false-positive activations (see also Bestmann et al., 2003). Here, a single TMS pulse coincided with the RF excitation pulse of the depicted section during finger tapping. In the absence of TMS, this task revealed localised activity in M1 and supplementary motor area (SMA). After TMS pulse interference large cortical areas appeared as activated even when excluding the perturbed images from the analysis. Additional subtle false-positive activations might be induced in adjacent brain sections due to imperfect slice excitation profiles (not shown). It has also been shown that MR images can be distorted up to 100 ms after application of a TMS pulse of approximately 250 μs duration (Shastri et al., 1999).

In order to accommodate the requirements of both rTMS and fMRI, two basic strategies emerge as feasible technical solutions. A first approach employs the use of short trains of rTMS at high frequencies such as 10 Hz, while deliberately sacrificing those images that are acquired during the administration of the rTMS train. This strategy is demonstrated in Fig. 2 and was originally chosen by Baudewig et al. (2001). It benefits from the fact that BOLD MRI responses exhibit a delayed maximum effect after about 4–6 s, so that perturbed images may be discarded from the analysis without afflicting images with relevant physiological information. The technique allows for high-frequency rTMS at the expense of restricted pulse train durations and/or MRI volume coverage.

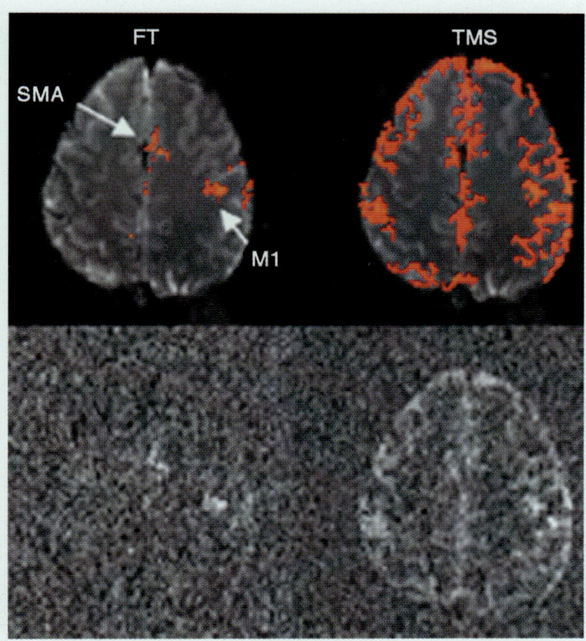

Fig. 1. Activation maps and (bottom) unthresholded maps of correlation coefficients obtained for right-hand finger tapping (FT) (left) in the absence and (right) in the presence of a single TMS pulse applied during RF excitation. Both maps were calculated using a boxcar reference function matching the FT protocol shifted by 4 s to account for hemodynamic response delays. TMS pulse application resulted in false-positive activations within the whole image section not due to decreased signal-to-noise ratio (Modified from Bestmann et al., 2003, with permission). M1: primary motor cortex, SMA: supplementary motor cortex.

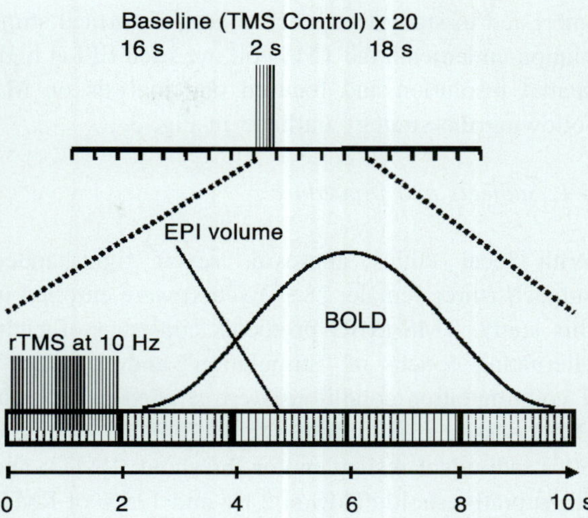

Fig. 2. Schematic outline of an event-related TMS-fMRI protocol using rTMS epochs of 2 s duration (10 Hz, 20 pulses) and control periods of 18 s in conjunction with multi-slice single-shot EPI (TR = 2000 ms, 20 sections). Although TMS results in image destruction of a whole EPI volume, subsequent volumes remain unperturbed, so that TMS-induced BOLD MRI responses are fully detected because of their hemodynamic delay.

Alternatively, rTMS and fMRI may be completely separated in time as proposed by Bohning et al. (1998, 1999, 2000, 2003). Though technically less intricate to implement, this approach is limited to rTMS at low frequencies on the order of 1–2 Hz. For example, as shown in Fig. 3, TMS pulses may be applied every 500 ms for 12 s. Thus, the maximum stimulation frequency is limited by the number of sections required for coverage of the respective brain region.

Summarising the technical requirements, there is a trade-off between optimal fMRI and rTMS protocols. For example, for high rTMS frequencies, it will be necessary to decrease the spatial resolution, increase the TR, or introduce gaps between sections in order to cover large brain regions. However, if high spatial resolution and large brain coverage is important, rTMS can only be applied at low frequencies of up to 2 Hz.

3. BOLD-sensitive fMRI of 2 Hz repetitive TMS

So far, most TMS-fMRI studies have focused on TMS-induced effects in the M1 hand area, which had been investigated in great detail by electrophysiological means (Rothwell 1997; Modugno et al., 2001; Di Lazzaro et al., 2002a, b; Fisher et al., 2002). Moreover, effective stimulation of M1 can be readily controlled by evoking a motor response in a contralateral muscle. Here, we present a combined rTMS-fMRI study in which sub- and suprathreshold rTMS was applied over the left M1 hand area at a frequency of 2 Hz. Because we were primarily interested to study the direct effects of cortical stimulation underneath the TMS coil, we used EPI at high spatial resolution and focused our analysis on M1 following the strategy outlined in Fig. 3.

3.1. Subjects and procedure

With local ethics approval, seven right-handed subjects (three female; 28 ± 3 years) were enrolled in this study. TMS-fMRI protocols consisted of eight alternating epochs of "stimulation" and "baseline". Two stimulation conditions were studied in separate fMRI sessions: (i) subthreshold rTMS at 2 Hz and 80% individual resting motor threshold (RMT); and (ii) suprathreshold rTMS at 2 Hz and 125% of RMT. In both cases, rTMS was applied for 12 s over the left M1 hand area, followed by a resting epoch of 18 s duration. In a separate session, subjects performed a simple finger tapping task with their right hand at a rate of 2 Hz. Each finger movement was cued by a TMS stimulus at 15% of stimulator output (ineffective TMS). This condition was introduced to identify the movement-related activation pattern in motor cortical areas. The order of experimental conditions was balanced among subjects.

Subjects were comfortably placed inside the MRI head coil with the TMS coil fixed over the left M1 hand area. They were instructed to relax their hand muscles throughout the experiment and keep their eyes closed. Accurate positioning of the TMS coil and determination of the RTM were again controlled with the subject placed inside the scanner, as well as after each session.

3.2. Interleaved TMS and fMRI

The implementation of interleaved TMS and fMRI was achieved following the recommendations given elsewhere (Shastri et al., 1999; Baudewig et al., 2000, Bestmann et al., 2003). Sixteen 4 mm thick axial EPI sections were acquired at 2.0 T (Siemens Vision, Erlangen, Germany; TR = 2000 ms, TE = 53 ms, flip angle = 70°, 128 × 128 matrix size, frequency-selective fat suppression, 2 × 2 mm² in-plane resolution). During stimulation epochs, 24 TMS pulses were applied every 500 ms, starting directly after the onset of the first image acquisition (compare Fig. 3) and timed in a way which strictly avoided direct interference with the RF excitation pulses of sections covering the frontal motor cortex.

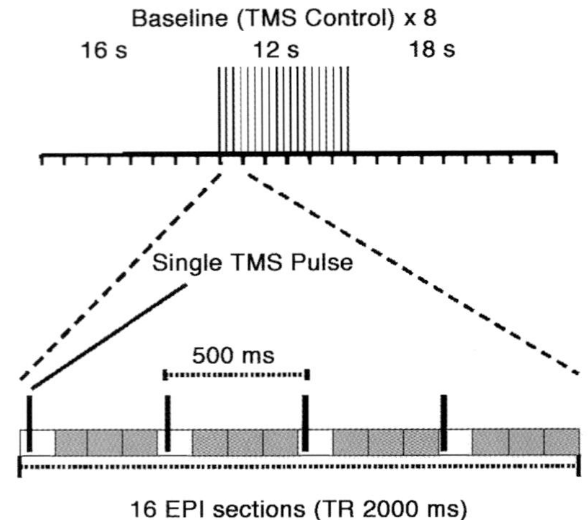

Fig. 3. Schematic outline of an interleaved TMS-fMRI protocol using single TMS pulses for a period of 12 s (2 Hz, 24 pulses) synchronised to EPI (TR = 2,000 ms, 16 sections). The protocol perturbs every fourth section and therefore restricts TMS applications to low frequencies.

The non-ferromagnetic TMS coil (figure-of-eight, 70 mm outer wing diameter) was connected to a Magstim Rapid stimulator (The Magstim Company, Wales, UK) outside the radio-frequency (RF) shielded cabin via an 8 m cable through an RF filter tube. A 5 V TTL pulse derived from the EPI sequence at the time of each RF excitation pulse was fed into the printer port of a personal computer with a DOS operating system. Accurate TMS triggering was achieved by an in-house developed C program. Stimulation was conducted at the optimal scalp site to elicit muscle twitches in the right hand muscles in five out of ten trials. The coil was oriented roughly perpendicular to the presumed line of the central sulcus and laterally oriented at a 45° angle away from the midline. The position was marked on the subject's head. Biphasic electrical pulses of approximately 250 μs duration induced a current that was directed in a posterior-to-anterior orientation.

3.3. *Data analysis*

A boxcar function reflecting the experimental protocol was shifted by 4 s to account for hemodynamic response delays. Activation maps were obtained in an user-independent manner as quantitative maps of correlation coefficients (in-house software). Correlation coefficients were re-scaled as percentile ranks of the noise distribution, based on the noise distribution of the histogram of each correlation coefficient map (adapted from Kleinschmidt et al., 1995). Pixels above the 99.99% percentile rank of the individual noise distribution were identified as activated (corresponding to an type-one error probability of $p < 0.0001$). Accepted pixels were iteratively appended by directly neighbouring pixels exceeding a 95% percentile rank of the noise distribution (corresponding to an type-one error probability of $p < 0.05$). Activation maps were colour coded and superimposed onto the individual EPI scans.

3.4. *Results*

In all seven subjects, finger tapping of the right hand evoked consistent increases in BOLD MRI signal in left M1 and SMA. Figure 4 shows two selected sections covering M1 and the auditory cortex (AUD), respectively, in a representative subject. In five subjects, suprathreshold TMS evoked similar but somewhat weaker responses in left M1 and SMA. During subthreshold TMS, however, no overt finger movements were visible and significant activations in left M1 could only be detected in a single subject, while in three subjects subtle BOLD MRI signal changes were observed in SMA. As can be seen from Fig. 4, prominent bilateral activations in AUD were observed in all conditions. They are presumably caused by the loud noise related to the discharge of the TMS coil, in concordance to previous reports (Bohning et al., 1998, 2000; Baudewig et al., 2001). Table 1 summarises activations in left M1, SMA and AUD in terms of number of activated pixels averaged across subjects.

3.5. *Discussion*

The present findings support previous observations on significant BOLD MRI responses in the stimulated

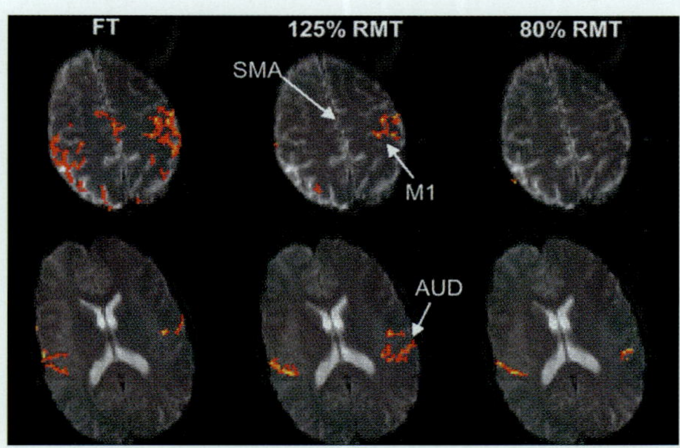

Fig. 4. Combined TMS-fMRI at 2.0 T. Two brain sections of a single subject obtained for (left) auditory cued right-hand finger tapping (FT), (middle) suprathreshold rTMS (125% resting motor threshold (RMT), 2 Hz, 12 s) over the left M1 hand area, and (right) subthreshold rTMS (80% RMT, 2 Hz, 12 s), in accordance with the TMS-fMRI protocol shown in Fig. 3 (control period 18 s). While suprathreshold TMS evoked similar responses in M1 as finger tapping, no significant activations were found after subthreshold stimulation. All conditions revealed bilateral activation in the auditory cortex (AUD).

M1 hand area after suprathreshold rTMS (Bohning et al., 1998, 1999, 2000, 2003; Baudewig et al., 2001; Kemna and Gembris, 2003). So far, however, all attempts failed to demonstrate a reliable change of the BOLD MRI signal in the stimulated M1 hand area after subthreshold TMS. For example, in a comparison of low-frequency (1 Hz) stimulation above and below RMT, Bohning et al. (1999) found significant M1 responses only after suprathreshold TMS. This is in agreement with a recent study by our group demonstrating the absence of TMS-induced activations in the stimulated M1 area after a 1 s train of subthreshold rTMS at 10 Hz (Baudewig et al., 2001). In the same study, a similar 1 s burst of rTMS at 10 Hz to the left lateral prefrontal cortex also failed to induce BOLD MRI signal changes in the stimulated prefrontal cortex even when using a "suprathreshold" intensity (as referred to M1). These results strongly suggest that the induction of a positive BOLD MRI response by suprathreshold TMS over M1 mainly reflects re-afferent feedback

TABLE 1

CORTICAL ACTIVATIONS FOR FINGER TAPPING AND RTMS OVER LEFT M1

Paradigm movement	FT yes	125% RMT yes	80% RMT no
Left M1	131 ± 64	64 ± 75	3 ± 8
SMA	85 ± 59	66 ± 87	14 ± 33
AUD	86 ± 35	143 ± 106	98 ± 102

Values are given as numbers of activated pixels (mean ± SD) averaged across subjects ($n = 7$). AUD: auditory cortex, M1: primary motor cortex, SMA: supplementary motor cortex. FT: finger tapping with rTMS at 15% stimulator output, 80% and 125% RMT: sub- and suprathreshold rTMS at 80% and 125% resting motor threshold, respectively.

activation caused by TMS-induced movements in the contralateral hand. This notion is also supported by Kemna and Gembris (2003), who showed significant BOLD MRI responses after suprathreshold TMS over M1, whereas TMS in slightly anterior or posterior locations neither resulted in muscle movements nor elicited BOLD MRI activations. The lack of BOLD MRI activations after subthreshold rTMS may be explained by the fact that activation of cortical output neurons or their axons contributes significantly more to the generation of a BOLD MRI signal change than activation of intracortical circuits, which are primarily targeted by subthreshold rTMS (Di Lazzaro et al., 1998). It may also be possible that the TMS-induced neuronal discharge is followed by inhibitory post-synaptic potentials that reduce cortical activity over a 100–200 ms period, so that the net physiological effect will be small and merely deviate from background activity levels.

Finally, in contrast to most other studies, Nahas et al. (2001b) reported BOLD MRI signal changes underneath the coil which were evoked by high intensity rTMS (120% RMT) over the left prefrontal cortex. This inconsistency of present fMRI observations of TMS-induced brain activations requires further detailed investigations both at sub- and suprathreshold stimulation intensities.

4. TMS during fMRI at 3.0 Tesla

MRI with respect to basic and clinical neuroscience shows a tendency toward the use of higher magnetic field strengths well above 1.5 T. This trend is partially based on expectations of increased BOLD MRI sensitivity. However, with regard to TMS-fMRI combinations, the forces exerted onto the TMS coil in cases where the magnetic field generated by the TMS coil and the static magnetic field of the MR scanner are not orthogonal substantially increase with field strength, and therefore, pose a major problem. While the corresponding increase of the discharge noise can effectively be filtered because of its high-frequency components, the mechanical vibrations are likely to exceed acceptable limits for the comfort of the subject. Therefore, possible solutions for very high fields of 4.0 T or above might only emerge from the development of novel dampened coils or cushioning material which do not increase the coil cortex distance. Alternatively, such studies will have to restrict TMS applications to subjects with very low stimulation thresholds.

Here, Fig. 5 shows preliminary data from a TMS experiment in a single subject at 3.0 T (Siemens Trio, Erlangen, Germany) using a specially strengthened TMS coil (The Magstim Company, Wales, UK). Repetitive TMS was applied at 4 Hz during the acquisition of five horizontal EPI sections covering M1 (TR = 2000 ms). Suprathreshold cortical stimulation induced localised activity in M1 and SMA, similar to activation after finger tapping and in agreement with the aforementioned results obtained at 2.0 T. Despite the general problems outlined above, this study demonstrates for the first time that TMS is technically feasible at a higher magnetic field strength, so that TMS-fMRI combinations may complement other high-field MRI approaches which aim at a better understanding of the functional connectivity of the human brain.

5. Conclusion

Since the initial report by Bohning et al. (1997), a number of combined TMS-fMRI studies have

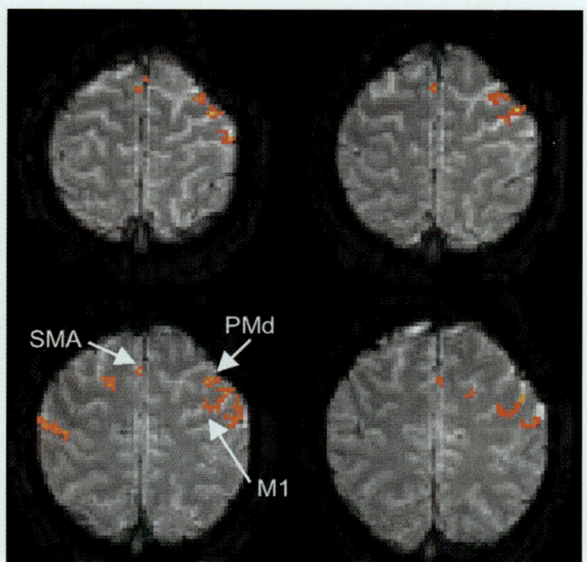

Fig. 5. Combined TMS-fMRI at 3.0 T. Four adjacent brain sections of a single subject showing activation obtained for suprathreshold rTMS (120% resting motor threshold (RMT), 2 Hz, 10 s) over the left M1 hand area, in accordance with the protocol shown in Fig. 3 (control period 20 s). Suprathreshold TMS evoked responses in M1, SMA and premotor cortex (PM) in agreement with the results obtained at 2.0 T (see Fig. 4).

demonstrated the technical feasibility of applying rTMS during functional MRI. Although cortical stimulation protocols need to be adapted to the scanning parameters and vice versa, event-related or interleaved strategies ensure successful brain imaging at the expense of some flexibility of the experimental procedures, e.g. with respect to volume coverage. Several technical issues remain to be optimised. This particularly applies to the design of smaller MR-compatible TMS coils which would allow for a much larger number of possible cortical areas to be stimulated within the restricting geometry of a MRI head coil. So far, certain brain regions, such as temporal lobe and parietal areas, remain largely inaccessible to TMS during fMRI.

The aforementioned difficulties most likely explain the limited number of groups performing TMS-fMRI studies to date. As far as experimental robustness is concerned, and despite the fact that sufficient MRI quality may be achieved by means of suitable experimental procedures, a reliable BOLD MRI response in directly stimulated areas remains to be demonstrated. In this regard, the electrophysiological data suggesting intracortical neuronal activity at subthreshold intensities (Ziemann et al., 1996; Di Lazzaro et al., 1998; Fisher et al., 2002) is at variance with fMRI data showing no consistent change in BOLD MRI activation. For the future use of combined rTMS-fMRI studies, it is therefore mandatory to explore this issue in more detail and to clarify whether TMS does or does not evoke a response in directly stimulated as well as connected cortical areas. Further insights are likely to be expected by expanding on the use of subthreshold TMS protocols, which have been shown by electrophysiological means to effectively target the cortex (Di Lazzaro et al., 1998, 2002b).

Acknowledgements

SB was supported by a grant from the Deutsche Forschungsgemeinschaft DFG GK-GRK 632/1-00. The authors are grateful to Anthony Thomas for providing the TMS coil.

References

Baudewig, J., Paulus, W. and Frahm, J. Artefacts caused by transcranial magnetic stimulation coils and EEG electrodes in T2*-weighted echo-planar imaging. *Magn. Reson. Imaging*, 2000, 18: 479–484.

Baudewig, J., Siebner, H.R., Bestmann, S., Tergau, F., Tings, T., Paulus, W. and Frahm, J. Functional MRI of cortical activations induced by transcranial magnetic stimulation (TMS). *NeuroReport*, 2001, 12: 3543–3548.

Bestmann, S., Baudewig, J. and Frahm, J. On the synchronization of transcranial magnetic stimulation and functional echo-planar imaging. *J. Magn. Reson. Imaging*, 2003, 17: 309–316.

Bohning, D.E., Pecheny, A.P., Epstein, C.M., Speer, A.M., Vincent, D.J., Dannels, W. and George, M.S. Mapping transcranial magnetic stimulation (TMS) fields in vivo with MRI. *NeuroReport*, 1997, 8: 2535–2538.

Bohning, D.E., Shastri, A., Nahas, Z., Lorberbaum, J.P., Andersen, S.W., Dannels, W.R., Haxthausen, E.U., Vincent, D.J. and George, M.S. Echoplanar BOLD fMRI of brain activation induced by concurrent transcranial magnetic stimulation. *Invest. Radiol.*, 1998, 33: 336–340.

Bohning, D.E., Shastri, A., McConnell, K.A., Nahas, Z., Lorberbaum, J.P., Roberts, D.R., Teneback, C., Vincent, D.J. and George, M.S. A combined TMS/fMRI study of intensity-dependent TMS over motor cortex. *Biol. Psychiat.*, 1999, 45: 385–394.

Bohning, D.E., Shastri, A., McGavin, L., McConnell, K.A., Nahas, Z., Lorberbaum, J.P., Roberts, D.R. and George, M.S. Motor cortex brain activity induced by 1-Hz Transcranial Magnetic Stimulation is similar in location and level to that for volitional movement. *Invest. Radiol.*, 2000, 11: 676–683.

Bohning, D.E., Shastri, A., Lomarev, M.P., Lorberbaum, J.P., Nahas, Z. and George, M.S. BOLD-fMRI response vs. transcranial magnetic stimulation (TMS) pulse-train length: Testing for linearity. *J. Magn. Reson. Imaging*, 2003, 17: 279–290.

Chen, R. Studies of human motor physiology with transcranial magnetic stimulation. *Muscle Nerve Suppl.*, 2000, 9: S26–32.

Di Lazzaro, V., Restuccia, D., Oliviero, A., Profice, P., Ferrara, L., Insola, A., Mazzone, P., Tonali, P. and Rothwell, J. C. Magnetic transcranial stimulation at intensities below active motor threshold activates intracortical inhibitory circuits. *Exp. Brain Res.*, 1998, 119: 265–268.

Di Lazzaro, V., Oliviero, A., Berardelli, A., Mazzone, P., Insola, A., Pilato, F., Saturno, E., Dileone, M., Tonali, P.A. and Rothwell, J.C. Direct demonstration of the effects of repetitive transcranial magnetic stimulation on the excitability of the human motor cortex. *Exp. Brain Res.*, 2002a, 144: 549–553.

Di Lazzaro, V., Oliviero, A., Mazzone, P., Pilato, F., Saturno, E., Dileone, M., Insola, A., Tonali, P.A. and Rothwell, J.C. Short-term reduction of intracortical inhibition in the human motor cortex induced by repetitive transcranial magnetic stimulation. *Exp. Brain Res.*, 2002b, 147: 108–113.

Fisher, R.J., Nakamura, Y., Bestmann, S., Rothwell, J.C. and Bostock, H. Two phases of intracortical inhibition revealed by transcranial magnetic threshold tracking. *Exp. Brain Res.*, 2002, 143: 240–248.

Ilmoniemi, R.J., Virtanen, J., Ruohonen, J., Karhu, J., Aronen, H.J., Naatanen, R. and Katila, T. Neuronal responses to magnetic stimulation reveal cortical reactivity and connectivity. *NeuroReport*, 1997, 8: 3537–3540.

Kemna, L.J. and Gembris, D. (2003) Repetitive transcranial magnetic stimulation induces different responses in different cortical areas: a functional magnetic resonance study in humans. *Neurosci. Lett.*, 336: 85–88.

Kleinschmidt, A., Requardt, M., Merboldt, K.D. and Frahm, J. On the Use of Temporal Correlation Coefficients for Magnetic Resonance Mapping of Functional Brain Activation. Individualized Thresholds and Spatial Response Delineation. *Intern. J. Imag. Sys. Technol.*, 1995, 6: 238–244.

Logothetis, N.K., Pauls, J., Augath, M., Trinath, T. and Oeltermann, A. Neurophysiological investigation of the basis of the fMRI signal. *Nature*, 2001, 412: 150–157.

Modugno, N., Nakamura, Y., MacKinnon, C.D., Filipovic, S.R., Bestmann, S., Berardelli, A. and Rothwell, J.C. Motor cortex excitability following short trains of repetitive magnetic stimuli. *Exp. Brain Res.*, 2001, 140: 453–459.

Nahas, Z., Teneback, C.C., Kozel, A., Speer, A.M., DeBrux, C., Molloy, M., Stallings, L., Spicer, K.M., Arana, G., Bohning, D.E., Risch, S.C. and George, M.S. Brain effects of TMS delivered over prefrontal cortex in depressed adults: role of stimulation frequency and coil-cortex distance. *J. Neuropsychiatry. Clin. Neurosci.*, 2001a, 13: 459–470.

Nahas, Z., Lomarev, M., Roberts, D.R., Shastri, A., Lorberbaum, J.P., Teneback, C., McConnell, K., Vincent, D.J., Li, X., George, M.S. and Bohning, D.E. Unilateral left prefrontal transcranial magnetic stimulation (TMS) produces intensity-dependent bilateral effects as measured by interleaved BOLD fMRI. *Biol. Psychiat.*, 2001b, 50: 712–720.

Rothwell, J.C. Techniques and mechanisms of action of transcranial stimulation of the human motor cortex. *J. Neurosci. Methods*, 1997, 74: 113–122.

Shastri, A., George, M.S. and Bohning, D.E. Performance of a system for interleaving transcranial magnetic stimulation with steady-state magnetic resonance imaging. *Electroenceph. Clin. Neurophysiol. Suppl.*, 1999, 51: 55–64.

Siebner, H.R. and Rothwell, J.C. Transcranial magnetic stimulation: new insights into representational cortical plasticity. *Exp. Brain Res.*, 2003, 148: 1–16.

Siebner, H.R., Peller, M., Willoch, F., Minoshima, S., Boecker, H., Auer, C., Drzezga, A., Conrad, B. and Bartenstein, P. Lasting cortical activation after repetitive TMS of the motor cortex: a glucose metabolic study. *Neurology*, 2000, 54: 956–963.

Strafella, A.P. and Paus, T. Cerebral blood-flow changes induced by paired-pulse transcranial magnetic stimulation of the primary motor cortex. *J. Neurophysiol.*, 2001, 85: 2624–2629.

Walsh, V. and Cowey, A. Transcranial magnetic stimulation and cognitive neuroscience. *Nat. Rev. Neurosci.*, 2000, 1: 73–79.

Ziemann, U. and Rothwell, J.C. I-waves in motor cortex. *J. Clin. Neurophysiol.*, 2000, 17: 397–405.

Ziemann, U., Rothwell, J.C. and Ridding, M.C. Interaction between intracortical inhibition and facilitation in human motor cortex. *J. Physiol.*, 1996, 496: 873–881.

Transcranial Magnetic Stimulation and Transcranial Direct Current Stimulation (Supplements to Clinical Neurophysiology, Vol. 56)
Editors: W. Paulus, F. Tergau, M.A. Nitsche, J.C. Rothwell, U. Ziemann, M. Hallett

Chapter 7

Applications of combined TMS–PET studies in clinical and basic research

Hartwig Roman Siebner[a,*], Martin Peller[a] and Lucy Lee[b]

[a]*Department of Neurology, Christian-Albrechts-University, D-24105 Kiel (Germany)*
[b]*Wellcome Department of Imaging Neuroscience, Institute of Neurology, University College, London WC1N 3BG (UK)*

1. Introduction

Transcranial magnetic stimulation (TMS) is the method of choice for non-invasive stimulation of the human cortex through the intact scalp. In contrast to other brain mapping techniques, TMS actually interacts with synaptic activity in the cortex. This opens up several interesting applications for studies of human brain function. First, TMS can detect changes in cortical excitability caused by a given intervention such as drug administration (see chapter by Ziemann) or by pathology (Ziemann, 1999). Second, TMS causes a temporary dysfunction in the stimulated cortex (Walsh and Rushworth, 1999; Pascual-Leone et al., 2000). The disruptive effect of TMS on cortical processing can be used to interfere with task performance when applied over relevant cortical areas (see chapter by Walsh). Third, TMS can be used to study the cortico-cortical and cortico-subcortical connections of the stimulated cortex. For example, TMS of the primary motor cortex and spinal nerve roots is well established in clinical neurology as a method of assessing the function of central motor pathways in patients with neurological disorders (Rothwell et al., 1999). Finally, TMS can be used to promote short-term functional reorganisation by applying repetitive TMS (rTMS) (Siebner and Rothwell, 2003).

Metabolic neuroimaging techniques, such as functional magnetic resonance imaging (fMRI) and positron emission tomography (PET), reveal regionally specific changes in synaptic activity during cognitive processes. Mapping these changes has significantly enhanced the understanding of human brain function. However, there are limitations associated with functional neuroimaging. Because subjects are usually scanned while they perform a specific task, many experiments rely heavily on the subject's ability and willingness to perform. More importantly, the presence of localised, task-related changes in metabolic activity does not necessarily imply that regionally specific synaptic activity is causally related to a particular cognitive process. The details of how and when an activated region contributes to the cognitive process remain unclear.

Until recently, the effects of TMS have been explored by measuring behavioural consequences of TMS such as motor evoked responses (MEPs), TMS-evoked phosphenes or disruptive effects of TMS on

* *Correspondence to*: Dr. Hartwig Roman Siebner, Christian-Albrechts-Universität Kiel, Niemannsweg 147, D-24105 Kiel, Germany.
Tel: ++ 49-4315972703; Fax: ++49-4315972712;
E-mail: h.siebner@neurologie.uni-kiel.de

task performance. By combining functional imaging techniques with TMS it is possible to image TMS-related effects in the targeted cortical area and to map the spread of TMS effects throughout the brain. Similarly, TMS provides a way to overcome some of the limitations of functional brain mapping. The aim of this chapter is to highlight how TMS and functional brain imaging can benefit from each other. First, we describe how "*on-line*" PET imaging during TMS can be used to assess the connectivity and excitability of the human cerebral cortex without requiring the subject to engage in any specific behaviour. Second, we will illustrate some of the ways in which TMS can be combined with "*off-line*" PET imaging to study acute reorganisation at a systems level in the intact human brain. Third, we will discuss the use of TMS as a method of exploring the functional relevance, and temporal involvement of regionally specific activity identified during functional neuroimaging experiments. Finally, we will consider how a combined TMS-PET approach may be used to investigate the pathophysiology of neuropsychiatric disorders.

This chapter will exclusively focus on the combination of TMS with PET imaging of regional cerebral blood flow (rCBF) and regional cerebral metabolic rate of glucose (rCMRglc), as the chapter by Bestmann et al. in this book deals with the combined use of TMS and fMRI. Despite limited temporal and spatial resolution, the combination of PET with TMS offers some methodological advantages over combined TMS-fMRI studies. Compared with TMS in the MRI scanner, the prerequisites for applying TMS in the PET scanner are relatively easy to establish. PET measurements give an estimate of regional synaptic activity over several tens of seconds ($H_2{}^{15}O$-PET) or minutes (^{18}FDG-PET). Combined TMS-PET studies can use the limited temporal resolution of PET as an advantage because a single PET scan will represent the summation of the effects of individual stimuli on regional synaptic activity. The major advantage of PET is that it is possible to make direct comparisons of synaptic activity between different scanning sessions. This makes PET ideally suited to comparing changes in activity as a result of different rTMS paradigms (alterations in intensity, frequency or sham stimulation) performed on separate days. Serial PET scanning can also be used to track the time-course of rTMS-induced effects either at rest or during a task.

2. "On-line" PET imaging during rTMS

If PET imaging of rCBF or rCMRglc is performed "*on-line*" (i.e. during TMS), it is possible to study the excitability of the stimulated cortex and to map functional intracerebral connections (Fig. 1).

Conventional TMS techniques, such as motor or phosphene thresholds are useful measurements of the excitability of primary motor and visual cortex. For the primary motor cortex, cortical excitability is usually assessed further "downstream" by measuring transcranially evoked motor responses (Rothwell et al., 1999). Combined PET-rTMS studies significantly extend the scope of currently available TMS techniques that probe cortical excitability in two ways: first, as a method of assessing the effects of stimulation in so called "silent areas" such as prefrontal cortex, and second, as a method of assessing the spatial extent of rTMS effects simultaneously across the whole brain.

Conventional TMS measures of cortical excitability are dependent on a number of factors, specifically the balance between activity in excitatory and inhibitory neuronal populations in the stimulated area, synaptic efficacy and the excitability of cortical outputs. Metabolic imaging techniques detect changes in net synaptic activity and do not distinguish between changes in activity of excitatory or inhibitory neurons. Additional TMS measurements of cortical excitability allow a better interpretation of data from metabolic imaging experiments in these terms.

In addition to local effects at the site of stimulation, TMS can cause both indirect (trans-synaptic) and direct (anterograde or retrograde) activation of cortico-cortical and cortico-subcortical pathways. This may result in modification of synaptic activity in connected areas. Since PET can detect regional changes in synaptic activity across the whole brain,

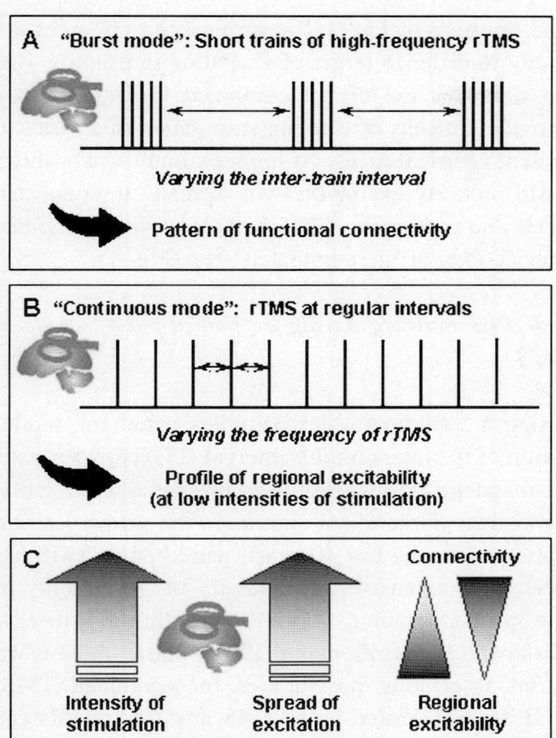

Fig. 1. PET imaging during TMS. (A) A "burst mode" of rTMS leads to a summation of cortical excitation and facilitates the excitation of cortico-cortical and cortico-subcortical interneurones. "Burst mode" rTMS is therefore suitable for exploring functional connections of the stimulated cortex (Paus et al., 1997; Paus et al., 1998). (B) During continuous rTMS, the excitatory effects of consecutive stimuli do not interact if rTMS is given at low intensities or frequencies ≤ 5 Hz. Such protocols selectively activate the area directly targeted with rTMS and can therefore be used to study the effect rTMS in specific cortical regions. (C) Both the temporal pattern of rTMS and the intensity of stimulation have an impact on the spread of excitation to connected areas. Higher stimulation intensities increase the probability of activating cortico–cortical and cortico–subcortical connections. Therefore, continuous rTMS at higher intensities represents another method of mapping the functional connections of the stimulated area.

imaging of rTMS-induced changes in rCBF or rCMRglc can be used to identify inter-regional connectivity of the stimulated cortex. In addition, PET can reveal changes in synaptic activity in areas that cannot be probed directly, such as basal ganglia.

2.1. PET imaging during short trains of rTMS

Using $H_2^{15}O$-PET, Paus et al. (1997) were the first to map the acute effects of rTMS on rCBF. In six healthy volunteers, they applied short trains of 10 Hz rTMS to the left frontal eye field (FEF). The number of stimulus trains was varied across PET scans, from 5 to 30 pulse trains. The rCBF in the stimulated FEF and anatomically connected visual areas in the superior parietal and medial parieto-occipital cortex showed a positive correlation with the number of TMS trains per PET scan, demonstrating functional cortico-cortical connectivity of the stimulated FEF (Paus et al., 1997). A second experiment on the same subjects in which an identical rTMS protocol was used to stimulate the primary left motor hand area ($M1_{HAND}$) confirmed the feasibility of "on-line" PET imaging as a method of mapping functional connections of the stimulated cortex (Paus et al., 1998). However, in contrast to rCBF changes induced by TMS to the FEF, rCBF changes in the stimulated $M1_{HAND}$ and remote anatomically connected areas were negatively correlated with the number of TMS trains per PET scan. Thus, an identical rTMS protocol delivered to the FEF or $M1_{HAND}$ induced either relative increases or decreases in rCBF at both the site of stimulation and in connected areas. This suggests that in addition to the rTMS protocol, intrinsic properties of the stimulated cortex may influence both local and remote effects on synaptic activity.

2.2. PET imaging during continuous rTMS

Siebner et al. performed a series of PET studies to image the acute effects of continuous rTMS to the left $M1_{HAND}$ (Siebner et al., 1998, 1999b, c, 2001a, b). A continuous train of irregular suprathreshold rTMS to the left $M1_{HAND}$ at an average rate of 2 Hz caused an increase of rCMRglc in the stimulated left $M1_{HAND}$ (extending into adjacent primary somatosensory cortex and caudal dorsal premotor cortex) (Siebner et al., 1998; Siebner et al., 2001). Additional increases in rCMRglc were observed in caudal supplementary motor area (SMA) and contralateral right dorsal premotor cortex (Siebner et al., 2001a).

rTMS-associated rCMRglc increases in the left $M1_{HAND}$ were smaller in magnitude than rCMRglc increases during voluntary imitation of rTMS-induced arm movements (Siebner et al., 1998). Focal rTMS of the $M1_{HAND}$ selectively activated executive frontal motor areas, whereas, voluntary movements activated both executive and higher-order motor areas involved in cognitive aspects of motor control (Siebner et al., 1998). This suggests that rTMS is capable of activating a subset of areas within the functional network subserving voluntary movements. Stimulation with subthreshold intensities (i.e. intensities that do not evoke a movement) also produced a focal increase in synaptic activity in the stimulated $M1_{HAND}$ (Siebner et al., 1999; Siebner et al., 2001). This excludes the possibility that activation of $M1_{HAND}$ merely reflects somatosensory stimulation caused by TMS-induced hand movements.

Siebner et al. (2001b) investigated rate-dependent functional activation of the left $M1_{HAND}$. Continuous trains of subthreshold rTMS (90% of active motor threshold) were given during $H_2^{15}O$-PET. Nine stimulation frequencies were used, ranging from 1 to 5 Hz. Compared to ineffective rTMS, subthreshold rTMS led to an increase in rCBF in the stimulated $M1_{HAND}$. The increase in rCBF showed a positive linear relationship with the frequency of rTMS, indicating a rate-dependent modulation of synaptic activity in the stimulated $M1_{HAND}$ (Siebner et al., 2001). No spread of activation to connected areas was observed at this low intensity (90% active motor threshold). The use of PET during continuous trains of rTMS demonstrates that changes in synaptic activity are restricted to the site of stimulation when very low stimulation intensities are used. Such protocols selectively activate the area directly targeted with rTMS and can therefore be used to study the effect rTMS in discrete cortical regions. (Fig. 1). One of the practical problems of selecting stimulation intensities for TMS relates to the fact that the threshold for activating cortico-cortical or cortico-subcortical connections is unknown for non-motor areas. Regionally specific properties of the stimulated cortex (Zilles et al., 2003) and differences in the spatial relationship between the cortical target area and the transducing coil mean that cortical areas are likely to differ in terms of excitation thresholds. It is possible that the use of combined PET-rTMS may provide a means of titrating stimulation intensities in "silent" cortical areas. At higher stimulus intensities, TMS-induced excitation will spread to connected areas and continuous rTMS will also reveal functional connections of the stimulated area (Fig. 1).

2.3. PET imaging during a "paired-pulse" mode of TMS

Using a conditioning-test stimulus paradigm, modulation of the interstimulus interval (ISI) between pairs of magnetic pulses, results in preferential activation of distinct intracortical circuits in the primary motor cortex. Over the last 10 years, paired-pulse TMS has been used extensively to quantify the excitability of the primary motor cortex in health and disease (Rothwell, 1999; Ziemann, 1999). Paired-pulse TMS offers interesting possibilities for combined TMS-PET studies. Paired-pulse TMS at different ISIs can be used to target distinct subsets of intracortical neurones, with different anatomical and functional connections. Specific effects at the site of stimulation and in connected areas can then be quantified by mapping changes in rCBF or rCMRglc.

Strafella and Paus (2001) assessed changes in rCBF induced by paired-pulse TMS of $M1_{HAND}$. PET scans were acquired during single-pulse TMS and paired-pulse TMS at ISIs of 3 ms and 12 ms. Relative changes in rCBF (i.e. rCBF during paired-pulse TMS minus rCBF during single-pulse TMS) were correlated with the degree of suppression and facilitation of EMG responses during paired-pulse TMS. Correlation analysis revealed different patterns of rCBF change during paired-pulse TMS depending on the ISI, lending further support to the notion that different sets of cortical interneurons generate paired-pulse inhibition and facilitation (Strafella and Paus, 2001).

2.4. Non-specific acute effects of rTMS

When TMS is given during PET imaging, it is important to remember that remote changes in rCBF may not always reflect inter-regional connectivity. For instance, the noise caused by the discharging magnetic coil induces a consistent activation of the auditory system (Siebner et al., 1999b). Since the coil is in contact with the head during rTMS, the click of the discharging coil is trans-mitted directly via bone conduction to the inner ear. Given the high intensity of the coil-generated click, it is not feasible to mask the acoustic input with white noise (Siebner et al., 1999b). In addition to auditory stimulation, the rapidly changing magnetic field may also stimulate afferent trigeminal nerve fibres, which in turn, activate the somatosensory system (Siebner et al., 1999a). An emotional response to rTMS (e.g. unpleasantness or discomfort) may also result in activation of the anterior insular or anterior cingulate cortex (Siebner et al., 2001). However, rCBF changes caused by sensory stimulation and rCBF changes directly induced by electrical cortex stimulation may be modulated in the same fashion by the parametric manipulation of the TMS varia-bles. In this case it will be impossible to disambiguate between specific and non-specific effects.

The significance of indirect brain stimulation via auditory and somatosensory afferents was demonstrated in an $H_2^{15}O$-PET study (Siebner et al., 1999c). In eight healthy subjects, changes in rCBF were measured during continuous trains of rTMS to the left $M1_{HAND}$ at 90% of resting motor threshold. Subjects were scanned three times during each of the following four conditions: (a) continuous 1 Hz rTMS, (b) continuous 3 Hz rTMS, (c) continuous 5 Hz rTMS, and (d) ineffective rTMS given at maximal stimulator output via a second coil, positioned 7 cm above the vertex. Focal rTMS at 90% resting motor threshold caused a relative increase in normalized rCBF in four brain regions ($p < 0.05$, corrected at a cluster level), including the stimulated left $M1_{HAND}$, right caudal SMA, and bilateral temporoparietal cortices (Fig. 2a). In the stimulated $M1_{HAND}$ 1 Hz rTMS had no effect on rCBF, whereas rTMS at 3 and 5 Hz resulted in a significant increase in rCBF (Fig. 2b). The remaining areas showed a different pattern of frequency-related changes (Fig. 2b). In contrast to rTMS of the $M1_{HAND}$, ineffective rTMS caused no somatosensory stimulation of afferent trigeminal nerve fibres. Moreover, it is likely that, due to additional bone conduction, rTMS of the $M1_{HAND}$ resulted in a greater auditory stimulation than ineffective stimulation. Therefore, it is possible that rCBF changes in the right SMA and temporoparietal areas reflects synaptic activity due to repetitive stimulation of the auditory and somatosensory system, rather than activation via cortical connections with the stimulated $M1_{HAND}$.

3. "Off-line" PET imaging of rTMS-induced regional plasticity

In the last decade, rTMS has been increasingly used to promote lasting changes in cortical function. Since rTMS can give rise to changes in excitability in connected cortical areas, rTMS represents a means of investigating plasticity within a distributed functional network (Siebner and Rothwell, 2003). In this context, PET provides a powerful means to characterise rTMS-induced re-organisation at a systems level. The pattern of re-organisation revealed by PET may be driven by two mechanisms. Re-organisation may be a direct consequence of the conditioning effects of rTMS on synaptic activity, both in directly stimulated and anatomically connected areas (i.e. stimulus driven re-organisation). Alternatively, re-organisation may reflect a dynamic response of those parts of a network that have not been affected by rTMS, for instance to compensate for lasting disruptive effects of rTMS (i.e. operational re-organisation in response to rTMS-induced modulation of synaptic efficacy).

Compared with PET studies of immediate effects of rTMS, PET studies that focus on lasting effects of rTMS have a methodological advantage because TMS and PET can be separated in space and time. By giving rTMS prior to imaging, the confounding effects of auditory and somatosensory stimulation can be avoided. Depending on the protocol of stimulation, the conditioning effects of rTMS last up to several hours and in these experiments TMS can be performed outside the PET scanner.

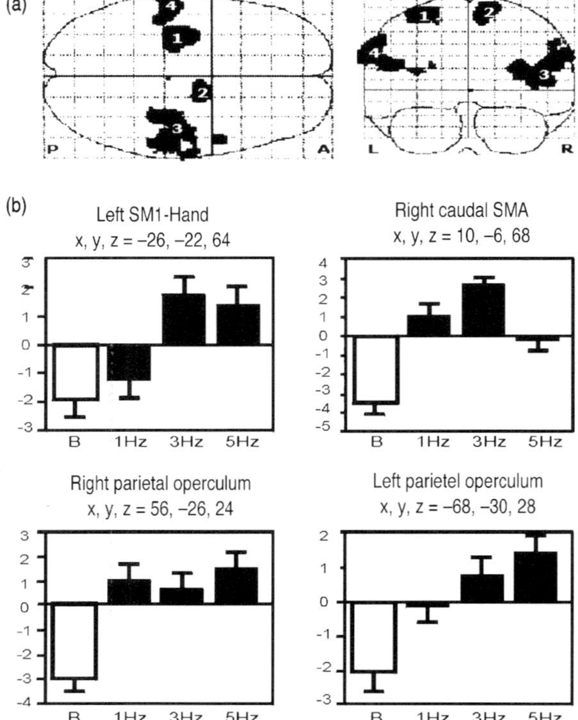

Fig. 2. Pattern of changes in normalized rCBF during continuous subthreshold rTMS of the left primary motor hand area ($M1_{HAND}$). (a) Axial and coronal projections of statistical parametric maps showing a relative increase in regional cerebral blood flow (rCBF) during effective rTMS of the left $M1_{HAND}$ compared with ineffective rTMS ($p <$ 0.001, uncorrected). Effective rTMS was given at an intensity of 90% of resting motor threshold and a frequency of 1 Hz, 3 Hz, or 5 Hz. Focal rTMS at 90% resting motor threshold caused a relative increase in normalized rCBF in four areas ($p < 0.05$, corrected at a cluster level): (1) the stimulated left primary motor hand area; (2) the right caudal supplementary area (SMA); (3) a right-hemispheric; and (4) a left-hemispheric temporoparietal cluster. The bilateral temporoparietal clusters included primary auditory cortex and secondary somatosensory cortex. (b) Bar charts illustrating region-specific profiles of rCBF changes for those voxels showing peak activation during effective rTMS at 1 Hz, 3 Hz, and 5 Hz compared with baseline (B). Each bar represents the mean percentage change in rCBF (± standard error) for each of the four conditions in healthy subjects. rCBF values given on the ord nate are adjusted to the mean.

3.1. PET imaging of lasting changes in baseline activity

PET imaging can be used to identify lasting changes in regional activity at "baseline" without requiring the subject to engage in any specific behaviour. Using ^{18}FDG-PET, Siebner et al. (2000) demonstrated a lasting increase in normalized rCMRglc in the stimulated left $M1_{HAND}$ after a conditioning session of 2250 stimuli of 5 Hz rTMS at 90% of resting motor threshold. Additional increases in normalized rCMRglc occurred in the caudal SMA and the right homologous $M1_{HAND}$ (Siebner et al., 2000). This study demonstrated a spread of conditioning effects from the site of stimulation to other executive motor areas, lasting for the duration of the experiment. In a follow-up study, Siebner et al. (2002a) used $H_2{}^{15}O$-PET to explore the time course of regional changes in synaptic activity in more detail. In this study, 30-s trains of 5 Hz rTMS were given to the left $M1_{HAND}$, with a stimulus intensity of 90% active motor threshold to minimize spread of conditioning effects to other motor areas. Repeated PET measurements revealed a selective increase in rCBF in the stimulated left $M1_{HAND}$ for an average of 8 min after a single rTMS train.

In addition to studies of rCBF and rCMRglc, radioligand-PET enables assessment of the effects of rTMS on neurotransmission. Using ^{11}C-raclopride PET, Strafella et al. (2001) measured changes in extracellular dopamine concentration in vivo following high-frequency rTMS of the left dorsolateral prefrontal cortex in healthy volunteers. Prefrontal rTMS led to a decrease in ^{11}C-raclopride binding in the left dorsal caudate nucleus when compared to rTMS of the left occipital cortex, indicating increased release of endogenous dopamine in the ipsilateral caudate nucleus after prefrontal rTMS (Strafella et al., 2001).

3.2. PET imaging of lasting changes in task-related activation

In addition to changes in baseline activity, repeated measurements of rCBF can reveal rTMS-induced changes in the magnitude of activation during a given task (e.g. finger movement). Although rTMS may exert substantial effects on regional rCBF at baseline, this does not necessarily mean that these changes are paralleled by changes in task-related activity or task performance. In addition, changes task-related activity may occur in different brain regions than changes in baseline activity. It is worth noting that the choice of the experimental task used during scanning will substantially influence the probability of detecting changes in task-related activation after rTMS. For instance, it may be difficult to demonstrate task-related changes in activation after rTMS if the brain regions targeted by rTMS are not crucial for the experimental task. Conversely, if the brain regions conditioned by rTMS are essential for the experimental task, participants may show a lasting change in performance. This will make it difficult to assign changes in task-related activations to the neuromodulatory effect of rTMS or to changes in task performance.

Using $H_2{}^{15}O$-PET, Lee et al. (2003) measured rCBF at rest and during freely selected finger movements after 30 min of 1 Hz rTMS to the left $M1_{HAND}$. Despite significant increases in synaptic activity as a result of 1 Hz rTMS (e.g. in the stimulated left $M1_{HAND}$), task performance was unaffected. A significant increase in movement-related activity in the right dorsal premotor cortex suggested that maintenance of task performance involved activation of premotor areas contralateral to the site of rTMS (Lee et al., 2003).

3.3. PET imaging of lasting changes in inter-regional coupling

Combined rTMS-PET studies can also be used to address how rTMS shapes functional integration between brain areas. Paus et al. (2001) used a combined TMS-PET method to explore how 10 Hz rTMS of the mid-dorsolateral frontal cortex modulates the functional connectivity of the stimulated area. In this study, conditioning rTMS caused a lasting change in regional excitability of the cortical target area as well as changes in *functional* connectivity between the target area and distant brain regions (Paus et al., 2001). The rTMS-related modulation of brain activity in the fronto-cingulate circuit was confirmed in a parallel experiment in rat cortex using electrical stimulation and field-potential recordings.

Lee et al. (2003) explored the conditioning effects of subthreshold 1-Hz rTMS on *effective* connectivity of the motor network. Using $H_2{}^{15}O$-PET, rCBF was mapped at rest and during freely selected finger movements after real and sham rTMS. Changes in effective connectivity within the motor network were assessed using the ‘Psychophysiological Interaction’ (PPI) method (Friston et al., 1997). The analysis of effective connectivity (PPI) demonstrated that the stimulated part of the left $M1_{HAND}$ became less responsive to inputs from premotor and mesial motor areas after 1 Hz rTMS, indicating a persisting lesion effect at the site of stimulation (Lee et al., 2003). Conversely, following rTMS there was increased coupling between an inferomedial portion of the left $M1_{HAND}$ and anterior motor areas (ipsilateral premotor and mesial motor cortex) during movement (Lee et al., 2003). This strengthening of functional coupling between premotor areas and non-stimulated parts of the left $M1_{HAND}$ was interpreted as a compensatory mechanism by which the motor system maintains functional integrity. Lee et al. (2003) proposed that these acute patterns of remapping provide a neuronal substrate for compensatory plasticity of the motor system in response to a focal lesion, such as stroke.

4. Probing the relevance of functional activations with TMS

PET and fMRI reveal regionally specific changes in synaptic activity associated with cognitive processes. Because TMS interferes with organised activity in the stimulated cortex, the disruptive effect of TMS (often referred to as a “virtual lesion”) can be used to test the functional relevance of task-related cortical activations (Walsh and Rushworth, 1999; Pascual-Leone et al., 2000). TMS provides a method with which to investigate how and when a cortical area, identified during a PET or fMRI study, is engaged during performance of a specific task or cognitive process. This approach can also be used to probe the functional relevance of cortical re-organisation after brain injury or in disease (Cohen et al., 1997; Johansen-Berg et al., 2002).

5. Combined TMS-PET studies in patients with neuropsychiatric disorders

To date, PET and single-photon emission computed tomography (SPECT) have mainly been used to assess the effects of repeated sessions of dorsolateral prefrontal rTMS on blood flow or glucose metabolism as a treatment for depression (Speer et al., 2000; Catafau et al., 2001; Mottaghy et al., 2002; Nadeau et al., 2002; Shajahan et al., 2002). These studies show that serial metabolic PET or SPECT studies provide important insight into the mechanism of action of rTMS and may help to predict antidepressant efficacy of different stimulation paradigms.

5.1. Serial PET studies in patients with major depression

Speer et al. (2000) performed serial measurements of rCBF in 10 patients with major depression at baseline and 3 days after 10 daily treatments with 20 Hz rTMS, and 10 daily treatments with 1 Hz rTMS, given in a counterbalanced order. TMS was administered over the left prefrontal cortex at 100% of resting motor threshold. 20 Hz rTMS was associated with increased rCBF bilaterally in the insula, basal ganglia, uncus, hippocampus, parahippocampus, thalamus and cerebellum. Increased rCBF was also seen bilaterally in the prefrontal and cingulate cortex (with larger changes in the left hemisphere) and in the left amygdala. In contrast, 1 Hz rTMS was associated with decreased rCBF in the right prefrontal cortex, left medial temporal cortex, left basal ganglia, and left amygdala. There was an inverse relationship between the changes in mood following the two rTMS frequencies: individuals who improved with one frequency worsened with the other.

Using HMPAO-SPECT, Nadeau et al. (2002) explored changes in rCBF after prefrontal 20 Hz rTMS (2000 stimuli per day for 10 days) in four men with major depression. Patients who responded to prefrontal rTMS had reduced blood flow in orbitofrontal cortex and/or anterior cingulate cortex when compared to non-responders. Mottaghy et al. (2002) used Tc99m-Bicisate-SPECT to evaluate whether rCBF measurements prior to rTMS reveal patterns of activity that may predict antidepressant efficacy of left dorsolateral prefrontal rTMS at 10 Hz (1600 stimuli per day; 5 days per week for 2 weeks). Before rTMS there was a significant left-right asymmetry, with more activity in the right hemisphere. Two weeks after treatment with rTMS this asymmetry was reversed. The rCBF at baseline in limbic structures was negatively correlated with the clinical outcome after rTMS, whereas rCBF in several neocortical areas showed a positive correlation.

5.2. Other applications of combined TMS-PET studies in patients

In addition to studies of antidepressant effects of prefrontal rTMS in depression, the combined TMS-PET approach represents a new method with which to study the pathophysiology of neuropsychiatric disorders. For instance, PET imaging during rTMS can be employed to investigate regional changes in excitability and connectivity in patients suffering from epilepsy or stroke. In addition, on-line PET imaging can be used to investigate the effects of centrally active drugs on regional excitability. Another interesting application is as a method of mapping patterns of acute functional reorganisation induced by a conditioning session of rTMS, i.e investigating changes in the plasticity of functional brain networks.

In healthy subjects and in patients with primary focal dystonia, Siebner et al. (2003) examined the pattern and time course of changes in rCBF produced by rTMS over the left dorsal premotor cortex. Subjects received 1800 stimuli of subthreshold 1 Hz rTMS (90% resting motor threshold) or sham stimulation to the left hemisphere. Afterwards, rCBF was measured by PET at rest and during performance of freely selected finger movement. In both groups, rTMS caused widespread bilateral decreases in synaptic activity in prefrontal, premotor and primary motor cortex and in the left putamen. Patients showed significantly greater suppression of synaptic activity in lateral and medial premotor areas, putamen and thalamus, indicating increased susceptibility to rTMS of the cortico-basal ganglia thalamic loop in focal arm dystonia. (Siebner et al., 2003).

6. Conclusion

The combined use of TMS and PET has considerably expanded the applications of TMS in basic neuroscience and clinical research. TMS during PET imaging provides a behaviour-independent assay of cortical excitability and connectivity. Mapping the conditioning effects of rTMS with PET provides a powerful approach with which to pinpoint neural substrates of compensatory plasticity in both healthy subjects and in disease states. The combination of rTMS with PET can also improve our understanding of the potential treatment effects of rTMS and reveal new insights into the pathophysiology of certain brain disorders.

Acknowledgements

H. Siebner was supported by the Deutsche Forschungsgemeinschaft (SI 738/1-1). L. Lee was supported by the Wellcome Trust.

References

Catafau, A.M., Perez, V., Gironell, A., Martin, J.C., Kulisevsky, J., Estorch, M., Carrio, I. and Alvarez, E. SPECT mapping of cerebral activity changes induced by repetitive transcranial magnetic stimulation in depressed patients. A pilot study. *Psychiatry Res.*, 2001, 106: 151–160.

Cohen, L.G., Celnik, P., Pascual-Leone, A., Corwell, B., Falz, L., Dambrosia, J., Honda, M., Sadato, N., Gerloff, C., Catala, M.D. and Hallett, M. Functional relevance of cross-modal plasticity in blind humans. *Nature*, 1997, 389: 180–183.

Friston, K.J., Buechel, C., Fink, G.R., Morris, J., Rolls, E. and Dolan, R.J. Psychophysiological and modulatory interactions in neuroimaging. *Neuroimage*, 1997, 6: 218–229.

Johansen-Berg, H., Rushworth, M.F., Bogdanovic, M.D., Kischka, U., Wimalaratna, S. and Matthews, P.M. The role of ipsilateral premotor cortex in hand movement after stroke. *Proc. Natl. Acad. Sci. U.S.A.*, 2002, 99: 14518–14523.

Lee, L., Siebner, H.R., Rowe, J.B., Rizzo, V., Rothwell, J.C., Frackowiak, R.S.J. and Friston, K. Changes in effective connectivity induced by 1 Hz rTMS to primary motor cortex. *J. Neurosci.*, 2003 (in press).

Mottaghy, F.M., Keller, C.E., Gangitano, M., Ly, J., Thall, M., Parker, J.A. and Pascual-Leone, A. Correlation of cerebral blood flow and treatment effects of repetitive transcranial magnetic stimulation in depressed patients. *Psychiatry Res.*, 2002, 115: 1–14.

Nadeau, S.E., McCoy, K.J., Crucian, G.P., Greer, R.A., Rossi, F., Bowers, D., Goodman, W.K., Heilman, K.M. and Triggs, W.J. Cerebral blood flow changes in depressed patients after treatment with repetitive transcranial magnetic stimulation: evidence of individual variability. *Neuropsychiatry Neuropsychol. Behav. Neurol.*, 2002, 15: 159–175.

Pascual-Leone, A., Walsh, V. and Rothwell, J. Transcranial magnetic stimulation in cognitive neuroscience – virtual lesion, chronometry, and functional connectivity. *Curr. Opin. Neurobiol.*, 2000, 10: 232–237.

Paus, T., Jech, R., Thompson, C.J., Comeau, R., Peters, T. and Evans, A.C. Transcranial magnetic stimulation during positron emission tomography: a new method for studying connectivity of the human cerebral cortex. *J. Neurosci.*, 1997, 17: 3178–3184.

Paus, T., Jech, R., Thompson, C.J., Comeau, R., Peters, T. and Evans, A.C. Dose-dependent reduction of cerebral blood flow during rapid-rate transcranial magnetic stimulation of the human sensorimotor cortex. *J. Neurophysiol.*, 1998, 79: 1102–1107.

Paus, T., Castro-Alamancos, M.A. and Petrides, M. Cortico-cortical connectivity of the human mid-dorsolateral frontal cortex and its modulation by repetitive transcranial magnetic stimulation. *Eur. J. Neurosci.*, 2001, 14: 1405–14011.

Rothwell, J.C. Paired-pulse investigations of short-latency intracortical facilitation using TMS in humans. *Electroencephalogr. Clin. Neurophysiol. Suppl.*, 1999, 51: 113–119.

Rothwell, J.C., Hallett, M., Berardelli, A., Eisen, A., Rossini, P. and Paulus, W. Magnetic stimulation: motor evoked potentials. The International Federation of Clinical Neurophysiology. *Electroencephalogr. Clin. Neurophysiol. Suppl.*, 1999, 52: 97–103.

Shajahan, P.M., Glabus, M.F., Steele, J.D., Doris, A.B., Anderson, K., Jenkins, J.A., Gooding, P.A. and Ebmeier, K.P. Left dorsolateral repetitive transcranial magnetic stimulation affects cortical excitability and functional connectivity, but does not impair cognition in major depression. *Prog. Neuro-psychopharmacol. Biol. Psychiatry*, 2002, 26: 945–954.

Siebner, H.R. and Rothwell, J. Transcranial magnetic stimulation: new insights into representational cortical plasticity. *Exp. Brain Res.*, 2003, 148: 1–16.

Siebner, H.R., Willoch, F., Peller, M., Auer, C., Boecker, H., Conrad, B. and Bartenstein, P. Imaging brain activation induced by long trains of repetitive transcranial magnetic stimulation. *NeuroReport*, 1998, 9: 943–948.

Siebner, H.R., Auer, C., Roeck, R. and Conrad, B. Trigeminal sensory input elicited by electric or magnetic stimulation interferes with the central motor drive to the intrinsic hand muscles. *Clin. Neurophysiol.*, 1999a, 110: 1090–1099.

Siebner, H.R., Peller, M., Willoch, F., Auer, C., Bartenstein, P., Drzezga, A., Schwaiger, M. and Conrad, B. Imaging functional activation of the auditory cortex during focal repetitive transcranial magnetic stimulation of the primary motor cortex in normal subjects. *Neurosci. Lett.*, 1999b, 270: 37–40.

Siebner, H., Takano, B., Peller, M., Bartenstein, P., Rossmeier, C., Weyh, T. and Conrad, B. Subthreshold repetitive transcranial magnetic stimulation induced a rate-dependent increase of regional cerebral blood flow in the stimulated primary motor cortex. *Clin. Neurophysiol.*, 1999c, 110(Suppl. 1): S81-S82.

Siebner, H.R., Peller, M., Willoch, F., Minoshima, S., Boecker, H., Auer, C., Drzezga, A., Conrad, B. and Bartenstein, P. Lasting cortical activation after repetitive TMS of the motor cortex: a glucose metabolic study. *Neurology*, 2000, 54: 956–963.

Siebner, H., Peller, M., Bartenstein, P., Willoch, F., Rossmeier, C., Schwaiger, M. and Conrad, B. Activation of frontal premotor areas during suprathreshold transcranial magnetic stimulation of the left primary sensorimotor cortex: a glucose metabolic PET study. *Hum. Brain Mapp.*, 2001a, 12: 157–167.

Siebner, H.R., Takano, B., Peinemann, A., Schwaiger, M., Conrad, B. and Drzezga, A. Continuous transcranial magnetic stimulation during positron emission tomography: a suitable tool for imaging regional excitability of the human cortex. *NeuroImage*, 2001b, 14: 883–890.

Siebner, H.R., Takano, B., Peller, M., Drzezga, A. Functional labelling of the human motor cortex by means of transcranial magnetic stimulation: a PET activation study. *Abstr. Soc. Neurosci.*, 2002, 32: 163.11 (Available on http://sfn.scholarone.com)

Siebner, H., Filipovic, S.R., Rowe, J.B., Cordivari, C., Gerschlager, W., Rothwell, J.C., Frackowiak, R. and Bhatia, K.P. Repetitive TMS to premotor cortex uncovers increased plasticity of the motor system in focal arm dystonia. *Brain*, 2003, submitted in revised version.

Speer, A.M., Kimbrell, T.A., Wassermann, E.M. J.D.R., Willis, M.W., Herscovitch, P. and Post, R.M. Opposite effects of high and low frequency rTMS on regional brain activity in depressed patients. *Biol. Psychiatry*, 2000, 48: 1133–1141.

Strafella, A.P. and Paus, T. Cerebral blood-flow changes induced by paired-pulse transcranial magnetic stimulation of the primary motor cortex. *J. Neurophysiol.*, 2001, 85: 2624–2629.

Strafella, A.P., Paus, T., Barrett, J. and Dagher, A. Repetitive transcranial magnetic stimulation of the human prefrontal cortex induces dopamine release in the caudate nucleus. *J. Neurosci.*, 2001, 21: RC157.

Walsh, V. and Rushworth, M. A primer of magnetic stimulation as a tool for neuropsychology. *Neuropsychologia*, 1999, 37: 125–135.

Ziemann, U. Intracortical inhibition and facilitation in the conventional paired TMS paradigm. *Electroencephalogr. Clin. Neurophysiol. Suppl.*, 1999, 51: 127–136.

Zilles, K., Palomero-Gallagher, N., Grefkes, C., Scheperjans, F., Boy, C., Amunts, K. and Schleicher, A. Architectonics of the human cerebral cortex and transmitter receptor fingerprints: reconciling functional neuroanatomy and neurochemistry. *Eur. Neuropsychopharmacol.*, 2002, 12: 587–599.

Section II

Animal Studies

Transcranial Magnetic Stimulation and Transcranial Direct Current Stimulation (Supplements to Clinical Neurophysiology, Vol. 56)
Editors: W. Paulus, F. Tergau, M.A. Nitsche, J.C. Rothwell, U. Ziemann, M. Hallett

Chapter 8

A coil for magnetic stimulation of the macaque monkey brain

Yukio Nonaka[a], Takuya Hayashi[b], Takashi Ohnishi[c], Shingo Okabe[d], Noboru Teramoto[b], Shoogo Ueno[e], Hiroshi Watabe[b], Hiroshi Matsuda[c], Hidehiro Iida[b] and Yoshikazu Ugawa[d]*

[a]*Neurology Division, Nihon Kohden Corporation,*
[b]*Department of Investigative Radiology, National Cardio-Vascular Center, Research Institute,*
[c]*Department of Radiology, National Center Hospital of Mental, Nervous and Muscular Disorders, National Center of Neurology and Psychiatry,*
[d]*Department of Neurology, Division of Neuroscience, Graduate School of Medicine, University of Tokyo, 7-3-1, Hongo, Bunkyo-ku, Tokyo 113-8655 (Japan)*
[e]*Bioimaging and Biomagnetics Laboratory, Department of Biomedical Engineering, Graduate School of Medicine, University of Tokyo, Tokyo (Japan)*

1. Introduction

Transcranial magnetic stimulation (TMS) has been used more than 15 years since its invention by Barker et al. (1985). We have two ways to specify a responsible brain structure for the elicited effect by TMS. One is to measure a specific response; such as motor evoked potential (MEP) or visual evoked potentials and so on. When we record MEPs elicited by TMS, even if TMS activates several other areas as well as the motor cortex, we can evaluate the effect of activation of the motor cortex or motor systems. Then it allows us to study the excitability of the central motor pathways even using non-focal simulation. The other way is to perform a localized stimulation of the brain. When we activate a localized area of the brain by TMS, we can evaluate the function of that area even by measuring some non-specific effects influenced by several factors. Focal stimulation has been partly accomplished by using a figure-of-eight coil (Ueno et al., 1988). The former strategy has been used in MEP studies and the latter in neuropsychological studies.

In recently advanced neuroimaging studies during or after single-pulsed TMS or repetitive TMS (rTMS), we should perform focal stimulation because we measure changes which are not specific to one neuronal system; such as blood flow or glucose metabolism. Moreover, combined TMS and neuroimaging studies in animals are expected to promote understanding of biological effect of TMS. However, it is well known that TMS is not able to induce enough currents to activate neurons within small

* *Correspondence to*: Dr. Y. Ugawa, Department of Neurology, Division of Neuroscience, Graduate School of Medicine, University of Tokyo, 7-3-1 Hongo, Bunkyo-ku, Tokyo 113-8655, Japan.
Tel: +81-3-5800-8672; Fax: +81-3-5800-6548;
E-mail: ugawa-tky@umin.ac.jp

volume structures. For example, spinal cord in the spinal canal can be activated by high voltage electrical stimulation (Ugawa et al., 1995) but cannot be activated by TMS, even though spinal roots are activated by TMS (Ugawa et al., 1989). The aims of this chapter are to make a special coil for TMS of the monkey brain, to compare induced currents in the phantom brain elicited by different coils and to confirm that with our coil, focal stimulation is achieved in the monkey brain using positron emission computed tomography (PET).

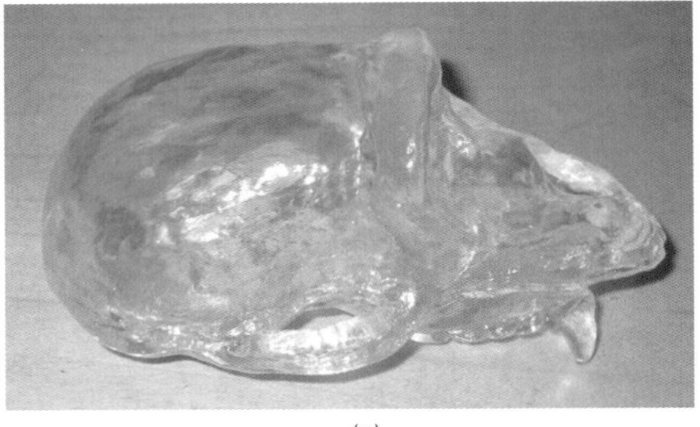

(a)

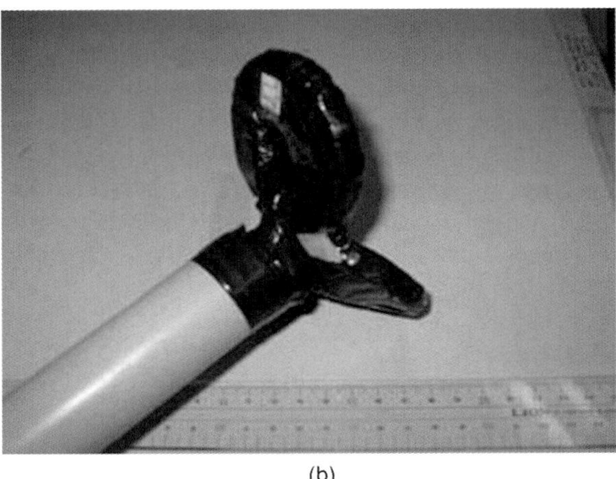

(b)

Fig. 1. A plastic skull model for the macaque monkey (a) and a coil made for stimulation of the macaque monkey brain (b).

2. Methods

We did two experiments in the present investigation: measurements of electric fields induced by single-pulsed TMS with three kinds of coils in the phantom brain, and measurement of glucose metabolism in a macaque monkey brain with the coil specially developed for the monkey brain stimulation by using ^{18}F-fluorodeoxyglucose (FDG)-PET. Magnetic stimulation was performed with a Magnetic Stimulator (AAA-15486, Nihon Kohden, Tokyo, Japan). This stimulator can produce both monophasic and biphasic repetitive stimuli. In the present experiments, we used a single-pulse monophasic stimulus in the former experiment and repetitive monophasic stimuli in the latter experiment.

2.1. TMS coils

We used three different magnetic coils in the first experiment. One is a special small double cone coil for stimulation of the macaque monkey (*Macaca fascicularis*) brain. We first made a plastic phantom of the skull of macaque monkeys with plastic based on magnetic resonance images (MRIs) of their skull and brain (Fig. 1a). Then, we made a small double cone coil (outer diameter of each coil, 62 mm). The angle between the two coils was fixed to fit the curvature of the skull over the motor cortex (135°) (Fig. 1b). Another one is a small flat figure-of-eight coil (outside diameter of each coil, 62 mm) which is similar to that often successfully used to activate the motor cortex in monkey experiments (Oliver et al., 2001). However, in such experiments, there must have been a craniotomy over the motor cortex in monkeys. Therefore, we do not know whether the motor cortex is able to be activated with this coil in monkeys with an intact skull (without a craniotomy). The other is a figure-of-eight coil (outer diameter of each coil, 92 mm) which is usually used for focal cerebral stimulation in humans. These coils were placed over the motor cortex. Posteriorly directed currents were induced at the center of the coil to elicit anteriorly directed currents under the coil in the phantom brain.

2.2. *Electric field measurements in the phantom brain*

The electric fields induced by TMS in the brain were measured with a probe made from a coaxial cable similar to those in previous reports (Maccabee et al., 1991; Kobayashi et al., 1997). The coaxial cable was passed through an acrylic tube and connected to an amplifier. The distal 5 mm of the outside insulation and shield of the cable were stripped to record the voltage drop between the cable shield and the bared distal tip. The distal end of the probe was bent at a right-angle and submerged in the saline solution. By dividing the voltage drop by 5 mm, we calculated the induced electric field (mV/mm or V/m). The probe was placed in the skull model filled with isotonic saline. Measurement was performed at 54 sites which were 1 cm apart from each other. All sites were 5 mm deep from the inner surface of the skull where the monkey cerebral cortex must be present judging from MRI images. All points were on a dome shaped surface. At each site, we measured the voltage drop in two directions; anterior-posterior and left-right directions. An amplitude and direction of the vector made by the voltage drops measured in two directions were calculated at each point. These amplitudes and directions were illustrated as contour map. We fixed 1 cm thick plasticine over the whole outer surface of the skull to mimic muscles attached to the monkey skull. Measurement was performed using the above three different coils. Measured electric fields were depicted in an unfolded view of the dome shaped inner surface of the skull. The amplitude of vectors was depicted by colors and their direction was depicted by arrows. The center of the coil was placed over the left motor cortex. The intensity was fixed at 35% of the maximum stimulator output in all experiments. The induced electric field in the monkey brain at this intensity was about 70 V/m under the center of the coil, which is almost the same as that induced in the human phantom brain by TMS at an intensity of the active motor threshold. These indicate that TMS with this intensity can definitely activate the cerebral cortex under the coil but induce no movements when monkeys relax their muscles. Therefore, it suggests that a small area must be activated with this stimulation. Based on this speculation, we set the intensity at 35% of the maximum stimulator output.

2.3. *PET measurements during rTMS with our special coil for the macaque monkey*

2.3.1. *Animal preparation*

One adult male cynomolgous monkey (*Macaca fascicularis*) with body weight of 4.9 kg took part in this study. The animal underwent two FDG PET scans under generalized anesthesia: one is the control condition in which sham rTMS was given and the other taken during real rTMS. Our procedures were performed according to guidelines for animal research on Human Care and Use of Laboratory Animals (Rockville, National Institute of Health/Office for Protection from Research Risks, 1996) and approved by the ethical committee for animal research at National Cardio-Vascular Center, Osaka, Japan.

2.3.2. *rTMS techniques*

We used the above mentioned coil developed for *Macaca fascicularis*. Stimulation parameters of rTMS were as follows: 20 trains of 5 Hz stimulation for 20 s were applied with an inter-train interval of 40 s over the right primary motor cortex (M1). In total, 2000 ($5 \times 20 \times 20$) stimuli were given. The intensity was set at 35% of the maximal stimulator output which was determined to mimic the active motor cortex threshold in the human brain. The coil position was centered over the target site, $x = 16$ mm, $y = 6$ mm, $z = 15$ mm in an anterior-posterior commissure (AC-PC) coordinate in a stereotaxic space of *Macaca fascicularis* brain (Martin et al., 2000) (corresponding to upper limb region of M1). This position was determined stereotaxically using T1-weighted magnetic resonance images (MRIs) obtained with inversion recovery-FSPGR sequence (TR = 9.4 ms, TE = 2.1 ms, TI = 600 ms) using a 3-Tesla MRI scanner (Signa LX VAH/I, GE, Milwaukee, USA).

2.3.3. PET acquisition

PET scans were performed on the ECAT EXACT HR PET scanner (Siemens-CTI, Knoxville, USA) at Bio-Functional Research Institute at National Cardiovascular Center. The spatial resolution is 3.8 × 3.8 × 4.7 mm. The monkey was positioned in the PET scanner with his head fixed in a molded polyurethane holder two hours after introduction of anesthesia when physiological state was kept stable and the effect of ketamine hydrochloride was withdrawn. A 15-min transmission scan for attenuation correction was performed with a rotating ^{68}Ge/^{68}Ga rod source. A 187 MBq of ^{18}F-FDG was injected intravenously over a 1-min period. ^{18}F-FDG accumulation in brain was quantified with a 2D-mode PET scanner six times (one frame: 5 min duration) 30–60 min after the tracer injection. We started 20 trains of rTMS at the beginning of tracer injection in the real stimulation condition. In the control condition, rTMS was done with a sham coil. PET data of ^{18}F-FDG radioactivity were reconstructed by filtered back projection with a matrix of 128 × 128 × 47 and a voxel size of 1.1 × 1.1 × 3.13 mm.

2.3.4. Data analysis

Voxel-based analysis was performed to test the difference of ^{18}F-FDG radioactivity between the real and sham stimulation conditions based on general linear model. PET images were summed and co-registered to the subject's MRI using mutual information algorithm (Ashburner et al., 1997). Then T1-weighted MRI images were transformed to a standard brain space of *Macaque fascicularis* (Martin and Bowden, 2000). This transformation was applied to co-register each PET frame data of ^{18}F-FDG radioactivity. The normalized images with six-frame data for each condition were compared voxel-wise by paired *t*-test. Statistical inferences were based on the theory of random Gaussian field theory (Friston et al., 1995). A contrast of conditions: rTMS minus control was regarded to show rTMS-induced activation and the statistically significant level was set at corrected p less than 0.05.

3. Results

Figure 2 shows the electric field maps of eddy currents in the phantom brain induced by three different coils.

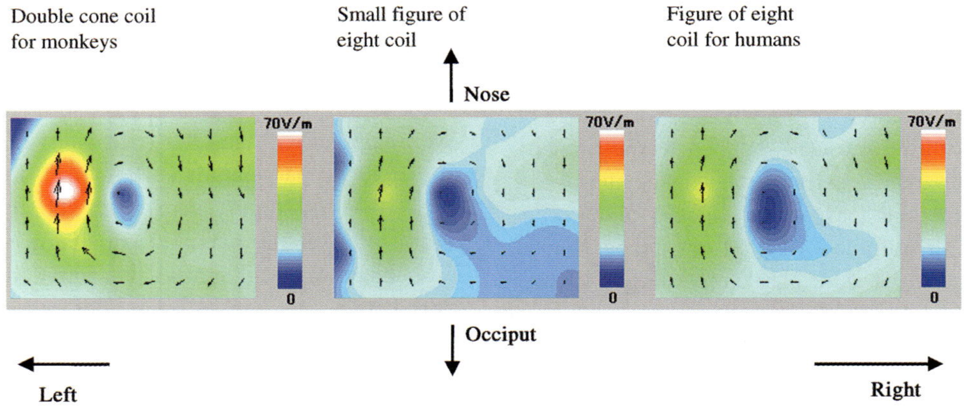

Fig. 2. The amounts of induced electric fields were depicted by colors on the inner surface of the skull. The dome shaped inner surface is unfolded and seen from above. Therefore, the top of the figure faces the nose, the bottom the occiput, the left the left side, and the right the right side. The amplitude of the vector calculated from the induced fields in two directions is depicted by colors and its direction by arrows. When stimulating with a coil for the macaque monkey brain, electric fields were maximal under the center of the coil and localized. Small oppositely directed currents were elicited in the right hemisphere. When using a small, flat figure-of-eight coil, low amount and diffuse fields were induced in the left hemisphere and almost no fields in the right hemisphere. Stimulation with a figure-of-eight coil for human brain elicited an electric field pattern similar to that by the flat small coil. The maximum fields were 70, 45 and 48 V/m, respectively.

With the coil for the macaque monkey brain (left), high amount, moderately localized electric fields were evoked. They were localized under the center of the coil. The highest amplitude was approximately 70 V/m just under the center of the coil. Small oppositely directed fields (0–30 V/m at maximum) were evoked in the contralateral hemisphere. Small currents at most 30 V/m, must have no biological effects when the threshold is about 70 V/m. This indicates that no activation occurs in the contralateral cortex or that the contralateral cortex is not stimulated. Therefore, we can say that the contralateral hemisphere was not practically affected by this stimulation even though small currents were actually elicited there. With a small flat figure-of-eight coil (middle), electric fields were less localized and smaller as compared with those evoked by the former coil. The maximum amplitude of 45 V/m was elicited under the center of the coil, which was about 65% of that evoked by the coil for the macaque monkey. With a coil for focal stimulation in humans (right), the map of electric fields was similar to that with a flat small figure-of-eight coil and the highest amplitude was 48 V/m (68% of that induced by the coil for macaque monkeys).

Figure 3 shows areas showing significant glucose metabolic increase in real stimulation with the coil for the macaque monkey as compared with sham stimulation. Glucose metabolism increased at multiple areas including the site of stimulation (right M1): the right primary motor, primary sensory and frontopolar cortices.

4. Discussion

It is well known that TMS can not induce enough currents to activate neurons within a small volume structure. However, rTMS was given to a rat brain by a 5 cm circular coil in some studies (Ji et al., 1998; Zangen and Hyodo, 2002). To find out an appropriate size and shape of the coil for focal stimulation of an animal brain, we investigated how induced currents are affected by the different stimulating coils.

The measurements of induced electric fields have shown that stronger, more localized fields were elicited with our monkey coil than with a flat, same-sized, figure-of-eight coil or with a larger coil for human brain stimulation. Moreover, a FDG-PET study has shown that localized activation was really accomplished in the monkey brain with this coil.

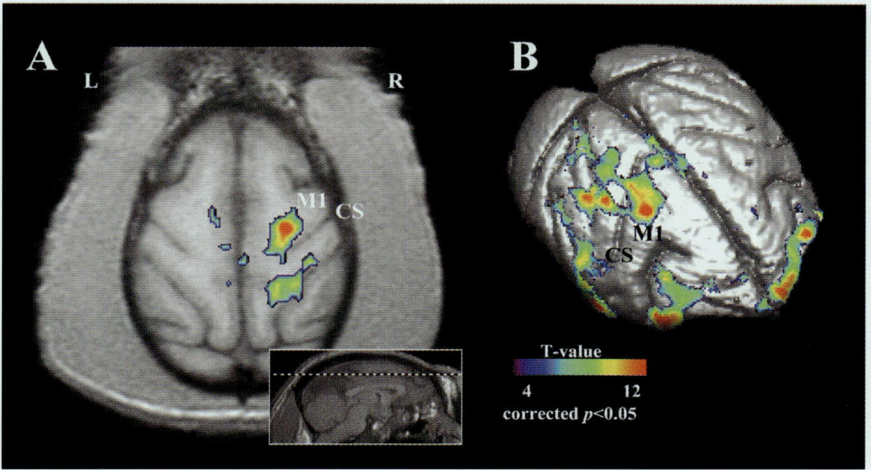

Fig. 3. Activated areas during rTMS over the right motor cortex with our coil. Activated foci were shown in t-values (rainbow color) overlaid on an axial slices of T1-weighted MRI image (A) and on the skull-stripped rendered brain (B). rTMS was given over the right M1. CS: central sulcus; M1: primary motor cortex.

Unfortunately we did not perform PET recordings during rTMS with the other two coils and could not compare PET results among different coils. Therefore, we can not say that more localized stimulation was performed with our coil in the monkey brain than with the other coils. However, we can say that focal stimulation is really achieved in the monkey brain with our coil. These results suggest that focal activation can be optimally achieved by a coil which fits to the animal skull strictly.

In conclusion, we recommend the use of an appropriate-sized double cone coil with its two wings fitting to the curvature of the skull in TMS experiments of animals.

Acknowledgements

A part of this work was supported by Research Project Grant-in-aid for Scientific Research No. 12680768 from the Ministry of Education, Science, Sports and Culture of Japan.

References

Ashburner, J. and Friston, K.J. Multimodal image coregistration and partitioning – A unified framework. *NeuroImage*, 1997, 6: 209–217.

Barker, A.T., Jalinous, R. and Freeston, I.L. Non-invasive stimulation of human motor cortex. *Lancet*, 1985, I: 1106–1107.

Friston, K.J., Holmes, A.P., Worsley, K.J., Poline, J.P., Frith, C.D. and Frackowiak, R.S.J. Statistical Parametric Maps in Functional Imaging: A General Linear Approach. *Hum. Brain Map.*, 1995, 2: 189–210.

Ji, R., Schelaepfer, T.E., Aizenman, C.D., Epsstein, C., Qiu, D., Huang, J.C. and Rupp, F. Repetitive transcranial magnetic stimulation activates specific regions in rat brain. *Proc. Nat. Acad. Sci.*, 1998, 95: 15635–15640.

Kobayashi, M., Ueno, S. and Kurokawa, T. Importance of soft tissue inhomogeneity in magnetic peripheral nerve stimulation. *Electroenceph. Clin. Neurophyiol.*, 1997, 105: 406–413.

Maccabee, P.J., Amassian, V.E., Eberle, L.P., Rudell, A.P., Cracco, R.Q., Lai, K.S. and Somasundarum, M. Measurement of the electric field induced into inhomogeneous volume conductors by magnetic coils: application to human spinal neurogeometry. *Electroenceph. Clin. Neurophyiol.*, 1991, 81: 224–237.

Martin, R.F. and Bowden, D.M. *Primate Brain Maps: Structure of the Macaque Brain*. Elsevier Science, 2000.

Oliver, E., Baker, S.N., Nakajima, K., Brocheir, T. and Lemon, R.N. Investigation into non-monosynaptic corticospinal excitation of macaque upper limb single motor units. *J. Neurophysiol.*, 2001, 86: 1573–1586.

Ueno, S., Tashiro, T. and Harada, K. Localized stimulation of neural tissues in the brain by means of paired configuration of time-varying magnetic fields. *J. App. Phys.*, 1988, 64: 5862–5864.

Ugawa, Y., Rothwell, J.C., Day, B.L., Thompson, P.D. and Marsden, C.D. Magnetic stimulation over the spinal enlargements. *J. Neurol. Neurosurg. Psychiatry*, 1989, 52: 1025–1032.

Ugawa, Y., Genba-Shimizu, K. and Kanazawa, I. Electrical stimulation of the human descending motor tracts at several levels. *Can. J. Neurol. Sci.*, 1995, 22: 36–42.

Zangen, A. and Hyodo, K. Transcranial magnetic stimulation induces increases in extracellular levels of dopamine and glutamate in the nucleus accumbens. *NeuroReport*, 2002, 18: 2401–2405.

Transcranial Magnetic Stimulation and Transcranial Direct Current Stimulation (Supplements to Clinical Neurophysiology, Vol. 56)
Editors: W. Paulus, F. Tergau, M.A. Nitsche, J.C. Rothwell, U. Ziemann, M. Hallett

Chapter 9

Neurophysiological characterization of magnetic seizure therapy (MST) in non-human primates

Sarah H. Lisanby[a,b,*], Tammy Moscrip[a], Oscar Morales[a,b], Bruce Luber[a], Charles Schroeder[c] and Harold A. Sackeim[a,b]

[a]*Magnetic Brain Stimulation Laboratory, Department of Biological Psychiatry, New York State Psychiatric Institute, New York, NY 10032 (USA)*
[b]*Department of Psychiatry, College of Physicians and Surgeons, Columbia University, New York, NY (USA)*
[c]*Nathan Kline Institute, Orangeberg, NY (USA)*

1. Introduction

Electroconvulsive therapy (ECT) remains an important treatment for psychiatric disorders, including severe major depressive episodes (American Psychiatric Association, 2001). Recent research in the field of ECT has demonstrated that seizures differ markedly in their therapeutic efficacy and side effect profile (Sackeim, 1986). This substantial body of work on the relationships among the parameters of the electrical stimulus used to elicit the seizure, the characteristics of the induced seizure, and clinical outcome supports the hypothesis that electrical current density and seizure initiation in prefrontal cortex are associated with the most effective forms of treatment. This suggests that strategies to focus current and seizure initiation in prefrontal cortex may enhance efficacy. Likewise, limiting current and seizure spread in medial temporal lobes might be expected to reduce side effects.

The application of an electrical stimulus across the scalp, as with conventional ECT, results in significant shunting of current through the scalp and skull and offers little control over the distribution of the induced electric field (Sackeim et al., 1994). Since magnetic fields pass through tissue without impedance, seizure induction using a rapidly alternating magnetic field offers the promise of more precise control over induced current and seizure initiation (Sackeim, 1994). Magnetic seizure therapy (MST) involves the induction of a seizure under general anesthesia using high intensities of repetitive transcranial magnetic stimulation (rTMS). We demonstrated the feasibility of MST in non-human primates (Lisanby et al., 2001c) and in patients with major depression (Lisanby et al., 2001, 2001b) using nonfocal stimulating coils, but no work to date has been done on refining MST technique to focus seizure initiation in targeted brain regions.

* *Correspondence to*: Dr. S.H. Lisanby, Magnetic Brain Stimulation Laboratory, Department of Biological Psychiatry, New York State Psychiatric Institute, 1051 Riverside Drive, Unit 126, New York, NY 10032, USA. Tel: (212) 543-5568; Fax: (212) 543-6056; E-mail: SHL24@columbia.edu

We hypothesize that seizure characteristics will differ as a function of the mode of seizure induction, and that it should be possible to create a magnetic form of convulsive therapy that preserves effects in prefrontal cortex, while limiting spread of the induced electric field and resultant seizure in medial temporal structures or other regions implicated in the adverse effects of ECT. Here, we present a model with which to test those hypotheses, and report the first data on the intracerebral spatial distribution of the electric field and the neurophysiological characteristics of electrically and magnetically induced seizures in non-human primates. The aim of this work is to inform the early stages of development of a novel putative therapeutic intervention for the treatment of major depression and other psychiatric disorders.

2. Background

2.1. Rationale for magnetic seizure therapy (MST)

Despite the continued development of novel anti-depressant medications, severe major depression remains an important public health concern, responsible for significant morbidity and mortality (American Psychiatric Association, 2001). A substantial proportion of patients fails to respond to currently available pharmacotherapy or cannot tolerate the side effects. ECT remains the only somatic treatment with proven efficacy in such patients. ECT is the most effective and rapidly acting treatment for MDE, but its use is limited by cognitive and other side effects. Retrograde amnesia, the most persistent adverse effect of ECT, usually improves during the first few months following ECT (American Psychiatric Association, 2001). Nonetheless, for many patients recovery is incomplete, with permanent amnesia for events that occurred close in time to the treatment (Donahue, 2000). Electrode placement and electrical dosage are strongly associated with the magnitude of acute, subacute, and long-term cognitive side effects (Sackeim, 1986; Sackeim et al., 1993, 2000; Lisanby et al., 2000). Several studies have shown that high dose right unilateral (RUL) ECT is as effective as bilateral (BL) ECT, but retains advantages in terms of lower cognitive side effects (McCall et al., 2000; Sackeim et al., 2000, 2001). Studies of regional brain activity following ECT suggest that prefrontal changes are associated with antidepressant efficacy while temporal changes are related to the amnestic side effects of the treatment (Sackeim et al., 1996; Luber et al., 2000). Such work suggests that it may be possible to begin to disentangle the antidepressant effects from the cognitive side effects of ECT through improved focusing and control over the induced seizure (Nobler et al., 2000).

While modifications in ECT technique (such as electrode placement, dosage, and the characteristics of the electrical stimulus) have reduced its side effects, amnesia remains a significant risk. This may be due to the fact that the site of seizure initiation and patterns of seizure spread, factors key to the efficacy and side effects of ECT (Sackeim et al., 1993, 2000; McCall et al., 2000), cannot be adequately controlled with current ECT technique (Sackeim, 1994; Sackeim et al., 1994). A form of convulsive therapy that retains the therapeutic efficacy of ECT, but with a better side effect profile, should substantially improve the quality of life for patients needing convulsive therapy and should increase access to effective treatment. MST is under development as a means of achieving that goal (Lisanby and Sackeim, 2001; Lisanby et al., 2001c, 2002).

While both MST and ECT induce seizures through electrical stimulation of the brain, the electric field induced by MST is more focal than that induced by ECT by virtue of the differing physics of direct electrical stimulation vs. indirect magnetic induction of electrical current (Lisanby et al., 1998a, b). The high impedance of the skull (Geddes and Baker, 1967; Rush and Driscoll, 1968; Driscoll, 1970) shunts the bulk of the electrical stimulus away from brain, resulting in a nonfocal, widespread intracerebral current distribution regardless of electrode placement. Measurements of shunting across the scalp and skull in humans (Smitt and Wegener, 1944; Law, 1993) and monkeys (Hayes, 1950) range from 80 to 97%. The topography of shunting varies considerably among individuals, due to differences in skull thickness and anatomy (Driscoll, 1970). Skull inhomogeneities, result in regional variability in current density (Hayes, 1950; Weaver et al., 1976; Law, 1993; Sackeim et al., 1994). Thus, highly variable and widespread current distribution is inherent in the application of an external electrical stimulus that must traverse the scalp, skull, and cerebral spinal fluid to reach brain.

Stimulating the brain with rTMS obviates many of the limitations of electrical stimulation by inducing intracerebral current non-invasively using rapidly alternating magnetic fields. Unlike electricity, magnetic fields pass through tissue without impedance, resulting in better control over the electrical field induced in the brain and presumably over the resultant seizure (Barker et al., 1985). The electric field induced by rTMS is capable of neural depolarization at a depth extending to about 2 cm below the scalp (i.e., gray-white matter junction), so direct effects are limited to the cortex (Epstein, 1990). In addition, depending principally on coil geometry, the magnetic field can be spatially targeted in cortical regions, offering further control over intracerebral current paths (Maccabee et al., 1990; Maccabee et al., 1991; Brasil-Neto et al., 1992; Mills et al., 1992). Thus, MST should offer more precise control over current paths than the transcranial application of electricity, opening the possibility of limiting seizure spread and thereby reducing side effects. Measurements in non-human primates with intracerebral multicontact electrodes presented in detail below and abstracted elsewhere (Lisanby et al., 1998b) support the hypothesis that MST-induced current and the resulting seizure are more focal than those obtained with electroconvulsive shock (ECS).

2.2. *Current state of development of MST*

All of the animal work on the development of MST to date has been in rhesus monkeys because it has not yet been possible to design a coil and device capable of magnetic seizure induction in an organism with a smaller brain. This is likely because the magnitude of the induced electric field is proportional to the size of the brain and the ratio between coil size and brain size (Weissman et al., 1992). The monkey model presents advantages in the study of the differential cognitive effects of MST and ECS (Moscrip et al., 2001).

We demonstrated the feasibility of using MST to induce seizures in non-human primates under the same general anesthesia as used for human ECT (Lisanby et al., 2001c) and studies are under way to investigate its neurobiological effects in comparison with ECS. Results of thorough, blinded neuropathological examination in 12 monkeys randomized to receive chronic treatment for 6 weeks with MST, ECS, or anesthesia-alone sham, demonstrated that both ECS and MST lack any evidence for neuropathological effects, supporting the safety of these interventions (Dwork et al., unpublished observations). Preliminary work suggests that the interventions differ in key measures of neural plasticity in the hippocampus (mossy fiber sprouting and cellular proliferation), consistent with MST having less of an effect on medial temporal structures than ECS (Lisanby et al., 2002, in press).

Initial human trials with MST showed that MST is feasible in the clinical setting (Lisanby et al., 2001) and provided early evidence for cognitive advantages, especially on tasks heavily reliant on hippocampal functioning (Lisanby et al., 2001b, in press). This preliminary clinical work also indicated that the MST device developed for use in the monkey was unable to achieve focal seizure induction in the prefrontal cortex at substantially suprathreshold levels in the human, which is thought to be critical to antidepressant efficacy of ECT, and by extension, MST. Studies presently underway will yield the first data on antidepressant efficacy, and device modifications are being piloted in an attempt to overcome output limitations.

Like rTMS, MST is not yet FDA approved and is presently at an early phase of investigation. As of this writing, a total of 16 non-human primates and 26 human patients with major depression have received MST worldwide. More work needs to be done to establish the proper parameters of stimulation, coil design and placement, and other factors, to determine whether it will have antidepressant action and to maximize its clinical utility.

This chapter presents three sets of data on the neurophysiological effects of magnetically and electrically induced seizures in rhesus monkeys generated during the original development of the MST device: (1) the efficiency of the MST waveform; (2) characterization of the electric fields induced in the brain with MST and ECS; and (3) analyses of the resultant seizures. The aim of these studies was to describe the relative characteristics of seizures induced with these two modalities, and test the hypothesis that focal cortical seizure induction with MST results in greater control over the induced electric field and patterns of seizure propagation.

3. Efficiency of the MST pulse width and waveform in inducing seizure

It has long been observed that the types of electrical current used with ECT vary in their efficiency in seizure induction and side effects. For example, sine wave ECT results in more severe short-term cognitive side effects than brief pulse ECT (Weiner et al., 1986). This difference is thought to be a consequence of the inefficient properties of the sine wave stimulus, which continues to stimulate neurons after they have been depolarized by the leading edge of the pulse (Sackeim et al., 1994). Neurophysiological studies suggest that the optimal pulse width (PW) for stimulating cortical neurons may be briefer than the 1–2 ms typically used in ECT (Sackeim et al., 1994). Briefer pulses have the advantage of more efficient neuronal excitation at a lower charge density because they are closer to the chronaxie, which describes the physiological relationship between PW and threshold current (Yuen et al., 1981). Briefer pulses also have a larger safety margin by virtue of their lower charge per phase (McCreery et al., 1990). A series of studies in animals and humans have found briefer PWs (in the range of 0.15–0.3 ms) to be more efficient in inducing seizure than the PWs commonly used with ECT (Liberson, 1948; Goldman, 1949; Woodbury and Davenport, 1952; Cronholm and Ottosson, 1963; Valentine et al., 1968; Robin and De Tissera, 1982; Hyrman et al., 1985; Lisanby et al., 1997). There are also suggestions that briefer PWs are associated with fewer cognitive side effects (Cronholm and Ottosson, 1963; Valentine et al., 1968). Recent work by our group indicates that, when given as a sufficient dosage above threshold, ultrabrief pulse RUL ECT can be as effective as conventional PW BL ECT when given at a dosage six times the seizure threshold, but retains significant advantages in terms of cognitive side effects (Sackeim et al., 2001).

The effective PW of the MST stimulus is in the ultra-brief range (0.3 ms), suggesting that MST may be more efficient in stimulating neurons, but also indicating that dosage above threshold may be critical to the efficacy of MST as it is with ultra-brief pulse ECT. However, it was not known whether the shape of the MST pulse (dampened cosine, compared with the square-wave of ECS) would affect its efficiency. Magnetic stimulators possess this unique waveform for reasons of efficiency in operation and charge recovery. Building a magnetic stimulator capable of inducing a square-wave electric pulse presented substantial technical challenges that would have been a barrier to the development of MST. We tested the relative efficiency of the MST and ECS waveforms in inducing seizure by comparing electrical seizure threshold with square wave ECS (given at a conventional and ultrabrief PW) with threshold titrated with the dampened cosine waveform of the MST device.

3.1. Methods

3.1.1. Subjects

All studies described in this chapter were approved by the Institutional Animal Care and Use Committees of New York State Psychiatric Institute and Columbia University. Two male rhesus monkeys (*Macaca mulatta*, weight 4 kg) were used in experiment I.

3.1.2. Design

Three conditions (0.15 ms PW ECS, 1.0 ms PW ECS, and ECS delivered with an MST-like waveform) were administered to each monkey in a counterbalanced order on separate days (12 replications for 0.15 ms PW, 14 for 1.0 ms PW, and two for MECS).

3.1.3. Anesthesia and monitoring
Pre-intervention sedation was achieved with ketamine 15 mg/kg i.m. Anesthesia for all conditions included methohexital (1 mg/kg i.v.) and succinylcholine (3.5 mg/kg i.v.). The monkeys were oxygenated (100% O_2 by face mask) until the return of spontaneous respirations. Just prior to the injection of succinylcholine, a tourniquet was placed on the left upper limb to block the distribution of the muscle relaxant. Adequacy of muscle relaxation was monitored with a peripheral nerve stimulator. A bite block was inserted in the mouth to protect the teeth. Anesthetic doses were adjusted based on earlier anesthetic response. As is common practice with clinical ECT, the anticholinergic agent atropine was administered on all threshold titration days to reduce seizure-induced secretions and protect the airway. Monkeys were shaved over the sites for ECS electrodes, bifrontomastoid scalp EEG, and distal legs for IV access. Physiological monitoring at each session included ECG, EEG, pulse oximetry, end-tidal Pco_2, and blood pressure. EEG data were digitized for quantitative analysis.

3.1.4. ECS
The bifrontotemporal ECS electrodes sites were cleaned with alcohol to remove scalp oils and abraded with Redux (ground quartz) paste to reduce impedance. ECS electrodes were positioned with the electrode center 0.75 in. above the mid-point of the line connecting the external canthus and tragus. Self-adhesive Thymapad electrodes (Somatics) were cut to 1.25 in. in diameter to approximate the electrode to skull diameter ratio for human ECT. The ECS stimulus was delivered with a human MECTA Model D device. This constant current device produces a bidirectional square-wave pulse.

3.1.5. ECS delivered with an MST-like waveform
An inductively coupled electrical stimulator was constructed by attaching six windings of copper wire to the surface of the MST coil (Magstim Company Limited, 5 cm diameter round coil), and using the electrical current induced in this wire to administer a transcranial electrical stimulation via ECS electrodes. This method delivers ECS with a waveform that matches the MST device (dampened cosine). The device was calibrated by measuring the voltage drop across a 10 Ω resistor to administer 0.8 A in the second phase of the pulse, since this is the phase thought to be effective in neuronal depolarization.

3.1.6. Seizure threshold (ST) titration
ST was determined using the ascending method-of-limits procedure, as is standard for human ECT (Sackeim et al., 1986). Frequency was fixed at 40 pulses per second (the 20 Hz setting on the MECTA device delivers 20 pulse pairs, or a total of 40 pulses per second). Current was fixed at 0.8 A. For square-wave ECS, PW was set at 1.0 ms for the conventional PW condition, and 0.15 ms for the ultrabrief PW condition. At each session, seizure threshold was titrated by progressively increasing stimulus duration from 0.5 to 2.0 s, in 0.25 s steps, at 20 s intervals. Incrementing train duration has been found to be more efficient than increasing other parameters with ECT (Devanand et al., 1998). The criterion for an adequate seizure was at least 10 s of convulsive motor activity, timed from the offset of stimulation. Twenty seconds is the conventional cutoff for clinical ECT. However, the average seizure duration in the rhesus monkey is shorter (17 ± 4 s) (Lisanby et al., 2001c). If a brief seizure was noted (< 10 s), re-stimulation at a higher stimulus intensity followed a 60–90 s pause to allow the immediate post-ictal refractory period to pass.

3.2. Results and discussion

ST differed across conditions ($F(2,4) = 154$, $p < 0.01$, Fig. 1). ST with the conventional 1.0 ms PW was significantly greater than ECS with an ultra-brief PW, and than ECS delivered with the MST-waveform (Tukey's posthoc t test, $p < 0.05$). The MST-waveform appeared to be as efficient as square-wave ECS with an ultra-brief PW, but a larger sample size would be required to provide proof of equivalency. The finding that briefer pulses are more efficient in inducing seizure is consistent with our preliminary data in humans

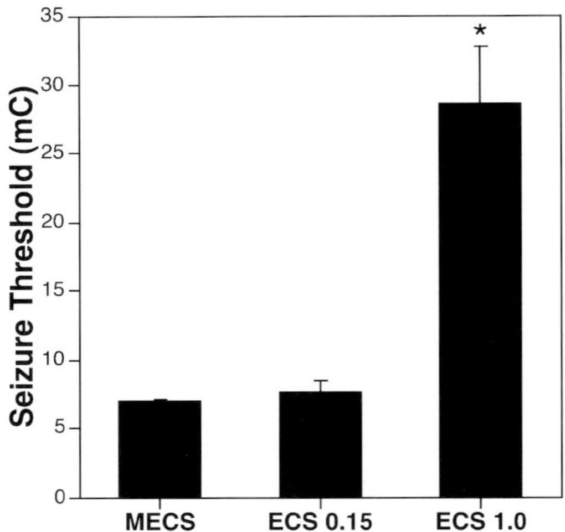

Fig. 1. Seizure threshold titrated with ECS administered with an MST-like dampened cosine waveform (MECS), or a conventional square-wave at a 0.15 or 1.0 ms pulse width. Seizure threshold differed across conditions ($F(2,4) = 154$, $p < 0.01$). *1.0 ms PW differed from the other two groups, $p < 0.05$.

contrasting PWs of 0.3 and 1.5 ms (Sackeim et al., 2001).

These findings suggest that the briefer PW delivered by MST devices is more efficient than the wider PW commonly used in ECT, consistent with the hypothesis that PW closer to the chronaxie should be more efficient (Yuen et al., 1981). This result supports the feasibility of magnetic seizure induction with the dampened cosine waveform, and also has broader implications for more optimal parameter selection for clinical ECT.

4. Intracerebral electric field distributions of MST and ECS

While theories about the mechanisms of action of ECT focus on the topography of the induced current paths, seizure initiation and the spatial distribution of the resultant neurophysiological changes, there is a critical absence of direct measurements of intracerebral current, patterns of seizure onset, and spatial distribution of neurophysiological alterations with ECT. Most of the existing data come from studies conducted over 50 years ago with sine wave ECT using intracerebral voltage measurements in cadavers (Smitt and Wegener, 1944; Lorimer et al., 1949). Driscoll developed a theoretical model that was tested with an electrolytic-tank preparation (Rush and Driscoll, 1968). Hayes (1950) conducted the only study to assess current paths in a live subject (Hayes, 1950). He used a single spider monkey, with limited intracerebral sampling in one plane obtained by progressively moving probes through the occipital protuberance and towards the supraorbital ridge. While this work has been influential, each set of studies was characterized by methodological shortcomings.

Similarly, most of the empirical data on induced charge density with TMS come from mathematical or saline-filled physical models (Weissman et al., 1992). Mathematical and physical models (Roth et al., 1991; Weissman et al., 1992; Cerri et al., 1995) indicate that the magnitude of induced current falls off exponentially with distance from the coil (Tofts, 1990), and the deepest penetration is thought to be near the gray-white junction (Epstein, 1990). Coil shape and angle of orientation are also thought to be important factors in determining field strength and physiological effects (Rösler, 1989; Cohen et al., 1990; Meyer et al., 1991a, b; Amassian et al., 1992; Mills et al., 1992; Maccabee et al., 1993).

Induced current depends on numerous factors, not all of which may be adequately modeled. Important factors are the conductivity of white matter, gray matter, and cerebrospinal fluid. Some models assign standard tissue conductivity values to concentric spheres (Roth et al., 1991) or fit these to segmented MRI scans (De Leo et al., 1992; Cerri et al., 1995) but local inhomogeneities and dynamic changes in tissue conductivity may affect the field distribution. Thus, there is a role for direct measurement of the MST and ECS-induced electrical field, not only to validate models, but also to provide data on irregularities due to factors influencing the coupling between the brain tissue and the magnetic pulse. This study compared the strength and distribution of the electric field induced by MST and ECS in rhesus monkeys to test the hypothesis that magnetic stimulation provides better control over the site and intensity of stimulation, factors thought to be central to the efficacy and side effects of ECT.

4.1. Methods

4.1.1. Subjects

Three male rhesus monkeys (weight 4 kg) implanted with multicontact intracerebral electrodes were used in experiment II.

4.1.2. Design

Each monkey received both ECS (MECTA SPECTRUM) and MST (Magstim MST device, 2.5 cm diameter figure-of-8 coil) using a variety of scalp placements in randomized order. As expected, preliminary testing revealed that both the magnitude and distribution of the electric field were identical for each pulse throughout a train of stimulation. Thus, subsequent measurements were made by administering single pulses rather than complete trains. This permitted data collection on each modality of stimulation in a single session (since trails were all subconvulsive) to reduce variability in experimental conditions across modalities. Three replications were acquired of each modality on each day, and averaged. Additionally, each modality was repeated on each of three separate testing days.

4.1.3. Intracerebral electrode implantation

The non-ferrous, MRI-compatible multicontact electrodes (Ad-Tech Co.) incorporated design features to minimize inductive artifact (current induced in the leads during magnetic stimulation): (1) lead wires from the indwelling electrodes were twisted to cancel magnetic flux, and (2) leads extended 23 inches beyond the scalp so that connector cables are remote from the magnetic field. In pilot testing, strong flux in the connector was the major source of artifact. Ten teflon-insulated 42-gauge nickel-chromium lead wires were encased in a 0.5 mm diameter polyamide plastic shaft. The shaft length was approximately 4 cm (individualized based upon pre-implantation MRI), with 4 mm spacing between contacts (0.5 mm length). These electrodes performed well in pilot testing of magnetically-induced current in saline models.

Multicontact linear arrays (10 recording sites per linear array, three arrays per monkey for a total of 30 recording sites) were chronically implanted in bilateral prefrontal cortex and hippocampus using standard stereotaxic techniques under anesthesia. Electrode position was verified with MRI in all three monkeys, and with neuropathology in one monkey. Non-ferrous titanium skull screws anchored an acrylic mound to the occipital operculum, which was used to fix the head during recording sessions. It also had a removable cap to house the electrode extensions between recording sessions. Intracerebral recordings began after a 3-week period post surgery to allow tissue to stabilize around the implanted electrodes. These procedures were designed to minimize the impact of the surgical implantation on current distributions, by using a single skull entry site in the occipital cortex, away from the site for seizure induction with MST and ECS.

4.1.4. MST device

To overcome the anticonvulsant effects of anesthesia, it was necessary to modify the commercially available magnetic stimulator to increase its output characteristics (Lisanby et al., 2001c). The peak induced magnetic field was 2 T at the coil surface. The pulse had a dampened cosine waveform with a width twice as wide as commercial rTMS devices. The device achieves a peak output of 60 Hz, 100% intensity, for 6.6 s (total of 400 pulses) by increasing the number of charging units to 16 from the usual four. This device has been capable of inducing seizures in all monkeys and humans tested to date, but trials in rodents have consistently been unsuccessful. The average MST threshold in monkeys was 105 ± 19 pulses, administered at a frequency of at least 40 Hz at 100% of maximal stimulator output.

4.1.5. Electric field measurements

All recordings were made under anesthesia (ketamine 15 mg/kg and xylazine 7 mg/kg i.m.). Inductive artifact was reduced by running all recording equipment through a line isolation unit, and by electrically linking the animal to building ground. Recordings were referenced to an extracranial needle electrode. Electrophysiological data were acquired with Tectronix AM-501 operational amplifiers. Voltages were digitized using a Datel PCI-416 A/D (Mansfield, MA), capable of sampling eight channels simultaneously at 250 k samples/s/channel. Digitized data were recorded using a Gateway P5-166 computer. The sampling rate allowed 4 μs time resolution, which was adequate to resolve the dampened cosine induced electrical signal of the MST pulse, and the square-wave of the ECS pulse (Fig. 2). The dampened cosine waveform of magnetically induced pulses could be distinguished from the sinusoidal capacitative artifact by adding the waveforms recorded with the direction of the induced current reversed (by flipping the round coil or rotating the figure-of-8 coil) since capacitative effects should not reverse with changes in pulse polarity. Using this method, artifact represented 13% of the signal. For magnetic trials, the amplitude was measured as the baseline-to-peak voltage of the second phase of the dampened cosine waveform. The amplitude in ECS trials was the height of the square-wave pulse.

4.2. Results

4.2.1. Pulse morphology

Intracerebral recordings of representative waveforms of individual ECS, TMS and MST pulses are presented in Fig. 2. While the ECT device delivers a square-wave, the pulse recorded from brain reveals a slight sloping at its peak, consistent with some degree of tissue capacitance. The waveform of TMS and MST pulses recorded from brain matches those recorded in saline-filled models. The MST pulse is identical to the TMS pulse, except for a slightly longer pulse width (0.2 vs. 0.4).

The polarity of the induced electrical pulse reversed when the figure-of-8 coil angle was rotated 180°, but the induced voltage retained the same absolute magnitude and spatial distribution (Fig. 2). A rotation of 90° resulted in an abolition of induced voltage to the level of artifact, as would be expected when the induced electric field vector is perpendicular (and thus, isoelectric) to the recording sites (Fig. 2). Pulses induced by round coils reversed polarity when the coil was flipped, and had opposite polarity on the

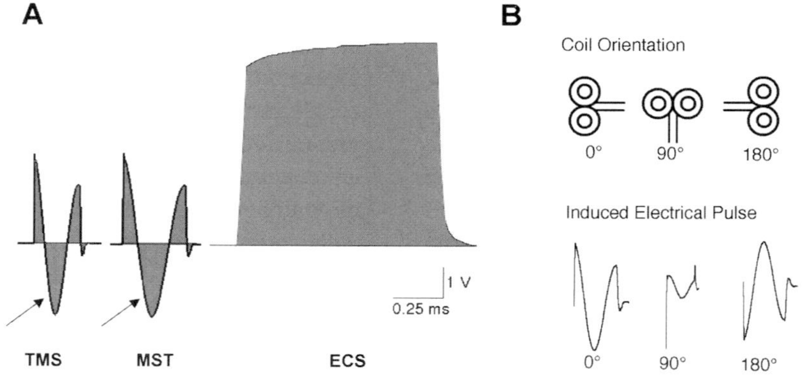

Fig. 2. (A) In vivo intracerebral recordings of the electrical pulses induced in the brain by conventional TMS, MST, and ECS. The typical ECS pulse is a square wave (1–2 ms in width), while the typical TMS pulse is a dampened cosine (0.2–0.3 ms in width). The MST pulse resembles the typical TMS pulse, but its width is doubled (0.4 ms). While the intensity of the TMS and MST pulse can be increased such that the peak-to-peak amplitude approximates that of ECS in superficial cortex, the area under the curve (shaded in gray) remains much greater with ECS. The sloped top of the ECS pulse likely represents tissue capacitance effects. The arrows indicate the second phase of the TMS and MST pulse, thought to be the most efficient in neuronal depolarization. (B) Rotating the figure-of-8 coil 180° results in a polarity reversal of the dampened cosine waveform. At 90° rotation, the waveform is dampened, as expected when the vector of the induced current is perpendicular (or isoelectric) to the recording electrodes.

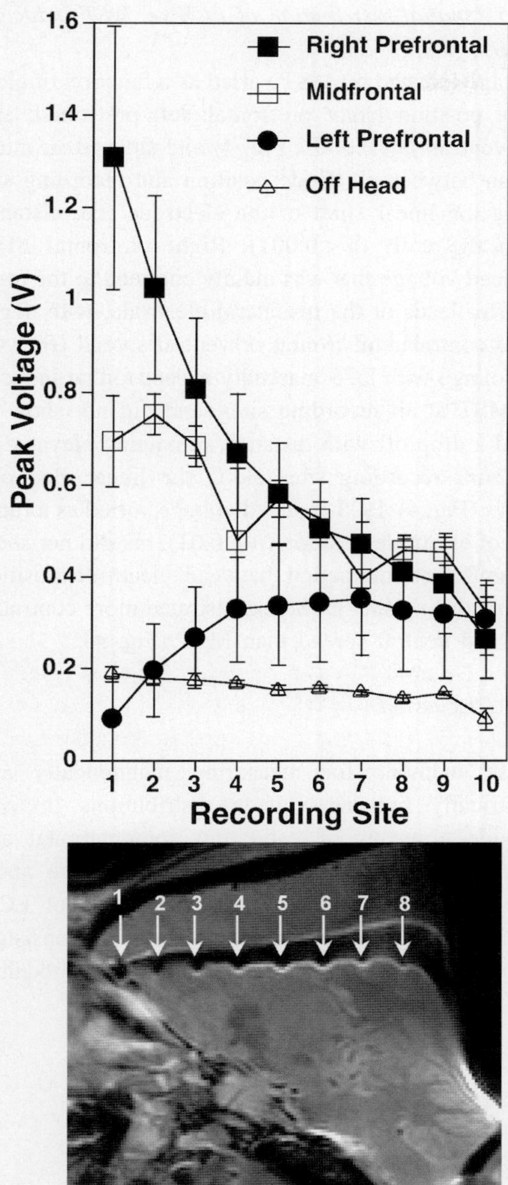

Fig. 3. (Top) Spatial distribution of the MST-induced electric field in vivo in the right prefrontal cortex as a function of figure-of-8 coil position (right prefrontal, midfrontal, left prefrontal, or off the head as a control). Peak voltage is plotted for each of 10 recording sites along a linear electrode array extending from anterior prefrontal cortex (site No. 1) to occipital cortex (site No. 10). Each data point represents the mean of four observations (two replications in each of two monkeys acquired on separate days). Induced voltage drops off with increasing distance from the coil. Recordings in right prefrontal are highest with the coil positioned adjacent to the electrode (black squares). When the coil is moved to midline frontal cortex (white squares), voltage drops by approximately 50%. When the coil is moved to the contralateral hemisphere (black circles), voltage drops to near noise levels (open triangles, recorded with the coil off the head). (Bottom) Sagittal MRI (7 T) of multicontact intracerebral electrodes chronically implanted in a rhesus monkey. Each electrode represents a linear array with 10 recording sites (visualized as swellings along the shaft of the electrode). Eight of the ten sites are visible on this image (white numbers). Artifact at the occipital pole is secondary to titanium screws that secured the implant.

two hemispheres, as expected due to the opposite flow of current in the two hemispheres induced by round coils. Likewise, reversing the polarity of the ECS electrodes resulted in a reversal of the polarity of the first pulse in the train of biphasic pulse pairs.

4.2.2. Effect of parameters of stimulation

The amplitude of individual pulses within ECS and MST trains showed little variation (mean CV = 2.4%), was unrelated to frequency of stimulation with ECS or MST, and was unrelated to pulse width. Pulses maintained the same amplitude throughout the duration of trains up to 6.6 s with no degradation as a function of train length. Pulse amplitude was linearly related to intensity of stimulation (MST: $r^2 = 0.96$, $p < 0.0005$; ECS: $r^2 = 0.99$. $p < 0.005$). As expected, there was a drop off in field strength with increasing distance from the coil (Fig. 3).

4.3.3. Effect of coil size and position

As predicted, the peak electric field varied as a function of coil size ($F(2,7) = 8.81$, $p < 0.01$). Average peak voltages were 3.6 ± 1.8, 3.0 ± 0.6, and 0.7 ± 0.2 V with the 5 cm round coil, 5 cm figure-of-8, and 2.5 cm figure-of-8, respectively. The spatial distribution of the electric field induced in the brain varied as a function of coil position (Fig. 3). Recordings in two monkeys, on each of two occasions, with three different coil positions for the figure-of-8 coil (right prefrontal, midline prefrontal, left prefrontal), revealed significant main effects of coil position ($F(2,28) = 55.7$, $p < 0.0001$) and an interaction between coil position and recording site (i.e. spatial distance from the coil along the linear shaft of the recording electrode, $F(9,29) = 12$, $p < 0.0001$). As shown in Fig. 3, when the coil was positioned over the right prefrontal cortex (near the recording electrodes), voltages were highest and showed the expected drop-off with distance. When the coil was moved to the contralateral hemisphere, amplitudes dropped. Mid-line coil placement resulted in intermediate values.

4.2.4. MST/ECS charge comparison

Table 1 presents calculations of induced charge based upon peak voltage measured over a known area in prefrontal cortex. While the intensity of the TMS and MST pulse can be increased such that the peak-to-peak amplitude approximates that of ECS in superficial cortex, the induced charge delivered by each pulse remains much greater with conventional ECS than MST by a factor of 7 (or a factor of 10 in the comparison between conventional ECS with commercially available rTMS devices). The charge per phase of MST is half that delivered by ultra-brief pulse ECS. These measurements in prefrontal cortex directly adjacent to the source of the stimulation are expected to underestimate the differences between MST and ECS in brain regions more remote from the site of transcranial stimulation (for example, see Fig. 4).

4.2.5. Spatial distribution of ECS vs. MST induced electric field

Voltage induced by MST varied as a function of electrode position (right prefrontal, left prefrontal, and left ventral; $p < 0.0001$; Fig. 4) and showed an interaction between electrode position and recording site along the linear shaft of the electrode (i.e. distance from the coil) ($p < 0.001$). Right prefrontal MST induced voltage that was mainly confined to the most anterior leads of the ipsilateral electrode, with negligible contralateral frontal or ventral spread (Fig. 4).

Voltage with ECS markedly exceeded that induced by MST at all recording sites, and did not show as rapid a drop-off with distance, remaining elevated in posterior recording sites along the linear electrode arrays (Fig. 4). ECS-induced voltage varied as a function of electrode position ($p < 0.01$), but did not show a significant interaction between electrode position and recording site. ECS demonstrated more contralateral and ventral spread than MST (Fig. 4).

4.3. Discussion

These methods for measuring magnetically and electrically induced voltage distributions in vivo provide a means of validating computational and in vitro models and have yielded new data about stimulation pathways in an animal model of ECT, rTMS, and MST. These measurements are consistent with predictions from prior experimental and modeling

TABLE 1

COMPARISON OF TMS AND ECS CHARGE CALCULATIONS IN PREFRONTAL CORTEX

	TMS	MST	Ultrabrief pulse ECS	ECS
Peak electric field	256 V/m	256 V/m	208 V/m	208 V/m
Current density	$\sigma \times 256$ V/m	$\sigma \times 256$ V/m	σ x 208 V/m	$\sigma \times 208$ V/m
Total pulse width	200 μs	400 μs	300 μs	1000 μs
Effective pulse width *	120 μs	200 μs	300 μs	1000 μs
Induced charge per phase**	$\sigma \times 0.02$ C/m^2	$\sigma \times 0.03$ C/m^2	$\sigma \times 0.06$ C/m^2	$\sigma \times 0.21$ C/m^2

All measurements recorded from the left dorsolateral prefrontal cortex of a live rhesus monkey.
* In the case of TMS and MST, effective pulse width refers to the second phase of the pulse.
** Since tissue conductivity (σ) was not known, table provides the relative values between MST and ECS, rather than absolute values.

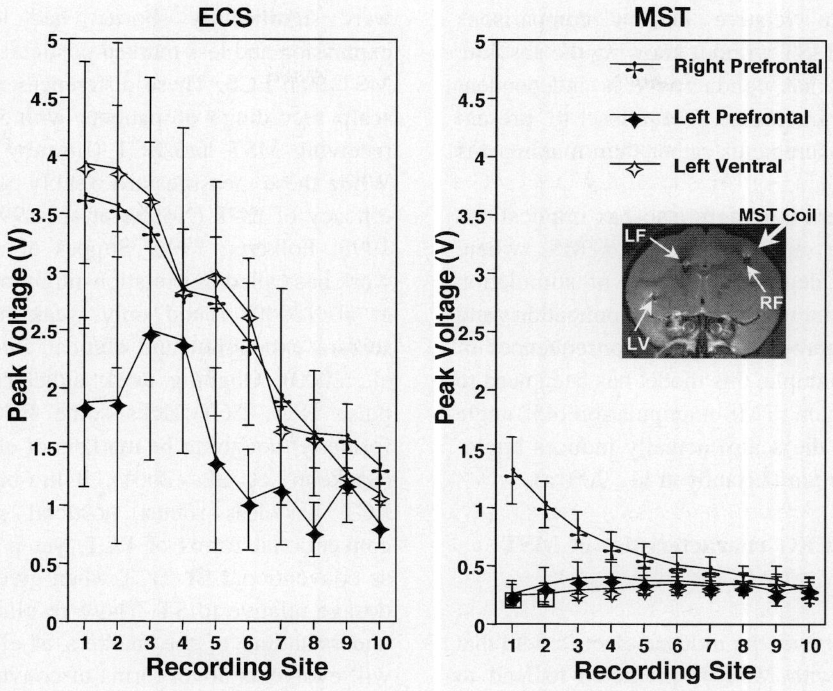

Fig. 4. Spatial distribution of MST and ECS induced electric field in three brain regions (left prefrontal cortex, right prefrontal cortex, and left ventral frontal cortex; see inset coronal MRI illustrating electrode positions). Each data point represents six observations (two replications in each of three monkeys acquired on separate days). MST was administered with a figure-of-8 coil on right prefrontal cortex (indicated by while arrow on inset MRI). Measurements with ECS were larger and more variable than with MST. With MST, induced voltage was confined to the most anterior three electrodes (recording sites 1–3) of the right prefrontal electrode with negligible spread to contralateral prefrontal or ventral regions, while ECS induces substantial voltage at all recording sites, including ventral regions and extending to parietal and occipital regions.

work. Specifically, they confirm the expected effects of stimulation parameters and coil factors (e.g. coil size, position, orientation, distance from the recording site). These results illustrate that rotating the figure-of-8 coil 180° does not alter the magnitude of the induced electric pulse, but reverses its polarity. Other work has shown that coil orientation has a profound impact upon physiological effects of TMS (e.g. Brasil-Neto et al., 1992; Mills et al., 1992). That work, together with our results, implicates the waveform polarity rather than the magnitude of induced voltage as being responsible for this effect. This further indicates that mere knowledge of the induced electric field strength is inadequate to predict the physiological effects of TMS without knowledge of waveform polarity relative to the target tracts being stimulated.

MST showed negligible spread to contralateral prefrontal or ventral regions, while ECS induces substantial voltage at most recording sites, including ventral regions and extending to parietal and occipital cortex. Comparisons between MST and ECS support the hypothesis that MST is more focal and less variable in its induced electric field than ECS, and supports the rationale for attempting seizure induction with MST as a means of limiting exposure of key brain regions to the direct effects of the induced electric field. Limitations in this work include the small sample size, and the fact that electric field rather than current was measured. However, current can be computed from the electric field and tissue conductivity. While conductivity was not measured in this experiment, it is nevertheless possible to make relative current comparisons between ECS and MST without knowing the absolute values, assuming that conductivity is independent of modality of stimulation. We chose to present direct voltage measurements rather than making this assumption.

This measurement paradigm also has implications for subconvulsive applications of rTMS, where knowledge of the degree of focality of stimulation is important to targeting rTMS application and interpreting the neurophysiological consequences of stimulation. For example, this model has been used to document that a sham rTMS manipulation (45° angle tilt of the coil off the scalp) actually induces appreciable voltage in brain (Lisanby et al., 2001a).

5. Intracerebral EEG characteristics of MST and ECS

The greater control over the induced electric field that can be achieved with MST is predicted to lead to greater specificity in the sites of seizure onset and patterns of seizure spread with MST compared with ECT. As an initial step in developing and characterizing seizures induced magnetically, we have started by examining the effects of seizures that generalize to the motor strip, as evidenced by motor convulsion. For clinical application, the ultimate goal would be to induce focal seizures that remain localized to the site of initiation and do not generalize, on the assumption that the site of seizure initiation is critical to efficacy. The availability of focal MST would provide the means for evaluating the relative roles of seizure initiation and spread in clinical effects (antidepressant efficacy and cognitive side effects).

Our preliminary studies in this area have revealed marked differences in the nature of the seizures induced by these two interventions in non-human primates and patients with major depression, even when comparing seizures that generalize to the motor strip. Scalp EEG recordings of seizures induced by MST and ECS were examined in 12 monkeys receiving chronic treatment with MST, ECS, or anesthesia-alone sham in a randomized, controlled design (Lisanby et al., 2002). Seizures were significantly shorter, had less robust ictal expression and less marked postictal suppression with MST than ECS. These differences were also seen in scalp recordings of patients with major depression receiving MST and ECT (Lisanby et al., in press). While these measures are weakly correlated with the efficacy of ECT (Nobler et al., 1993; Krystal et al., 1995; Folkerts, 1996; Suppes et al., 1996) recent work has called this relationship into question. Nobler et al. (2000) found only weak relations between seizure expression and clinical outcome (Nobler et al., 2000). Ongoing work indicates that ultra-brief pulse RUL ECT lacks some EEG characteristics formerly thought to be markers of effective treatment (Sackeim et al., 2001). Ultra-brief pulse RUL ECT has less robust postictal suppression than conventional forms of ECT, yet it was as effective as conventional BL ECT when given at an adequate dosage relative to ST. These results suggest that our understanding of the markers of effective treatment will evolve as novel forms of convulsive therapy are developed and tested.

In addition to differences in the quality of seizure expression, it was predicted that MST and ECS would differ in their spatial distribution. In Experiment III, we tested the hypothesis that MST induced seizures would be more localized to site of seizure onset than those induced with ECT.

5.1. Methods

5.1.1. Design

To compare MST and ECS in focality of seizure expression, ictal power was measured in 3 monkeys with intracerebral electrodes. ECS and MST were administered to each of four scalp positions in a randomized, within-subject crossover design, with two replications of each of eight conditions on separate days (16 sessions per monkey). ECS was delivered in the BL, bifrontal (BF), RUL and left unilateral (LUL) placements. MST was delivered with a 5 cm round coil on vertex (analog to BL); and 5 cm figure-of-8 coil on midline prefrontal cortex (analog to BF) or left or right prefrontal cortex (analog to LUL and RUL). In all cases, generalized seizures of at least 10 s in motor manifestations were induced, as observed in a non-paralyzed limb.

5.1.2. EEG acquisition and analysis

Electrophysiological data were acquired with electrically-isolated bioamplifiers (SA Instruments, San Diego, California), bandpass filtered from 0.3 Hz to 100 Hz, and digitized at 1 kHz. EEG was recorded from the thirty intracerebral sites, referenced to the left mastoid. Artifact-free data were subjected to a fast Fourier transformation using 1 s epochs with overlapping 0.5 s windows, starting immediately after the termination of the MST or ECT stimulus and continuing until 15 s after there was clear termination of the seizure on any recording site. Average power (μV^2) in each of four frequency bands (delta 1–3.5 Hz, theta 3.5–7.5 Hz, alpha 7.5–12.5 Hz, beta 12.5–29.5 Hz) was calculated for each channel, separately for the ictal and postictal periods. A repeated measures MANOVA was performed on the log mean EEG power in the 30 sites during the ictal period, using factors of treatment type and band. Significant main effects were followed up with post-hoc ANOVAs and paired *t*-tests, as appropriate. Tests of significance were two-tailed, with an α of 0.05.

5.2. Results and discussion

5.2.1. Comparison of ictal expression in prefrontal cortex with ECS and MST

MANOVA across the 10 recording sites in the left prefrontal cortex electrode, eight conditions, and four frequency bands revealed that ECS induced greater ictal activity than MST ($F(1,160) = 285$, $p < 0.0001$). The degree of ictal expression differed as a function of scalp position of stimulation ($F(3,160) = 3.62$, $p < 0.01$), and there was an interaction between modality (ECS vs MST) and scalp position (BL, BF, RUL, LUL) ($F(3,160) = 5.96$, $p < 0.0007$). As predicted, MST showed more differentiation in ictal expression as a function of the site of stimulation (e.g. bilateral and midline placements inducing more ictal activity in prefrontal cortex than unilateral placements) than ECS did.

5.2.2. Prefrontal and hippocampal involvement in seizure expression with MST and ECS

Data from one monkey with electrodes positioned in the hippocampus as well as prefrontal cortex are presented in Fig. 5. Comparison of simultaneously recorded global ictal power in prefrontal cortex and hippocampus revealed significant main effects of modality (ECS > MST, $F(1,12) = 81.2$, $p < 0.0001$), recording site (frontal > hippocampal, $F(1,12) = 6.2$, $p < 0.03$) and an interaction between modality and site ($F(1,12) = 7.0$, $p < 0.02$). As shown in Fig. 5, seizure expression was as robust in hippocampus as prefrontal cortex with ECS, but markedly less robust in hippocampus than prefrontal cortex with MST. Seizures lasted longer by an average of 6 s in hippocampus than in prefrontal cortex with ECS, but not with MST (modality by site interaction $F(1,11) = 6.3$, $p < 0.03$). This continued seizure expression in hippocampus following the termination of prefrontal seizure expression in prefrontal cortex is clearly visualized in the raw EEG data presented in Fig. 5 as a high frequency component of the seizure that is sustained following the termination of the high amplitude lower frequency component that is associated with the motor convulsion. These data fit with the hypothesis that MST seizures are more localized to superficial cortex and show a relative sparing of hippocampus. As well, they suggest that, with ECS, seizure shutdown is more efficient and rapid at the site of seizure initiation.

5.2.3. Association between induced electric field and ictal characteristics

To test the hypothesis that the characteristics of the seizure are contingent upon the spatial distribution of the induced electric field that induced it, intracerebral recordings of induced voltage and ictal EEG at the identical recording sites were analyzed in one subject, with 16 ictal recording sessions on separate days. Repeated measures ANOVA on ictal expression across the four frequency bands, revealed main effects of induced voltage ($F(1,163) = 12.2$, $p < 0.0006$), modality (ECS vs. MST, $F(1,163) = 52.6$, $p < 0.0001$), an interaction between induced voltage and modality ($F(1,163) = 11.8$, $p < 0.0008$), and an inter-

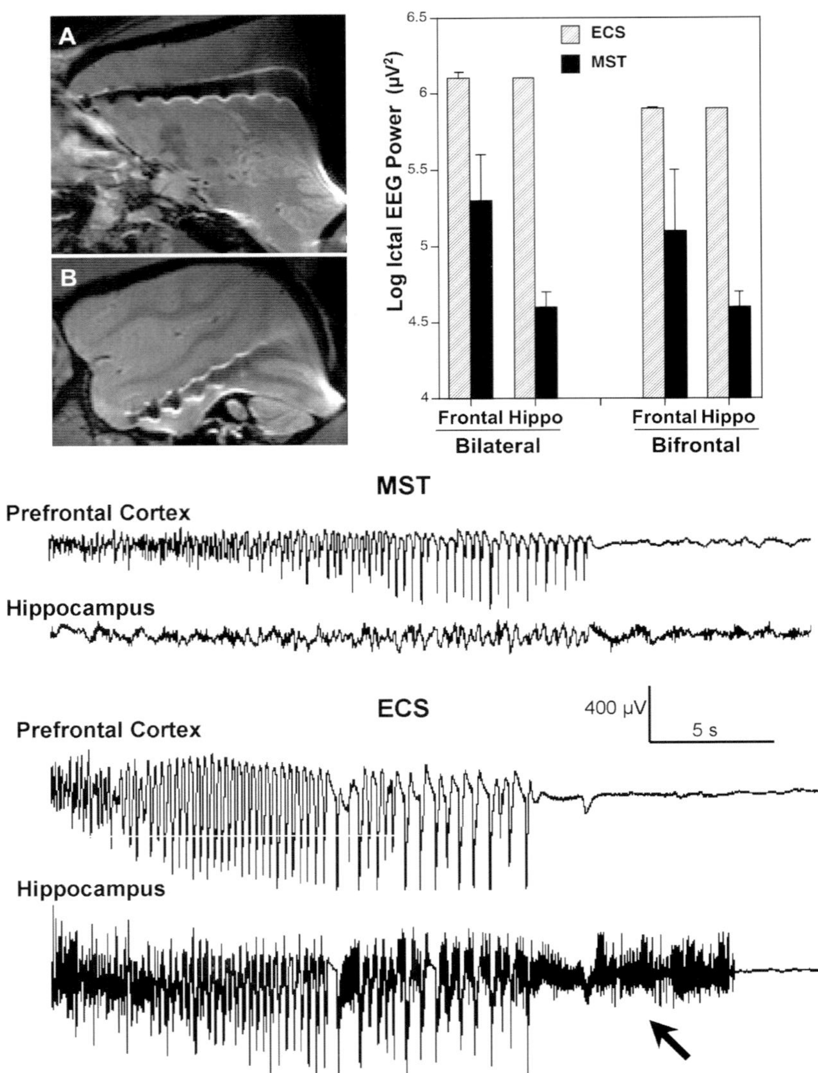

Fig. 5. Ictal EEG characteristics of seizures induced by MST and ECS in prefrontal cortex and hippocampus of a rhesus monkey. (Top left) Inset shows positions of linear electrode arrays extending to prefrontal cortex (A) and hippocampus (B). (Top right) Bar graph depicts global ictal power in prefrontal cortex and hippocampus during ECS and MST administered bilaterally and bifrontally. Ictal expression is significantly lower with MST than ECS in all cases. While ictal expression is high in both prefrontal cortex and hippocampus with ECS, MST demonstrates less involvement of hippocampus than frontal regions. (Bottom) Simultaneous recordings in prefrontal cortex and hippocampus during MST and ECS induced seizures. ECS seizures show overall greater amplitude than MST, and involvement of hippocampus is as robust as prefrontal cortex. In fact, high frequency ictal activity continues in hippocampus following the termination of the seizure in prefrontal cortex with ECS (black arrow), not seen with MST.

action between frequency band and induced voltage ($F(3,161) = 5.9$, $p < 0.0008$). Induced voltage was a significant predictor of ictal expression for MST ($F(1,75) = 12.7$, $p < 0.0006$), but not for ECS. The association between induced voltage and ictal expression for MST was mainly seen in the delta frequency band ($r^2 = 0.40$, $p < 0.0002$ for RUL; $r^2 = 0.15$, $p < 0.04$ for LUL; $r^2 = 0.32$, $p < 0.002$ for BL MST). For ECS, induced voltage was correlated with ictal expression only for the RUL placement ($r^2 = 0.43$, $p < 0.0001$ for RUL; $r^2 = -0.27$, NS for LUL, and $r^2 = 0.00$, NS for BL ECS). These results support the hypothesis that with MST, ictal expression is related to the spatial distribution of the induced electric field. It is not surprising that this association is less strong with ECS, since ECS seizures generalize more robustly away from the site of initial seizure onset. Future analyses examining only the initial phase of seizure onset may help to shed light on that issue.

6. Conclusions

The rationale behind attempting to improve upon ECT through inducing the seizures magnetically hinges on the supposition that the magnetic stimulus would yield better control over the magnitude and distribution of electrical current induced in the brain, and of the site of onset and patterns of spread of the resultant seizure. Presented here is a non-human primate model for the characterization of the neurophysiological effects of MST and ECS-induced seizures to test that premise. Results from three preliminary studies employing this model support the notion that, relative to ECS, MST yields better control over intracerebral patterns of electric field distribution and seizure generalization. These two factors are considered to be central to the efficacy and side effects of convulsive therapy. The enhanced control that MST provides opens the door to improving the risk/benefit ratio of this highly effective treatment for mood disorders.

The finding that the pulse width of the MST waveform is more efficient in inducing seizure than that used in conventional ECT has implications for future ECT device design. Indeed, newer models of commercially available ECT devices now offer an extended parameter range making ultrabrief pulse ECT more widely available.

Measurements of the electric field induced in the brain with MST illustrate the exquisite dependence of induced field on coil size, shape, orientation, location, and distance from the recording site. This highlights the importance of rigorous control over coil placement, both in terms of reproducibility and anatomical precision, in rTMS studies of neurophysiological processes and treatment of clinical conditions. The fact that coils with a smaller diameter and focal design (figure-of-8 as opposed to round) induce less voltage in the brain helps to explain why it has not yet been possible to induce a seizure in prefrontal cortex using a focal coil in humans under anesthesia.

As expected, MST-induced voltage was lower in magnitude and more restricted to regions near the site of stimulation than that obtained with ECS, supporting the hypothesis that MST would be a more focal form of brain stimulation than ECS. Preliminary data suggest that the induced electric field has a demonstrable impact on ictal expression. This was most clearly seen with MST and highlights the importance of control over this factor in designing a more focal form of convulsive therapy. Indeed, there is evidence that MST induced seizures are less robust overall, and generalize less to hippocampus and other ventral and medial structures. The unexpected preliminary observation that ECS-induced seizures have a longer duration in hippocampus than in prefrontal cortex is intriguing and should be examined in a larger sample size.

In addition to these electrophysiological differences between MST and ECS in deeper brain structures, there are suggestions that the two modalities differ in neuroendocrine, neuroplastic, and cognitive measures. For example, MST seizures do not elicit as robust a prolactin surge as ECS, suggesting less of an effect on diencephalic activity (Morales et al., 2003). The modalities also appear to differ in the degree of mossy fiber sprouting and cellular proliferation in the dentate gyrus, which is much more robust with ECS as might be predicted based upon its greater involvement of the hippocampus in spread of current and induced seizure (Lisanby et al., 2002, in press). Studies in the neurophysiological and anatomical consequences of seizures may shed light on the pathogenesis of these neuroplastic changes that are seen in response to antidepressant treatments and in models of epilepsy. Finally, preliminary human work has demonstrated differences between MST and ECT in acute cognitive side effects, especially on tasks that rely on the integrity of hippocampal networks, however the interpretation of this work is complicated by differences in dosage above threshold that could be achieved with the two modalities (Lisanby et al., 2001b).

An important limitation in the work presented is that multiple repeated measures were obtained in a small sample size. In part, this is related to the fact that animal MST work is presently restricted to monkeys due to the limitations in the strength of the magnetic field that can be induced in a small brain with relatively large coils. The creation of coils and devices powerful enough to induce seizures in smaller animals (which could be studied in larger sample sizes) would represent a significant advance in the ability to characterize the neurophysiological, anatomical, and behavioral effects of MST. The creation of more powerful devices and smaller coils will also assist with the goal of accomplishing seizure induction in prefrontal cortex using a focal coil, which has not yet been possible in the human under anesthesia due to present limits in device output. Much future work will be needed to examine how best to take advantage of the relative focality offered by MST, and determine the clinical significance of the neurophysiological differences between MST and ECT in the treatment of major depression.

Acknowledgements

Supported in part by grants K08 MH01577 and R01 MH60884 from the National Institute of Mental Health, Rockville, MD, the Stanley Foundation, and a Paul Beeson Physician Faculty Scholars Award from the American Federation for Aging Research.

Thanks go to Drs. Vahe Amassian, Joseph Arezzo, and Reza Jalinous for helpful scientific input; and Mr. Edward Kwon, Michael Crupain, and Carlos Niko Reyes for expert technical assistance.

References

Amassian, V.E., Eberle, L., Maccabee, P.J. and Cracco, R.Q. Modeling magnetic coil excitation of human cerebral cortex with a peripheral nerve immersed in a brain-shaped volume conductor: The significance of fiber bending in excitation. *Electroencephalogr. Clin. Neurophysiol.*, 1992, 85: 291–301.

American Psychiatric Association. *The Practice of ECT: Recommendations for Treatment, Training and Privileging (2nd ed.)*, American Psychiatric Press, Washington, D.C., 2001.

Barker, A.T., Jalinous, R. and Freeston, I.L. Non-invasive magnetic stimulation of human motor cortex. *Lancet*, 1985, 1: 1106–1107.

Brasil-Neto, J.P., Cohen, L.G., Panizza, M., Nilsson, J., Roth, B.J. and Hallett, M. Optimal focal transcranial magnetic activation of the human motor cortex: effects of coil orientation, shape of the induced current pulse, and stimulus intensity. *J. Clin. Neurophysiol.*, 1992, 9(1): 132–136.

Cerri, G., De Leo, F., Moglie, F. and Schiavoni, A. An accurate 3-D model for magnetic stimulation of the brain cortex. *J. Med. Eng. Technol.*, 1995, 19: 7–16.

Cohen, L.G., Roth, B.J., Nilsson, J., Dang, N., Panizza, M., Bandinelli, S., Friauf, W. and Hallett, M. Effects of coil design on delivery of focal magnetic stimulation: Technical considerations. *Electroenceph. Clin. Neurophysiol.*, 1990, 75: 350–357.

Cronholm, B. and Ottoson, J.O. Ultrabrief stimulus technique in electroconvulsive therapy. II. Comparative studies of therapeutic effects and memory disturbances in treatment of endogenous depression with the Elther ES electroshock apparatus and Siemens Konvulsator III. *J. Nerv. Ment. Dis.*, 1963, 137: 268–276.

De Leo, R., Cerri, G., Balducci, D., Moglie, F., Scarpino, O. and Guidi, M. Computer modelling of brain cortex excitation by magnetic field pulses. *J. Med. Eng. Technol.*, 1992, 16(4): 149–156.

Devanand, D.P., Lisanby, S.H., Nobler, M.S. and Sackeim, H.A. The relative efficiency of altering pulse frequency or train duration when determining seizure threshold. *J. Ect.*, 1998, 14: 227–235.

Donahue, A.B. Electroconvulsive therapy and memory loss: a personal journey. *J. Ect.*, 2000, 16(2): 133–143.

Driscoll, D.A. An investigation of a theoretical model of the human head with application to current flow calculations and EEG interpretation. Ph.D. Thesis. University of Vermont, 1970.

Epstein, C.M. Localizing the site of magnetic brain stimulation in humans. *Neurol.*, 1990, 40: 666–670.

Folkerts, H. The ictal electroencephalogram as a marker for the efficacy of electroconvulsive therapy. *Eur. Arch. Psychiatry Clin. Neurosci.*, 1996, 246: 155–164.

Geddes, L.A. and Baker, L.E. The specific resistance of biological material – A compendium of data for the biomedical engineer and physiologist. *Med. Biol. Engng.*, 1967, 5: 271–293.

Goldman, D. Brief stimulus electric shock therapy. *J. Nerv. Ment. Dis.*, 1949, 110: 36–45.

Hayes, K.J. The current path in ECS. *Arch. Neurol. Psychiatry*, 1950, 63: 102–109.

Hyrman, V., Palmer, L.H., Cernik, J. and Jetelina, J. ECT: the search for the perfect stimulus. *Biol. Psychiatry*, 1985, 20(6): 634–645.

Krystal, A.D., Weiner, R.D. and Coffey, C.E. The ictal EEG as a marker of adequate stimulus intensity with unilateral ECT. *J. Neuropsychiatry. Clin. Neurosci.*, 1995, 7(3): 295–303, 0895–0172.

Law, S.K. Thickness and resistivity variations over the upper surface of the human skull. *Brain Topography*, 1993, 6: 99–109.

Liberson, W.T. Brief stimulus therapy: Physiological and clinical observations. *Am. J. Psychiatry*, 1948, 105: 28–29.

Lisanby, S.H. Update on magnetic seizure therapy (MST): A novel form of convulsive therapy. *J. Ect.*, 2002, 18: 182–188.

Lisanby, S.H. and Sackeim, H.A. New developments in convulsive therapy for major depression. *Epilepsy and Behavior*, 2001, 2: S68–73.

Lisanby, S.H. and Sackeim, H.A. Transcranial magnetic stimulation and electroconvulsive therapy: similarities and differences. In: A. Pascual-Leone, N. Davey, J. Rothwell, E. Wassermann and B.K. Puri (Eds.), *Handbook of Transcranial Magnetic Stimulation*. Arnold Publishers, London, UK, 2002: 376–395.

Lisanby, S.H., Luber, B., Osman, M., Finck, D., Dichter G, Fitzsimons, L. and Sackeim, H. The effect of pulse width on seizure threshold during electroconvulsive shock (ECS). *Convul. Ther.*, 1997, 13: 56.

Lisanby, S.H., Luber, B., Schroeder, C., Osman, M., Finck, D., Jalinous, R., Amassian, V.E., Arezzo, J. and Sackeim, H.A. Intracerebral measurement of rTMS and ECS induced voltage in vivo. *Biol. Psychiatry*, 1998a, 43: 100S.

Lisanby, S.H., Luber, B.L., Schroeder, C., Osman, M., Finck, D., Amassian, V.E., Arezzo, J. and Sackeim, H.A. rTMS in primates: Intracerebral measurement of rTMS and ECS induced voltage in vivo. *Electroencephalogr. Clin. Neurophysiol.*, 1998b, 107: 79P.

Lisanby, S.H., Maddox, J.H., Prudic, J., Devanand, D.P. and Sackeim, H.A. The effects of electroconvulsive therapy on memory of autobiographical and public events. *Arch. Gen. Psychiatry*, 2000, 57(6): 581–590.

Lisanby, S.H., Gutman, D., Luber, B., Schroeder, C. and Sackeim, H.A. Sham TMS: intracerebral measurement of the induced electrical field and the induction of motor-evoked potentials. *Biol. Psychiatry*, 2001a, 49: 460–463.

Lisanby, S.H., Luber, B., Barroilhet, L., Neufeld, E., Schlaepfer, T. and Sackeim, H.A. Magnetic seizure therapy (MST): Acute cognitive effects of MST compared with ECT. *J. Ect.*, 2001b, 17: 77A.

Lisanby, S.H., Luber, B., Finck, A.D., Schroeder, C. and Sackeim, H.A. Deliberate seizure induction with repetitive transcranial magnetic stimulation. *Arch. Gen. Psych.*, 2001c, 58: 199–200.

Lisanby, S.H., Schlaepfer, T.E., Fisch, H.-U. and Sackeim, H.A. Magnetic seizure induction for the treatment of major depression. *Arch. Gen. Psychiatry*, 2001d, 58: 303–305.

Lisanby, S.H., Luber, B., Kwon, E., Crupain, M. and Sackeim, H.A. Physiological characteristics of magnetic seizure therapy (MST) induced seizures in nonhuman primates and patients with major depression. *Biol. Psychiatry*, 2002a, 51: 43S.

Lisanby, S.H., Sackeim, H.A., Dwork, A., Underwood, M.D., Wang, X., Kassir, S.A., Luber, B. and Arango, V. Effects of electrically- and magnetically-induced seizures on synaptic remodeling and cellular proliferation in the primate hippocampus. American College of Neuropsychopharmacology, 41st Annual Meeting, Scientific Abstracts, San Juan, Puerto Rico, 2002b.

Lisanby, S.H., Luber, B., Schlaepfer, T.E. and Sackeim, H.A. Safety and feasibility of magnetic seizure therapy (MST) in major depression: Randomized within-subject comparison with electroconvulsive therapy. *Neuropsychopharmacology,* in press.

Lisanby, S.H., Sackeim, H.A., Dwork, A., Underwood, M.D., Wang, X., Kassir, S.A., Luber, B. and Arango, V. Effects of electroconvulsive shock and magnetic seizure therapy on mossy fiber sprouting and cellular proliferation in the primate hippocampus. *Biol. Psychiatry*, in press, Abstract.

Lorimer, F.M., Segal, M.M. and Stein, S.N. Path of current distribution in brain during electro-convulsive therapy: Preliminary report. *EEG Clin. Neurophysiol.*, 1949, 1: 343–348.

Luber, B., Nobler, M.S., Moeller, J.R., Katzman, G.P., Prudic, J., Devanand, D.P., Dichter, G.S. and Sackeim, H.A. Quantitative EEG during seizures induced by electroconvulsive therapy: Relations to treatment modality and clinical features. II. Topographic analyses. *J. Ect.*, 2000, 16: 229–243.

Maccabee, P.J., Eberle, L., Amassian, V.E., Cracco, R.Q., Rudell, A. and Jayachandra, M. Spatial distribution of the electric field induced in volume by round and figure '8' magnetic coils: relevance to activation of sensory nerve fibers. *Electroencephalogr. Clin. Neurophysiol.*, 1990, 76: 131–141.

Maccabee, P.J., Amassian, V.E., Eberle, L.P., Rudell, A.P., Cracco, R.Q., Lai, K.S. and Somasundaram, M. Measurement of the electric field induced in inhomogeneous volume conductors by magnetic coils: application to human spinal neurogeometry. *Electroencephalogr. Clin. Neurophysiol.*, 1991, 81: 224–237.

Maccabee, P.J., Amassian, V.E., Eberle, L.P. and Cracco, R.Q. Magnetic coil stimulation of straight and bent amphibian and mammalian peripheral nerve in vitro: Locus of excitation. *J. Physiol.* (Lond), 1993, 460: 201–219.

McCall, W.V., Reboussin, D.M., Weiner, R.D. and Sackeim, H.A. Titrated moderately suprathreshold vs fixed high-dose right unilateral electroconvulsive therapy: acute antidepressant and cognitive effects. *Arch. Gen. Psychiatry*, 2000, 57(5): 438–444.

McCreery, D.B., Agnew, W.F., Yuen, T.G.H. and Bullara, L. Charge density and charge per phase as cofactors in neural injury induced by electrical stimulation. *IEE Trans. Biomed. Eng.*, 1990, 37: 996–1001.

Meyer, B.U., Britton, T.C., Kloten, H., Steinmetz, H. and Benecke, R. Coil placement in magnetic brain stimulation related to skull and brain anatomy. *Electroencephalogr. Clin. Neurophysiol.*, 1991a, 81(1): 38–46.

Meyer, B.U., Diehl, R., Steinmetz, H., Britton, T.C. and Benecke, R. Magnetic stimuli applied over motor and visual cortex: influence of coil position and field polarity on motor responses, phosphenes, and eye movements. *Electroencephalogr. Clin. Neurophysiol.*, 1991b, (Suppl.), 43: 121–34

Mills, K.R., Boniface, S.J. and Schubert, M. Magnetic brain stimulation with a double coil: the importance of coil orientation. *Electroencephal. Clin. Neurophysiol.*, 1992, 85: 17–21.

Morales, O., Luber, B., Kwon, E., Ellsasser, R., Sackeim, H.A. and Lisanby, S.H. Prolactin response to convulsive therapy: Magnetic seizure therapy (MST) vs. electroconvulsive shock (ECS) in nonhuman primates. *J. Ect.*, 2003, 19: 58A

Moscrip, T.D., Terrace, H.S., Sackeim, H.A. and Lisanby, S.H. The Cognitive Effects of ECS and MST in Rhesus Monkeys. *Society for Neuroscience*, 2001: Abstract.

Nobler, M.S., Sackeim, H.A., Solomou, M., Luber, B., Devanand, D.P. and Prudic, J. EEG manifestations during ECT: effects of electrode placement and stimulus intensity. *Biol. Psychiatry*, 1993, 34(5): 321–330.

Nobler, M.S., Luber, B., Moeller, J.R., Katzman, G.P., Prudic J., Devanand, D.P., Dichter, G.S. and Sackeim, H.A. Quantitative EEG during seizures induced by electroconvulsive therapy: Relations to treatment modality and clinical features. I. Global analyses. *J. Ect.*, 2000, 16: 211–228.

Robin A and De Tissera S.A. double-blind controlled comparison of the therapeutic effects of low and high energy electroconvulsive therapies. *Br. J. Psychiatry*, 1982, 141: 357–366.

Rösler, K.M. Significance of shape and size of the stimulating coil in magnetic stimulation of the human motor cortex. *Neuroscience Letters*, 1989, 100: 347–352.

Roth, B.J., Saypol, J.M., Hallett, M. and Cohen, L.G. A theoretical calculation of the electric field induced in the cortex during magnetic stimulation. *Electroencephalogr. Clin. Neurophysiol.*, 1991, 81: 47–56.

Rush, S. and Driscoll, D. Current distribution in the brain from surface electrodes. *Anesth. Anal.*, 1968, 47: 717–723.

Sackeim, H.A. Acute cognitive side effects of ECT. *Psychopharm. Bull.*, 1986, 22: 482–484.

Sackeim, H.A. Magnetic stimulation therapy and ECT. *Convulsive Ther.*, 1994, 10: 255–258.

Sackeim, H.A., Decina, P., Prohovnik, I., Portnoy, S., Kanzler, M. and Malitz, S. Dosage, seizure threshold, and the antidepressant efficacy of electroconvulsive therapy. *Ann. NY Acad. Sci.*, 1986, 462: 398–410.

Sackeim, H.A., Prudic, J., Devanand, D.P., Kiersky, J.E., Fitzsimons, L., Moody, B.J., McElhiney, M.C., Coleman, E.A. and Settembrino, J.M. Effects of stimulus intensity and electrode placement on the efficacy and cognitive effects of electroconvulsive therapy. *N. Engl. J. Med.*, 1993, 328(12): 839–846.

Sackeim, H.A., Long, J., Luber, B., Moeller, J.R., Prohovnik, I., Devanand, D.P. and Nobler, M.S. Physical properties and quantification of the ECT stimulus: I. Basic principles. *Convuls. Ther.*, 1994, 10(2): 93–123.

Sackeim, H.A., Luber, B., Katzman, G.P., Moeller, J.R., Prudic, J., Devanand, D.P. and Nobler, M.S. The effects of electroconvulsive therapy on quantitative electroencephalograms. Relationship to clinical outcome. *Arch. Gen Psychiatry*, 1996, 53(9): 814–824.

Sackeim, H.A., Luber, B., Moeller, J.R., Prudic, J., Devanand, D.P. and Nobler, M.S. Electrophysiological correlates of the adverse cognitive effects of electroconvulsive therapy. *J. Ect.*, 2000a, 16(2): 110–120.

Sackeim, H.A., Prudic, J., Devanand, D.P., Nobler, M.S., Lisanby, S.H., Peyser, S., Fitzsimons, L., Moody, B.J. and Clark, J. A prospective, randomized, double-blind comparison of bilateral and right unilateral electroconvulsive therapy at different stimulus intensities. *Arch. Gen. Psychiatry*, 2000b, 57(5): 425–434.

Sackeim, H.A., Prudic, J., Nobler, M.S., Lisanby, S.H., Devanand, D.P. and Peyser, S. Ultra-brief Pulse ECT and the Affective and Cognitive Consequences of ECT. *J. Ect.*, 2001, 17: 77.

Smitt, J.W. and Wegener, C.F. On electric convulsive therapy with particular regard to a parietal application of electrodes, controlled by intracerabral voltage measurements. *Acta Psychiatr. Neurol.*, 1944, 19: 529–549.

Suppes, T., Webb, A., Carmody, T., Gordon, E., Gutierrez-Esteinou, R., Hudson, J.I. and Pope, H.G. Jr. Is postictal electrical silence a predictor of response to electroconvulsive therapy? *J. Affect. Disord.*, 1996, 41: 55–58.

Tofts, P.S. The distribution of induced currents in magnetic stimulation of the nervous system. *Phys. Med. Biol.*, 1990, 35: 1119–1128.

Valentine, M., Keddie, K.M. and Dunne, D. A comparison of techniques in electro-convulsive therapy. *Br. J. Psychiatry*, 1968, 114(513): 989–996.

Weaver, L., Williams, R. and Rush, S. Current density in bilateral and unilateral ECT. *Biol. Psychiatry*, 1976, 11(3): 303–312.

Weiner, R.D., Rogers, H.J., Davidson, J.R. and Squire, L.R. Effects of stimulus parameters on cognitive side effects., 1986, *Ann. NY Acad. Sci.* 462: 315–325.

Weissman, J.D., Epstein, C.M. and Davey, K.R. Magnetic brain stimulation and brain size: Relevance to animal studies. *Electroencephalogr .Clin. Neurophysiol.*, 1992, 85: 215–219.

Woodbury, L.A. and Davenport, V.D. Design and use of a new electroshock seizure apparatus, and analysis of factors altering seizure threshold and pattern. *Arch. Int. Pharmacodyn.*, 1952, 92: 97–107.

Yuen, G.H., Agnew, W.F., Bullara, L.A., Jacques, S. and McCreery, D.B. Histological evaluation of neural damage from electrical stimulation: Considerations for the selection of parameters for clinical application. *Neurosurgery*, 1981, 9: 292–299.

Transcranial Magnetic Stimulation and Transcranial Direct Current Stimulation (Supplements to Clinical Neurophysiology, Vol. 56)
Editors: W. Paulus, F. Tergau, M.A. Nitsche, J.C. Rothwell, U. Ziemann, M. Hallett

Chapter 10

rTMS as treatment strategy in psychiatric disorders – neurobiological concepts

Martin E. Keck

Max Planck Institute of Psychiatry, Kraepelinstr. 2–10, D-80804 Munich (Germany)

1. Introduction

It is important to note that the effects obtained by use of repetitive transcranial magnetic stimulation (rTMS) do not occur on the basis of the magnetic field applied, but are achieved by the electric field induced that ultimately leads to neuronal depolarisation. A charge is moved across the excitable neuronal membranes, creating a transmembrane potential. If sufficient, this causes membrane depolarisation and initiates an action potential, which then propagates along the nerve (Barker and Jalinous, 1985). rTMS can activate the output and input connections of any area of the cortex. This implies that the effects induced are not necessarily limited to the cortical area targeted by rTMS but that changes can also occur at distant interconnected sites in the brain. The threshold for producing effects at a distance depends on the intensity of stimulation (e.g. Padberg et al., 2002b; review: Siebner and Rothwell, 2003).

As a measure for the strength of TMS applied in preclinical and clinical studies, the biological efficacy of the stimulus in the individual subject rather than the output of a given stimulation device is critical (Keck et al., 1998; Wassermann, 1998). Therefore, the intensity of TMS is typically given as a multiple or percentage of the threshold intensity for evoking a small motor evoked potential in a relaxed hand muscle (Rossini et al., 1994). It is of note that the strength of association between motor threshold reflecting motor cortex excitability and thresholds for neuronal depolarisation in other cortical regions is unknown. However, to date there is no method for determining stimulus strength in other brain areas more relevant for psychiatric disorders, e.g. mood circuitries (Siebner and Rothwell, 2003). Motor threshold can also be determined in rodents and should be a prerequisite for conducting basic research in these animals (Jennum and Klitgaard, 1996; Linden et al., 1999; Müller et al., 2000b; Luft et al., 2001).

1.1. rTMS encounters psychiatry

rTMS holds the potential of being able to selectively modulate activity in brain circuitries involved in pathological processes such as depression, mania, obsessive-compulsive disorder, post-traumatic stress disorder and schizophrenia (e.g. Hoflich et al., 1993; Pascual Leone et al., 1996; Greenberg et al., 1997; Grisaru et al., 1998a, b; McCann et al., 1998; Cohen

* *Correspondence to*: Dr. Martin E. Keck, Max Planck Institute of Psychiatry, Kraepelinstr. 2–10, D-80804 Munich, Germany.
Tel: ++49-89-30622-233; Fax: ++49-89-30622-569;
E-mail: keck@mpipsykl.mpg.de

et al., 1999; George et al., 1999, 2000; Padberg et al., 1999, 2002a, b; Berman et al., 2000; Grunhaus et al., 2000; Rollnik et al., 2000). The largest single area of TMS research in psychiatry, however, has been the exploration of possible therapeutic effects of cortical, usually prefrontal, stimulation on symptoms of major depression (review: Padberg and Möller, 2003).

To use rTMS optimally, it is most important to know how it is acting in brain tissue, i.e. knowledge concerning the putative neurobiological changes underlying the observed clinical effects is essential. The limitations of human research necessitate preclinical studies in suitable animal models and basic studies at the cellular and molecular level for a better understanding of how the induced intracerebral current density is regulated and which regulatory elements might serve as potential treatment targets.

1.2. Problems with rodent studies

Animal models are indispensable tools in the search to identify new psychiatric treatments (e.g. Müller et al., 2002). In the vast majority of rodent studies, however, the entire brain is likely to be stimulated due to the usage of commercially obtained stimulation coils (review: Belmaker and Grisaru, 1998; Siebner and Rothwell, 2003). It is, therefore, difficult to relate the effects measured to specific neuronal circuits. Like in clinical studies, another problem arises from the sham stimulation conditions used, which in some cases are likely to elicit biologically active conductive patterns (e.g. Loo et al., 1999). Further, the question of whether or not the animals were trained and handled (to exclude the possibility of being stressed due to the stimulation procedure per se or by the necessity to restrain them) is of importance especially for the interpretation of the neuroendocrine and behavioural data.

The pioneering studies from the Belmaker group in rodents have demonstrated that chronic rTMS has an antidepressant-like effect in rats, e.g. on apomorphine-induced stereotypy and electroconvulsive shock thresholds (Fleischmann et al., 1995); the latter finding has been replicated (Ebert and Ziemann, 1999). However, in these studies, stimulation patterns used were not tested to be analogous to those used under clinical conditions and the effects observed were most probably due to a stimulation of the entire rat brain (review: Belmaker and Grisaru, 1998). Although in most cases not anatomically precise (Herwig et al., 2001), in clinical studies rTMS effects most probably relate to frontal forebrain stimulation (review: Lisanby et al., 2002; Padberg and Möller, 2003). Consequently, to reliably investigate the underlying neurobiological effects in animal models, the adoption of equivalent stimulation conditions is indispensable. It is worth noting that magnetic stimulation of rodent brains is not diffuse by necessity (Siebner and Rothwell, 2003). One possibility of working around these problems is to calculate the spatial distribution of current density induced in both the rat and human brain and to adjust the stimulation parameters accordingly.

The coil and stimulation parameters used in the studies conducted at our laboratory (Post et al., 1999; Keck et al., 2000a, c, 2001a, 2002a; Czeh et al., 2002; Müller et al., 2000b) were selected according to an exact characterization of the conductive phenomena elicited by rTMS in both human and rat brain. This enabled us to accurately adapt the experimental set-up in order to achieve a stimulation pattern which is analogous to the one used in patients during standard clinical treatment. The results of the above procedure show that our experimental set-up allows to obtain a stimulation pattern which exhibits a definite peak in the left frontal region as desired (e.g. Keck et al., 2000a, c, 2001a). It is, therefore, justified to interpret subsequently collected data as related to selective stimulation of this brain area.

1.3. Appropriate rodent models

To obtain predictions about the clinical condition in human depression, an animal model of depressive-like behaviour with face, construct and predictive validity should be used (e.g. Geyer and Markou, 1995; Holsboer, 1999a; Muller and Keck, 2002). Accordingly, our experiments aimed at investigating the neuroendocrine and behavioral impact of rTMS of left frontal brain regions in an appropriate animal model that reflects significant psychopathological features of human depression. We, therefore, characterized the effects of rTMS on the regulation of HPA system activity, stress coping and anxiety-related behavior in two Wistar rat lines selectively bred for high (HAB) and low (LAB) anxiety-related behavior under a regimen adapted from clinical conditions. These two rat breeding lines differ not only in their inborn anxiety, but also in their stress coping strategies and their hypothalamic-pituitary-adrenocortical (HPA) system susceptibility to external stressors (Liebsch et al., 1998a, b; Landgraf et al., 1999; Henniger et al., 2000; Ohl et al., 2001). Moreover, HAB and LAB rats differ markedly in their reactivity to acute benzodiazepine treatment (Liebsch et al., 1998b), treatment with the high affinity corticotropin releasing hormone (CRH) one receptor antagonist R121919, and chronic paroxetine treatment (Keck et al., 2001b, 2003a, b).

2. Behavioural effects: changes in stress coping strategies

Chronic rTMS treatment in the above-mentioned psychopathological animal model under stimulation conditions adapted from hospital use (e.g. George et al., 1999) induced profound changes in acute stress coping strategies, as revealed by the forced swim test (Keck et al., 2001a). The occurrence of changes towards more active coping strategies during exposure to modified versions of the Porsolt's swim test has frequently been shown to predict the antidepressant efficacy of a drug when administered to patients suffering from depression (review: Borsini and Meli, 1988; Cryan et al., 2002). Therefore, the reported behavioral effects of rTMS support a potential antidepressant efficacy of this treatment. This rTMS induced shift in HAB animals towards active stress coping was markedly higher than has previously been reported in commercially obtained rats, i.e. "normal" rats (Zyss et al., 1997; Keck et al., 2000a). Thus, we could demonstrate that rTMS-induced effects are not only present in the HAB rat line but are even amplified in the genetically predisposed animal model. In contrast, rTMS-treated LAB animals, innately displaying rather active stress coping abilities, were unaffected (Liebsch et al., 1998a, b). Our findings that chronic rTMS differentially affected the coping abilities of HAB and LAB rats, indicate that these treatment induced changes are determined by both the rats innate emotionality and coping strategy. Consequently, it is tempting to extrapolate the results obtained in the present study to the clinical condition. Indeed, it should be emphasized that antidepressant treatment strategies such as psychopharmacological agents exert marked beneficial actions in depressed individuals only, but have no mood elevating effects in healthy controls.

As both the dopamine content in brain homogenates (Ben-Shachar et al., 1997) and in hippocampal, striatal and accumbal microdialysates (Keck et al., 2000c, 2002a) have been found to be elevated after acute rTMS, it is tempting to relate the decrease in rTMS-induced immobility time to these findings (e.g. Borsini and Meli, 1988). A further explanation of the increase in active stress coping is concluded from our finding of a significant increase in brain-derived neurotrophic factor (BDNF) mRNA and protein in specific areas of the rat brain after chronic rTMS (Muller et al., 2000b). In line with this finding is the observation that local infusion of high concentrations of BDNF into the mid-brain exerts antidepressant-like effects in the forced swim test (Siuciak et al., 1997).

These findings extend former reports of reduced immobility in mice (Fleischmann et al., 1995; 25 Hz) and rats (Zyss et al., 1997; 50 Hz). However, in these pioneering studies the distribution pattern of intracerebral current density is unclear and most probably the whole brain has been stimulated electrically (Belmaker and Grisaru, 1998). Recently, effects in the forced swim test obtained with frequencies ranging from 1 Hz to 25 Hz were found to be comparable to those seen with the antidepressant imipramine (Sachdev et al., 2002). In this study, the various frequencies of rTMS did not demonstrate a significant differential acute antidepressant effect but the findings suggest that the antidepressant effect of the higher frequencies is likely to be sustained (Sachdev et al., 2002).

Although most clinical trials have focused on the treatment of major depression, increasing attention has been paid to anxiety disorders in recent years. It was shown, however, that chronic rTMS (20 Hz) had no effect on the behavior of rats in the elevated plus-maze and social interaction tests (Keck et al., 2000a). These tests have been validated for the detection of emotional responses to anxiogenic and anxiolytic substances. The observed lack of an anxiolytic effect of rTMS is consistent with the finding that benzodiazepine-binding characteristics were found to be unchanged after chronic rTMS treatment (Ben-Shachar et al., 1999; Keck et al., 2000a), suggesting that 20 Hz rTMS might not be beneficial in treating anxiety-related behavior. In contrast, most recently, it was demonstrated that rTMS applied with 25 Hz exerts anxiolytic effects in rats pointing out that such therapeutic effects might depend on the stimulation frequency (Kanno et al., 2003).

3. Attenuation of the stress-induced activity of the HPA system

Profound changes in HPA system regulation are a common feature in major depression. Previously, we provided data that normalization of an initial aberrancy might be predictive of a favourable antidepressant drug treatment response. Moreover, persistent HPA abnormality correlates with therapy resistance or relapse (review: Keck and Holsboer, 2001; Zobel et al., 2001). Therefore, a hypothesis relating stress hormone dysregulation to causality of depression was submitted suggesting that antidepressants may act through normalization of these HPA changes (review: Holsboer, 2000). Indeed, findings of blunted hormone responses to stress have been obtained in rats after chronic treatment with various antidepressants (review: Reul et al., 2000). Thus, this neuroendocrine system was hypothesized to be a common denominator for clinically efficacious antidepressant treatments (Holsboer and Barden, 1996). In line with the above are the findings on rTMS induced changes in stress-induced corticotropin (ACTH) and corticosterone plasma levels both in commercially obtained rats (Keck et al., 2000a; Czeh et al., 2002) and – to a higher extent – in a psychopathological animal model (Keck et al., 2001a) suggesting that chronic rTMS of frontal brain regions attenuates the stress-induced activity of the HPA system. Moreover, basal corticosterone plasma concentrations were reported to be lowered after a single rTMS (15 Hz) application (Hedges et al., 2002).

Within the limits of neuroendocrine HPA regulation it seems clear that corticosteroids suppress CRH and vasopressin (AVP) expression (the main ACTH secretagogues at the level of the anterior pituitary) through activation of hypothalamic glucocorticoid receptors (review: De Kloet et al., 1998). The mechanism underlying HPA hyperdrive in depression is not yet firmly established, but clinical studies in patients and probands with high genetic risk are consistent with decreased glucocorticoid receptor and mineralocorticoid receptor function, rendering the cortisol-mediated negative feedback on CRH and AVP expression insufficient (Lopez et al., 1998; review: Holsboer, 2000). Several groups have shown that treatment of rats with various antidepressant drugs increases the binding capacity and gene expression of mineralocorticoid and glucocorticoid receptors in the hippocampus as well as other limbic and cortical brain areas (Brady et al., 1991; Seckl and Fink, 1992; Reul et al., 2000). Thus, the effects of antidepressants on these receptors may be a key phenomenon in the readjustment of HPA regulation in major depression. To date, it is unclear whether or not in the case of rTMS HPA system regulation is changed due to alterations in mineralocorticoid and glucocorticoid receptor function, or if the blunted stress-induced HPA system activity is achieved via different mechanisms leading to a decrease in CRH and AVP gene expression. Most likely rTMS-induced changes in the neuroendocrine regulation occur at the hypothalamic level (Keck et al., 2000a, 2001a) and the findings of a specific activation in terms of immediate-early gene expression in the paraventricular nucleus of the hypothalamus in response to acute rTMS support this notion (Ji et al., 1998). Similarly, changes in the dynamic release patterns of AVP and specific amino acids in this hypothalamic region have been reported (Keck et al., 2000c). The observation of an rTMS induced blunted HPA activity is also interesting in light of findings suggesting that the prefrontal cortex may participate in the regulation of the neuroendocrine response to stressful stimuli and, in particular, can inhibit HPA system response to stress, i.e. CRH and AVP synthesis and release (e.g. Diorio et al., 1993). Accordingly, projections of the prefrontal cortex to the perinuclear area of the hypothalamic paraventricular nucleus have been demonstrated (Hurley et al., 1991; Takagishi and Chiba, 1991), and major depression is known to be frequently accompanied by frontal cortex dysfunction (review: Soares and Mann, 1997). Therefore, we hypothesize that rTMS-induced stimulation of frontal brain regions may normalize aberrant neuronal circuit functioning, subsequently leading to a readjustment in hypothalamic CRH and AVP synthesis and release (Post and Keck, 2001). Thus, in the case of anti-depressant drug treatment and chronic rTMS, the neuroendocrine endpoint (i.e. normalization of HPA system function via regulation of CRH and AVP gene expression) might be reached through different pathways.

4. Intracerebral neurochemical changes in response to rTMS

Behavioral alterations and changes in HPA system activity are likely to be mediated through local changes in neurotransmitter, neuromodulator release and gene expression. Selected local neurotransmitter/neuromodulator systems might be particular candidates for rTMS induced changes in interneuronal communication. In this context it is important to note that these substances become only biologically active after their release into the extracellular space (Landgraf, 1995). Microdialysis is a method to reliably detect changes in extracellular bioactive substances in vivo (review: Horn and Engelmann, 2001). This technique provides a direct approach to monitor changes in interneuronal communication by monitoring the fluctuation of local, extracellular concentrations of neurotransmitters/neuromodulators in freely moving animals.

As outlined later, using the microdialysis technique, a differentiated modulatory effect of acute rTMS on the dynamics of release patterns of selected neurotransmitter/neuromodulator systems was demonstrated (Levkovitz et al., 1999; Gur et al., 2000; Keck et al., 2000c, 2002a; Kanno et al., 2003).

4.1. Intracerebral release pattern of vasopressin

There is increasing evidence that neuropeptides are preferentially released and exert their main actions when neurons are strongly activated and under pathological conditions (review: Hökfelt et al., 2000). Accordingly, hyperactivity of central neuropeptidergic circuits such as AVP and CRH neuronal systems is thought to play a causal role in the etiology and symptomatology of affective disorders (Hökfelt et al., 2000; Holsboer, 2000). In support of this, after prolonged stress, AVP is increasingly expressed and released from hypothalamic neurons in both humans and rodents (Antoni, 1993; Keck et al., 2000b). Similarly, a markedly increased synthetic activity of hypothalamic AVP neurons has been described in depressed patients (Purba et al., 1996). Most recently, administration of a non-peptide AVP V_{1b} receptor antagonist was shown to display anxiolytic and antidepressant-like effects in rodents (Griebel et al., 2002). The neuropeptide AVP triggers a variety of central effects on neuroendocrine, autonomic, emotional and cognitive functions (Antoni, 1993; Landgraf et al., 1998; Raber, 1998). Moreover, AVP has been shown to exert behavioural effects such as, for example, increased anxiety following intracerebroventricular administration, and to increase CRH-induced ACTH secretion from pituitary corticotrope cells (Antoni, 1993; Bhattacharya et al., 1998; Landgraf et al., 1998; Insel and Young, 2000). In this context it is of interest to note that AVP released into the portal blood is likely to become the primary secretagogue of ACTH in affective disorders, herewith contributing markedly to HPA system dysregulation (Von Bardeleben and Holsboer, 1989; Müller et al., 2000a; Keck et al., 2002b). The observation that long-term rTMS of frontal brain regions in rats induced an attenuated HPA system response to stress, therefore, may be related to changes in intra-paraventricular nucleus release of AVP (Keck et al., 2000a, 2001a; Czeh et al., 2002).

Indeed, a continuous decrease in AVP release of up to 50% in response to acute rTMS was reported to occur in this nucleus (Keck et al., 2000c). Additional indirect evidence for AVP playing a role in affective disorders derives from the finding that fluoxetine treatment leads to a reduction in cerebrospinal fluid (CSF) concentrations of AVP in patients with major depression (De Bellis et al., 1993). Most recently, in our laboratory it was shown that long-term treatment with the antidepressant paroxetine is able to decrease hypothalamic AVP mRNA expression in rats (Keck et al., 2003b). This phenomenon was accompanied by an increase in active stress coping and a normalization of HPA system regulation (Keck et al., 2003b). These findings suggest that the AVPergic system is likely to be critically involved in the behavioural and neuroendocrine effects of antidepressant treatment. The mechanism of action of both rTMS and paroxetine on AVP gene regulation and release render AVPergic neuronal circuits a promising target for the development of more causal antidepressant treatment strategies.

4.2. Intracerebral release pattern of amino acids

Amino acids in the brain act as neurotransmitters and neuromodulators and have been implicated in the metabolism and turnover rate of monoamines and in HPA system dysregulation (e.g. Garcia de Yebenes Prous et al., 1978; Raber, 1998). In response to acute rTMS an increase of distinct amino acids in the hypothalamic paraventricular nucleus, which is likely to reflect specific biological effects, was reported (Keck et al., 2000c). The observed changes in amino acids level are substance-specific, as in the hypothalamic paraventricular nucleus only taurine, serine, and aspartate, but not γ-aminobutyric acid (GABA), glutamate, glutamine, and arginine concentrations in the extracellular fluid were elevated in response to rTMS (Keck et al., 2000c).

In the hypothalamic supraoptic nucleus, taurine of glial origin is involved in the inhibition of AVPergic neurons (Deleuze et al., 1998; Engelmann et al., 2001). Hence, the increased extracellular concentration of the inhibitory amino acid taurine may have contributed to the decrease in intra-paraventricular AVP release after rTMS (Keck et al., 2000c). In contrast, the finding of an increase in intra-paraventricular serine and aspartate release is difficult to interpret and needs further investigation. In patients suffering from bipolar affective disorder (Fekkes et al., 1994) and in a subgroup of depressed patients that were non-responders to treatment with antidepressants (Maes et al., 1998), decreased plasma levels of aspartate and serine were described. Accordingly, serine has been reported to be elevated in CSF samples from patients receiving antidepressants (Pangalos et al., 1992).

4.3. rTMS and monoamines: focus on dopamine

Although converging lines of evidence such as the delayed onset of action common to all antidepressant drugs have led us beyond the monoaminergic synapse for strategies to improve antidepressant therapy, an increase of disposition of biogenic amines accompanies the therapeutic effects of most antidepressant treatments (for review: Blier and De Montigny, 1994; Holsboer, 1995). Previous studies using brain homogenates, however, revealed conflicting results on the effects of rTMS of the entire rat brain on monoaminergic transmission (Ben-Shachar et al., 1997, 1999). Dynamic release patterns of monoamines in response to acute rTMS (20 Hz) of frontal brain regions were first monitored in the hippocampus as specific effects of chronic rTMS in hippocampal areas have been reported previously (Hausmann et al., 2000; Müller et al., 2000b; Doi et al., 2001). Interestingly, we found a selective stimulation of hippocampal dopamine release, but not serotonin or noradrenaline release (Keck et al., 2000b; Fig. 1). Therefore, the dopaminergic system appeared to be one of the primary candidate neurotransmitter systems which is directly and selectively modulated by rTMS of frontal brain regions. It has been demonstrated that the prefrontal cortex has dense efferent projections to both the ventral tegmental area (VTA) and the substantia nigra, i.e. the regions of origin of the mesolimbic and mesostriatal dopaminergic pathways (Fig. 1; Sesack and Pickel, 1992). These neuroanatomical connections

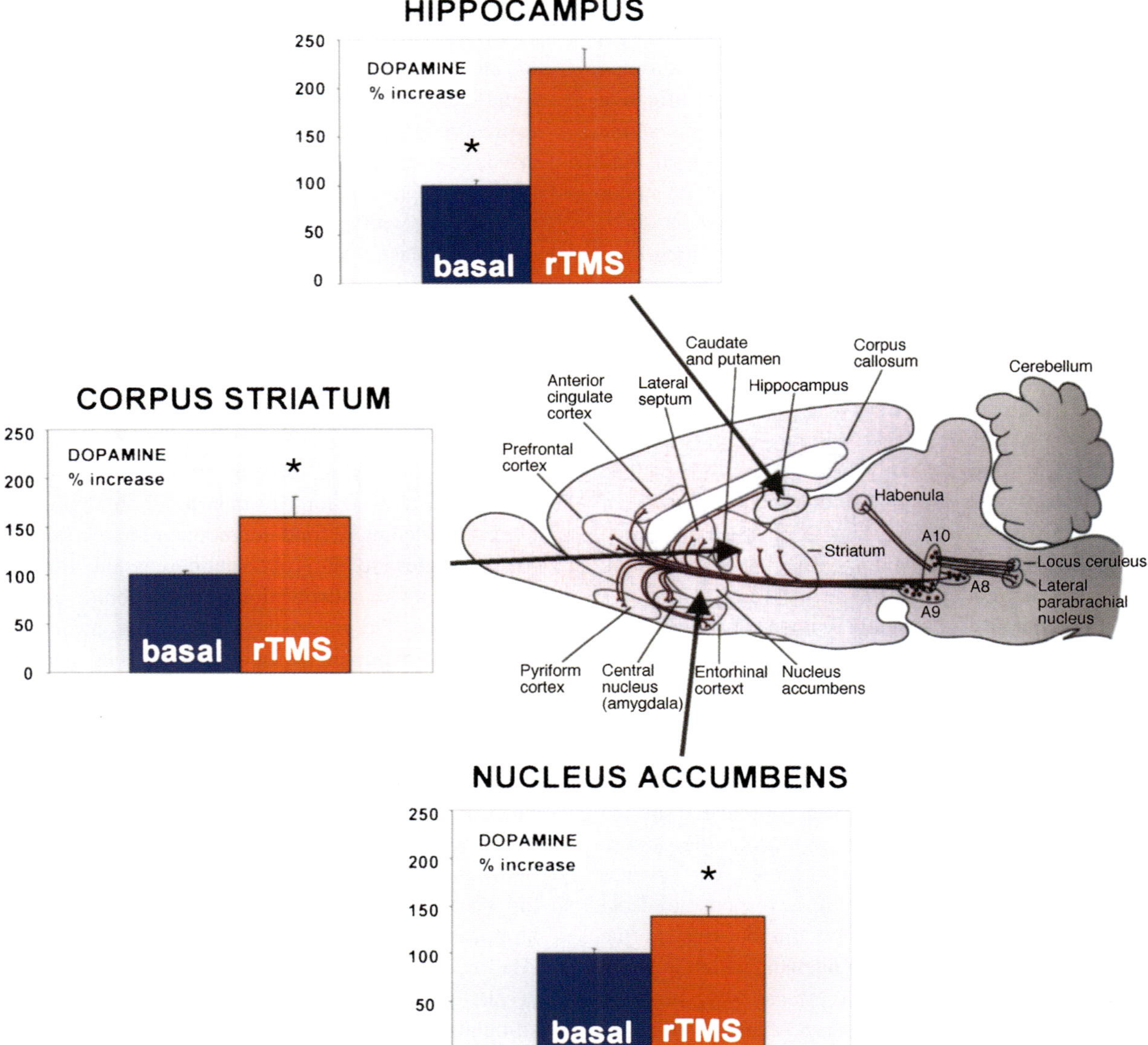

Fig. 1. Effects of 20 trains (1,000 stimuli) of repetitive transcranial magnetic stimulation (rTMS; 20 Hz) and sham stimulation on the dopamine content of 30-min dialysates collected consecutively from the dorsal hippocampus, dorsal striatum and nucleus accumbens shell of male Wistar rats. Data are maximum increase expressed as percentage of baseline ± SEM. The schematic drawing represents a transversal rat brain section showing the mesolimbic and mesostriatal dopaminergic projections originating primarily from cell groups in the ventral tegmental area (A10 cell group), with smaller contributions from the substantia nigra (A9 cell group) $*P < 0.05$ vs. sham stimulation (Keck et al., 2002a).

may explain how stimulation of frontal brain regions enhances dopamine efflux in axon terminal areas originating from mesencephalic dopaminergic cell groups. Apart from the hippocampus, the ventral (i.e. nucleus accumbens) and dorsal striatum receive dense dopaminergic projections from the VTA and substantia nigra, respectively (review: Fibiger, 1995; Feldman et al., 1997) and, therefore, might be candidate regions for possible rTMS induced changes in interneuronal communication. Consistent with the hypothesis that stimulation of frontal brain regions by rTMS may increase dopaminergic neurotransmission in areas other than the hippocampus, it has been reported that direct electrical stimulation of the prefrontal cortex enhances dopamine release in the dorsal striatum and nucleus accumbens (e.g. Taber and Fibiger, 1995; You et al., 1998). In support of this assumption we found that rTMS applied under the same conditions increased dopamine release also in the striatum and the nucleus accumbens septi (Fig. 1; Keck et al., 2002a). In this respect, the nucleus accumbens septi is of particular interest as it is a major component of the neural circuitry of reward and incentive motivation, which most likely is dysfunctional not only in depression but also in schizophrenia leading to negative symptoms such as anhedonia and loss of interest (review: Fibiger et al., 1995). Indeed, preliminary clinical evidence suggests that rTMS might be able to improve negative symptoms in patients suffering from schizophrenia (Cohen et al., 1999; Nahas et al., 2000).

Taken together, the existence of psychiatric syndromes associated with impaired dopamine neurotransmission, i.e. depression, mania, and schizophrenia (Holsboer, 1995) with a suggested therapeutic effect of rTMS (e.g. Pascual-Leone et al., 1996; Grisaru et al., 1998a, b; Nahas et al., 2000; Rollnik et al., 2000), indicates that the effect of rTMS on dopaminergic activity might be of particular relevance to elucidate its mechanism of action. Interestingly, recent evidence from a clinical study supports our finding of an rTMS-induced increase in dopamine release (Strafella et al., 2001) and beneficial effects have been reported in the treatment of patients suffering from Parkinson's disease (Siebner and Rothwell, 2003).

Other studies reported effects of rTMS on the brain serotonergic and noradrenergic systems: Levkovitz et al. (1999) demonstrated lasting effects of chronic rTMS (25 Hz) on reactivity of the rat's hippocampus to electrode stimulation of its main excitatory afferent pathway, i.e. the perforant path. A long-lasting reduction in noradrenergic and serotonergic functions in the hippocampus of chronically treated rats was reported and animals showed significant changes in motility in an open field as well as an increase in pain sensitivity (Levkovitz et al., 1999). Further, 7 days of rTMS (25 Hz) did not affect single population spikes but caused an increase in paired-pulse inhibition. This effect, which was still evident 3 weeks after the last series of daily rTMS, could also be obtained after a 7-day series of treatment with the antidepressants desipramine and mianserine (Levkovitz et al., 2001). The efficacy of rTMS in modulating inhibitory circuits of the hippocampus, however, was found to be drastically reduced in aged rats (Levkovitz and Segal, 2001). This finding may contribute to the understanding of the reduced antidepressant efficacy of rTMS in aged patients (Mosimann et al., 2002). Taken together, the data reported by the Levkovitz group suggest that rTMS (25 Hz) affects local inhibitory circuits more than the main excitatory afferent to the hippocampus. The modulation of local inhibition reported may either be a direct action by increasing the efficacy of inhibition pre- or postsynaptically, or an indirect one by reducing the efficacy of GABAergic modulators, e.g. serotonin (Levkovitz and Segal, 2001).

Kole et al. (1999) monitored a selective increase in 5-HT_{1A} binding sites in the frontal cortex, the cingulate cortex, and the anterior olfactory nucleus in response to a single train of rTMS (20 Hz). As corticosteroids are well known to play an inhibitory role in 5-HT_{1A} mRNA and protein expression (Chalmers et al., 1993; review: Chaouloff, 1995), this finding is in line with the observation of an attenuated stress-induced HPA system activity in response to rTMS (Keck et al., 2000a, 2001a; Czeh et al., 2002). 5-HT uptake sites, however, showed no changes after a single train of rTMS (20 Hz) (Kole et al., 1999). While most antidepressant drugs typically upregulate postsynaptic 5-HT_2 receptors, Ben-Shachar et al. (1999) found postsynaptic 5-HT_{2A} receptors to be downregulated in the frontal cortex and striatum after 10 days of rTMS (15 Hz). By use of in vivo microdialysis of the prefrontal cortex combined with challenges with a 5-HT_{1A} receptor agonist or a 5-HT_{1B} receptor antagonist subsequent to 10 days of rTMS (15 Hz), subsensitivity of presynaptic serotonergic autoreceptor activity was demonstrated, revealing thus parallels to other antidepressant treatments (Gur et al., 2000). In a recent study, 3 days of rTMS (25 Hz) were shown to be able to reduce stress-induced increase in serotonin release in frontal cortical regions (Kanno et al., 2003). However, like in the other studies showing an influence of rTMS on brain serotonergic systems, rats had to be restrained during stimulation (Kole et al., 1999; Belmaker et al., 2000; Gur et al., 2000). Therefore, it is difficult to distinguish between pure rTMS-related effects and effects secondary to the stress of restraint necessary for treatment. These findings suggest, however, that the serotonergic system might be influenced at various levels in response to rTMS under certain conditions.

4.4. rTMS-induced increase in BDNF

BDNF belongs to the family of neurotrophins and was shown to be involved in survival and differentiation in specific areas of the central nervous system as well as in regulating neuronal connectivity and synaptic plasticity (Lewin and Barde, 1996). BDNF, which is expressed at high levels in the adult hippocampus, can be upregulated by electrical stimulation (Balkowiec and Katz, 2000) and plays a role in hippocampal long-term potentiation (Chen et al., 1999). Interestingly, Wang et al. (1996) observed both long-term potentiation and long-term depression-like changes after rTMS in the gerbil auditory cortex. Chronic rTMS treatment increased BDNF mRNA and protein level in specific areas of rat brains, namely in the CA3 region of the hippocampal pyramidal cell layer and in the granule cell layer of the dentate gyrus (Müller et al., 2000b). Therefore, rTMS might be a stimulus for the release of endogenous BDNF comparable to the effect of direct electrical stimulation in neuronal cells (Balkowiec and Katz, 2000).

Furthermore, it is noteworthy that after chronic rTMS treatment BDNF mRNA and protein expression are increased in exactly the same brain regions as observed after ECT and antidepressant drug treatment (Nibuya et al., 1995, 1996). These findings suggest that a common molecular mechanism may underlie different antidepressant treatment strategies. This again might be achieved via attenuation of HPA system activity that occurs both in response to long-term rTMS and antidepressant drug treatment (Keck et al., 2000a, 2001a; Reul et al., 2000; Czeh et al., 2002), as it has been shown that glucocorticoid and mineralocorticoid receptors participate in the control of neurotrophic factor gene expression (Hansson et al., 2000).

5. RTMS and adult neurogenesis: unexpected findings

It is widely accepted that chronic stress increases the risk of developing and is associated with affective disorders (Kendler et al., 1999). Stress-induced structural remodelling in the adult hippocampus may provide a cellular basis for understanding the impairment of neural plasticity in depressive illness. Accordingly, reversal of structural remodelling might be a desirable goal for an antidepressant therapy. Proliferation and maturation of functional neurons have been demonstrated to occur at a significant rate in the adult hippocampus in many different mammalian species including humans (Van Praag et al., 2002). Moreover, adult neurogenesis is an extremely dynamic process that is regulated in both a positive and negative manner by neuronal activity and environmental factors (Gould et al., 2000). Exposure to psychotropic drugs or stress regulates the rate of neurogenesis in adult brain, suggesting a possible role for neurogenesis in the pathophysiology and treatment of neurobiological illnesses such as depression and post-traumatic stress disorder (Duman et al., 1999, 2001). In this context, a hypothesis relating stress hormone dysregulation to causality of depression was proposed (Holsboer, 2000). In line with the above are the findings on chronic rTMS-induced changes in stress-induced ACTH and corticosterone plasma levels in rats providing evidence that rTMS of frontal brain regions attenuates the stress-induced activity of the HPA system (Keck et al., 2000a, 2001a; Czeh et al., 2002). In a study designed to examine the effects of concomitant rTMS treatment on plasma stress hormone levels and on neurogenesis in the hippocampal dentate gyrus of the adult rat during chronic psychosocial stress, rTMS (20 Hz) normalized the stress-induced elevation of plasma ACTH and corticosterone (Czeh et al., 2002). An important finding of this study is that the effect of rTMS on plasma stress hormone levels did not parallel the effects on hippocampal neurogenesis: rTMS normalized the stress-induced changes in HPA system activity but had no consistent effect on the stress-induced suppression of hippocampal neurogenesis. In fact, the survival rate of the 5-bromo-2′-deoxyuridine (BrdU)-labelled neurons decreased, whereas the proliferation rate of hippocampal progenitor cells was only mildly increased by concomitant rTMS. However, when applied outside the context of psychosocial stress, rTMS had no substantial effect on hippocampal neurogenesis (Czeh et al., 2002). Recent studies demonstrated that single and multiple electroconvulsive shocks significantly and dose-dependently increased adult hippocampal neurogenesis in rats and it was hypothesized that this might be an important neurobiological element underlying the clinical effects of electroconvulsive treatment (Madsen et al., 2000; Scott et al., 2000). Similarly, treatment with various types of antidepressant drugs augmented neurogenesis (Malberg et al., 2000; Duman et al., 2001). It should be emphasized, however, that all these studies were conducted on otherwise undisturbed, non-stressed animals. Another possible explanation for the discrepancies in neurobiological findings between electroconvulsive shock, drug treatment, and rTMS might be that these treatment strategies may have different effects on various neurobiological circuitries (Post and Keck, 2001). Recent evidence supports the view that serotonin may stimulate granule cell production (Brezun and Daszuta, 2000a, b), whereas depletion of serotonin reduces neurogenesis (Brezun and Daszuta, 1999). Consistently, treatment with the serotonin reuptake inhibitor fluoxetine increased neurogenesis (Malberg et al., 2000). This increase in hippocampal cell proliferation is likely to be mediated, at least in part, by action at the 5-HT_{1A} receptor (Jacobs et al., 1998). Therefore, the findings that neither intrahippocampal release of serotonin (Keck et al., 2000c) nor hippocampal 5-HT_{1A} receptor number and affinity (Kole et al., 1999) are changed in response to rTMS (20 Hz) presumably also explain why rTMS had no stimulating effect on hippocampal cell proliferation in either stressed or unstressed animals.

Although the definite task of newly generated hippocampal neurons is not yet known, several lines of evidence suggest that they may play an important role in learning (Shors et al., 2001). Thus, theoretically, rTMS when applied during chronic stress might impair cognitive function via suppressing neurogenesis. However, it has been shown that long-term rTMS treatment did not affect cognitive outcome as assessed in the Morris water-maze task (Post et al., 1999), which is considered a good indicator of hippocampal function. Hence, it is unlikely that chronic rTMS (20 Hz) of frontal brain regions impairs learning and memory performance, and evidence from clinical studies supports this view (Lisanby et al., 2002; review: Padberg and Möller, 2003).

6. Conclusion

Though there are many caveats when trying to relate modulatory effects of rTMS in the rodent brain to rTMS effects in humans, the preclinical findings provide, at least in part, an explanation for the possible neurobiological mechanisms underlying the therapeutic effects reported in numerous clinical trials. There is accumulating evidence that acute rTMS (20 Hz) of frontal brain regions leads to alterations in mesolimbic and mesostriatal release patterns of dopamine in vivo. Dopamine-active antidepressant treatment strategies may be of particular benefit in a subgroup of patients with a low level of dopamine function, as reflected by symptoms such as anhedonia, marked psychomotor retardation or concomitant Parkinson's disease. Therefore, with respect to the design of clinical trials, the identification of such patients with a putative deficit in dopaminergic neurotransmission related to psychopathology might lead to a better antidepressant efficacy of rTMS beyond the only moderate and rather short-lived therapeutic effects reported so far. In support of this hypothesis are findings that depressed patients suffering from psychotic symptoms (reflecting dopaminergic hyperactivity) poorly respond to rTMS (Grunhaus et al., 2000). In addition, rTMS-induced modulation of dopaminergic neurotransmission in brain circuitries, relevant to incentive motivation, might represent a new approach to the treatment of substance abuse-related disorders which is currently under investigation at the Max Planck Institute of Psychiatry.

In accordance with clinical studies (review: Padberg and Möller, 2003), the rodent studies available so far support the notion that rTMS is a safe technique even when used chronically (Post et al., 1999; Müller et al., 2000b; Liebetanz et al., 2003). Based on current validation studies, however, it seems premature for rTMS to be approved for routine clinical use. Current challenges in the field include determining the influence of varying stimulation parameters (e.g. the duration of treatment, the total number of magnetic stimuli applied, the stimulation frequency and precise localization of the stimulation coil). This should enable us to better characterize the neurobiological effects of TMS responsible for its therapeutic efficacy and to separate myth from reality.

Acknowledgements

The transcranial magnetic stimulation studies at the Max Planck Institute of Psychiatry in Munich are supported by the German Federal Research Ministry within the promotional emphasis "*Competence Nets in Medicine*" (Kompetenznetz Depression and Suizidalität; subproject 4.5). The author would like to acknowledge the excellent scientific work of Drs. Mario Engelmann, Karl Ebner, Angelika Erhardt, Rainer Landgraf, Marianne B. Müller, Frauke Ohl, Anke Post, Inge Sillaber, Nicola Toschi, and Tobias Welt. The stimulation device was generously provided by Medtronic, Dusseldorf, Germany.

References

Antoni, F.A. Vasopressinergic control of pituitary adrenocorticotropin secretion comes of age. *Front. Neuroendocrinol.*, 1993, 14: 76–122.

Balkowiec, A. and Katz, D.M. Activity-dependent release of endogenous brain-derived neurotrophic factor from primary sensory neurons detected by ELISA in situ. *J. Neurosci.*, 20: 7417–7423.

Barker, A.T. and Jalinous, R. Non-invasive stimulation of the human motor cortex. *Lancet*, 1985, 1: 1106–1107.

Belmaker, R.H. and Grisaru, N. Magnetic stimulation of the brain in animal depression models responsive to ECS. *J. Ect.*, 1998, 14: 194–205.

Belmaker, R.H., Einat, H., Levkovitz, Y., Segal, M. and Grisaru, N. TMS effects in animal models of depression and mania: Implications of hippocampal electrophysiology. In: M.S. George and R.H. Belmaker (Eds.), *Transcranial Magnetic Stimulation in Neuropsychiatry*. American Psychiatric Press, Inc., Washington DC., 2000: 99–114.

Ben-Shachar, D., Belmaker, R.H., Grisaru, N. and Klein, E. Transcranial magnetic stimulation induces alterations in brain monoamines. *J. Neural Transm.*, 1997, 104: 191–197.

Ben-Shachar, D., Gazawi, H., Riboyad-Levin, J. and Klein, E. Chronic repetitive transcranial magnetic stimulation alters β-adrenergic and 5-HT_2 receptor characteristics in rat brain. *Brain Res.*, 1999, 816: 78–83.

Berman, R.M., Narasimhan, M., Sanacora, G., Miano, A.P., Hoffman, R.E., Hu, X.S., Charney, D.S. and Boutros N.N. A randomized clinical trial of repetitive transcranial magnetic stimulation in the treatment of major depression. *Biol. Psychiat.*, 2000, 47: 332–337.

Bhattacharya, S.K., Bhttacharya, A. and Chakrabarti, A. Anxiogenic activity of intraventricularly administered arginine-vasopressin in the rat. *Biogenic Amines*, 1998, 14: 367–385.

Blier, P. and De Montigny, C. Current advances and trends in the treatment of depression. *Trends Pharmacol. Sci.*, 1994, 15: 220–226.

Borsini, F. and Meli, A. Is the forced swimming test a suitable model for revealing antidepressant activity? *Psychopharmacol.*, 1988, 94: 147–160.

Brady, L.S., Whitfield, H.J. Jr., Fox, R.J., Gold, P.W. and Herkenham, M. Long-term antidepressant administration alters corticotropin-releasing hormone, tyrosine hydroxylase, and mineralocorticoid receptor gene expression in rat brain: Therapeutic implications. *J. Clin. Invest.*, 1991, 87: 831–837.

Brezun, J.M. and Daszuta, A. Depletion in serotonin decreases neurogenesis in the dentate gyrus and the subventricular zone of adult rats. *Neuroscience*, 1999, 89: 999–1002.

Brezun, J.M. and Daszuta, A. Serotonin may stimulate granule cell proliferation in the adult hippocampus, as observed in rats grafted with foetal raphe neurons. *Eur. J. Neurosci.*, 2000a, 12: 391–396.

Brezun, J.M. and Daszuta, A. Serotonergic reinnervation reverses lesion-induced decreases in PSA-NCAM labeling and proliferation of hippocampal cells in adult rats. *Hippocampus*, 2000b, 10: 37–46.

Chalmers, D.T., Kwak, S.P., Mansour, A., Akil, H. and Watson, S.J. Corticosteroids regulate brain hippocampal 5-HT1A receptor mRNA expression. *J. Neurosci.*, 1993, 13: 914–923.

Chaouloff, F. Regulation of 5-HT receptors by corticosteroids: where do we stand? *Fund. Clin. Pharmacol.*, 1995, 9: 219–233.

Chen, G., Kolbeck, R., Barde, Y.A., Bonhoeffer, T. and Kossel, A. Relative contribution of endogenous neurotrophins in hippocampal long-term potentiation. *J. Neurosci.*, 1999, 19: 7983–7990.

Cohen, E., Bernardo, M., Masana, J., Arrufat, F.J., Navarro, V., Valls-Solé, J., Boget, T., Barrantes, N., Catarineu, S., Font, M. and Lomena, F.J. Repetitive transcranial magnetic stimulation in the treatment of chronic negative schizophrenia: a pilot study. *J. Neurol. Neurosurg. Psychiat.*, 1999, 67: 129–130.

Crawley, J.N. and Corwin, R.L. Biological actions of cholecystokinin. *Peptides*, 1994, 5: 731–755.

Cryan, J.F., Markou, A. and Lucki, I. Assessing antidepressant activity in rodents: recent developments and future needs. *Trends Pharmacol. Sci.*, 2002, 23: 238–245.

Czeh, B., Welt,T., Fischer, A.K., Erhardt, A., Schmitt, W., Muller, M.B., Toschi, N., Fuchs, E. and Keck, M.E. Chronic psychosocial stress and concomitant repetitive transcranial magnetic stimulation: effects on stress hormone levels and adult hippocampal neurogenesis. *Biol. Psychiat.*, 2002, 52: 1057–1065.

De Bellis, M.D., Gold, P.W., Geracioti, T.D. Jr., Listwak, S.J. and Kling, M.A. Association of fluoxetine treatment with reductions in CSF concentrations of corticotropinreleasing hormone and arginine vasopressin in patients with major depression. *Am. J. Psychiatry*, 1993, 150: 656–667.

De Kloet, E.R., Vreugdenhil, E., Oitzl, M.S. and Joels, M. Brain corticosteroid receptor balance in health and disease. *Endocr. Rev.*, 1998, 19: 269–301.

Deleuze, C., Duvoid, A. and Hussy, N. Properties and glial origin of osmoticdependent release of taurine from the rat supraoptic nucleus. *J. Physiology*, 1998, 507: 463–471.

Diorio, D., Viau, V. and Meaney, M.J. The role of the medial prefrontal cortex (cingulate gyrus) in the regulation of hypothalamic-pituitary-adrenal response to stress. *J. Neurosci.*, 1993, 13: 3839–3847.

Doi, W., Sato, D., Fukuzako, H. and Takigawa, M. c-Fos expression in rat brain after repetitive transcranial magnetic stimulation. *NeuroReport*, 2001, 12: 1307–1310.

Duman, R.S., Malberg, J. and Thome, J. Neural plasticity to stress and antidepressant treatment. *Biol. Psychiat.*, 1999, 46: 1181–1191.

Duman, R.S., Malberg, J. and Nakagawa, S. Regulation of adult neurogenesis by psychotropic drugs and stress. *J. Pharmacol. Exp. Ther.*, 2001, 299: 401–407.

Ebert, U. and Ziemann, U. Altered seizures susceptibility after high-frequency transcranial magnetic stimulation in rats. *Neurosci. Lett.*, 1999, 273: 155–158.

Engelmann, M., Ludwig, M., Singewald, N., Ebner, K., Sabatier, N., Lubec, G., Landgraf, R. and Wotjak, C.T. Taurine selectively modulates the secretory activity of vasopressin neurons in conscious rats. *Eur. J. Neurosci.*, 2001, 14: 1047–1055.

Fekkes, D., Pepplinkhuizen, L., Verheij, R. and Bruinvels, J. Abnormal plasma levels of serine, methionine, and taurine in transient acute polymorphic psychosis. *Psychiatry Res.*, 1994, 51: 11–18.

Feldman, R.S., Meyer, J.S. and Quenzer, L.F. *Principles of Neuropsychopharmacology*. Sunderland, Sinauer, Mass., 1997.

Fibiger, H. C. Neurobiology of depression: focus on dopamine. *Depress. Mania*, 1995, 49: 117.

Fleischmann, A., Prolov, K., Abarbanel, J. and Belmaker, R.H. The effect of transcranial magnetic stimulation of rat brain on behavior: models of depression. *Brain Res.*, 1995, 699: 130–132.

Fleischmann, A., Sternheim, A., Etgen, A.M., Li, C., Grisaru, N. and Belmaker, R.H. Transcranial magnetic stimulation downregulates beta-adrenoreceptors in rat cortex. *J. Neural. Transm.*, 1996, 103: 1361–1366.

Fleischmann, A., Hirschmann, S., Dolberg, O.T., Dannon, P.N. and Grunhaus, L. Chronic treatment with repetitive transcranial magnetic stimulation inhibits seizure induction by electroconvulsive shock in rats. *Biol. Psychiat.*, 1999, 45: 759–763.

Fujiki, M. and Steward, O. High frequency transcranial magnetic stimulation mimics the effects of ECS in upregulation astroglia gene expression in the murine CNS. *Mol. Brain Res.*, 1997, 44: 301–308.

Garcia de Yebenes Prous, J., Carlsson, A. and Mena Gomez, M. The effect of taurine on motor behavior, body temperature, and monoamine metabolism in rat brain. *Naunyn Schmiedebergs Arch. Pharmacol.*, 1978, 304: 95–99.

George, M.S., Wassermann, E.M. and Post, R.M. Transcranial magnetic stimulation: a neuropsychiatric tool for the 21st century. *J. Neuropsychiat. Clin. Neurosci.*, 1996, 8: 373–382.

George, M.S., Lisanby, S. and Sackeim, H.A. Transcranial magnetic stimulation. *Arch. Gen. Psychiat.*, 1999, 56: 300–311.

George, M.S. and Belmaker, R.H. Historical overview. In: M.S. George and R.H. Belmaker (Eds.), *Transcranial Magnetic Stimulation in Neuropsychiatry*. American Psychiatric Press, Inc., Washington DC., 2000a: 1–12.

George, M.S., Nahas, Z., Molloy, M., Speer, A.M., Oliver, N.C., Li, X.B., Arana, G.W., Risch, S.C. and Ballenger, J.C. A controlled trial of daily left prefrontal cortex TMS for treating depression. *Biol. Psychiat.*, 2000b, 48: 962–970.

Geyer, M.A. and Markou, A. Animal models of psychiatric disorders. In: F.E. Bloom and D.J. Kupfer (Eds.), *Psychopharmacology: The Fourth Generation of Progress*. Raven Press, New York, 1995: 787–798.

Glue, P., Costello, M.J., Pert, A., Mele, A. and Nutt, D.J. Regional neurotransmitter responses after acute and chronic electroconvulsive shock. *Neuropsychopharmacol.*, 1990, 100: 60–65.

Gould, E., Tanapat, P., Rydel T. and Hastings, N. Regulation of hippocampal neurogenesis in adulthood. *Biol. Psychiat.*, 2000, 48: 715–720

Grafman, J. and Wassermann, E. Transcranial magnetic stimulation can measure and modulate learning and memory. *Neuropsychologia*, 1999, 37: 159–167.

Grafman, J., Pascual-Leone, A., Alway, D., Nichelli, P., Gomez-Tortosa, E. and Hallett, M. Induction of a recall deficit by rapid-rate transcranial magnetic stimulation. *NeuroReport*, 1994, 5: 1157–1160.

Greenberg, B.D., George, M.S., Martin, J.D., Benjamin, J., Schlaepfer, T.E., Altemus, M., Wassermann, E.M., Post, R.M. and Murphy, D.L. Effect of prefrontal repetitive transcranial magnetic stimulation in obsessive-compulsive disorder: a preliminary study. *Am. J. Psychiat.*, 1997, 154: 867–869.

Griebel, G., Simiand, J., Serradeil-Le Gal, C., Wagnon, J., Pascal, M., Scatton, B., Maffrand, J.P. and Soubrié, P. Anxiolytic- and antidepressant-like effects of the non-peptide vasopressin V_{1b} receptor antagonist, SSR 149415, suggest an innovative approach for the treatment of stress-related disorders. *Proc. Natl. Acad. Sci. USA*, 2002, 99: 6370–6375.

Grisaru, N., Chudakov, B., Yaroslavsky, Y. and Belmaker, R.H. Transcranial magnetic stimulation in mania: A controlled study. *Am. J. Psychiat.*, 1998b, 155: 1608–1610.

Groenewegen, H.J., Wright, C.I. and Uylings, H.B.M. The anatomical relationship of the prefrontal cortex with limbic structures and the basal ganglia. *J. Psychopharmacol.*, 1997, 11: 99–106.

Grunhaus, L., Dannon, P.N., Schreiber, S., Dolberg, O.H., Amiaz, R., Ziv, R. and Lefkifker, E. Repetitive transcranial magnetic stimulation is as effective as electroconvulsive therapy in the treatment of nondelusional major depressive disorder: an open study. *Biol. Psychiat.*, 2000, 47: 314–324.

Gur, E., Lerer, B., Dremencov, E. and Newman, M.E. Chronic repetitive transcranial magnetic stimulation induces subsensitivity of presynaptic serotonergic autoreceptor activity in rat brain. *NeuroReport*, 2000, 11: 2925–2929.

Hallett, M. Transcranial magnetic stimulation and the human brain. *Nature*, 2000, 406: 147–150.

Hansson, A.C., Cintra, A., Belluardo, N., Sommer, W., Bhatnagar, M., Bader, M., Ganten, D. and Fuxe, K. Gluco- and mineralocorticoid receptor-mediated regulation of neurotrophic factor gene expression in the dorsal hippocampus and the neocortex of the rat. *Eur. J. Neurosci.*, 2000, 12: 2918–2934.

Hausmann, A., Weis, C., Marksteiner, J., Hinterhuber, H. and Humpel, C. Chronic repetitive transcranial magnetic stimulation enhances c-fos in the parietal cortex and hippocampus. *Mol. Brain. Res.*, 2000, 76: 355–362.

Hedges, D.W., Salyer, D.L., Higginbotham, B.J., Lund, T.D., Hellewell, J.L., Ferguson, D. and Lephart, E.D. Transcranial magnetic stimulation (TMS) effects on testosterone, prolactin, and corticosterone in adult male rats. *Biol. Psychiat.*, 2002, 51: 417–421.

Henniger, M.S.H., Ohl, F., Hölter, S.M., Weissenbacher, P., Toschi, N., Lorscher, P., Wigger, A., Spanagel, R. and Landgraf, R. Unconditioned anxiety and social behaviour in two rat lines selectively bred for high and low anxiety-related behaviour. *Behav. Brain Res.*, 2000, 111: 153–163.

Herwig, U., Padberg, F., Unger, J., Spitzer, M. and Schönfeldt-Lecuona, C. Transcranial magnetic stimulation in therapy studies: examination of the reliability of "standard" coil positioning by neuronavigation. *Biol. Psychiatr.*, 2001, 50: 58–61.

Höflich, G., Kasper, S., Hufnagel, A., Ruhrmann, S. and Möller, H.J. Application of transcranial magnetic stimulation in treatment of drug-resistant major depression – a report of two cases. *Hum. Psychopharmacol.*, 1993, 8: 361–365.

Hökfelt, T., Broberger, C., Xu, Z.Q.D., Sergeyev, V., Ubink, R. and Diez, M. Neuropeptides – an overview. *Neuropharmacology*, 2000, 39: 1337–1356.

Holsboer, F. Neuroendocrinology of mood disorders. In: F.E. Bloom and D.J. Kupfer (Eds.), *Psychopharmacology: The Fourth Generation of Progress*. Raven Press, New York, 1995: 957–968.

Holsboer, F. The rationale for corticotropin-releasing hormone receptor (CRH-R) antagonists to treat depression and anxiety. *J. Psychiatr. Res.*, 1999a, 33: 181–214.

Holsboer, F. Animal models of mood disorders. In: D.S. Charney, E.J. Nestler and B.S. Bunney (Eds.), *Neurobiology of Mental Illness*. Oxford University Press, New York, 1999b: 317–322.

Holsboer, F. The corticosteroid receptor hypothesis of depression. *Neuropsychopharmacol.*, 2000, 23: 477–501.

Holsboer, F. and Barden, N. Antidepressants and hypothalamic-pituitaryadrenocortical regulation. *Endocr. Rev.*, 1996, 17: 187–205.

Honig, A., Bartlett, J.R., Bouras, N. and Bridges, P.K. Amino acid levels in depression: a preliminary investigation. *J. Psychiatr. Res.*, 1989, 22: 159–164.

Horn, T.F.W. and Engelmann, M. In vivo microdialysis for nonapeptides in rat brain – a practical guide. *Methods*, 2001, 23, 41–53.

Hurley, K.M., Herbert, H., Moga, M.M. and Saper, C.B. Efferent projections of the infralimbic cortex of the rat. *J. Comp. Neurol.*, 1991, 308: 249–276.

Insel, T.R. and Young, L.J. Neuropeptides and the evolution of social behavior. *Curr. Opin. Neurobiol.*, 2000, 10: 784–789.

Jacobs, B.L., Tanapat, P., Reeves, A.J. and Gould, E. Serotonin stimulates the production of new hippocampal granule neurons via the $5HT_{1A}$ receptor in the adult brain. *Soc. Neurosci. Abs.*, 1998, 24: 796.6.

Jennum, P. and Klitgaard, H. Repetitive transcranial magnetic stimulations of the rat. Effect of acute and chronic stimulations on pentylenetetrazole-induced clonic seizures. *Epil. Res.*, 1996, 23: 115–122.

Ji, R.R., Schlaepfer, T.E., Aizenman, C.D., Epstein, C.M., Qiu, D., Huang, J.C. and Rupp, F. Repetitive transcranial magnetic stimulation activates specific regions in rat brain. *Proc. Natl. Acad. Sci. USA*, 1998, 95: 15635–15640.

Kanno, M., Matsumoto, M., Togashi, H., Yoshioka, M. and Mano, Y. Effects of repetitive transcranial magnetic stimulation on behavioral and neurochemical changes in rats during an elevated plus-maze test. *J. Neurol. Sci.*, 2003: in press.

Keck, M.E. and Holsboer, F. Hyperactivity of CRH neuronal circuits as a target for therapeutic interventions in affective disorders. *Peptides*, 2001, 22: 835–844.

Keck, M.E., Pijnappels, M., Schubert, M., Colombo, G., Curt, A. and Dietz, V. Stumbling reactions in man: influence of corticospinal input. *Electroencephalogr. Clin. Neurophysiol.*, 1998, 109: 215–223.

Keck, M.E., Engelmann, M., Müller, M.B., Henniger, M.S.H., Hermann, B., Rupprecht, R., Neumann, I.D., Toschi, N., Landgraf, R. and Post, A. Repetitive transcranial magnetic stimulation induces active coping strategies and attenuates the neuroendocrine stress response in rats. *J. Psychiatr. Res.*, 2000a, 34: 265–276.

Keck, M.E., Hatzinger, M., Wotjak, C.T., Holsboer, F., Landgraf, R. and Neumann, I.D. Ageing alters intrabypothalamic release patterns of vasopressin and oxytocin in rats. *Eur. J. Neurosci.*, 2000b, 12: 1487–1494.

Keck, M.E., Sillaber, l., Ebner, K., Welt, T., Toschi, N., Kaehler, S.T., Singewald, N., Philippu, A., Elbel, G.K., Wotjak, C.T., Holsboer, F., Landgraf, R. and Engelmann, M. Acute transcranial magnetic stimulation of frontal brain regions selectively modulates the release of vasopressin, biogenic amines and amino acids in the rat brain. *Eur. J. Neurosci.*, 2000c, 12: 3713–3720.

Keck, M.E., Welt, T., Post, A., Müller, M.B., Toschi, N., Wigger, A., Landgraf, R., Holsboer, F. and Engelmann, M. Neuroendocrine and behavioral effects of repetitive transcranial magnetic stimulation in a psychopathological animal model are suggestive of antidepressant-like effects. *Neuropsychopharmacol.* 2001a, 24: 337–349.

Keck, M.E., Welt, T., Wigger, A., Renner, U., Engelmann, M., Holsboer, F. and Landgraf, R. The anxiolytic effect of the CRH' receptor antagonist R121919 depends on innate emotionality in rats. *Eur. J. Neurosci.*, 2001b, 13: 373–380.

Keck, M.E., Welt, T., Müller, M.B., Erhardt, A., Ohl, F., Toschi, N., Holsboer, F. and Sillaber, I. Repetitive transcranial magnetic stimulation increases the release of dopamine in the mesolimbic and mesostriatal system. *Neuropharmacology*, 2002a, 43: 101–109.

Keck, M.E., Wigger, A., Welt, T., Müller, M.B., Gesing, A., Reul, J.M.H.M., Holsboer, F., Landgraf, R. and Neumann, I.D. Vasopressin mediates the response of the combined dexamethasone/CRH test in hyper-anxious rats: implications for pathogenesis of affective disorders. *Neuropsychopharmacol.*, 2002b, 26: 94–105.

Keck, M.E., Welt, T., Müller, M.B., Landgraf, R. and Holsboer, F. The high-affinity non-peptide CRH1 receptor antagonist R121919 attenuates stress-induced alterations in plasma oxytocin, prolactin, and testosterone in rats. *Pharmacopsychiatry*, 2003a, 36: 27–31.

Keck, M.E., Welt, T., Müller, M.B., Uhr, M., Ohl, F., Wigger, A., Toschi, N., Holsboer, F. and Landgraf, R. Reduction of hypothalamic vasopressinergic hyperdrive contributes to clinically relevant behavioral and neuroendocrine effects of chronic paroxetine treatment in a psychopathological rat model. *Neuropsychopharmacol.*, 2003b, 28: 235–243.

Kendler, K.S., Karkowski, L.M. and Prescott, C.A. Causal relationship between stressful life events and the onset of major depression. *Am. J. Psychiatr.*, 1999, 156: 837–841.

Kimbrell, T.A., Little, J.A., Dunn, R.T., Frye, M.A., Greenberg, B.D., Wassermann, E.M., Repella, J.D., Danielson, A.L., Willis, M.W., Benson, B.E., Speer, A.M., Osuch, E., George, M.S. and Post, R.M. Frequency dependence of antidepressant response to left prefrontal repetitive transcranial magnetic stimulation (rTMS) as a function of baseline cerebral glucose metabolism. *Biol. Psychiat.*, 1999, 46: 1603–1613.

Kolbinger, H.M., Höflich, G., Hufnagel, A., Moller, H.J. and Kasper, S. Transcranial magnetic stimulation (TMS) in the treatment of major depression – a pilot study. *Hum. Psychopharmacol.*, 1995, 10: 305–310.

Kole, M.H.P,, Fuchs, E., Ziemann, U., Paulus, W. and Ebert, U. Changes in 5-HT1A and NMDA binding sites by a single rapid transcranial magnetic stimulation procedure in rats. *Brain Res.*, 1999, 826: 309–312.

Landgraf, R. Intracerebrally released vasopressin and oxytocin: measurement, mechanisms and behavioural consequences. *J. Neuroendocrinol.*, 1995, 7: 243–253.

Landgraf, R., Wotjak, C.T., Neumann, I.D. and Engelmann, M. Release of vasopressin within the brain contributes to neuroendocrine and behavioral regulation. In: J.P.H. Burbach and D. De Wied (Eds.), *Progress in Brain Research*. I.J.A. Urban, Elsevier, Amsterdam, 1998, 119: 201–220.

Landgraf, R., Wigger, A., Holsboer, F. and Neumann, I.D. Hyperreactive hypothalamo-pituitary-adrenocortical (HPA) axis in rats bred for high anxiety-related behavior. *J. Neuroendocrinol.*, 1999, 11: 405–407.

Levkovitz, Y. and Segal, M. Aging affects transcranial magnetic modulation of hippocampal evoked potentials. *Neurobiol. Aging*, 2001, 22: 255–263.

Levkovitz, Y., Marx, J., Grisaru, N. and Segal, M. Long-term effects of transcranial magnetic stimulation on hippocampal reactivity to afferent stimulation. *J. Neurosci.*, 1999, 19: 3198–3203.

Levkovitz, Y., Grisaru, N. and Segal, M. Transcranial magnetic stimulation and antidepressive drugs share similar cellular effects in rat hippocampus. *Neuropsychopharmacol.*, 2001, 25: 608–618.

Lewin, G.R. and Barde, Y.A. Physiology of neurotrophins. *Ann. Rev. Neurosci.*, 1996, 19: 289–317.

Liebetanz, D., Fauser, S., Michaelis, T., Czeh, B., Watanabe, T., Paulus, W., Frahm, J. and Fuchs, E. Safety aspects of chronic low-frequency transcranial magnetic stimulation based on localized proton magnetic resonance spectroscopy and histology of the rat brain. *J. Psychiatr. Res.*, 2003, 37: 277–286.

Liebsch, G., Linthorst, A.C.E., Neumann, I.D., Reul, J.M.H.M., Holsboer, F. and Landgraf, R. Behavioral, physiological, and neuroendocrine stress responses and differential sensitivity to diazepam in two Wistar rat lines selectively bred for high and low anxiety-related behavior. *Neuropsychopharmacol.*, 1998a, 19: 381–396.

Liebsch, G., Montkowski, A., Holsboer, F. and Landgraf, R. Behavioural profiles of two Wistar rat lines selectively bred for high or low anxiety-related behaviour. *Behav. Brain Res.*, 1998b, 94: 301–310.

Linden, R.D., Zhang, Y.P., Burke, D.A., Hunt, M.A., Harpring, J.E. and Shields, C.B. Magnetic motor evoked potential monitoring in the rat. *J. Neurosurg.*, 1999, 91: 205–210.

Lisanby, S.H., Kinnunen, L.H., Crupain, M.J. Applications of TMS to therapy in psychiatry. *J. Clin. Neurophysiol.*, 2002, 19: 344–360.

Loo, C.K., Taylor, J.L., Gandevia, S.C., McDarmont, B.N., Mitchell, P.B. and Sachdev, P.S. Transcranial magnetic stimulation (TMS) in controlled treatment studies: are some "sham" forms active? *Biol. Psychiat.*, 2000, 47: 325–331.

Lopez, J.F., Chalmers, D.T., Little, K.Y. and Watson, S.J. Regulation of serotonin 1A, glucocorticoid, and mineralocorticoid receptor in rat and human hippocampus: implications for the neurobiology of depression. *Biol. Psychiat.*, 1998, 43: 547–573.

Luft, A.R., Kaelin-Lang, A., Hauser, T.K., Cohen, L.G., Thakor, N.V. and Hanley, D.F. Trancranial magnetic stimulation in the rat. *Exp. Brain Res.*, 2001, 140: 112–121.

Madsen, T.M., Treschow, A., Bengzon, J., Bolwig, T.G., Lindvall, O. and Tingstrom, A. Increased neurogenesis in a model of electroconvulsive therapy. *Biol. Psychiat.*, 2000, 47: 1043–1049.

Maes, M., Verkerk, R., Vandoolaeghe, E., Lin, A. and Scharpe, S. Serum levels of excitatory amino acids, serine, glycine, histidine, threonine, taurine, alanine and arginine in treatment-resistant depression: modulation by treatment with antidepressants and prediction of clinical responsivity. *Acta Psychiat. Scand.*, 1998, 97: 302–308.

Malberg, J.E., Eisch, A.J., Nestler, E.J. and Duman, R.S. Chronic antidepressant treatment increases neurogenesis in adult rat hippocampus. *J. Neurosci.*, 2000, 20: 9104–9110.

Mosimann, U.P., Marre, S.C., Werlen, S., Schmitt, W., Hess, C.W., Fisch, H.U. and Schlaepfer, T.E. Antidepressant effects of repetitive transcranial magnetic stimulation in the elderly: correlation between effect size and coil-cortex distance. *Arch. Gen. Psychiat.*, 2002, 59: 560–561.

Müller, M.B. and Keck, M.E. Genetically engineered mice for studies of stress-related clinical conditions. *J. Psychiatr. Res.*, 2002, 36: 53–76.

Müller, M.B., Landgraf, R. and Keck, M.E. Vasopressin, major depression, and hypothalamic-pituitary-adrenocortical desensitization. *Biol. Psychiat.*, 2000a, 47: 330–333.

Müller, M.B., Toschi, N., Kresse, A.E., Post, A. and Keck, M.E. Long-term repetitive transcranial magnetic stimulation increases the expression of brain-derived neurotrophic factor and cholecystokinin mRNA, but not neuropeptide tyrosine mRNA in specific areas of rat brain. *Neuropsychopharmacol.*, 2000b, 23: 205–215.

Müller, M.B., Holsboer, F. and Keck, M.E. Genetic modification of corticosteroid receptor signaling: novel insights into pathophysiology and treatment strategies of human affective disorders. *Neuropeptides*, 2002, 36: 117–131.

Nahas, Z., Molloy, M., Risch, S.C. and George, M.S. TMS in schizophrenia. In: M.S. George and R.H. Belmaker (Eds.), *Transcranial Magnetic Stimulation in Neuropsychiatry*. American Psychiatric Press, Inc., Washington DC, 2000: 237–252.

Nibuya, M., Morinobu, S. and Duman, R.S. Regulation of BDNF and trkB mRNA in rat brain by chronic electroconvulsive seizure and antidepressant drug treatments. *J. Neurosci.*, 1995, 15: 7539–7547.

Nibuya, M., Nestler, E. and Duman, R.S. Chronic antidepressant administration increases the expression of cAMP response element binding protein (CREB) in rat hippocampus. *J. Neurosci.*, 1996, 16: 2365–2372.

Ohl, F., Toschi, N., Wigger, A., Henniger, M.S.H. and Landgraf, R. Dimensions of emotionality in a rat model of innate anxiety. *Behav. Neurosci.*, 2001, 115: 429–436.

Padberg, F. and Möller, H.J. Repetitive transcranial magnetic stimulation: Does it have potential in the treatment of depression? *CNS Drugs*, 2003, 17: 383–403.

Padberg, F., Zwanzger, P., Thoma, H., Kathmann, N., Haag, C., Greenberg, B.D., Hampel, H. and Möller, H.J. Repetitive transcranial magnetic stimulation (rTMS) in pharmacotherapy-refractory major depression: comparative study of fast, slow and sham rTMS. *Psychiatry Res.*, 1999, 88: 163- 171.

Padberg, F., Schüle, C., Zwanzger, P., Baghai, T., Ella, R., Mikhaiel, P., Hampel, H., Möller, H.J. and Rupprecht, R. Relation between responses to repetitive transcranial magnetic stimulation and partial sleep deprivation in major depression. *J. Psychiatr. Res.*, 2002a, 36: 131–135.

Padberg, F., Zwanzger, P., Keck, M.E., Kathmann, N., Mikhaiel, P., Ella, R., Rupprecht, P., Thoma, H., Hampel, H., Toschi, N. and Möller, H.J. Repetitive transcranial magnetic stimulation (rTMS) in major depression: Relation between efficacy and stimulation intensity. *Neuropsychopharmacol.*, 2002b, 27: 638–645.

Pangalos, M.N., Malizia, A.L., Francis, P.T., Lowe, S.L., Bertolucci, P.H., Procter, A.W., Bridges, P.K., Bartlett, J.R. and

Bowen, D.M. Effect of psychotropic drugs on excitatory amino acids in patients undergoing psychosurgery for depression. *Br. J. Psychiat.*, 1992, 160: 638–642.

Pascual-Leone, A., Rubio, B., Pallardo, F. and Catala, M.D. Rapid-rate transcranial magnetic stimulation of left dorsolateral prefrontal cortex in drug-resistant depression. *Lancet*, 1996, 348: 233–237.

Petty, F. GABA and mood disorders: a brief review and hypothesis. *J. Affect. Disord.*, 1995, 34: 275–281.

Platt, J.E. and Stone, E.A. Chronic restraint stress elicits a positive antidepressant response on the forced swim test. *Eur. J. Pharmacol.*, 1982, 82: 179–181.

Post, A. and Keck, M.E. Transcranial magnetic stimulation as a therapeutic tool in psychiatry: what do we know about the neurobiological mechanisms? *J. Psychiat. Res.*, 2001, 35: 193–215.

Post, A., Müller, M.B., Engelmann, M. and Keck, M.E. Repetitive transcranial magnetic stimulation in rats: evidence for a neuroprotective effect in vitro and in vivo. *Eur. J. Neurosci.*, 1999, 11: 3247–3254.

Purba, J.S., Hoogendijk, W.J.G., Hofman, M.A. and Swasb, D.F. Increased number of vasopressin- and oxytocin-expressing neurons in the paraventricular nucleus of the hypothalamus in depression. *Arch. Gen. Psychiat.*, 1996, 53: 137–143.

Raber, J. Detrimental effects of chronic hypothalamic-pituitary-adrenal axis activation. From obesity to memory deficits. *Mol. Neurobiol.*, 1998, 18: 1–22.

Reul, J.M.H.M., Gesing, A., Droste, S., Stec, I.S.M., Weber, A., Bachmann, C., Bilang-Bleuel, A., Holsboer, F. and Linthorst, A.C.E. The brain mineralocorticoid receptor: greedy for ligand, mysterious in function. *Eur. J. Pharmacol.*, 2000, 405: 235–249.

Rollnik, J.D., Huber, T.J., Mogk, H., Siggelkow, S., Kropp, S., Dengler, R., Emrich, H.M. and Schneider, U. High frequency repetitive transcranial magnetic stimulation (rTMS) of the dorsolateral prefrontal cortex in schizophrenic patients. *Neuroreport*, 2000, 11: 4013–4015.

Rossini, P.M. and Rossi, S. Clinical applications of motor evoked potentials. *Electroencephalogr. Clin. Neurophysiol.*, 1998, 106: 180–194.

Rossini, P.M., Barker, A.T., Berardelli, A., Caramia, M.D., Caruso, G., Cracco, R.Q., Dimitrijevic, M.R., Hallett, M., Katayama, Y., Lucking, C.H., Denoordhout, A.L.M., Marsden, C.D., Murray, N.M.F., Rothwell, J.C., Swash, M. and Tomberg, C. Non-invasive electrical and magnetic stimulation of the brain, spinal cord and roots – basic principles and procedures for routine clinical application – report of an IFCN commitee. *Electroencephalogr. Clin. Neurophysiol.*, 1994, 91: 79–92.

Sachdev, P.S., McBride, R., Loo, C., Mitchell, P.M., Malhi, G.S. and Croker, V. Effects of different frequencies of transcranial magnetic stimulation (TMS) on the forced swim test model of depression in rats. *Biol. Psychiat.*, 2002, 51: 474–479.

Scott, B.W., Wojtowicz, J.M. and Burnham, W.M. Neurogenesis in the dentate gyrus of the rat following electroconvulsive shock seizures. *Exp. Neurol.*, 2000, 165: 231–236.

Seckl, J.R. and Fink, G. Antidepressants increase glucocorticoid and mineralocorticoid receptor mRNA expression in rat hippocampus in vivo. *Neuroendocrinology*, 1992, 55: 621–626.

Sesack, S.R. and Pickel, V.M. Prefrontal cortex efferents in the rat synapse on unlabeled neuronal targets of catecholamine terminals in the nucleus accumbens septi and on dopamine neurons in the ventral tegmental area. *J. Comp. Neurol.*, 1992, 320: 145–160.

Shimohama, S., Tamura, Y., Akaike, A., Tsukahara, T., Ohara, O., Watanabe, S. and Kimura, J. Brain-derived neurotrophic factor pretreatment exerts a partially protective effect against glutamate-induced neurotoxicity in cultured rat cortical neurons. *Neurosci. Lett.*, 1993, 164: 55–58.

Shors, T.J., Miesegaes, G., Beylin, A., Zhao, M., Rydel, T. and Gould, E. Neurogenesis in the adult is involved in the formation of trace memories. *Nature*, 2001, 410: 372–376.

Siebner, H.R. and Rothwell, J. Trancranial magnetic stimulation: new insights into representational cortical plasticity. *Exp. Brain Res.*, 2003, 148: 1–16.

Siuciak, J.A., Lewis, D.R., Wiegand, S.J. and Lindsay, R.M. Antidepressant-like effect of brain-derived neurotrophic factor (BDNF). *Pharmacol. Biochem. Behav.*, 1997, 56: 131–137.

Soares, J.C. and Mann, J.J. The functional neuroanatomy of mood disorders. *J. Psychiatr. Res.*, 1997, 31: 393–432.

Steward, O., Kelly, M.S. and Torre, E.R. The process of reinnervation in the dentate gyrus of adult rats: temporal relationship between changes in the levels of glial fibrillary acidic protein (GFAP) and GFAP mRNA in reactive astrocytes. *Exp. Neurol.*, 1993, 124: 167–183.

Strafella, A.P., Paus, T., Barrett, J. and Dagher, A. Repetitive transcranial magnetic stimulation of the human prefrontal cortex induces dopamine release in the caudate nucleus. *J. Neurosci.*, 2001, 21: RC157, 1–4,.

Taber, M.T. and Fibiger, H.C. Electrical stimulation of the prefrontal cortex increases dopamine release in the nucleus accumbens of the rat: modulation by metabotropic glutamate receptors. *J. Neurosci.*, 1995, 15: 3896–3904.

Takagishi, M. and Chiba, T. Efferent projections of the infralimbic (area 25) region of the medial prefrontal cortex in the rat: an anterograde tracer PHA-L study. *Brain Res.*, 1991, 566: 26–39.

Van Praag, H., Schinder, A.F., Christie, B.R., Toni, N., Palmer, T.D. and Gage, F.H. Functional neurogenesis in the adult hippocampus. *Nature*, 2002, 415: 1030–1034.

Von Bardeleben, U. and Holsboer, F. Cortisol response to a combined dexamethasone-human corticotropin-releasing hormone (CRH) challenge in patients with depression. *J. Neuroendocrinol.*, 1989, 1: 485–488.

Wang, H., Wang, X. and Scheich, H. LTD and LTP induced by transcranial magnetic stimulation in auditory cortex. *Neuroreport*, 1996, 7: 521–525.

Wassermann, E.M. Risk and safety of repetitive transcranial magnetic stimulation: report and suggested guidelines from the International Workshop on the Safety of Repetitive Transcranial

Magnetic Stimulation, June 5–7, 1996. *Electroencephalogr. Clin. Neurophysiol.*, 1998, 108: 1–16.

Wotjak, C.T., Kubota, M., Liebsch, G., Montkowski, A., Holsboer, F., Neumann, I. and Landgraf, R. Release of vasopressin within the rat paraventricular nucleus in response to emotional stress: a novel mechanism of regulating adrenocorticotropic hormone secretion? *J. Neurosci.*, 1996, 16: 7725–7732.

Yoshida, K., Higuchi, H., Kamata, M., Yoshimoto, M., Shimizu, T. and Hishikawa, Y. Dopamine releasing response in rat striatum to single and repeated electroconvulsive shock treatment. *Prog. Neuro-Psychopharmacol. Biol. Psychiat.*, 1997, 21: 707–715.

You, Z.B., Tzschentke, T.M., Brodin, E. and Wise, R.A. Electrical stimulation of the prefrontal cortex increases cholecystokinin, glutamate, and dopamine release in the nucleus accumbens: an in vivo microdialysis study in freely moving rats. *J. Neurosci.*, 1998,18: 6492–6500.

Zobel, A.W., Nickel, T., Sonntag, A., Uhr, M., Holsboer, F. and Ising M Cortisol response in the combined dexamethasone/CRH test as predictor of relapse in patients with remitted depression: a prospective study. *J. Psychiatr. Res.*, 2001, 35: 83–94.

Zyss, T., Gorka, Z., Kowalska, M. and Vetulani, J. Preliminary comparison of behavioral and biochemical effects of chronic transcranial magnetic stimulation and electroconvulsive shock in the rat. *Biol. Psychiat.*, 1997, 42: 920–924.

Section III

Motor Control

Transcranial Magnetic Stimulation and Transcranial Direct Current Stimulation (Supplements to Clinical Neurophysiology, Vol. 56)
Editors: W. Paulus, F. Tergau, M.A. Nitsche, J.C. Rothwell, U. Ziemann, M. Hallett

Chapter 11

Motor cortical and other cortical interneuronal networks that generate very high frequency waves

Vahe E. Amassian[a,b,*] and Mark Stewart[a]

Departments of [a]Physiology and Pharmacology and [b]Neurology, State University of New York, Downstate Medical Center, Brooklyn, NY 11203 (USA)

1. Introduction

Among neocortical areas, the motor cortex early presented a favorable opportunity of applying the "black box" approach in analyzing the functions of the complex cortical synaptic network. Some of its output neurons, projecting in "pure culture" in the pyramidal tract (PT) and relatively accessible in the lateral corticospinal tract (CT), readily permitted population and single fiber recording of the I responses. From such PT and CT recordings, inferences could be made as to the direct and synaptic bases for the descending volleys, with subsequent testing of the hypotheses by recording intra- and extracellularly within the motor cortex. Furthermore, the study of the relationship of PT unit activity to behavior in the awake monkey as pioneered by Evarts (1968) provided a crucial guide to identifying the physiological significance of the output neuronal activities.

A remarkable feature of the human motor cortex is that single, brief electrical or magnetic stimuli can elicit periodic, high frequency (above 500 Hz) waves in the major, fast conducting output neuron of the system, the large pyramidal tract (PT) or corticospinal tract (CT) neuron. Such periodic responses were first recorded in animal preparations and identified as directly (D), and indirectly (I), excited PT or CT neurons (Patton and Amassian, 1954, 1960; Kernell and Wu, 1967; Rosenthal et al., 1967). In human recordings, D and I discharges in the CT were correctly inferred from measurements of muscle response latencies to anodic and magnetic stimulation and from discrete latency jumps in single motor units (review: Rothwell et al., 1991). Subsequently, the validity of these inferences was confirmed by recordings from the spinal cord (Boyd et al., 1986; Katayama et al., 1988; Matsuma and Shimazu, 1989; Berardelli et al., 1990; Burke et al., 1990, 1992, 1993; Deletis, 1993, 1994; Fujiki et al., 1996; Kaneko et al., 1996; Nakamura et al., 1996; Deletis and Kothbauer, 1998; Di Lazzaro et al., 1998; Amassian and Deletis, 1999). The existence of very high frequency CT responses to a single, brief cortical stimulus raises several questions, including: (1) how widespread are such high frequency CT activities in mammalian forms? (2) what is their synaptic (or membrane) basis?

* *Correspondence to*: Professor Vahe E. Amassian, Department of Physiology and Pharmacology, SUNY Downstate Medical Center, 450 Clarkson Avenue, Box 31, Brooklyn, NY 11203, USA.
Tel: 718-270-3900; Fax: 718-270-3103;
E-mail: mark@theta.hippo.hscbklyn.edu

(3) how widespread are they in other neocortical neuronal systems? (4) are comparable activities present in archicortex, i.e. hippocampus and related structures? Finally, (5) what is the possible physiological significance of such high frequency neocortical activity when it is most easily elicited by unphysiological stimuli such as electrical or magnetic pulses?

2. Phylogeny of D and I waves in the CT and PT

A comparison of D and I waves in the anesthetized rat, cat, monkey and human reveals an increasing trend in higher forms towards sharp definition of each wave in the D-multiple I wave complex when appropriately recorded (Fig. 1). Optimal population recording from the PT or CT depends on blocking conduction in the fibers to avoid phase cancellation in less than perfectly synchronized discharges; blocking conduction converts the classical (+ – +) potential change in the volume conductor into a usually longer lasting and higher amplitude positive wave. Furthermore, the reference electrode must be sufficiently distant from the focal electrode to avoid differentiating the response and thereby artificially creating the appearance of separate waves (Fehlings et al., 1988; cf. Stewart et al., 1990).

In humans, whether lightly anesthetized or awake, the separate identities of I_1, I_2, I_3, etc. are very clear despite conduction in the CT fibers from cerebral cortex to cervical and thoracic cord, a distance several orders of magnitude greater than in the animal recordings described below (Katayama et al., 1988; Burke et al., 1990; Deletis and Kothbauer, 1998; Di Lazzaro et al., 1998; Deletis et al., 2001b). Such findings do not reflect a human CT conduction velocity higher than in all other species, nor can they be explained by a narrower band of responding CT fibers. In rare blocked conduction recordings in a human, the predominantly positive D wave recorded from the cervical and thoracic spinal cord had durations of 2.8 and 2.2 ms, respectively (Matsuma and Shimazu, 1989; Katayama et al., 1994). Thus, a transient stimulus elicits an extraordinary periodic synchronization of CT neuronal excitation in the human.

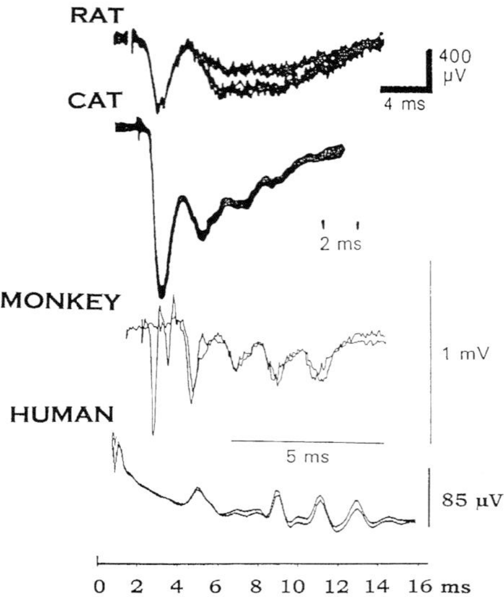

Fig. 1. Phylogenetic trend in I waves in PT and CT. In each recording, the small initial deflection is an electric stimulus artifact. Positivity of the focal electrode indicated by downward deflection of the sweep. From top to bottom, recordings are from rat, cat, monkey and human. Rat: five superimposed CT responses recorded with a 125 µm Teflon insulated tungsten wire at the level of C_1–C_2 following focal stimulation of motor cortex. Rat under urethane anesthesia. The initial D wave is followed 4 ms later by a much broader I wave; superimposed is the increased I wave after topically applying pentylentetrazol to the motor cortex. Reproduced from Stewart et al. (1990). Cat: D followed by three I waves recorded from medullary pyramid. Cat under dial anesthesia. Reproduced from Patton and Amassian (1954). Monkey: D wave followed by three I waves recorded from medullary pyramid and 22 mm distally from lateral CT. At each of the pyramidal and CT recording sites, 18 responses were averaged. The gain of the PT recording was increased ×1.26 and the D waves were superimposed in the CT recording showing that I wave synchrony and periodicity are conserved despite the 22 mm additional conduction distance. Reproduced from Amassian et al. (1987). Human: superimposed epidural recordings from midthoracic level of a patient undergoing scoliosis surgery. Focal anode at C_z and cathode at F_z. Stimulating pulse was 750 V given at 0 ms. The D wave peaks at 4 ms, is followed by clear I wave peaks at 9, 11 and 13 ms. I_1 at 7 ms is virtually absent because monosynaptically excitatory parietal corticocortical afferents would not be optimally stimulated by this stimulating montage (cf. C_z vs. P_z). Reproduced from Deletis (1993).

Similarly, the I waves remain clearly separated after conduction in the anesthetized monkey (Amassian et al., 1987), but it should be noted that the responses (as in lower forms) were recorded over much shorter conduction distances than in the human thoracic spinal cord. In the anesthetized cat, at least two I waves are readily observed following the D wave, but typically the earliest part of an I wave takes off from the antecedent I wave, without an intervening return to baseline. However, in cats under chloralose, a convulsant anesthetic (Patton and Amassian, 1954), or after a seizure has been induced (Berlin and Amassian, 1965), the I wave complex is prolonged and the separate identity of the I components tends to be obscured.

In the rat, the I wave complex in the CT is a broad positive wave, without obvious differentiation into separate I components. A possible factor in the differing I wave appearance in the rat is the much smaller diameter of the CT fibers, which rarely exceed 5 μm, with a maximum conduction velocity of 18 m/s (Stewart et al., 1990). By contrast, the conduction velocity of CT fibers in cat, monkey and human is at least three times greater. Conduction delays in the slower fibers in a given D or I discharge would increase relative to that in the fastest fibers as a function of the distance traveled, thereby tending to increase the duration of the D and I wave components. The absolute increase in duration would be augmented given the slower CT fiber spectrum in the rat; an increased duration of the I wave components would lead to some merging of the I wave components. However, in the rat, the D wave despite its slow conduction velocity, is clearly defined in the CT recorded at the C_1-C_2 level. If, as proved in the monkey, CT fibers discharging during D and I waves have comparable conduction velocities, then I wave components should also be readily identifiable within the overall I wave of the rat; their nearly complete merging in a broad I wave implies a relative lack of synchronized excitation of periodically discharging CT neurons during each response. Further evidence of a differing property of CT discharge in the rat is provided by the twofold increase in D-I wave interval (4 ms) as compared with that in higher forms (1.3–2.0 ms). (This is discussed in Section 3.3.3.)

3. Synaptic vs. intrinsic membrane basis of high frequency PT and CT response

The high frequency periodic PT or CT response to a single electrical or magnetic stimulus might reflect: (a) the direct membrane response of CT neurons; (b) the postsynaptic response of CT neurons to the presynaptic volley, or (c) the response to repeated excitations by a cortical interneuronal network. The analysis of PT or CT high frequency periodic waves first requires determining whether the individual neurons respond repetitively at similar high frequencies, or during only one I wave or some of the I waves. In the cat, partial occlusion occurring between a D wave elicited by a second electrical stimulus given during I_1 and I_2 implies that the same CT neurons can discharge during the D and an I wave, a deduction confirmed by single unit recording in the cat and monkey. In the cat, the unit D-I and I discharge frequency reached 680 Hz (Fig. 9C in Patton and Amassian, 1954). With high intensity cortical stimulation, Kernell and Wu (1967) showed a CT fiber in the monkey could discharge during the D wave and each of the four I waves at even higher frequency. Nevertheless, it is clear that not all I activation of units in cat and monkey is preceded by D activation, which evidently depends on matching the site of stimulation to that of the CT neuron (Patton and Amassian, 1954). Summarizing, the high frequency population CT response is composed of neurons responding: (a) only in the D wave; (b) during D and one or more I waves; and (c) only during one or more I waves.

3.1. Direct CT membrane response to an electrical or magnetic stimulus

The direct membrane response of PT neurons is best tested by intracellularly injected current. Significantly, such experiments by many investigators do not reveal a preferred period equaling that of the I wave, or its first harmonic, but always evidence gradable intervals as a function of depolarizing current intensity (e.g. Koike et al., 1970).

Extracellular cortical stimulation as a test of CT neuronal membrane function necessarily carries the risk also of activating other neurons, with added transynaptic activation of the CT neuron. Historically, surface anodic stimulation of motor cortex in monkeys was shown to excite directly neurons at lower threshold than that eliciting I discharge (Hern et al., 1962), but the D activity was recorded in responses conducted past the electrode, i.e. any I wave amplitude was underestimated unless CT conduction was blocked. The difference in threshold between D and I excitation by focal anodic stimulation is quite small (< 15%) when CT conduction is blocked (Amassian et al., 1987). With focal cathodic stimulation, I activation has a slightly lower threshold (by 10%) than for D activation, but the I threshold would clearly be influenced by anesthetic level. D activation requires a 50% increase in pulse intensity over that needed with focal anodic stimulation. More significantly, unlike with focal anodic stimulation, the monkey D wave elicited by a given focal cathodal stimuli is highly variable, leading to the conclusion that surface anodic stimulation excites CT axons at a distance from synapses on the CT neurons, i.e. in the white matter, while surface cathodal stimulation excites them near the initial segment (IS) or neighboring membrane (Amassian et al., 1990).

With surface bipolar stimulation, i.e. using an interpolar distance of several mm, the difference in threshold between D and I activation is further lessened. With threshold surface stimulation, the initial discharge of individual units 'jumps' between direct and earliest I latency. Intracellular recording in the cat revealed that D activation occurred when the prestimulus membrane potential was depolarized by ongoing synaptic activity; when the prestimulus membrane potential was more polarized, an I response was mediated by an EPSP elicited by the stimulus (Rosenthal et al., 1967).

Appropriately oriented (lateral-sagittal) magnetic stimuli at threshold elicit a 'pure' D wave in blocked monkey population CT fibers and in single CT fibers recordings (Amassian et al., 1990). Although recordings from the human CT are predominantly from unblocked fibers, the D/I wave ratio is clearly larger with a latero-medial (L-M) than with a postero-anterior (P-A) induced field (e.g. Kaneko et al., 1996), again confirming that D and I wave activation are differentially affected by using the appropriate orientation of the electric field.

In conclusion, at least in higher mammals, D activation unaccompanied by I wave can be elicited by direct electrical or magnetically induced activation of the PT membrane, thereby yielding no evidence of an intrinsic high frequency periodicity.

3.2. Postsynaptic CT neuronal membrane response to an afferent volley

The I wave periodicity could arise from the postsynaptic effect of a single presynaptic volley (Phillips, 1987), with prolonged transmitter induced multiple conductance increases (e.g. Na^+, K^+, Ca^{2+}), with or without electrogenic "boosting" in dendrites [e.g. fast prepotentials (Spencer and Kandel, 1957)]. Mammalian synapses elsewhere have long been known to grade latency, frequency and number of repetitive discharges as a function of stimulus intensity, e.g. at ascending levels in the neuraxis, e.g. ventroposterior thalamic neurons (Rose and Mountcastle, 1954) and archicortical neurons (Section 5). Thus, if I waves resulted from transmitter release by a single afferent volley, their periodicity would be expected to change as a function of the size of the afferent volley. For this test, candidate powerful excitatory sources for CT neurons include: (1) corticocortical fiber projections; (2) thalamic ventrolateral (VL) and ventroanterior (VA) projections; (3) thalamic ventroposterior (VP) projections; (4) motor cortical recurrent collaterals. The critical question is whether a given I wave period is conserved despite manipulation of the intensity, or the site of stimulation or the level of wakefulness.

3.2.1. Corticocortical projections

Evidence has long been available that single electrical pulses applied to parietal or premotor cortex of monkeys can elicit multiple I waves (Patton and Amassian, 1954, 1960); the anatomical projections underlying such activation of motor cortex were demonstrated by Pandya and Kuypers (1969). However, a hitherto unemphasized aspect of the I wave responses is the extraordinary conservation of the basic I wave period throughout a range of stimulus intensities eliciting a just suprathreshold to a seven-fold increase in I wave amplitude (Fig. 2). Similarly, altering the site of stimulation through parietal-to-motor-to-premotor cortex elicits major changes in relative amplitudes of the D and the multiple I waves, without a major change in the I wave periodicity (Fig. 3). Remarkably, the pattern of the I waves may increment during the response (as in Figs. 2 and 3), or decrement gradually or show a drastically reduced I_2 at some sites of stimulation with increased amplitude of later I waves (Fig. 3). Such differential amplitude changes in the periodic I wave responses are hard to reconcile with the post-synaptic action of a single presynaptic volley.

In humans, the role of corticocortical inputs to motor cortex has been investigated with TMS. A magnetic stimulus via a round coil at the vertex or via a figure-of-8 coil with junction parasagittally located and inducing a P-A directed electric field, typically elicits a hand muscle CMAP 1–2 ms later than the response to electrical anodic stimulation (reviewed by Rothwell et al., 1991). The latency difference is still greater with an A-P induced electric field (Sakai et al., 1997). The latency difference between electrical and magnetic stimulation can be demonstrated in single motor unit recordings (Rothwell et al., 1991), i.e. it does not depend on a difference in conduction velocity in the motoneurons responding to the two types of stimulation. Nor does the difference in latency reflect a peculiarity of magnetic stimulation because with the coil windings oriented latero-sagittally, CMAP latency can be equalized to that with electrical focal anodic stimulation (Amassian et al., 1989). Werhahn et al. (1994) established that the orientation of the induced electrical field was the crucial determinant of whether D activation (latero-medial; L-M field) or I activation (P-A field) of CT neurons occurs. The advent of direct recording of human D and I waves has given important confirmation of these inferences from EMG recordings (e.g. Kaneko et al., 1996).

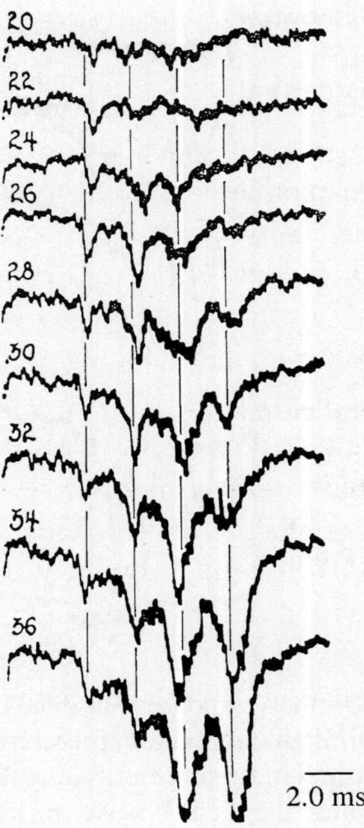

Fig. 2. Medullary PT responses in monkey to premotor cortical stimulation by electrical pulses at increasing intensity. Intensity in arbitrary units. Dial anesthesia. Reproduced from Patton and Amassian (1954), with addition of alignment lines related to corresponding I waves.

The evidence so far presented does not identify which portion of the corticocortical neuron has the lowest threshold to such sTMS stimulation. Two types of experiment implicate nodes of myelinated axons as the portions most readily excited. Barker et al. (1991) measured the chronaxie of neurons excited with the round coil at the vertex and found it approximated that of peripheral alpha motor axons. Rothwell et al. (1992) showed that facilitation of a near-threshold magnetic pulse (which induced an L-M directed field) by a focal anodic pulse had a decay time constant of 80–100 μs, again approximating that of peripheral alpha motor axons. Thus, the brevity of the time constant identified that nodal membrane was the portion excited. Subsequent modeling with peripheral nerve

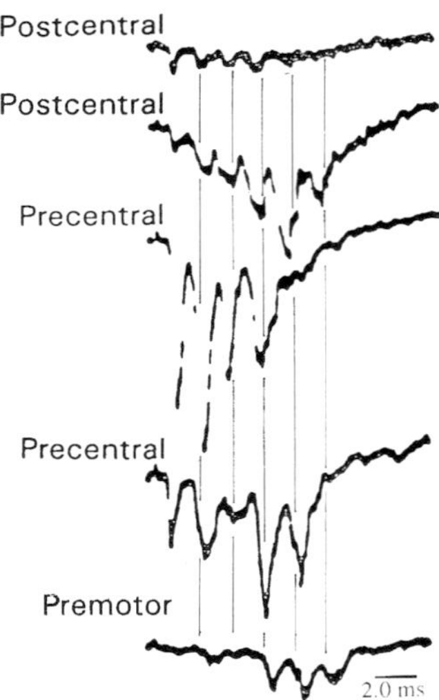

Fig. 3. Corticospinal responses in monkey to electrical stimulation of different postcentral, precentral and premotor sites. Dial anesthesia. At precentral stimulation sites, the D wave preceding the first I wave is large. The early I waves from the premotor site are very small. Records reproduced from responses in map in Patton and Amassian (1960) with addition of alignment lines related to corresponding I waves.

in a skull (Amassian et al., 1992) or a trough volume conductor (Maccabee et al., 1993) implied that a bend in a central axon created a low threshold point for membrane current exit and was therefore referred to as "bend" excitation. The complex neuropil of human motor cortex contains numerous myelinated axons (Braitenberg, 1961), the largest axons issuing presumably from the largest cortical neurons, the Betz cells. Despite the different orientations of Betz cells and the nearby portions of their axons in the anterior bank of the central sulcus, the gyral crown and the posterior bank of the precentral sulcus, excitation of CT neurons by the induced P-A field is typically indirect; such failure of direct excitation of the largest cortical axons by sTMS argues strongly against excitation by sTMS of any smaller myelinated fibers or neurons within the gray matter.

The bend superficially into motor cortex of corticocortical U fibers derived from other cortical areas, e.g. parietal and premotor areas, would constitute low threshold points for excitation. Classically, linear axons are best excited at the negative spatial derivative of the electric field; when using a figure-of-8 coil, the negative spatial derivative is near one of the bifurcations of the two coils, but bend excitation occurs optimally at the peak of the electric field near the midjunction (Maccabee et al., 1993). In agreement, when a figure-of-8 coil induces a P-A electric field, optimal hand muscle activation occurs when its midjunction and not the bifurcation of the coils is near the central sulcus. Confirmation of the excitatory efficacy in the human of both parietal and premotor corticocortical inputs was secured by demonstrating FDI facilitation with sTMS pulses applied through separate coils on each of parietal and premotor areas (Amassian et al., 1997). Thus, even when the coil is over motor cortex, with a P-A induced electric field the lowest threshold motor responses most likely result from corticocortical fiber excitation. However, it must be emphasized that when a just suprathreshold TMS pulse is followed 1 ms later by a subthreshold pulse, facilitation of the motor response most likely reflects activation within gray matter near the initial segment (IS) region, whose threshold was lowered by EPSPs resulting from corticocortical excitation by the first TMS pulse (Amassian et al., 1998; Ziemann et al., 1998a).

3.2.2. Thalamic VL-VA N projections

Powerful activation of feline PT neurons by stimulation of thalamic nuclei VL-VA has long been known (Brookhart and Zanchetti, 1956; Cohen et al., 1962; Schlag and Balvin, 1964) and contrasted with the weaker activation by "non-specific" thalamic nuclear stimulation (Nacimiento et al., 1964; Purpura et al., 1964). Studies on the synaptology of PT neuronal activation by VL-VA disclosed that the earliest transynaptic discharges by large PT neurons are monosynaptic; with stronger stimulation, additional activation occurs after delays of 1.2 ms in the sleeping cat (Weiner and Amassian, 1967) and 1.3–1.8 ms, in either locally anesthetized cats or those anesthetized with chloralose or pentobarbital (Amassian and Weiner, 1966). Single PT unit recordings showed the period of the double discharges

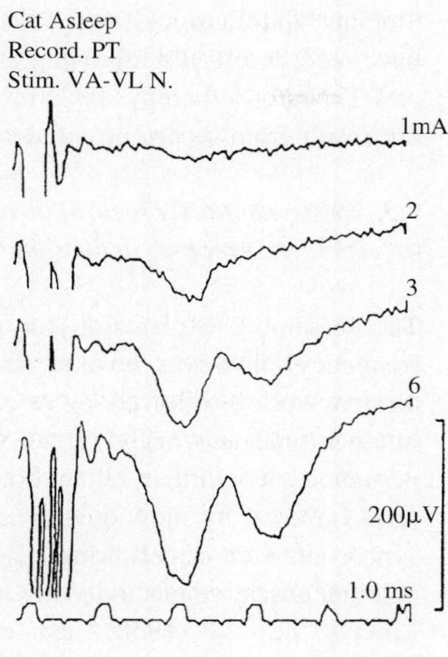

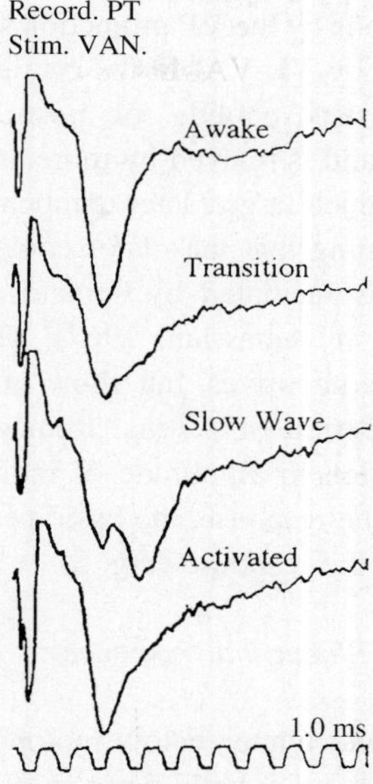

Fig. 4. Medullary PT responses in chronically implanted cat to thalamic N. stimulation. Left: cat asleep; electrical stimuli at increasing intensity (1–6 mA) delivered to N. ventralis lateral-anterior (VL-VA N.). At 3 mA, a disynaptic PT response is added to the monosynaptic response and present with weaker stimuli. Each trace shows the average of 200 responses. Stimulation rate 1 Hz. Right: differential effect of behavioral states on monosynaptic and disynaptic PT responses to same intensity electrical pulses delivered to dorsal VA N. at 1 per 2 s. Reproduced from Weiner and Amassian (1967). (Simultaneous electrocorticogram, eye movement and neck electromyogram records in cited reference.)

corresponds to the interval between the monosynaptic and the delayed waves, indicating that the delayed transynaptic wave did not reflect monosynaptically activated slow PT neurons. Could the delayed i.e. second PT wave or unit firing reflect a prolonged excitatory conductance change initiated by a single presynaptic input? As with a corticocortical volley, the interval between monosynaptic and delayed wave is minimally affected when the stimulus intensity is increased (Fig. 4). More significantly, changes in behavioral state from wakefulness through sleep stages differentially affect the monosynaptic and the delayed wave; the monosynaptic PT wave reached maximum amplitude during wakefulness and activated sleep, while during slow wave sleep, the monosynaptic wave was reduced and the delayed PT wave markedly increased. Such behavior is more readily explained by independent control of the excitability of PT and motor cortical interneurons during the wakefulness-sleep cycle, than by invoking the action of a single presynaptic volley on the PT neuronal membrane. It may be noted that VL-VA stimulation can monosynaptically activate motor cortical neurons that could not be labeled PT neurons by antidromic activation of the PT. While the existence of such neurons is essential for the 'interneuron' hypothesis, further proof that those recorded were excitatory rather than inhibitory is needed. Summarizing, the delayed wave has the properties expected of disynaptic activation of PT neurons.

The number of PT wave responses to VL-VA stimulation is strikingly fewer than with corticocortical stimulation (cf. Figs. 2, 3 vs. 4). The ubiquitous occurrence in PT neurons of an IPSP with a latency of 3 ms or more following VL-VA stimulation (e.g. Nacimiento et al., 1964) provides a ready explanation for the fewer relayed waves in this response.

3.2.3. Thalamic VP projections

Activation of PT neurons by the VP projection system is more complex than by VL-VA. In the cat, a small initial component resists cooling of post-dimple somatosensory area I and is relayed by more anterior cortex; however, the much larger, later component, is clearly reduced indicating that the major component of the PT response is mediated by somatosensory cortical relay (Fig. 1 in Amassian, 1967). The PT responses are not smooth waves, but show multiple components, with a period of 1.7 ms. Remarkably, despite marked variation in amplitude of individual wave components in the response, the basic period is conserved throughout the response (Fig. 5).

3.2.4. Postsynaptic CT neuronal response to recurrent collaterals

A stimulus to the white matter below motor cortex generates only a D wave, i.e. antidromic invasion of recurrent PT collaterals of fast PT neurons could not account for the I wave sequence (Patton and Amassian, 1954). Numerous studies (Phillips, 1956; Stefanis and Jasper, 1964; Takahashi et al., 1967) have recorded IPSPs following antidromic activation of PT neurons thereby explaining why I waves do not result from recurrent collateral action.

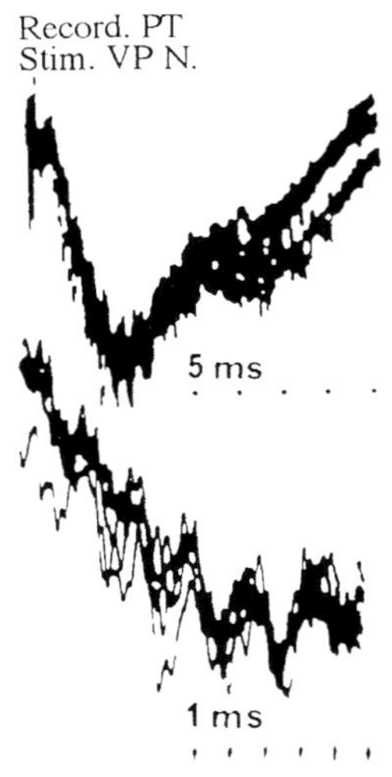

Fig. 5. Medullary PT responses of cat to electrical stimulation of ventralis posterior nucleus (VPN.). Chloralose anesthesia. Five superimposed traces at slow (above) and fast (below) sweep speeds showing conservation of period despite markedly differing number of responding PT fibers. Reproduced from Amassian and Weiner (1966).

3.3. Postsynaptic CT neuronal response to periodic or repetitive synaptic activation

The remaining explanation for multiple, very high frequency PT waves invokes first excitation by the afferent volley followed by re-excitation by a local interneuronal network (Fig. 6). Conservation of the periodicity would then reflect both the timing boundaries imposed by individual synaptic delays and the synchronization of cell firing. The meticulous tracing of intracortical connectivity in Golgi preparations by Lorente de Nó (1938) had earlier provided an anatomical basis for impulse flow from superficial to deep laminae, however, whether the connectivities were excitatory or inhibitory could not then be established by histological examination.

3.3.1. The I_1 discharge

The first I response in individual CT fibers occurs 1.2–1.6 ms later than the D discharge following a threshold stimulus to feline motor cortex, the discharge “jumping” between D and I latencies (Watson and Amassian, 1961). Initially, this suggested that an excitatory interneuron was interposed between the stimulated presynaptic input and the CT neuron, analogous to the Bishop and Clare (1953) proposal for visual cortical connectivity (see Section 4.1). Subsequently, intracellular recording revealed the slow EPSP rise to firing level (13.5 ± 4.1 V/s; mean, S.D.) in PT and uninvaded motor cortical neurons (Rosenthal et al., 1967). Furthermore, the D-I interval distributions in both invaded and uninvaded neurons were similar, i.e. no evidence of an intermediately activated group of motor cortical neurons was found. Thus, the I_1 discharge is monosynaptically mediated, i.e. by afferent fibers connecting with the CT neuron.

3.3.2. The I_2 discharge

The initial intracellular recordings of uninjured PT neurons (Phillips, 1956) and those of subsequent

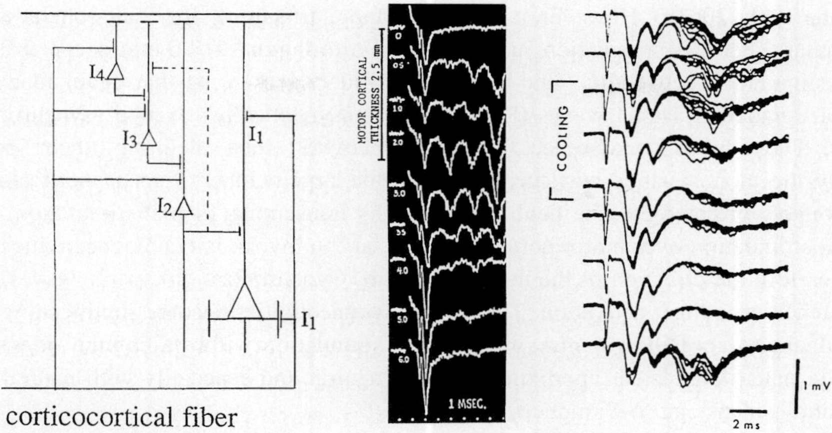

Fig. 6. Vertical organization of interneuronal chain exciting CT neurons revealed by intracortical stimulation and surface cooling of simian motor cortex. Right: 10 superimposed CT traces before, during and after cooling pial surface. Pentobarbital anesthesia. Focal cathode approximately 1 mm posterior to cooling probe. Current intensity 4.3 mA, 100 μs pulse duration. Middle: CT responses to microelectrode stimulation at the surface, within and below motor cortex at the indicated depths. Dial anesthesia. Left: diagram indicating a possible vertically oriented excitatory interneuronal chain capable of generating multiple, high frequency I waves following corticocortical afferent excitation. The dotted line indicates the possibility of "closed" chain functioning for which evidence is currently lacking. Inhibitory neurons are not shown but play an essential role in limiting the number of I waves. I_1 discharge relates to parietal, but not premotor corticortical input. Right record reproduced from Amassian et al., 1987; middle record reproduced from Patton and Amassian, 1954; left record reproduced from Amassian and Deletis, 1999.

investigators show partial destruction of the EPSP following the action potential of e.g. ≥ 70 mV; this implies the need for additional synaptic excitation of the PT neuron for the I_2 discharge as evidenced by a second EPSP in a few recordings on slower displays (Rosenthal et al., 1967). The I_2 discharge markedly differs from the I_1 in: (a) preferentially responding to microstimulation of superficial laminae (e.g. III) rather than lamina V; (b) preferentially reducing by progressive cooling of the pial surface; and (c) displaying greater variability to a given motor cortical stimulus (Fig. 6). Presumably, the increased variability of I_2 reflects the greater excitability changes of the cortical interneuron compared with that of the larger PT neuron.

3.3.3. The I_3 and later discharges

Further discharges follow the I_1 or I_2 discharges with characteristic I wave periodicity. The I_3 discharges share similar properties with I_2 including mediation by superficial laminae, sensitivity to pial cooling and variability in excitability. Taken together, these properties support the hypothesis of a vertically oriented excitatory network of motor cortical neurons, which generates I_2, I_3 and later I waves, the activity spreading from superficially located neurons to CT neurons.

Perhaps analogous to the I_3 delay with premotor stimulation in higher forms is the unusually long D-I interval (4 ms) in the CT system of the adult rat. Possible explanations for the rodent long D-I interval include: the absence of excitatory inputs directly impinging on CT neurons; this is most unlikely given that Lorente De Nó's (1938) Golgi studies were done on rodents. The problem arises of assigning excitatory synaptic potencies to a histologically determined, laminar distribution of inputs. Possibly, monosynaptic contacts on rat CT neurons are too weak to secure discharge, amplification of the input by cortical interneurons being a necessary condition to reach firing level.

In humans, electrical stimulation of motor cortex elicits an I wave sequence comparable to that recorded in monkeys (Deletis et al., 2001b). However, a peculiarity of transcranial electrical stimulation, usually related to bipolar stimulation between C3 and C4, is the small size of I_1 relative to later I waves (Fig. 1; Burke et al., 1990). The reduced I_1 may reflect failure to excite optimally the monosynaptic corticocortical inputs by a transversely oriented electric field. With magnetic twin coil stimulation over motor cortex, its orientation and therefore the direction of the induced field affects the latency of indirect activation. Thus, a P-A induced field elicits an FDI response with I_1 latency, especially when angulated approximately at 90° to the central sulcus; an A-P induced field elicits an I_2 mediated response (Sakai et al., 1997); such differences in FDI responses can be reproduced by parietal and premotor stimulation, respectively (Rothwell and Amassian, unpublished observations). Furthermore, other sites of parietal TMS elicit FDI responses with I_3 latency. The I_1 response of FDI to human parietal lobe stimulation is at least partly mediated by CT neurons among the largest in the responding population (Amassian et al., 1999), implying that such cortical neurons do not obey the Size Principle of alpha motoneurons (Henneman, 1981). Furthermore, the alpha motoneurons responding to the I_1 discharge are among the fastest and earliest recruited in the pool, again conflicting with the Size Principle (Amassian et al., 2000). Significantly, individually stimulated motor axons supplying thenar muscles showed no correlation between twitch or tetanic tension amplitudes and axonal conduction velocity (Thomas et al., 1990); thus, early voluntarily recruited motor axons could have both fast conduction velocities and elicit weak tensions.

The issue of the remarkable synchronicity of CT fiber discharge in I waves in the human and monkey has not been directly addressed. Significant factors include: (a) the synchronicity of activation by the afferent input especially corticocortical fibers; and (b) the lateral connectivities of excitatory cells in the network. With transcranial stimulation, evidently a large, but precisely unknown number of corticocortical afferent are most likely excited synchronously. Even with a silver ball electrode of typical dimensions, e.g. 1 mm diameter, the stimulus spread from the surface of the half-sphere (1.6 mm^2) on the pia to lamina V 2.0 mm deeper has increased manyfold (e.g. 4×), so that again many CT neurons are transynaptically excited synchronously, with the network then defining their periodicity. Given the large number of corticocortical afferents activated by transcranial or pial stimulation, it seems unnecessary to invoke lateral connectivities as an explanation of synchronization in I waves. However, such connectivities become significant with microelectrode stimulation within a column or within an excitatory neuron and especially with natural stimulation.

3.3.4. Relationships between neurohistology and I wave network

Clearly, the laminar distribution of synaptic inputs to motor cortex is of major importance in attempting to explain the generation of I waves by a vertically oriented network. Unfortunately, full agreement is lacking between the histological studies, which is only partly explicable by the differing techniques used. Thus, Lorente de Nó (1938) using Golgi preparations, Goldman and Nauta (1977) tracing degenerating boutons following cortical lesions and Szentagothai (1978), all show a wide laminar distribution of corticocortical terminals. However, Chang (1951) found such fibers terminated mainly in the superficial layers as did Jones et al. (1975) regarding somatosensory cortex. Even if corticocortical endings were distributed in all laminae, it would not follow that the excitatory weights of the endings were uniform. For example, premotor area projections could end on large CT neurons, but might be ineffective, e.g. through low transmitter quantal release or failure of invasion as compared with securely activating an excitatory interneuron. This could account for I_2 discharge mediating the initial FDI response to premotor TMS. However, a second TMS pulse to premotor or SMA cortex after an 1.5 ms interval revealed facilitation of the FDI response with I_2 latency to the first pulse, i.e. monosynaptic action occurred (Rothwell and Amassian, unpublished observations); this finding implies that if premotor input has endings on CT neurons, they are ineffective when carrying a single volley. The I_1 discharge can be selectively elicited without D activation in cat and monkey by stimulating with bipolar microwires inserted close to lamina V; the tangentially oriented electric field produced by such stimulation implies activation of tangentially oriented fibers, most likely the inner layer of Baillarger, which contains myelinated axons (Amassian et al., 1987). Remaining to be established is whether an electric field near lamina V elicits an I_1 discharge by exciting branches of entering cortico-cortical fibers or descending excitatory projections of neurons in superficial laminae.

3.4. The possible role of inhibitory cortical neurons in I wave periodicity

Cortical EPSPs have a longer duration (e.g. > 10 ms, Creutzfeldt et al., 1967) than that of the I wave sequence (e.g. 6 ms). Their duration and persistence, despite PT cell discharge in a study in the monkey (Fig. 3 in Ghosh and Porter, 1988), seemed to conflict with the network re-excitation hypothesis (Ziemann and Rothwell, 2000). The elegant remedy proposed envisaged activation of local inhibitory neurons by collaterals of the excitatory network neurons so that each I discharge was followed by an IPSP. However, an unimpaired PT action potential partially destroys the EPSP, so that another EPSP is required for the next discharge (Section 3.3.2). In the Ghosh and Porter (1988) recording, the PT action potentials were < 50 mV, but Stefanis and Jasper (1964) illustrate that deterioration of a feline PT action potential (from 72 to 50 mV in their Fig. 14) then resulted in failure of the action potential to reduce the EPSP. Given the partially depolarized resting membrane potentials in the simian recordings, if an IPSP had occurred following the PT action potential, it should have been magnified, but was absent.

An important finding by Ziemann et al. (1998b) disclosed that Lorazepam, a GABA potentiator, reduced facilitation at I wave periods in the twin pulse paradigm described by Tokimura et al. (1996). Remarkably, the reduced I wave facilitation was unaccompanied by an increased I wave period. Furthermore, there was no significant elevation in resting motor threshold, i.e. there was no evidence of potentiation of tonic inhibitory neuronal activity that could have accounted for the reduced I waves. Put another way, ongoing inhibitory neuronal activity may not be significant enough to set motor cortical excitability (cf. Ziemann and Rothwell, 2000). However, the second stimulus probably had both excitatory and inhibitory actions with the result of summation of these inputs shifting towards less excitation because of potentiation of GABA induced IPSPs.

Summarizing, despite the likely importance of inhibitory neurons in the normal functioning of motor cortex, their crucial role in the conserved periodicity of I waves to single stimuli is not supported by the available evidence. However, a single stimulus to motor cortex elicits excitation followed by a large IPSP, which most likely accounts for the ending of the I wave sequence (Amassian et al., 1987).

3.5. The relationship of in vivo experiments on higher mammalian I waves to those on neocortical slices

The use of electrophysiological techniques in studying neocortical and mature slices from rat and guinea pig brain has led to extraordinary advances in understanding of physical properties and membrane conductances as a function of identified portions of the cortical neuron (Feldmeyer and Sakmann, 2000). Their relevance to this survey is whether they advance an understanding of I waves, especially the remarkable conservation of periodicity. The difficulties in relating in vivo and slice data include: (1) The phylogenetic trend in I wave periodicity and synchronization implies that slices from lower mammalian forms may lack the substrate for generating 600 Hz synchronous activity. (2) While neurons in slices can readily be identified as pyramidal, or smaller GABAergic neurons, the subcortical targets of specific pyramidal neurons are unknown. By contrast, PT and CT neurons in vivo are relatively easily identified and their relationship to I waves is thereby established. Furthermore, while very fast PT neurons contribute to I waves, there is no evidence that the much more numerous slow PT neurons share their I wave periodicity. (3) In Section 3, the differences in responses to a number of anatomically defined afferent or antidromic inputs are described. Seeking correlations between such in vivo data and the effects of stimulating, e.g. white matter fibers in a slice becomes problematic.

3.5.1. Relationships at the cellular level

Recording from individual neurons in neocortical slices has facilitated a finer differentiation of types of cellular responses to injected current or transsynaptic stimulation with histological identification of the cell. McCormick et al. (1985) differentiated regular spiking from fast spiking cells with significantly briefer action potentials and rarer bursting cells. The fast spiking cells had a clear afterhyperpolarization and discharged with a prolonged high frequency discharge, with the period increasing from 3–90 ms. Such cells were most likely inhibitory GABAergic interneurons. The regular spiking cells were probably pyramidal cells, but fired at rates below 600 Hz; they lacked an after-hyperpolarization as compared with layer V pyramidal cells in somatomotor cortex (cf. Thomson and Deuchars, 1994). Bursting cells responded to a white matter stimulus with a prolonged high frequency discharge with increasing periods upwards of 2.7 ms in their records. Thus, in no category of the neocortical cells sampled was there evidence of a conserved 600 or even 300 Hz periodicity.

3.5.2. Relationships between cells

Intracellular recordings from pairs of large, lamina V neurons in rat sensorimotor cortex have revealed powerful excitatory connections between them (Thomson and Deuchars, 1994). A single axon may elicit an EPSP of up to 9 mV and spike discharge in a recipient cell in the deeper laminae of the same column, but laterally, the connections are weaker. If both pyramidal cells were PT neurons, this excitatory connection in vitro would conflict with the in vivo findings in cat and primates. However, the rodent PT neurons have much smaller axons than those of cats and primates and may share some of the properties of small feline PT neurons whose recurrent collaterals are excitatory to large PT neurons (Takahashi, 1965). If so, such recurrent excitatory action may contribute to the delayed rodent broad I wave in vivo.

Twin cell recordings also showed that a pyramidal neuron could elicit an EPSP in an inhibitory interneuron but rarely by the first discharge, a marked facilitation occurring with a second discharge. Such behavior resembles the need in cats for multiple antidromic PT volleys to elicit significant IPSPs in PT neurons (Phillips, 1959; Stefanis and Jasper, 1964; Pollen and Ajmone-Marijan, 1965). Thomson and Deuchars clearly envisage an excitatory network of pyramidal neurons, but at present do not provide a basis for conserved 600 Hz periodicity.

A study of connectivity in rodent barrel cortex disclosed that axonal distributions of layer IV spiny stellate neurons were distributed locally and vertically to laminar III and II, while those of lamina V pyramidal neurons were distributed both vertically, locally and horizontally (Feldmeyer and Sakmann, 2000). The spiny stellate projections locally and towards laminar III and II were considered to amplify thalamocortical input, while the lamina V pyramids, given their long dendrites and wider lateral connections, were considered integrative. Certainly, the in vitro observations support the notion of early spread of afferent activity towards the surface of SI.

The quality of the data yielded from recordings from neocortical slices is such that an understanding of higher mammalian I waves would advance significantly if in vivo and in vitro findings could be better correlated. For example, labeling both afferent sources and output, e.g. PT, neurons before preparing the slice from higher mammals might permit rigorous testing of the excitatory network hypothesis and a much deeper understanding of its synaptology.

4. The neocortical distribution of periodic high frequency waves

A difficulty in comparing the findings on the very high frequency, periodic output of motor cortex to that in other cortical areas, such as somatosensory, visual, auditory or association, is the lack of experiments in which the activities of the identified output neurons or fiber pathways are recorded following single electrical stimuli to the area and the synchronicity of such activity defined. Only rarely has a cortical output neuron other than PT been shown to respond with an I wave period after cortical stimulation. A corticothalamic projection neuron was shown to give "jumping" latencies between I type activations (Steriade and Yossif, 1977). Despite this limitation, very high frequency waves have long been identified in sensory receiving cortex such as visual and somatosensory areas to afferent input. While the emphasis in Section 3 has been on activity spreading through a vertically oriented interneuron chain from superficial to deep laminae, the reverse direction of spread dominates early activation of the sensory receiving areas.

4.1. Visual cortex

Bishop and Clare (1953) recorded a highly periodic sequence of waves from feline visual cortex following single stimuli to the optic nerve or radiations. Significantly, the periodicity was conserved with radiation stimulation, thereby identifying it as cortical in origin rather than depending on repetitive thalamic discharge (cf. Curio, 2000). Large and small deflections alternated, the period between large deflections being 1.5 ms (Fig. 7, left). The large and small deflections were attributed to discharge of pyramidal and Golgi type II neurons, respectively. Such configurations of evoked cortical responses are

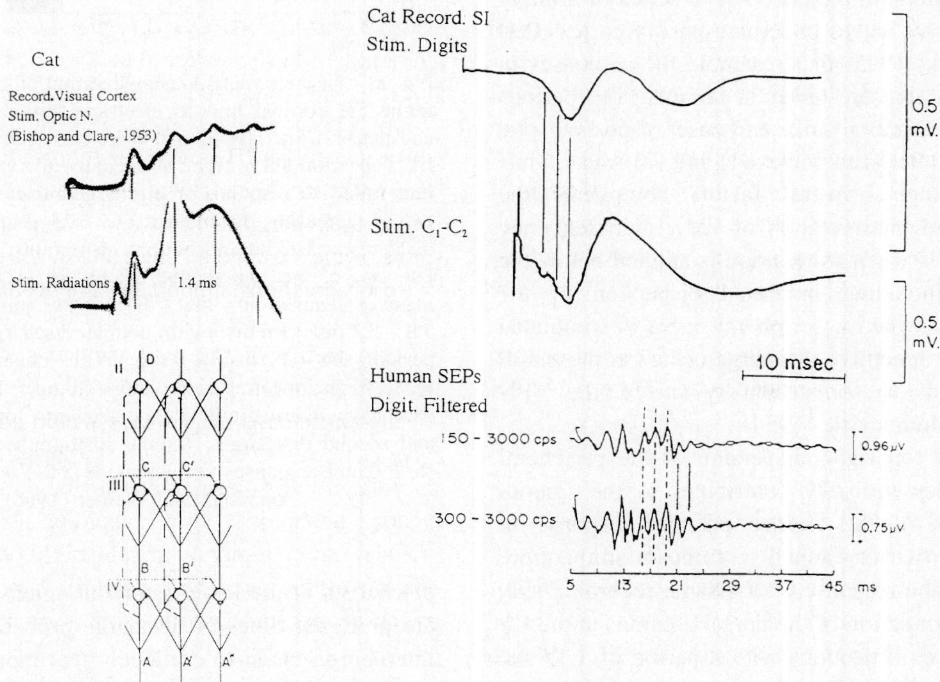

Fig. 7. Very high frequency waves in feline visual and somatosensory cortical receiving areas. Left (above and middle): Visual cortical responses to an electrical stimulus to optic nerve (N), and radiations, respectively. Only in these records is positivity upwards. Pentobarbital anesthesia. Bottom: diagram showing inferred spread of activity from lamina IV to lamina II neurons. Reproduced from Bishop and Clare (1953). Right: top, somatosensory area I (SI) response to an electrical stimulus to the paw (above) and to the dorsal columns at C_1-C_2 (below). Periodic deflections (1.3 ms) are not distinguishable with paw stimulation, but are distinguishable with C_1-C_2 stimulation. Reproduced from Amassian et al. (1964). Bottom: digital filtering of human somatosensory evoked potentials (SEPs) reveals in the restricted high frequency band recording a period of 1.8 ms. Median nerve stimulation at motor threshold. Contralateral recording 2 cm posterior to C_3 or C_4-shoulder. Reproduced from Maccabee et al. (1986) with additional alignments.

readily observed under barbiturate anesthesia, making it more likely that the large deflections reflect summed external fields of synchronized EPSPs, rather than action potentials (Amassian et al., 1964). Regardless of the membrane explanation of the large deflections, their period (666 Hz) resembles that of I waves. Significantly, Bishop and Clare (1953) attributed the high frequency periodicity to a vertically oriented interneuron chain distributed from lamina IV through III to II, a model entirely consistent with Lorente De Nó's (1938) histological observations.

4.2. *Somatosensory cortex*

Stimulation of the thalamic ventroposterior nucleus (VPN) radiations in the cat elicits a series of initially surface positive waves in somatosensory cortex (Perl and Whitlock, 1995) that resemble the responses in visual cortex, but are fewer in number. The periods between the radiation spike and onset of postsynaptic wave (1) and between waves (1) and (2) was 1.6 ms. Not surprisingly, several factors complicate the recording and interpretation of very high frequency cortical waves when stimulation is applied below the radiations, including increased dispersion of the afferent input when a peripheral nerve is stimulated and gradable repetitive discharge occurs at the major thalamic relay to somatosensory cortex, the VPN (Rose and Mountcastle, 1954).

In Fig. 7 top right, dispersion of the peripheral afferent volley probably contributes to the smooth configuration of the surface positive response in feline somatosensory area I to forepaw stimulation; by contrast, the response, at the same recording site, to central stimulation of the dorsal columns at the C_1-C_2 level shows inflections with a period of 1.35 ms. In the cat, the problems associated with subcortical stimulation are avoided by stimulating somatosensory area I at several intensities and recording from an individual unit in somatosensory area II (SII). Despite a change in the stimulus intensity applied to SI, the very brief periodicity of discharge is conserved (Fig. 8). Significantly, the consistently occurring second discharge of the unit at the higher stimulus intensity occurs at the same latency as the late initial

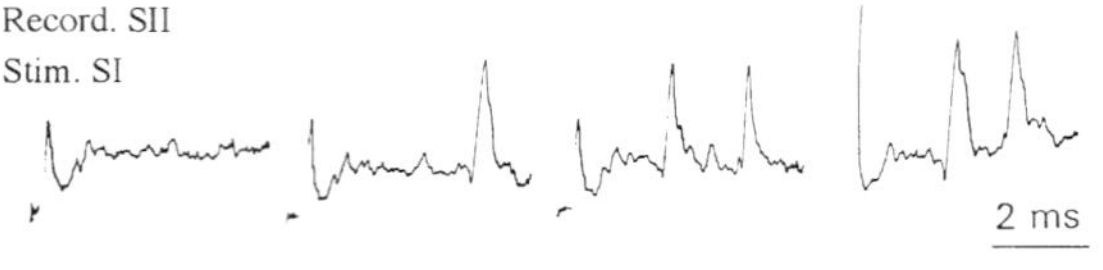

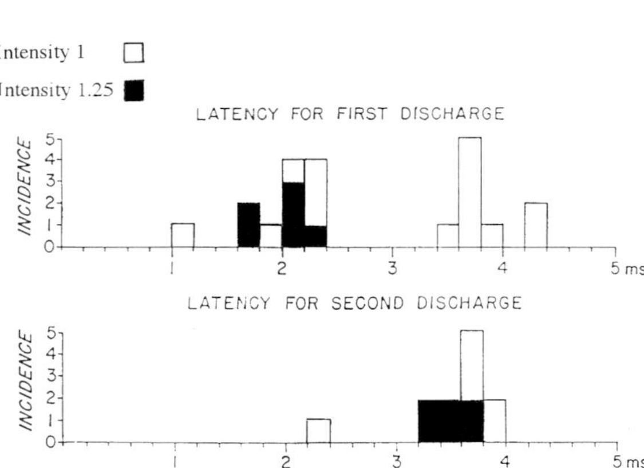

Fig. 8. Discontinuous latency distribution of responses by feline SII cortical unit to electrical stimulus to SI. Dial anesthesia. Unit was 530 μm deep, corresponding to lamina III. Top: from left to right, at intensity of 1 (arbitrary units), unit failed to respond, or discharged once or discharged twice; increasing the intensity to 1.25 resulted in double discharges. Middle and bottom histograms: distribution of latencies of first and second discharges. At intensity of 1, mean latencies of first discharges jumped between 3.8 – 2.2 ms = 1.6 ms; with double discharges, the mean period = 3.8 – 2.2 ms = 1.6 ms. With intensity increased to 1.25, the mean period = 3.5 – 2.0 ms = 1.5 ms, i.e. an excitatory interneuronal delay accounts for delayed first and second discharges. Similar histograms are illustrated for PT unit responses to thalamic N VL-VA stimulation in Amassian and Weiner (1966).

discharges at the lower, stimulus intensity, i.e. there are preferred times of discharge probably set by the interneuron chain to corticocortical input.

In humans, despite the factor of dispersion with peripheral stimulation, high pass filtering the somatosensory evoked response revealed very high frequency waves (Cracco and Cracco, 1976). Replacing analog by digital filtering (Maccabee et al., 1986) further improved the display of the very high frequency components with a period of 1.7 ms; only those with a latency < 20 ms are clearly subcortically generated (Fig. 7, bottom right). Hashimoto et al. (1996)

recorded similar very high frequency (300–900 Hz) responses to median nerve stimulation in the magnetoencephalogram, which were especially prominent when the humans were awake. They suggested that such responses reflected monosynaptic transmission to GABAergic inhibitory interneurons of high frequency thalamocortical discharges. However, potentials recorded at the scalp are unlikely to be directly affected by the 'closed' electric field of small inhibitory interneurons (cf. pyramidal neuronal contributions). The difficulty presented in interpreting very high frequency cortical waves following peripheral stimulation in the human is in separating periodicities that reflect input periodicities in far-field potentials and cortical responses to repetitive discharge of sensory relays from those intrinsic to the cortical network, however stimulated. Clearly, a 600 Hz periodicity present in scalp recordings before the presumed latency of transmission by the thalamocortical input reflects subcortical events, such as impulse conduction in ascending fibers plus monosynaptic relay, totaling 1.5–2 ms. Ideally, a single stimulus to the human internal capsule fibers during depth stimulation might be tested to see if the motor cortical network generates a 600 Hz response (cf. Bishop and Clare, 1953). Less invasively, the effect on the 600 Hz rhythm of changing peripheral stimulus intensity should be tested to determine if subcortical components alter their period while those believed to be postsynaptic cortical conserve the 600 Hz period.

Physiological evidence of spread of activity from the main sites of specific thalamocortical termination in lamina IV and lower III of somatosensory cortex towards the surface was initially obtained from unit recording. Latencies of responses of superficial units in lamina II and III to peripheral stimuli were usually increased as compared with deeper units (Amassian, 1953; cf. Mouncastle, 1957; Doetsch and Towe, 1976; Towe et al., 1976). The initial interpretation of the increased latency was ambiguous because they might result either from transynaptic spread from specific or nonspecific afferent input. However, when the surface positive response in somatosensory cortex to peripheral stimulated is recorded with a fine glass microelectrode at successive depths, reversal commences in the superficial laminae. An apparent velocity of spread towards the surface was calculated at 0.03–0.1 m/s (Amassian et al., 1964); this velocity range is close to that (0.01–0.02 m/s) for transynaptic spread of activity in the isolated cortical slab (Burns, 1950), leading to the conclusion that an excitatory interneuron chain mediated the spread of activity superficially. Notably, evidence is still lacking that the output neurons of sensory receiving cortex discharge synchronously at the fixed high frequency period of the evoked surface responses.

Summarizing, the similarity of the frequency bands in awake humans, anesthetized cats and cats under local anesthesia and with different types of afferent stimulation suggests that sensory receiving neocortex has an excitatory interneuronal network that is comparable to that in motor cortex for generating very high frequency periodic waves.

5. Activities of hippocampal and parahippocampal cortex

Given its simpler histological structure, an archicortex study might be expected to help understand the development of neocortical I waves. For example, hippocampal pyramidal cells have excitatory interconnections, a variety of patterns of firing and also their collaterals excite inhibitory neurons. Several types of high frequency activity can also be generated by synchronous activity in hippocampal and parahippocampal cortices. However, no records are available of output responses by the population of fornix fibers to single electrical stimuli to hippocampal cortex, thereby precluding a direct comparison with the synchronized discharges in PT or CT population responses. Nevertheless, many other activities of neocortex and hippocampal cortex can be compared.

At lower frequencies than the I waves discussed above, activity in the 40–100 Hz range, often called gamma activity, arises from different intrinsic and synaptic mechanisms in different archicortical and isocortical areas (Traub et al., 1999, for review). Voltage dependent, intrinsic 40–100 Hz activity was described in thalamic and cortical cells (Llinás et al.,

1991). Fast $GABA_A$ receptor mediated connections of inhibitory interneurons can synchronize cells of a cortex over remarkably wide areas to produce gamma oscillations in a population of neurons.

A higher frequency oscillation at about 200 Hz (Buzsáki et al., 1992; Ylinen et al., 1995), occurs spontaneously at the beginning of synchronous population events in the hippocampal formation called "sharp waves" (Buzsáki, 1986). Several cycles of this high frequency oscillation (a "ripple") occur within the single population spike in field potential recordings. In an area such as CA1, the 200 Hz activity is associated with low rates of firing by pyramidal cells and high rates of firing (e.g. up to 200 Hz) by interneurons. The synchrony that permits these oscillations to appear in field recordings depends on inhibitory interneurons. A recent model of these oscillations suggests an important role for axo-axonic gap junctions between pyramidal cells as an additional synchronizing influence (Draguhn et al., 1998; Traub and Bibbig, 2000). In the parahippocampal region (entorhinal cortex and parts of the subicular complex), single neurons can fire multiple times during the 200 Hz activity (Funahashi and Stewart, 1997, 1998). These cells may be able to synchronize each other through conventional fast glutamatergic synapses. Interestingly, 200 Hz is about the frequency of firing within the intrinsic burst events seen in many hippocampal pyramidal cells. Orthodromic or antidromic activation (cf. CT neurons) of some populations of burst capable neurons, such as those in the rat subiculum, can produce synchronous field events consisting of several spikes at about 200 Hz (Stewart, 1997). Burst firing neurons exhibit these firing frequencies in response to depolarizing current injection in intracellular recordings. Cells that do not possess voltage dependent burst firing can discharge at similarly high (200 Hz) frequencies in response to strong orthodromic activation or depolarizing current injection (Stewart, 1997). In entorhinal cortex, where neurons of superficial and deep cortical layers can re-excite each other, the 200 Hz ripple activity appeared to depend on intact superficial – deep cell interactions (Stewart, 1999). It is not clear, however, if the oscillations result from a re-activation of cells in a superficial – deep circuit at 200 Hz. Rather, the cells, which lost the ability to oscillate, may simply have had a critical excitatory input removed, resulting in a decreased depolarization of these cells. However, it is emphasized that the interval between discharges is gradable as a function of intensity of both orthodromic or injected current intensity.

Finally, the higher frequency type of activity, called very high frequency or fast ripples has a frequency that can reach 500 Hz, i.e. comes closest to the frequency range of I wave responses to a single stimulus. Fast ripples have been recorded in rat and human hippocampus, but only in "abnormal" tissue. Rats treated with kainic acid, a chronic seizure model, and humans with epilepsy have been found to have fast ripples in field recordings (Bragin et al., 1999), suggesting that these higher frequency oscillations may reflect burst firing by hippocampal pyramidal cells. By contrast, during the 200 Hz activity, inhibitory interneurons not only help synchronize the 200 Hz activity, but limit the responses of pyramidal cells to the orthodromic inputs triggering the sharp waves. The fast 500 Hz ripple results when inhibition is compromised or not activated and hippocampal pyramidal cells can then discharge at such high frequencies. Even then, the field potentials are not comparably synchronized to those of the I waves. Recently, evidence of gap junctions that couple axons of hippocampal pyramidal cells has been presented and shown to be sufficient for synchronizing the highest frequency activity (> 100 Hz) generated by these projection neurons (Traub et al., 1999; Traub and Bibbig, 2000). Evidence of such a mechanism in other cortical regions has not been published.

The behavior of subicular neurons may be the most relevant to the more complicated circuitry of isocortex because they resemble isocortical pyramidal cells in some of their properties (Stewart and Wong, 1993). Whereas burst firing subicular pyramidal cells will generate a synchronous multi-peaked field potential in response to antidromic stimulation, orthodromic inputs can activate either single spikes or bursts of action potentials depending on the location of the input and the strength of the input. Orthodromic

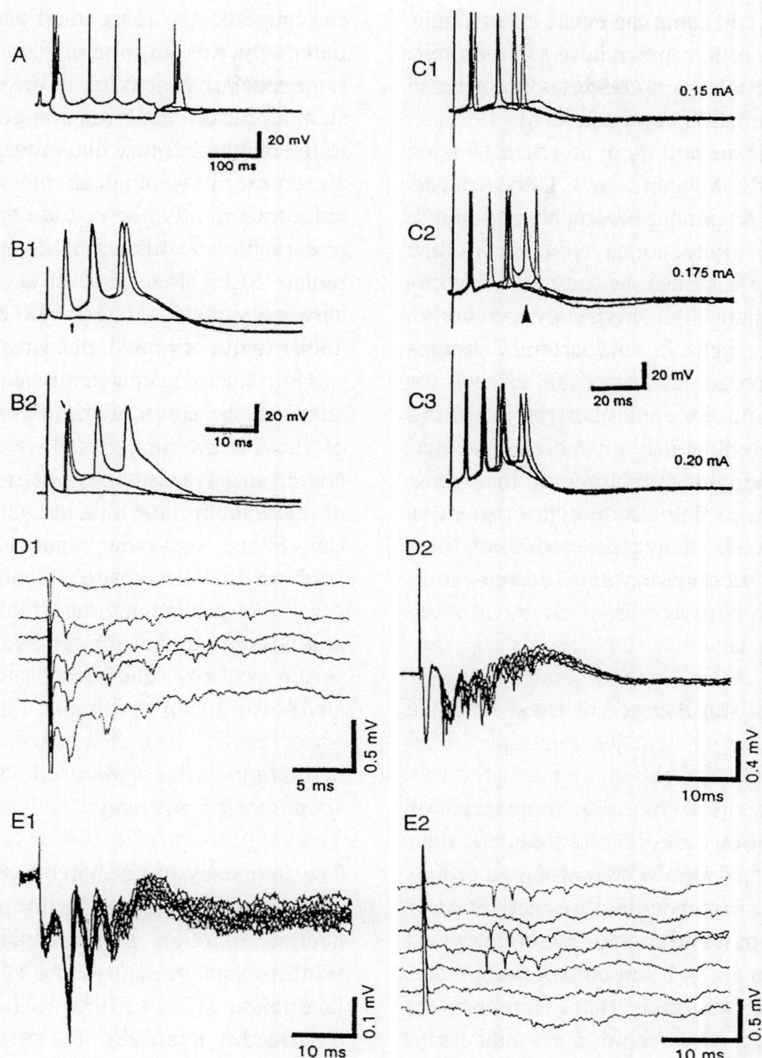

Fig. 9. High frequency discharges by rat subicular neurons. Subicular pyramidal neurons can discharge with bursts of action potentials that can be synchronous in response to orthodromic and antidromic stimulation. A: Superimposed responses by a subicular pyramidal neuron to depolarizing and hyperpolarizing current injection through a recording electrode. The cell's response to depolarizing current injection was an initial burst of action potentials followed by a series of simple action potentials. The burst event can also be trigged at the break of a hyperpolarizing current pulse. B: Antidromic responses by a burst firing neuron show that these cells can discharge multiple spikes at threshold (B1) or single spikes (B2) to a single stimulus pulse. C: Responses by a subicular burst firing neuron to three different orthodromic stimulus intensities show changes in the interspike interval and a switch from evoked single spikes to evoked burst responses. Arrow head in C2 shows the late slow component characteristic of a burst response. D: Extracellular recordings of orthodromic responses in subiculum. Intensity series (D1) shows minimal variation in the interval between first and second events, but more variation in intervals between later events. This is seen also in the set (D2) of superimposed traces at a single intensity where the first (directly activated) peak exhibits essentially no temporal jitter, but subsequent peaks show progressive variability in timing. E: Orthodromic activation from CA1 produces consistent synchronous responses at one intensity (E1).

A burst firing single unit is shown in E2. Calibrations are shown in the figure. Reproduced from Stewart (1997).

inputs ending near the cell soma can evoke either single spikes or bursts of action potentials. Orthodromic inputs to the more distal apical dendrites favor burst firing (Fig. 9; Stewart, 1997; Funahashi et al., 1999).

Summarizing, while the 500 Hz or more frequencies characterizing normal I waves in the CT are reached in hippocampus and parahippocampal structures, especially in seizure-prone cortex, frequencies are usually lower. Unlike CT neurons, antidromic stimulation may also elicit high frequency discharge. Furthermore, when repetitive discharge of hippocampal and parahippocampal neurons is elicited by orthodromic stimulation, excepting bursting cells, the rate of discharge is continuously gradable rather than being conserved or changing in multiples of the I wave period. Burst cells can exhibit a stereotyped pattern of waves at about 200 Hz that characteristically desynchronize so that successive waves decrement in amplitude. They are best synchronized by afferent activation near the soma.

6. The physiological significance of the I wave periodicity

During voluntary activities, the mean frequencies of discharge of CT neurons are several-fold less than that of I waves. Thus, Evarts (1968) when recording PT units in monkeys responding to various load conditions opposing movements described a range of mean frequencies up to 147 impulses/s, but in the majority the rate was less than 100/s. Humphrey et al. (1970) more commonly recorded PT unit mean frequencies of, or slightly above 200/s. The least interspike interval could be as brief as 1.5 ms (Evarts, 1968), or 4–5 ms (Porter, 1972), but the fact that the mean rates rarely exceeded one-third that of the I waves implies that most interspike intervals during physiological CT activity are longer than the I wave period of 1.5–2.0 ms. Part of the discrepancy between CT discharge rate during physiological activity and I waves is explained by the fact that a given CT neuron does not necessarily discharge during each I wave, thus yielding interspike intervals that are small multiples of the basic I wave period (e.g. Fig. 7 in Amassian et al., 1990); however, at best this factor can only account for a small part of the discrepancy. Inevitably, the question arises whether the very high frequency of I activity is an experimental artefact stemming from applying a large, brief electrical field to the cerebral cortex, thus revealing little or nothing about the physiological functioning of the grey matter. Currently, the counter to such criticism is the remarkable identification of similar periodicities in human SEPs (Maccabee et al., 1986) and magnetoencephalograms (Hashimoto et al., 1996; Curio, 2000) with peripheral electrical stimulation.

The physiological significance of I wave periodicity may be considered at two levels. The precision of the I wave period (or its harmonics) may: (1) confer an advantage in alpha motoneuron excitation or even help discriminate between the effects of CT fibers supplying several alpha motoneuron pools or their intermediary spinal interneurons; and (2) reflect a computational function in motor cortex and possibly other cortical areas, the high frequency period possibly functioning as a clock activated by any powerful input drive.

6.1. The possible influence of I wave periodicity on spinal cord processing

The frequency of discharge by CT neurons has long been known to influence discharge by alpha motoneurons through temporal summation of EPSPs (Phillips and Porter, 1977). However, the temporal facilitation of each EPSP to each D wave that they described is less clear. The oft-reproduced recording of 'D' activity in the CT and apparently incrementing alpha motoneuron EPSPs (e.g. Fig. 3.14 in Phillips and Porter, 1977) clearly shows the intrusion of I waves during the CT train of impulses, thereby evidencing facilitation in the motor cortex and multiplication of the CT discharge. The CT activity was conducted past their recording site, thereby underestimating I activity by a factor of 3.3 (Amassian and Deletis, 1999), i.e. I activity was still more prominent than in the cited figure. Nevertheless, whether or not each EPSP is augmented at the alpha motoneuron does not diminish the major importance of their temporal summation.

The possibility that a frequency coding in CT discharge might influence alpha motoneuron firing was explored in cats and monkeys by Brookhart (1952). In monkeys, the duration of a train of electrical stimuli (0.2 ms pulses) required to activate distal muscles fell as their frequency was increased until approximately 100 Hz, after which there was little reduction at higher frequencies tested up to 400 Hz. For proximal muscles, a longer duration pulse (1.5 ms), which was shown to activate also smaller PT fibers yielded similar results, but the use of the briefer stimulus caused the loss of the sharp reduction in train duration near 100 Hz. Nowhere was there an indication that the precision of I wave periodicity in the PT stimulation played an important role in securing a motor response. Significantly, the 100 Hz rate in Brookhart's study is remarkably close to the upper mean rates of 100 Hz usually found in discharge of PT neurons during 'voluntary' movements.

Porter (1972) demonstrated in monkeys that the timing of 4–5 ms interspike intervals in motor cortical unit discharge was related to the latency of response in a reaction time paradigm; an earlier timing of such brief intervals accompanied brevity in latency. While indicating the importance of timing in temporal facilitation, the I wave periodicity was not implicated in securing the early motor responses. Given the long duration of the alpha motoneuron time constant (3–4 ms), it seems unlikely that frequencies slightly below or above that of I waves or their harmonics could be significant at this anatomical level. However, a more precise timing requirement for temporal summation in spinal interneuronal systems is not excluded by these studies. Unlike motor cortical neurons, alpha motoneurons discharge at frequencies an order of magnitude lower than that of I waves, and continuously grade the frequency of discharge. The time parameters of resulting muscle contraction bear still less relation to I wave frequency.

6.2. The possible relation of I wave periodicity to a clock in cerebral cortex

We have described above the remarkable difference between usually continuously gradable interspike intervals at ascending somatosensory neuronal levels as functions of stimulus intensity vs. conservation of the I wave periodicity of motor cortical output. Such transformation leads to the hypothesis that the stable high frequency of I waves reflects a time quantizing or 'clock' property of the excitatory interneuronal chain in motor cortex and probably sensory receiving cortex, if not throughout the neocortex. The 'clock' would be programmable in the sense that powerful excitation by an electrical or magnetic pulse, or possibly by significant afferent stimulation would increase cortical interneuronal activity in the network and initiate clock activity. If coinciding with the clock period, other afferent inputs could preferentially sum, with subsequent transmission and synchronization of discharges. A minimal test of such a network property is whether a second stimulus reveals facilitation at the clock period or its harmonics. This was confirmed in the human by the two near-threshold magnetic pulse paradigm, which revealed the peaks of facilitation required by the hypothesis at the I wave periods (Tokimura et al., 1996; Ziemann et al., 1998). Such an interneuronal network might be expected to 'resonate' when driven by a longer train of weaker stimuli with the appropriate period; this was confirmed in humans (Fig. 10) with trains of three to four magnetic stimuli at periods of 1.5–1.7 ms (Amassian et al., 1996). Weak focal anodic stimuli which generate mainly D waves do not elicit such facilitation indicating that it is occurring in the motor cortical network rather than in the spinal cord.

It would be of interest if the increased PT discharge during voluntary movement by monkeys had interspike intervals or expectation density functions that were multiples of the I wave periodicity. If so, their significance would reflect computational functions in the motor cortex rather than coding for selective downstream action on alpha motoneurons (see Section 6.1). Finally, the phylogenetic trend towards increasingly precise firing periodicity in the excitatory interneuronal network, exemplified by that found in human motor cortex and possibly other neocortical areas may not be surprising if related to the functional including computing capacities of the human cerebral cortex. Thus, the properties of the high

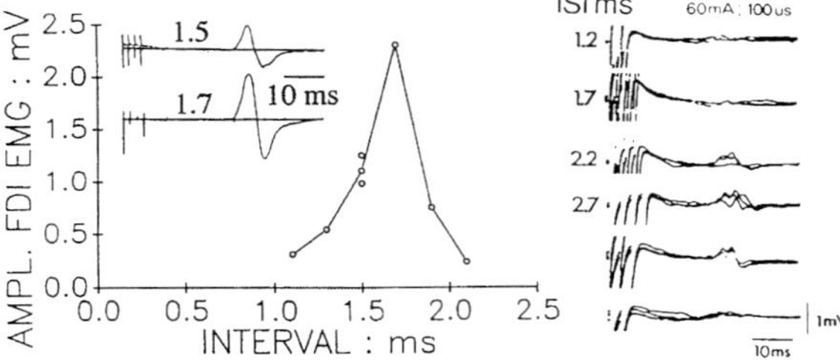

Fig. 10. Optimal periodicity of repetitive TMS and focal anodic stimulation are compared for hand muscle responses in same awake subject. EMG recording from first dorsal interosseous (FDI) muscle. Left: Average of 10 FDI responses plotted as a function of interstimulus interval (ISI) in a four pulse TMS train. To control for drift in motor cortical excitability, three separate averages were recorded at 1.5 ms ISI during the session. TMS was applied with coil windings over hand area. Optimal period 1.7 ms in this subject. Inset shows summed FDI responses at 1.5 and 1.7 ms ISI. Right: Superimposed FDI responses to focal anodic stimulation over hand area at indicated strength and pulse duration. Four pulses at ISI of 1.2 and 1.7 ms are ineffective, but are increasingly effective at 2.2 and 2.7 ms, at which interval three pulses are sufficient. While the optimal facilitation at 1.7 ms with TMS reflects the properties of the excitatory interneuronal chain, the optimal period for facilitation with a focal anodic train reflects delayed recovery of CT axons to direct electrical stimulation (Deletis et al., 2001a). Reproduced from Amassian and Deletis, 1999.

frequency excitatory cortical network revealed by transient stimulation might serve pragmatically in investigating human disease states, e.g. Alzheimer disease, where brain functioning impairment includes that of cerebral cortex.

Summary

A remarkable feature of motor cortical organization in higher mammals is that a brief electrical stimulus elicits in the pyramidal tract and corticospinal tract an unrelayed direct (D) wave followed by multiple indirect (I) waves at frequencies as high as 500–700 Hz. This review presents some conclusions regarding very high frequency synchronous activity in mammalian cortex: (1) Synchrony in repetitive I discharges is extraordinary in humans and monkeys, less in cats and still less in rats, being there represented by a delayed broad wave; such phylogenetic trends have important implications for the suitability of lower mammalian species for studies of high frequency cortical networks in the human brain; (2) The evidence from microstimulation at different cortical depths and pial cooling favors a vertically oriented chain of interneurons that centripetally excite corticospinal neurons as the basis for inter-I wave periodicity and synchrony; (3) Significantly, the I wave periodicity is conserved despite wide changes in stimulus parameters; (4) Synchronous high frequency activity similar to that of I waves can be recorded from other neocortical areas such as visual and somatosensory cortex; however, evidence is still lacking that the output neurons of these cortical regions have synchronized discharges comparable to I waves; (5) In limbic cortices, the frequency of synchronous neural activity is lower than that in motor cortex or related cortices and periodicity is not conserved with changes in stimulus parameters, indicating a lack of the neocortical interneuronal substrate in limbic cortex; (6) We propose that the very high frequency synchronous activity of motor cortical output reflects a computational function such as a "clock," quantizing times at which inputs would interact preferentially yielding synchronous output discharges. Such circuitry, if a general feature of neocortex, would facilitate rapid communication of significant computations between cortical regions.

References

Amassian, V.E. Evoked single cortical unit activity in the somatic sensory area. *Electroenceph. Clin. Neurophysiol.*, 1953, 5: 415–438.

Amassian, V.E. Discussion in: M.D. Yahr and D.P. Purpura (Eds.), *Neurophysiological Basis of Normal and Abnormal Motor Activities*. Raven Press, New York, 1967: 288–292.

Amassian, V.E. and Deletis, V. Relationships between animal and human corticospinal responses. In: W. Paulus, M. Hallett, P.M. Rossini and J.C. Rothwell (Eds.), Transcranial magnetic stimulation. *Electroenceph. Clin. Neurophysiol.* (Suppl.). Elsevier, New York, 1999, 51: 79–92.

Amassian, V.E. and Weiner, H. Monosynaptic and polysynaptic activation of pyramidal tract neurons by thalamic stimulation.

In: D.P. Purpura and M.D. Yahr (Eds.), *The Thalamus*, Columbia University Press, New York, 1966: 255–282.

Amassian, V.E., Waller, H.J. and Macy, J., Jr. Neural mechanism of the primary somatosensory evoked potential. *Ann. N.Y. Acad. Sci.*, 1964, 112: 5–32.

Amassian, V.E., Stewart, M.S., Quirk, G.J. and Rosenthal, J.L. Physiological basis of motor effects of a transient stimulus to cerebral cortex. *Neurosurgery*, 1987, 20: 74–93.

Amassian, V.E., Cracco, R.Q. and Maccabee, P.J. Focal stimulation of human cerebral cortex with the magnetic coil: A comparison with electrical stimulation. *Electroenceph. Clin. Neurophysiol.*, 1989, 74: 401–416.

Amassian, V.E., Quirk, G. and Stewart, M. A comparison of corticospinal activation by magnetic coil and electrical stimulation of monkey motor cortex. *Electroenceph. Clin. Neurophysiol.*, 1990, 77: 390–401.

Amassian, V.E., Eberle, L., Maccabee, P.J. and Cracco, R.Q. Modeling magnetic coil excitation of human cerebral cortex with a peripheral nerve immersed in a brain-shaped volume conductor: The significance of fiber bending in excitation. *Electroenceph. Clin. Neurophysiol.*, 1992, 85: 291–301.

Amassian, V.E., Cracco, R.Q., Maccabee, P.J., Vergara, M., Hassan, N., Eberle, L. and Rothwell, J.C. Spatial facilitation of human motor responses by near-threshold magnetic stimulation of parietal and frontal areas. *J. Physiol. (Lond.)*, 1997, 504: 115.

Amassian, V.E., Rothwell, J.C., Cracco, R.Q., Maccabee, P.J., Vergara, M., Hassan, N. and Eberle, L. What is excited by near-threshold twin magnetic stimuli over human cerebral cortex? *J. Physiol. (Lond.)*, 1998, 506: 122.

Amassian, V.E., Rothwell, J.C. Ziemann, U., Meyer, B.U., Cracco, R.Q, Trompetto, C., Ashby, P. and Lalli, S. Do human large corticospinal neurons obey the size principle? *J. Physiol.*, 1999, 521: 47.

Amassian, V.E., Lalli, S., Rothwell, J.C., Cracco, R.Q. and Gerschlager, W. Size relationships in mono- and polysynaptic excitation of human corticospinal neurons. *J. Physiol. (Lond.)*, 2000, 527: 134.

Barker, A.T., Garnham, C.W. and Freeston, I.L. Magnetic nerve stimulation: the effect of waveform on efficiency, determination of neural membrane time constants and the measurement of stimulator output. In: W.J. Levy, R.Q. Cracco, A.T. Barker and J. Rothwell (Eds.), Magnetic motor stimulation: Basic principles and clinical experience. *EEG* (Suppl. 43). Elsevier Scientific Publ., BV, New York, 1991: 227–248.

Berardelli, A., Inghilleri, M., Cruccu, G. and Manifredi, M. Descending volley after electrical and magnetictranscranial in man. *Neurosci. Let.*, 1990, 112: 54–58.

Berlin, L. and Amassian, V.E. Pyramidal tract responses during seizures. *Electroenceph. Clin. Neurophysiol.*, 1965, 19: 587–597.

Bishop, G.H. and Clare, M. Sequence of event in optic cortex response to volleys of impulses in the radiation. *J. Neurophysiol.*, 1953, 16: 490–498.

Boyd, S.G., Rothwell, J.C., Cowan, J.A., Webb, P.J., Morley, T., Asselman, P. and Marsden, C.D. A method of monitoring function in corticospinal pathways during scoliosis surgery with a note on motor conduction velocities. *J. Neurol. Neurosurg. Psychiat.*, 1986, 49: 251–257.

Bragin, A., Engel, J., Jr., Wilson, C.L., Fried, I. and Mathern, G.W. Hippocampal and entorhinal cortex high-frequency oscillations (100–500 Hz) in human epileptic brain and in kainic acid-treated rats with chronic seizures. *Epilepsia*, 1999a, 40: 127–137.

Bragin, A., Engel, J., Jr., Wilson, C.L., Vizentin, E. and Mathern, G.W. Electrophysiologic analysis of a chronic seizure model after unilateral hippocampal KA injection. *Epilepsia*, 1999b, 40: 1210–1221.

Braitenberg, V. A note on myeloarchitectonus. *J. Comp. Neurol.*, 1962, 118: 141–156.

Brookhart, J.M. A study of corticospinal activation of motor neurons. *Res. Publ. Ann. Nerv. Ment. Dis.*, 1952, 30: 157–173.

Brookhart, J.M. and Zanchetti, A. The relation between electrocortical waves and responsiveness of the cortico-spinal system. *Electroceph. Clin. Neurophysiol.*, 1956, 8: 427–444.

Burke, D., Hicks, R.G. and Stephen, P.H. Corticospinal volleys evoked by anodal and cathodal stimulation to the human motor cortex. *J. Physiol. (Lond.)*, 1990, 425: 283–299.

Burke, D., Hicks, R. and Stephen, J. Anodal and cathodal stimulation of the upper-limb area of the human motor cortex. *Brain*, 1992, 115: 1497–1508.

Burke, D., Hicks, R., Gandevia, S.C., Stephen, J., Woodforth, I. and Crawford, M. Direct comparison of corticospinal volleys in human subjects to transcranial magnetic and electrical stimulation. *J. Physiol. (Lond.)*, 1993, 470: 383–393.

Burns B.D. Some properties of the cat's isolated cerebral cortex. *J. Physiol. (Lond.)*, 1950, 111: 50–68.

Buzsaki, G. Hippocampal sharp waves: their origin and significance. *Brain Res.*, 1986, 398: 242–252.

Buzsaki, G., Horvath, Z., Urioste, R., Hetke, J., and Wise, K. High-frequency network oscillation in the hippocampus. *Science*, 1992, 256: 1025–1027.

Chang, H-T. Cortical response to activity of callosal neurons. *J. Neurophysiol.*, 1953, 16: 117–144.

Cohen, B. Housepian, E.M. and Purpura, D.P. Intrathalamic regulation of activity in a cerebellocortical projection pathway. *Expt. Neurol.*, 1962, 6: 492–506.

Cracco, R.Q. and Cracco, J.B. Somatosensory evoked potential in man: far-field potentials: *Electroenceph. Clin. Neurophysiol.*, 1976, 41: 460–466.

Creutzfeldt, O.D., Lux, H.D. and Watanabe, S. Electrophysiology of cortical nerve cells. In: D.P. Purpura and M.D. Yahr (Eds.), *The Thalamus*. Columbia University Press, New York, 1964: 209–235.

Curio, G. Linking 600-Hz "spike-like" EEG/MEG wavelets (and bursts) to cellular substrates. Concepts and caveats. *J. Clin. Neurophysiol.*, 2000, 17: 377–396.

Deletis, V. Intraoperative monitoring of the functional integrity of the motor pathways. In: O. Devinsky, A. Beric and M. Dogali (Eds.), *Advances in Neurology: Electrical and Magnetic Stimulation of the Brain*. Raven Press, New York, 1993: 201–214.

Deletis, V. Evoked potentials. In: C.L. Lake (Ed.), *Clinical Monitoring for Anesthesia and Critical Care*. Saunders, Philadelphia, 1994: 288–314.

Deletis, V. and Kothbauer, K. Intraoperative neurophysiology of the corticospinal tract. In: E. Stalberg, H.S. Sharma, Y. Olsson (Eds.), *Spinal Cord Monitoring*. Springer, New York, Wien, New York, 1998: 421–444.

Deletis, V., Isgum, V. and Amassian, V.E. Neurophysiological mechanisms underlying motor evoked potentials in anesthetized humans. Part 1. Recovery time of corticospinal tract direct waves elicited by pairs of transcranial electrical stimuli. *Clin. Neurophysiol.*, 2001a, 112: 438–444.

Deletis, V., Rodi, Z. and Amassian, V.E. Neurophysiological mechanisms underlying motor evoked potentials in anesthetized humans. Part 2. Relationship between epidurally and muscle recorded MEPs in man. *Clin. Neurophysiol.*, 2001b, 112: 445–452.

Di Lazzaro, Di. V., Oliviero, A., Profice, P., Saturno, E., Pilato, F., Insola, A., Mazzone, P., Tonali, P. and Rothwell, J.C. Comparison of descending volleys evoked by transcranial magnetic and electric stimulation in conscious humans. *Electroenceph. Clin. Neurophysiol.*, 1998, 109: 397–401.

Doetsh, G.S. and Towe, A.L. Response properties of distinct neuronal subsets of hindlimb sensorimotor cerebral cortex of the domestic cat. *Exp. Neurol.*, 1976, 53: 520–547.

Draguhn, A., Traub, R.D., Schmitz, D. and Jefferys, J.G.R. Electrical coupling underlies high-frequency oscillations in the hippocampus in vitro. *Nature*, 1998, 394: 189–1992.

Evarts, E.V. Relation of pyramidal tract activity to force exerted during voluntary movement. *J. Neurophysiol.*, 1968, 31: 14–27.

Fehlings, M.G., Tator, C.H., Linden, D. and Piper, I.R. Motor and somatosensory evoked potentials recorded from the rat. *Electroenceph. Clin. Neurophysiol.*, 1988, 69: 65–78.

Feldmeyer, D. and Sackmann, B. Synaptic efficacy and reliability of excitatory connections between the principal neurons of the input (layer 4) and output (layer 5) of the neocortex. *J. Physiol. (Lond.)*, 2000, 525: 31–39.

Fujiki, M., Isono, M., Hori, S. and Ueno, S. Corticospinal direct response to transcranial magnetic stimulation in humans. *Electroenceph. Clin. Neurophysiol.*, 1996, 101: 48–57.

Funahashi, M. and Stewart, M. Presubicular and parasubicular cortical neurons of the rat: functional separation of deep and superficial neurons in vitro. *J. Physiol. (Lond.)*, 1997, 501: 37–403.

Funahashi, M. and Stewart, M. Properties of cortical gamma-frequency oscillations initiated by propagating population bursts in rat brain slices. *J. Physiol. (Lond.)*, 1998, 510: 191–208.

Funahashi, M., Harris, E. and Stewart, M. Re-entrant activity in a presubiculum – subiculum circuit generates epileptiform activity in vitro. *Brain Res.*, 1999, 849: 139–146.

Ghosh, S. and Porter, R. Corticocortical synaptic influences on morphologically identified pyramidal neurons in motor cortex of the monkey. *J. Physiol. (Lond.)*, 1988, 400: 617–629.

Goldman, P.S. and Nauta, W.J.H. Columnar distribution of cortico-cortical fibers in the frontal association, limbic and motor cortex of the developing rhesus monkey. *Brain Res.*, 1977, 122: 393–413.

Hashimoto, I. Mashiko, T. and Imada, T. Somatic evoked high-frequency magnetic oscillations reflect activity of inhibitory interneurons in the human somatosensory cortex. *Electroenceph. Clin. Neurophysiol.*, 1996, 100: 189–203.

Henneman, E. Recruitment of motoneurons: The size principle. In: J.E. Desmedt (Ed.), Motor unit types, Recruitment and plasticity in health and disease. *Prog. Clin. Neurophysiol.*, 1981, 9: 26–60, Basel, Karger.

Hern, J.E.C., Landgren, S., Phillips, C.G. and Porter, R. Selective excitation of corticofugal neurones by surface-anodal stimulation of the baboon's motor cortex. *J. Physiol. (Lond.)*, 1962, 161: 73–90.

Humfrey, D.R., Schmidt, E.M. and Thompson, W.D. Predicting measures of motor performance from multiple cortical spike trains. *Science*, 1970, 179: 758–762.

Jones, E.G., Burton, H. and Porter, R. Commissural and cortico-cortical "columns" in the somatic/sensory cortex of primates. *Science*, 1975, 190: 572–574.

Kaneko, K., Kawai, S., Fuchigami, Y., Morieta, H. and Ofuji, A. The effect of current direction induced by transcranial magnetic stimulation on the corticospinal excitability in human brain. *Electroenceph. Clin. Neurophysiol.*, 1996, 101: 478–482.

Katayama, Y., Tsubokawa, T., Maejima, S., Hirayama, T. and Yamamoto, T. Corticospinal direct response in humans: identification of the motor cortex during intracranial surgery under general anesthesia. *J. Neurol. Neurosurg. Psychiat.*, 1988, 51: 50–59.

Kernell, D. and Wu, C.P. responses of the pyramidal tract to stimulation of the baboon's motor cortex. *J. Physiol. (Lond.)*, 1967, 191: 653–672.

Koike, H., Mano, N., Okada, Y. and Oshima, T. Repetitive impulses generated in fast and slow pyramidal tract cells by intracellularly applied current steps. *Exp. Brain Res.*, 1970, 11: 263–281.

Llinás, R.R., Grace, A.A. and Yarom, Y. In vitro neurons in mammalian cortical layer 4 exhibit intrinsic oscillatory activity in the 10- to 50- Hz frequency range. *Proc. Nat. Acad. Sci. (USA)*, 1991, 88: 897–901.

Lorente De Nó, R. Cerebral cortex: architecture, intracortical connections, motor projections. In: J.E. Fulton (Ed.), *Physiology of the Nervous System*. Oxford Univ. Press, New York, 1938.

Maccabee, P.J., Hassan, N.F., Cracco, R.Q. and Schiiff, J.A. Short latency somatosnsory and spinal evoked potentiaal: Power spectra and comparison between high pass analog and digital filter. *Electroenceph. Clin. Neurophysiol.*, 1986, 65: 177–187.

Maccabee, P.J., Amassian, V.E., Eberle, L.P. and Cracco, R.Q. Magnetic coil stimulation of straight and bent amphibian and mammalian peripheral nerve in-vitro: Locus of excitation. *J. Physiol.* (*Lond.*), 1993, 460: 201–219.

Matsuma, H. and Shimazu, A. Intraoperative spinal cord monitoring using electric responses to stimulation of caudal spinal cord or motor cortex. In: J.E. Desmedt (Ed.), *Neuromonitoring in Surgery*. Elsevier Science Publishing, 1989: 175–190.

McCormick, D.A., Connors, B.W., Lighthall, J.W. and Prince, D.A. Comparative electrophysiology of pyramidal and sparsely spiny stellate neurons of the neocortex. *J. Neurophysiol.*, 1985, 54: 782–806.

Mountcastle, V.B. Modality and topographic properties of single neurons of cat's somatic sensory cortex. *J. Neurophysiol.*, 1957, 20: 408–434.

Muller, R. A quarter century of place cells. *Neuron*, 1996, 17: 813–822.

Nacimiento, A.C., Lux, H.D. and Creuzfeldt, O.D. Postsynaptische Potentiale von Nervenzellen des motorischen Cortex nach elektrisher Reizung spezifischer und unspezifisher Thalamuskerne. *Arch. Ges. Physiol.* Pflugers, 1964, 281: 152–169.

Nakamura, H., Kitagawa, H., Kawaguchi, Y. and Tsuji, H. Direct and indirect activation of human corticospinal neurons by transcranial magnetic and electrical stimulation. *Neurosci. Lett.*, 1996, 210: 45–48.

Pandya, D.N. and Kuyers H.G.J.M. Cortico-cortical connections in the rhesus monkey. *Brain Res.*, 1969, 13: 13–36.

Patton, H.D. and Amassian, V.E. Single- and multiple-unit analysis of cortical stage of pyramidal tract activation. *J. Neurophsiol.*, 1954, 17: 39–58.

Patton, H.D. and Amassian, V.E. The pyramidal tract: its excitation and functions. In: J. Field (Ed.), *Handbook of Physiology*, Section 1, Vol. II. American Physiological Society, Washington, D.C., 1960: 837–861.

Pedroarena, C. and Llinás, R. Dendritic calcium conductances generate high-frequency oscillation in thalamocortical neurons. *Proc. Natl. Acad. Sci. USA*, 1997, 94: 724–728.

Perl, E.R. and Whitlock, D.G. Potentials evoked in cerebral somatsensory region. *J. Neurophysiol.*, 1955, 18: 486–501.

Phillips, C.G. Cortical motor threshold and the thresholds and distribution of excited Betz cells in the cat. *Quart. J. Exp. Physiol.*, 1956, 41: 70–84.

Phillips, C.G. Actions of antidromic pyramidal volleys on single Betz cells in the cat. *Quart. J. Exp. Physiol.*, 1959, 44: 1–25.

Phillips, C.G. Epicortical electrical mapping of motor areas in primates. Motor areas of the cerebral cortex. In: G. Bock, M.O Connor and J. Marsh (Eds.), *Ciba Sypmposium 132.* Wiley, Chichester, 1987: 5–16.

Phillips, C.G. and Porter, R. Corticospinal neurones: Their role in movement. *Monograph of the Physiological Society*, No. 14. Academic Press, London, 1977.

Pollen, D.A. and Ajmone-Marsan, C. Cortical inhibitory postsynaptic potentials and strychninization. *J. Neurophysiol.*, 1965, 28: 342–358.

Porter, R. Relationship of the discharge of cortical neurons to movement in free-to-move monkeys. *Brain Res.*, 1972, 40: 39–43.

Purpura, D.P., Shofer, R.J. Musgrave, F.S. Cortical intracellular potentials during augmenting and recruiting responses: II. Patterns of synaptic activities in pyramidal and nonpyramidal tract neurons. *J. Neurophysiol.*, 1964, 27: 133–151.

Rose, J.E. and Mountcastle, V.B. Activity of single neurons in the tactile thalamic region of the cat in response to a transient peripheral stmulus. *John Hopk. Hosp. Bull.*, 1954, 94: 238–282.

Rosenthal, J., Waller, H.J. and Amassian, V.E. An analysis of the activation of motor cortical neurons by surface stimulation. *J. Neurophysiol.*, 1967, 30: 849–858.

Rothwell, J.C., Thompson, P.D., Day, B.L., Boyd, S. and Marsden, C.D. Stimulation of the human motor cortex through the scalp. *Exp. Physiol.*, 1991, 76: 159–200.

Rothwell, J.C., Day, B.L. and Amassian, V.E. Near threshold electrical and magnetic transcranial stimuli activate overlapping sets of cortical neurons in humans. *J. Physiol.* (*Lond.*), 1992, 452: 109.

Sakai, K., Ugawa, Y., Terao, Y., Hanajima, R., Furabayashi, T. and Kanazawa, I. Preferential activation of different I waves by transcranial magnetic stimulation with a figure-of-eight shaped coil. *Exp. Brain Res.*, 1997, 113: 24–32.

Schiller, J., Schiller, Y., Stuart, G. and Sakmann, B. Calcum action potentials restricted to distal apical dendrites of rat neocortical pyramidal neurons. *J. Physiol.* (*Lond.*), 1997, 505: 605–616.

Schlag, J.E. and Balvin, R. Sequence of events following synaptic and electrical excitation of pyramidal neurons of the motor cortex. *J. Neurophysiol.*, 1994, 27: 334–365.

Spencer, W.A. and Kandel, E.R. Electrophysiology of hippocampal neurons. IV. Fast prepotentials. *J. Neurophysiol.*, 1961, 24: 272–285.

Stefanis, C. and Jasper, H. Recurrent collateral inhibition in pyramidal tract neurons. *J. Neurophysiol.*, 1964, 27: 855–877.

Steriade, M. and Yossif, G. Afferent and recurrent collateral influences on cortical somatosensory neurons. *Exp. Neurol.*, 1977, 56: 334–360.

Stewart, M. Antidromic and orthodromic responses by subicular neurons in rat brain slices. *Brain Res.*, 1997, 769: 71–85.

Stewart, M. Columnar activity supports propagation of population bursts in slices of rat antorhinal cortex. *Brain Res.*, 1999, 830: 274–284.

Stewart, M. and Wong, R.K.S. Intrinsic properties and evoked responses of guinea pig subicular neurons in vitro. *J. Neurophysiol.*, 1993, 70: 232–245.

Stewart, M., Quirk, G.J. and Amassian, V.E. Corticospinal responses to electrical stimulation of motor cortex in the rat. *Brain Res.*, 1990, 508: 341–344.

Szentagothai, J. The neuron network of the cerebral cortex: A functional interpretation. *Proc. Roy. Soc. Lond.*, 1978, B201: 219–248.

Takahashi, K. Slow and fast groups of pyramidal tract cells and their respective membrane properties. *J. Neurophysiol.*, 1965, 28: 908–924.

Thomas, C.K., Johansson, R.S., Westling, G. and Bigland-Ritchie, B. Twotch properties of human thenar motor units measured in response to intraneural motor-axon stimulation. *J. Neurophysiol.*, 1990, 64: 1339–1346.

Thomson, A.M. and Deuchars, J. Temporal and spatial properties of local circuits in neocortex. *Trends Neurosci.*, 1994, 17: 119–126.

Tokimura, H., Ridding, M.C., Tokimura, Y., Amassian, V.E. and Rothwell, J.C. Short latency facilitation between pairs of threshold magnetic stimuli applied to human motor cortex. *Electroenceph. Clin. Neurophysiol.*, 1996, 101: 263–272.

Towe, A.L., Patton, H.D. and Kennedy, T.T. Response properties of neurons in the pericruciate cortex of the cat following electrical stimulation of the appendage. *Exp. Neurol.*, 1964, 10: 325–344.

Traub, R.D. and Bibbig, A. A model of high-frequency ripples in the hippocampus based on synaptic coupling plus axon-axon gap junctions between pyramidal cells. *J. Neurosci.*, 2000, 20: 2086–2093.

Traub, R.D., Schmitz, D., Jeffreys, J.G. and Draguhn, A. High-frequency population oscillations are predicted to occur in hippocampal pyramidal neuronal networks interconnected by axoaxonal gap junctions. *Neurosci.*, 1999, 92: 407–426.

Watson, D.E. and Amassian, V.E. Synaptic organization of motor cortex. *The Physiologist*, 1961, 4: 131.

Weiner, H. and Amassian, V.E. Monosynaptic and disynaptic discharge of pyramidal tract neurons during sleep and wakefulness. In: *Psicofisiologia Del Sonno E'Del Sogno*. Bertini, Med. Vita e pensiero, Milan, 1970: 40–47.

Werhahn, K.J., Fong, J.K., Meyer, B.U., Priori, A., Rothwell, J.C., Day, B.L. and Thompson, P.D. The effect of magnetic coil orientation on the latency of surface EMG and single motor unit responses in the first dorsal interosseous muscle. *Electroencephal. Clin. Neurophysiol.*, 1994, 93: 138–146.

Ylinen, A., Bragin, A., Nadasdy, Z., Jando, G., Szabo, I., Sik, A. and Buzsaki, G. Sharp wave-associated high-frequency oscillation (200 Hz) in the intact hippocampus: network and intracellular mechanisms. *J. Neurosci.*, 1995, 15: 30–46.

Ziemann, U. and Rothwell, J.C. I-waves in motor cortex. *J. Clin. Neurophysiol.*, 2000, 17: 397–405.

Ziemann, U., Tergau, F., Wassermann, E.M., Wischer, S., Hildebrandt, J. and Paulus, W. Demonstration of facilitatory I-wave interaction in the human motor cortex by paired transcranial magnetic stimulation. *J. Physiol. (Lond.)*, 1998a, 511: 181–190.

Ziemann, U., Tergau, F., Wischler, S., Hilderbrandt, J. and Paulus, W. Pharmacological control of facilitatory I-wave interaction in the human motor cortex. A paired transcranial magnetic stimulation study. *Electroenceph. Clin. Neurophysiol.*, 1998b, 109: 127–135.

Transcranial Magnetic Stimulation and Transcranial Direct Current Stimulation (Supplements to Clinical Neurophysiology, Vol. 56)
Editors: W. Paulus, F. Tergau, M.A. Nitsche, J.C. Rothwell, U. Ziemann, M. Hallett

Chapter 12

Generation of I waves in the human: spinal recordings

V. Di Lazzaro[a,*], A. Oliviero[a], P. Mazzone[b], F. Pilato[a], E. Saturno[a], M. Dileone[a] and P.A. Tonali[a]

[a] *Department of Neurology, Università Cattolica, L.go A. Gemelli 8, 00168 Rome (Italy)*
[b] *Neurosurgery CTO, Via S. Nemesio 21, 00145 Rome (Italy)*

1. Introduction

Experimental studies in animals have shown that in response to a single electrical stimulus to the motor cortex, an electrode placed in the medullary pyramid or on the dorsolateral surface of the cervical spinal cord records a series of high frequency waves (Patton and Amassian, 1954). The earliest wave that persisted after cortical depression and after cortical ablation was thought to be generated from direct activation of the fast pyramidal tract neuron axons and was termed "D" wave (Patton and Amassian, 1954). The later waves that required intact gray matter, were thought to originate from indirect, trans-synaptic, activation of pyramidal tract neurons and were termed "I" waves (Patton and Amassian, 1954). Recordings from individual pyramidal tract axons showed that a given axon may give both a D and a subsequent I wave discharge.

Recently, the technique of direct recording of epidural activity in conscious humans has shown that monophasic magnetic stimulation with a figure-of-8 coil, inducing posterior-anterior current in the brain, evokes a high-frequency (approximately 700 Hz) repetitive discharge of corticospinal axons (Nakamura et al., 1996; Di Lazzaro et al., 1998a, b).

Thus, transcranial magnetic stimulation, similar to the direct stimulation of the exposed motor cortex in animals produces a series of high frequency waves. What is the origin of this repetitive discharge in humans?

We have had the opportunity to perform a series of direct recordings of the corticospinal volley evoked by transcranial stimulation from the cervical epidural space of conscious patients with chronically implanted spinal electrodes. These recordings provide insights about the physiological basis of the excitatory phenomena produced by transcranial stimulation.

2. Output of the motor cortex produced by transcranial stimulation

Transcranial stimulation can evoke several different kinds of descending activities depending on the type of stimulation: magnetic or electrical (Di Lazzaro et al., 1998a, b), and, in the case of magnetic stimulation, on the direction of the induced current in the brain (Di Lazzaro et al., 1998b, 2001a), the intensity of the stimulus (Di Lazzaro et al., 1998a), the phases of the stimulating current (monophasic or

* *Correspondence to*: Dr. Vincenzo Di Lazzaro, Dipartimento di Neurologia, Università Cattolica, L.go A. Gemelli 8, 00168 Rome, Italy.
Tel: + 39 06 3015 4435; Fax: + 39 06 3550 1909;
E-mail: vdilazzaro@rm.unicatt.it

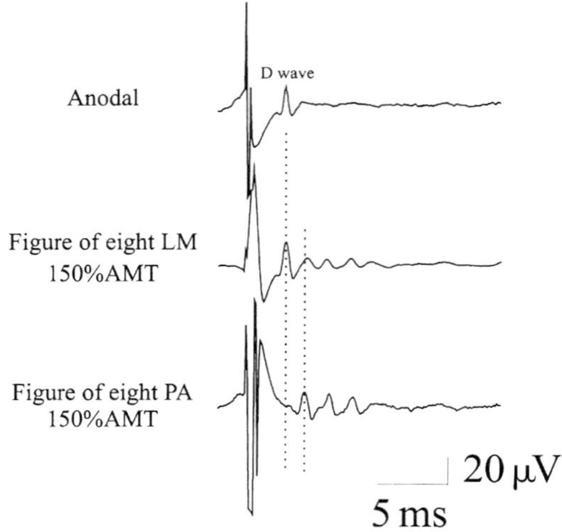

Fig. 1. Averaged descending volleys evoked at suprathreshold intensity by electrical anodal, LM magnetic stimulation, and PA magnetic stimulation in one conscious patient with no central nervous system abnormality. Electrical anodal stimulation evokes a single short latency descending volley (D wave). PA transcranial magnetic stimulation recruits three descending volleys (I waves) the earliest of which appears 1.2 ms later than the D wave evoked by anodal stimulation. LM transcranial magnetic stimulation recruits both D and I waves.

biphasic) (Di Lazzaro et al., 2001b), and the shape of the coil (Di Lazzaro et al., 2002a). The output also depends upon the motor area of the brain stimulated (upper or lower limb area) (Di Lazzaro et al., 2001c).

Some techniques evoke a very stereotyped output in all subjects, while the output may be more variable using different techniques.

The techniques that evoke invariably the same output in all subjects are: anodal stimulation and magnetic stimulation with an 8-shaped coil with a posterior-to-anterior or a lateral-to-medial induced monophasic current.

Electrical (anodal) stimulation of the upper limb motor area evokes at the level of the high cervical cord a single negative wave (Fig. 1) with a latency of 2–2.6 ms. This short latency of the wave evoked by anodal stimulation suggests that it originates from direct activation of corticospinal axons and that it is the equivalent of the D wave described by Patton and Amassian (1954) after direct stimulation of the exposed motor cortex in monkeys.

The lowest threshold volley recruited by magnetic stimulation with a posterior-to-anterior (PA) induced current in the brain has a latency which is 1–1.4 ms longer than the volley recruited by electrical anodal stimulation (Fig. 1) (Di Lazzaro et al., 1998a). This volley increases in size, and is followed by later volleys as the intensity of stimulation is increased. The inter-peak interval between the waves evoked by magnetic stimulation is about 1.4 ms with a periodicity of about 700 Hz. At a stimulus intensity of about 180–200% active motor threshold an earlier small wave appears. This wave has the same latency as the D wave evoked by electrical stimulation.

Changing the orientation of the figure-of-8 coil such that currents in the brain are induced in a lateral-to-medial (LM) direction, both an earliest volley with the same latency of the D wave evoked by electrical anodal stimulation and the later volleys preferentially evoked by PA magnetic stimulation are evoked (Fig. 2).

When the direction of the induced current in the brain is reversed from the usual posterior-to-anterior direction to an anterior-to-posterior (AP) direction, in some subjects magnetic stimulation recruits only some later waves, with approximately the same latency of the later waves evoked by PA magnetic stimulation, but without the preceding earlier waves evoked by PA stimulation (Fig. 2).

When magnetic stimulation is performed using a circular coil centered over the vertex, the earliest volley recorded by the epidural electrode has a latency of about 0.2 ms longer than the LM or anodal D wave (Fig. 3) (Di Lazzaro et al., 2002). This "delayed" D wave can also be evoked by different techniques of transcranial stimulation, like monophasic AP stimulation (Di Lazzaro et al., 2001a) and biphasic magnetic stimulation (Di Lazzaro et al., 2001b). The second volley evoked by magnetic stimulation with a circular coil centered over the vertex has the same latency as the lowest threshold volley evoked by PA magnetic stimulation. At suprathreshold intensities later volleys can be recruited;

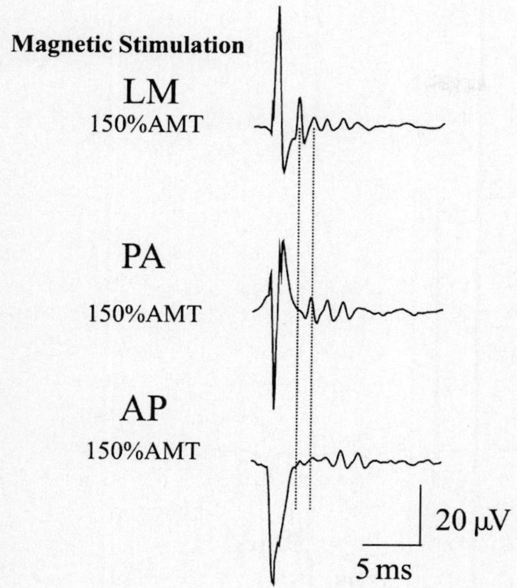

Fig. 2. Averaged descending volleys evoked at suprathreshold intensity by LM magnetic stimulation, PA magnetic stimulation and AP magnetic stimulation in one conscious patient with no abnormality of central nervous system. LM transcranial magnetic stimulation recruits both D and I waves. PA transcranial magnetic stimulation recruits three descending volleys (I waves) and a small D wave. AP transcranial magnetic stimulation recruits only later I waves.

these waves, in some cases, may have a latency that is outside the periodicity of the waves evoked by PA magnetic stimulation. At higher intensities the later waves evoked by non-focal magnetic stimulation are similar to those evoked by PA magnetic stimulation.

3. Changes in the output of the motor cortex produced by changes in cortical excitability

An increase in cortical excitability produced by voluntary contraction has no effect on the amplitude of the descending wave evoked by anodal stimulation (Di Lazzaro et al., 1999) (Fig. 4).

In contrast with the D wave evoked by electrical anodal stimulation and the D wave at the same latency evoked by LM magnetic stimulation, the slightly delayed D wave evoked by a circular coil centered over the vertex is facilitated by an increase in cortical excitability produced by voluntary contraction (Fig. 3). These features suggest that this delayed D wave is initiated closer to the cell body of the pyramidal neurons than the conventional D wave evoked by anodal or LM magnetic stimulation, perhaps at the initial segment rather than at some distance down the axon.

Changes in cortical excitability produce changes in the output of the motor cortex to PA magnetic stimulation. An increase in cortical excitability produced by voluntary contraction of the tested muscle results in an increase in the output of the motor cortex to magnetic stimulation. Voluntary contraction increases the size and number of epidural volleys evoked by a given intensity of magnetic stimulation and the amplitude of the descending waves is higher during activity (particularly during maximum contractions) than at rest (Fig. 4). The effect can be substantial: maximum contraction can increase the total amplitude of the volleys by 50%. This large effect on the size of descending waves is not paralleled by a comparable effect on the threshold for evoking recognisable activity after transcranial magnetic stimulation. The increase in cortical excitability has only a small effect on the threshold for descending activity and only in a minority of subjects (Di Lazzaro et al., 1998a). The limited effect of increase in cortical excitability produced by voluntary contraction on the threshold for descending activity suggests that the elements activated by PA magnetic stimulation of the upper limb area have a relatively constant threshold. The likely explanation is that magnetic stimulation activates cortical axons at some distance from the cell body so that the threshold is unaffected by synaptic activity.

The opposite effect on the output of the motor cortex is observed when the activity of intracortical inhibitory circuits of the cerebral cortex is potentiated through a pharmacological enhancement of inhibitory GABAergic activity. This can be obtained after benzodiazepine administration. After lorazepam the output of the motor cortex to transcranial magnetic stimulation is reduced with a pronounced suppression of later waves (Fig. 4) (Di Lazzaro et al., 2000a).

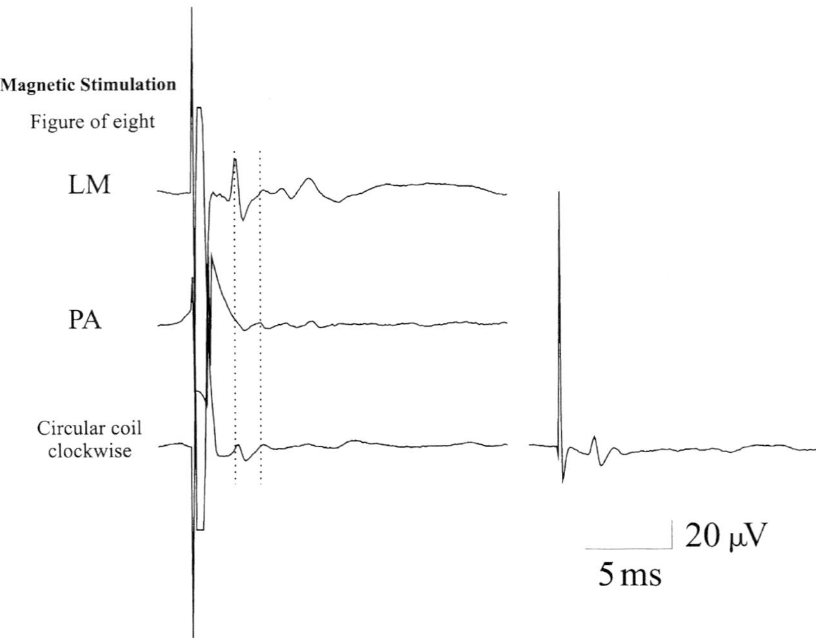

Fig. 3. Averaged descending volleys evoked at suprathreshold intensity by LM magnetic stimulation, PA magnetic stimulation and magnetic stimulation with a circular coil centered over the vertex in one conscious patient with no abnormality of central nervous system. Epidural volleys evoked by a circular coil centered over the vertex are recorded both at rest (left) and during maximum voluntary contraction (right). LM transcranial magnetic stimulation recruits a D wave and I waves. PA transcranial magnetic stimulation I waves. Transcranial magnetic stimulation with a circular coil centered over the vertex recruits a descending wave that has a latency about 0.2 ms longer than the D wave evoked by LM magnetic stimulation. There is a clear enhancing effect of maximum voluntary contraction on the amplitude of the "delayed" D wave evoked by the circular coil (increase of about 100%).

4. Which elements are activated by different forms of transcranial stimulation?

The fact that the earliest wave evoked by electrical anodal stimulation is not modified by changes in cortical excitability produced by voluntary contraction supports the hypothesis that it is due to activation of corticospinal axons in the sub-cortical white matter at some distance from the cell body and corresponds to the D wave described by Patton and Amassian (1954) (Fig. 5).

The slightly delayed D wave evoked by a circular coil centered over the vertex, by AP magnetic stimulation and by biphasic stimulation, appears to be sensitive to the level of cortical excitability. Therefore, we propose that it is initiated closer to the cell body of the pyramidal neurons than the conventional D wave evoked by anodal or LM magnetic stimulation, perhaps at the initial segment rather than at some distance down the axon (Fig. 5).

The lowest threshold volley evoked by PA magnetic stimulation, which has a latency that is 1–1.4 ms longer than the D wave evoked by electrical anodal stimulation as well as the following waves that are recruited at increasing intensities are influenced by the level of cortical excitability. Indeed, an increase or a decrease in cortical excitability are paralleled by an increase or a decrease of these waves. The longer latency of the lowest threshold volley evoked by PA magnetic stimulation, that is consistent with a synaptic delay (Ziemann and Rothwell, 2000), together with its sensitivity to

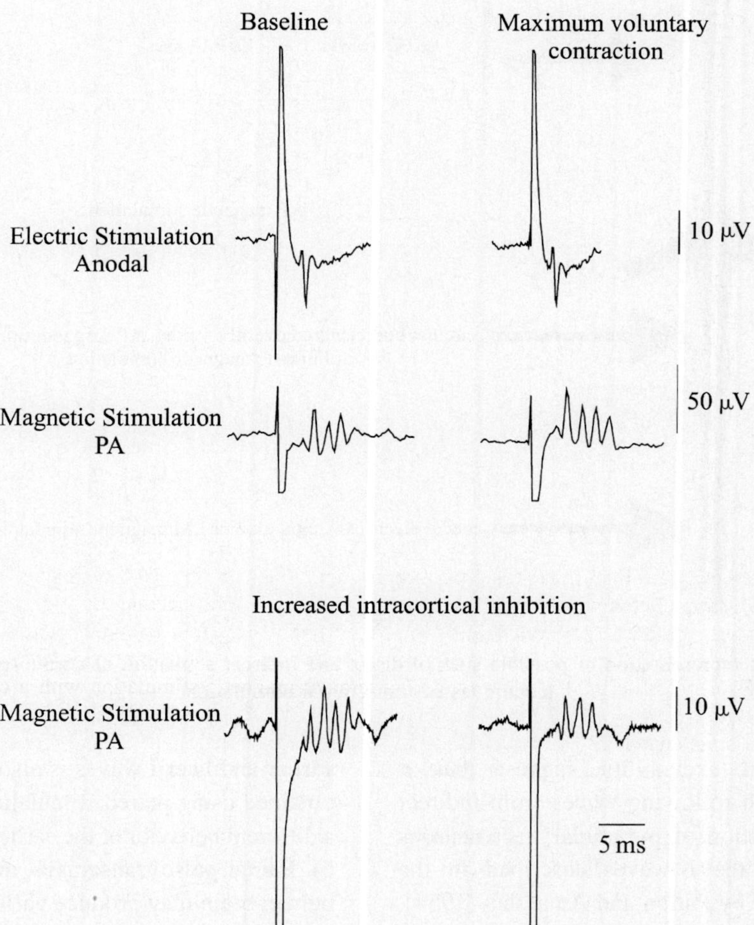

Fig. 4. Effects of changes in cortical excitability on the output of the motor cortex after transcranial electric and magnetic stimulation. Upper traces: descending volleys evoked by electric anodal stimulation, at rest and during maximum voluntary contraction in one subject. Voluntary contraction at maximum strength does not modify D wave amplitude. Middle traces: descending volleys evoked by PA transcranial magnetic stimulation with a figure-of-8 coil at rest and during maximum voluntary contraction in one subject. At rest the magnetic stimulus evokes a small D wave and three I waves, during maximal voluntary contraction the size of the waves increases and a fourth I wave becomes visible. Lower traces: descending volleys evoked by PA transcranial magnetic stimulation with a figure-of-8 coil, at baseline and 2 h after a single oral dose of 2.5 mg lorazepam. The earliest, low amplitude, wave has the same latency as the lowest threshold volley evoked by anodal stimulation (not illustrated) and therefore it is a D wave, later waves represent I waves. The D and I1 waves are unaffected by lorazepam in contrast later I waves which are smaller after lorazepam (adapted from Fig. 1 of Di Lazzaro et al., 2000a).

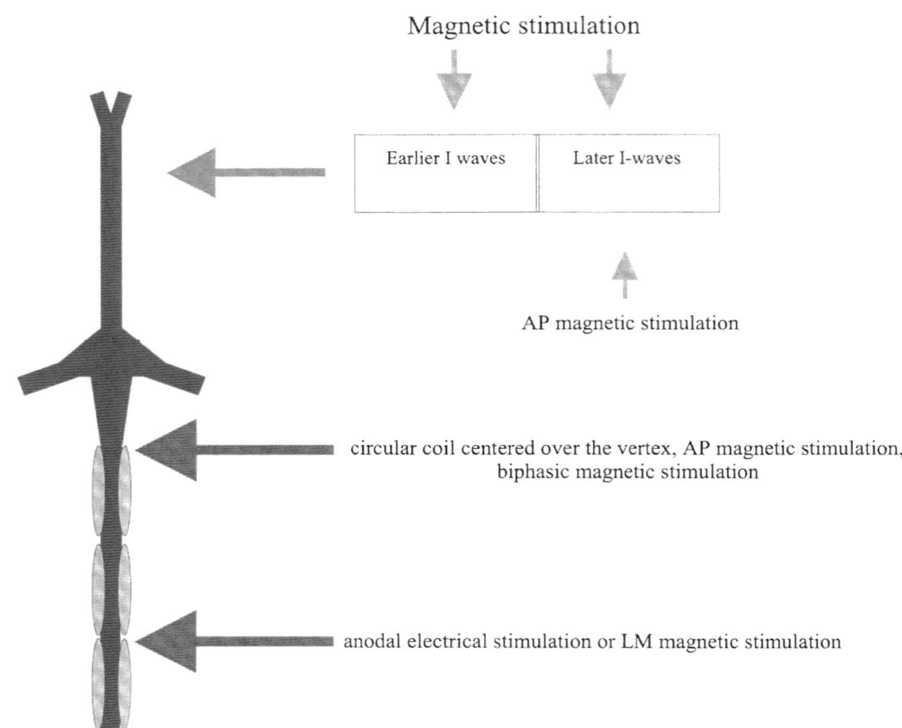

Fig. 5. Diagrammatic representation of possible sites of direct and indirect activation of corticospinal cells using different techniques of transcranial stimulation.

changes in cortical excitability suggest that it originates along with following waves from indirect trans-synaptic activation of pyramidal tract neurons and correspond to the I waves described in the experimental studies by Patton and Amassian (1954). They presumably originate from the activation of cortico-cortical axons projecting to the corticospinal cells. The fact that later I waves can be evoked in isolation in a few subjects using AP magnetic stimulation (Di Lazzaro et al., 2001a), suggests that probably there are two different and independent cortical mechanisms responsible for the generation of earlier and later I waves (Fig. 5).

5. Changes in the output of the motor cortex produced by paired stimulation protocols

The hypothesis of the existence of two independent cortical mechanisms responsible for the generation of earlier and later I waves is also supported by the data obtained using paired stimulation protocols that show a different behavior of the earlier and late I waves (Fig. 6). Paired pulse transcranial magnetic stimulation of human brain may produce various forms of inhibitory phenomena. In the motor cortex, three main types of inhibitory effects have been described. One is a short latency, low threshold inhibition that is believed to involve the $GABA_A$ receptor (Kujirai et al., 1993; Ziemann et al., 1996a, b; Di Lazzaro et al., 1998c, 2000). The second is a high threshold, long lasting inhibition that may involve $GABA_B$ receptors (Roick et al., 1993; Nakamura et al., 1997; Siebner et al., 1998; Werhahn et al., 1999; Sanger et al., 2001; Di Lazzaro et al., 2002b). The third inhibitory protocol is the interhemispheric inhibition produced via a transcallosal pathway on one hemisphere by a magnetic stimulus given 6–30 ms earlier over the opposite hemisphere (Ferbert et al., 1992; Di Lazzaro

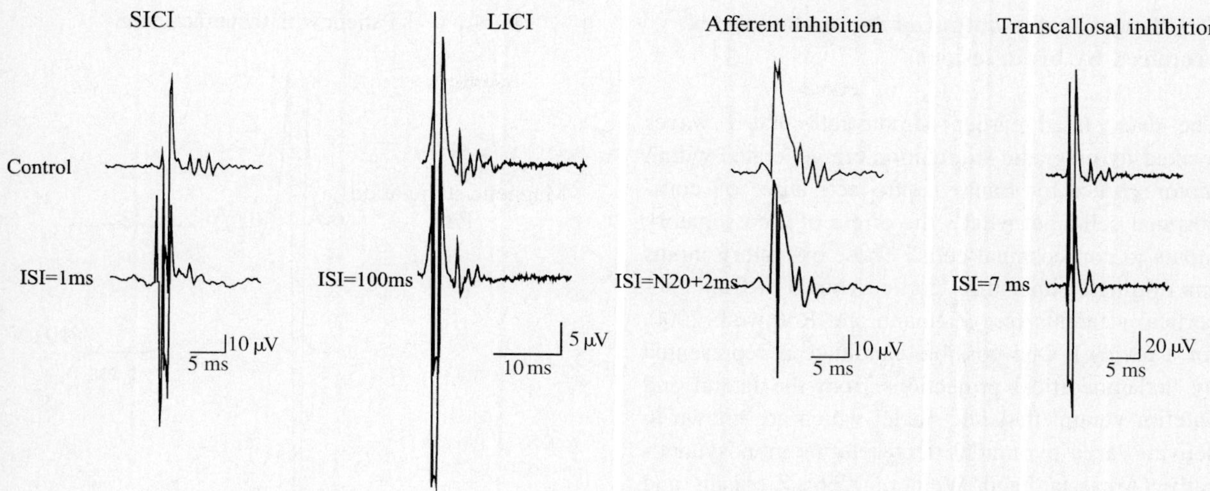

Fig. 6. Epidural volleys by single and paired cortical stimulation (SICI, LICI, transcallosal inhibition) and by cortical stimulation conditioned by median nerve stimulation (short latency afferent inhibition). SICI (short latency intracortical inhibition) is performed using a conditioning stimulus below threshold for obtaining motor responses in active hand muscles and a test suprathreshold magnetic stimulus given 1 ms later. The test stimulus alone (control, upper trace) evokes multiple descending waves (four waves). When both stimuli are delivered all the descending waves except the I1 are suppressed (lower trace). LICI (long latency intracortical inhibition) uses a suprathreshold conditioning stimulus and a test stimulus of the same intensity given 100 ms later. The conditioning stimulus alone (control, upper trace) evokes multiple descending waves (four waves), while the output of the motor cortex produced by the test stimulus delivered 100 ms later is clearly inhibited (lower trace). The latest I wave (I4 wave) is clearly suppressed and there is a slight inhibition of the I2 and I3 waves, whereas the I1 wave is not affected. Short latency afferent inhibition is performed by coupling transcranial magnetic stimulation with peripheral nerve stimulation. Single pulse magnetic stimulation evokes three I waves (control, upper trace). When cortical stimulation is conditioned with an electrical stimulus delivered to the median nerve at the wrist at an interstimulus interval corresponding to the latency of N20 wave of somatosensory evoked potential plus 2 ms, the later I wave (I3 wave) is suppressed while the I1 wave is not affected (lower trace). Transcallosal inhibition is obtained when the magnetic test stimulus over one motor cortex is preceded by a conditioning stimulus applied to the opposite hemisphere 7 ms earlier. The test stimulus alone (control, upper trace) evokes multiple descending waves (three waves) When both stimuli are delivered the latest (I3) wave is suppressed, the second (I2) wave is slightly inhibited while the earliest (I1) wave is not modified (lower trace).

et al., 1999b). The direct recording of the cortical output produced by all these protocols of cortical inhibition has shown that only later I waves are suppressed whereas earlier I waves are not affected (Fig. 6) (Di Lazzaro et al., 1998c, 1999b, 2002b). The same behavior of earlier and later I waves is observed using a different protocol of cortical inhibition based on coupling transcranial magnetic stimulation with peripheral nerve stimulation (Tokimura et al., 2000). The motor responses evoked by magnetic stimulation of the motor cortex can be suppressed by electrical stimulation of the median nerve if the time interval between stimulation of median nerve and motor cortex is 2–8 ms longer than the time needed by the peripheral nerve afferent inputs to reach the cortex (Tokimura et al., 2000). This effect, named short latency afferent inhibition of the motor cortex, is produced by interactions within the cerebral cortex (Tokimura et al., 2000) and the inhibitory effect only involves later I waves (Fig. 6). The implication of all these studies is that there are differences in some of the cortical structures involved in producing the early and late I waves and that these can be targeted differentially by several conditioning procedures.

6. Changes in the output of the motor cortex produced by brain lesions

The data stated earlier demonstrate that I waves evoked by magnetic stimulation are generated within motor cortex by transsynaptic activation of corticospinal cells, but what's the origin of the excitatory inputs to corticospinal cells? These excitatory inputs can originate either from corticocortical or from subcortical afferents (see Ziemann and Rothwell, 2000, for a review). One possible candidate is represented by thalamocortical projections from the lateral and anterior ventral thalamic nuclei which are known to activate large pyramidal tract neurons monosynaptically (Amassian and Weiner, 1966; Ziemann and Rothwell, 2000). However, experimental data in the cat suggest that projections from the thalamus are not essential for the production of I waves (Amassian et al., 1987). We have had the opportunity to evaluate directly the role of thalamocortical projections in the generation of I waves by recording directly the output of the motor cortex in one patient with thalamic lesions who had a high cervical epidural electrode (Di Lazzaro et al., 2002b). The patient was a 63-year-old woman with a left hemiparkinsonism associated with minimal dystonic findings and of a right pyramidal and parkinsonian syndrome. The MR of the brain of this patient showed multiple subcortical vascular lesions. At the level of the thalamus of the right side there were multiple non-acute lesions with lacunar lesions located in the lateral portion, and gliotic changes in the medial portion. The right thalamic lesion was associated with an extensive destructive lesion of the right putamen due to old hemorrhagic events. In this patient, PA magnetic stimulation of the right motor cortex at 110% resting motor threshold intensity evoked a completely normal descending activity with three I waves and a small D wave (Fig. 7). Therefore, projections from the thalamus to the motor cortex seem not be involved in the generation of I waves that more probably originate through the activation of corticocortical connections.

In this patient we observed that the amount of long latency intracortical inhibition was more pronounced than in subjects with no abnormality of the CNS.

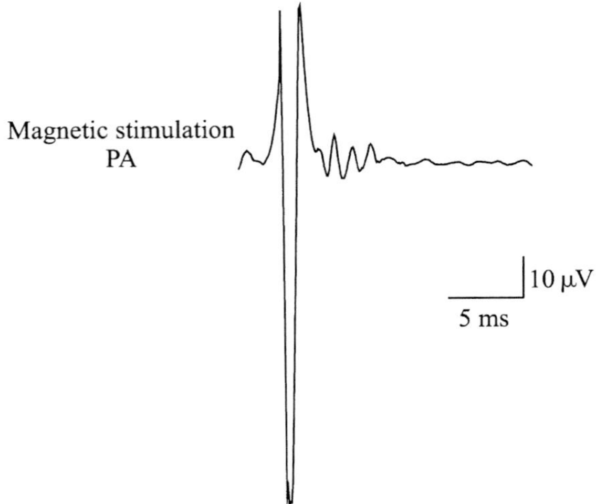

Fig. 7. Epidural volleys by magnetic stimulation of the right motor cortex in a patient with a lesion of the right motor thalamus and of the right putamen. Magnetic motor cortex stimulation evokes a fully normal descending volley with multiple descending waves (three I waves and a small D wave).

Using this protocol of cortical inhibition we observed that all the I waves were suppressed including the earliest one. Only the small D wave was not substantially modified.

A more pronounced suppression of the output of the motor cortex after long latency paired stimulation has also been reported in a different pathological condition. Chen et al. (1999) recorded epidural volleys evoked by paired suprathreshold magnetic stimulation at long interstimulus intervals in a single patient who had suffered avulsion of the brachial plexus, and found that all volleys were suppressed, including the initial D wave. Because Chen et al. (1999) used a large round coil the D wave they evoked was the "delayed" D wave that originates close to the cell body and for this reason is affected by changes in the excitability of pyramidal neurons.

Therefore, the data in these two patients suggest that the behavior of earlier, and late, I waves during paired stimulation may be different in some pathological conditions. Indeed, in both patients the epidural recordings are consistent with a direct inhibition of the corticospinal cells produced by the first conditioning stimulus. In contrast, the differential behavior of earlier and later I waves in subjects with no abnormality of the CNS is more consistent with an indirect inhibition of pyramidal cells, acting upstream to the pyramidal cells on the mechanism generating the later I waves. The source of the direct inhibition of pyramidal cells observed in the two patients might be represented by the chandelier cells that project to the initial segment of the axons of pyramidal cells or by the basket cells that give rise to a "basket" of terminals around the cell bodies of pyramidal neurons. Both of these cells have powerful effects on the output of the pyramidal neurons. It can be hypothesised that these inhibitory cells become accessible to transcranial stimulation in pathological conditions only, at least in the range of stimulus intensities commonly used.

7. Neurotransmitters involved in I wave generation

It has been hypothesised that GABAergic connections may be involved in the generation of I waves (Ziemann and Rothwell, 2000). This hypothesis has been supported by the direct recording of epidural volleys after lorazepam that showed that drugs potentiating $GABA_A$ function produce a suppression of later I waves (Di Lazzaro et al., 2000a) (Fig. 4).

The role of different neurotransmitters in the generation of I waves has been evaluated in several studies (Di Lazzaro et al., 2000, 2003), but inferences about the role of various neurotransmitters have been indirect since all these studies were based on EMG measures of responses to transcranial magnetic stimulation. The changes in the motor responses evoked by transcranial magnetic stimulation observed after different pharmacological manipulations suggest that I waves may be generated by glutamatergic circuits of the motor cortex (Ziemann et al., 1998; Di Lazzaro et al., 2003) that are modulated by GABAergic (Ziemann et al., 1996a; Di Lazzaro et al., 2000; Ilic et al., 2002), cholinergic (Di Lazzaro et al., 2000; Liepert et al., 2001); and noradrenergic (Ilic et al., 2003) connections.

References

Amassian, V.E. and Weiner, H. Monsynaptic and polysynaptic activation of pyramidal tract neurons by thalamic stimulation. In: D.P. Purpura and M.D. Yahr (Eds.), *The Thalamus*. Columbia University Press, New York, 1966: 255–282.

Amassian, V.E., Stewart, M., Quirk, G.J. and Rosenthal, J.L. Physiological basis of motor effects of a transient stimulus to cerebral cortex. *Neurosurgery*, 1987, 20: 74–93.

Chen, R., Lozano, A.M. and Ashby, P. Mechanism of the silent period following transcranial magnetic stimulation. Evidence from epidural recordings. *Exp. Brain Res.*, 1999, 128: 539–542.

Di Lazzaro, V., Restuccia, D., Oliviero, A., Profice, P., Ferrara, L., Insola, A., Mazzone, P., Tonali, P. and Rothwell, J.C. Effects of voluntary contraction on descending volleys evoked by transcranial stimulation in conscious humans. *J. Physiol.* (*Lond.*), 1998a, 508: 625–633.

Di Lazzaro, V., Oliviero, A., Profice, P., Saturno, E., Pilato, F., Insola, A., Mazzone, P., Tonali, P. and Rothwell, J.C. Comparison of descending volleys evoked by transcranial magnetic and electric stimulation in conscious humans. *Electroencephalogr. Clin. Neurophysiol.*, 1998b, 109: 397–401.

Di Lazzaro, V., Restuccia, D., Oliviero, A., Profice, P., Ferrara, L., Insola, A., Mazzone, P., Tonali, P. and Rothwell, J.C. Magnetic transcranial stimulation at intensities below active motor threshold activates intracortical inhibitory circuits. *Exp. Brain Res.*, 1998c, 119: 265–268.

Di Lazzaro, V., Oliviero, A., Profice, P., Insola, A., Mazzone, P., Tonali, P. and Rothwell, J.C. Effects of voluntary contraction on descending volleys evoked by transcranial electrical stimulation over the motor cortex hand area in conscious humans. *Exp. Brain Res.*, 1999a, 124: 525–528.

Di Lazzaro, V., Oliviero, A., Profice, P., Insola, A., Mazzone, P., Tonali, P. and Rothwell, J.C. Direct demonstration of interhemispheric inhibition of the human motor cortex produced by transcranial magnetic stimulation. *Exp. Brain Res.*, 1999b, 124: 520–524.

Di Lazzaro, V., Oliviero, A., Meglio, M., Cioni, B., Tamburrini, G., Tonali, P. and Rothwell, J.C. Direct demonstration of the effect of lorazepam on the excitability of the human motor cortex. *Clin. Neurophysiol.*, 2000a, 111: 794–799.

Di Lazzaro, V., Oliviero, A., Profice, P., Pennisi, M.A., Di Giovanni, S., Zito, G., Tonali, P. and Rothwell, J.C. Muscarinic receptor blockade has differential effects on the excitability of intracortical circuits in the human motor cortex. *Exp. Brain Res.*, 2000b, 135: 455–461.

Di Lazzaro, V., Oliviero, A., Saturno, E., Pilato, F., Insola, A., Mazzone, P., Profice, P., Tonali, P. and Rothwell, J.C. The effect on corticospinal volleys of reversing the direction of current induced in the motor cortex by transcranial magnetic stimulation. *Exp. Brain Res.*, 2001a, 138: 268–273.

Di Lazzaro, V., Oliviero, A., Mazzone, P., Insola, A., Pilato, F., Saturno, E., Accurso, A., Tonali, P. and Rothwell, J.C.

Comparison of descending volleys evoked by monophasic and biphasic magnetic stimulation of the motor cortex in conscious humans. *Exp. Brain Res.*, 2001b, 141: 121–127.

Di Lazzaro, V., Oliviero, A., Profice, P., Meglio, M., Cioni, B., Tonali, P. and Rothwell, J.C. Descending spinal cord volleys evoked by transcranial magnetic and electrical stimulation of the motor cortex leg area in conscious humans. *J. Physiol.*, 2001c, 537: 1047–1058.

Di Lazzaro, V., Oliviero, A., Pilato, F., Saturno, E., Insola, A., Mazzone, P., Tonali, P.A. and Rothwell, J.C. Descending volleys evoked by transcranial magnetic stimulation of the brain in conscious humans: effects of coil shape. *Clin. Neurophysiol.*, 2002a, 113: 114–119.

Di Lazzaro, V., Oliviero, A., Mazzone, P., Pilato, F., Saturno, E., Insola, A., Visocchi, M., Colosimo, C., Tonali, P.A. and Rothwell, J.C. Direct demonstration of long latency cortico-cortical inhibition in normal subjects and in a patient with vascular parkinsonism. *Clin. Neurophysiol.*, 2002b, 113: 1673–1679.

Di Lazzaro, V., Oliviero, A., Profice, P., Pennisi, M.A., Pilato, F., Zito, G., Dileone, M., Nicoletti, R., Pasqualetti, P. and Tonali, P.A. Ketamine increases human motor cortex excitability to transcranial magnetic stimulation. *J. Physiol.*, 2003, 547: 485–496.

Ferbert, A., Priori, A., Rothwell, J.C., Day, B.L., Colebatch, J.G. and Marsden, C.D. Interhemispheric inhibition of the human motor cortex. *J. Physiol.*, 1992, 453: 525–546.

Ilic, T.V., Meintzschel, F., Cleff, U., Ruge, D., Kessler, K.R. and Ziemann, U. Short-interval paired-pulse inhibition and facilitation of human motor cortex: the dimension of stimulus intensity. *J. Physiol.*, 2002, 545: 153–167.

Ilic, T.V., Korchounov, A. and Ziemann, U. Methylphenidate facilitates and disinhibits the motor cortex in intact humans. *Neuroreport*, 2003, 14: 773–776.

Kujirai, T., Caramia, M.D., Rothwell, J.C., Day, B.I., Thompson, P.D., Ferbert, A., Wroe, S., Asselman, P. and Marsden, C.D. Cortico-cortical inhibition in human motor cortex. *J. Physiol. (Lond.)*, 1993, 471: 501–520.

Liepert, J., Schardt, S. and Weiller, C. Orally administered atropine enhances motor cortex excitability: a transcranial magnetic stimulation study in human subjects. *Neurosci. Lett.*, 2001, 300: 149–152.

Nakamura, H., Kitagawa, H., Kawaguchi, Y. and Tsuji, H. Direct and indirect activation of human corticospinal neurons by transcranial magnetic and electrical stimulation. *Neurosci. Lett.*, 1996, 210: 45–48.

Nakamura, H., Kitagawa, H., Kawaguchi, Y. and Tsuji, H. Intracortical facilitation and inhibition after transcranial magnetic stimulation in conscious humans. *J. Physiol. (Lond.)*, 1997, 498.3: 817–823.

Patton, H.D. and Amassian, V.E. Single- and multiple-unit analysis of cortical stage of pyramidal tract activation. *J. Neurophysiol.*, 1954, 17: 345–363.

Roick, H., Von Giesen, H.J., Benecke, R. On the origin of the postexcitatory inhibition seen after transcranial magnetic brain stimulation in awake human subjects. *Exp. Brain Res.*, 1993, 94: 489–498.

Sanger, T.D., Garg, R.R. and Chen, R. Interaction between two different inhibitory systems in the human motor cortex. *J. Physiol. (Lond.)*, 2001, 530: 307–317.

Siebner, H.R., Dressnandt, J., Auer, C. and Conrad, B. Continuous intrathecal baclofen infusions induced a marked increase of the transcranially evoked silent period in a patient with generalized dystonia. *Muscle Nerve*, 1998, 21: 1209–1212.

Tokimura, H., Di Lazzaro, V., Tokimura, Y., Oliviero, A., Profice, P., Insola, A., Mazzone, P., Tonali, P. and Rothwell, J.C. Short latency inhibition of human hand motor cortex by somatosensory input from the hand. *J. Physiol.*, 2000, 523: 503–513.

Werhahn, K.J., Kunesch, E., Noachtar, S., Benecke, R. and Classen, J. Differential effects on motorcortical inhibition induced by blockade of GABA uptake in humans. *J. Physiol.*, 1999, 517: 591–597.

Ziemann, U. and Rothwell, J.C. I waves in motor cortex. *J. Clin. Neurophysiol.*, 2000, 17: 397–405.Ziemann, U., Lonnecker, S., Steinhof, B.J. and Paulus, W. The effect of lorazepam on the motor cortical excitability in man. *Exp. Brain Res.*, 1996a, 109: 127–135.

Ziemann, U., Lonnecker, S., Steinhoff, B.J. and Paulus, W. Effects of antiepileptics drugs on motor cortex excitability in humans: a transcranial magnetic stimulation study. *Ann. Neurol.*, 1996b, 40: 367–378.

Ziemann, U., Chen, R., Cohen, L.G. and Hallett, M. Dextromethorphan decreases the excitability of the human motor cortex. *Neurology*, 1998, 51: 1320–1324.

Transcranial Magnetic Stimulation and Transcranial Direct Current Stimulation (Supplements to Clinical Neurophysiology, Vol. 56)
Editors: W. Paulus, F. Tergau, M.A. Nitsche, J.C. Rothwell, U. Ziemann, M. Hallett

Chapter 13

Surround inhibition

Mark Hallett

Human Motor Control Section, NINDS, NIH, Bethesda, MD 20892–1428 (USA)

1. Introduction

A basic operational principle of the central nervous system is that any activation, considered either at the level of a single neuron or group of neurons, is the net result of an interplay between excitatory and inhibitory influences. There are many types of excitatory and inhibitory mechanisms. With respect to inhibition, in particular, there are a large number of types of inhibitory neurons and many types of connections (Somogyi et al., 1998). Transcranial magnetic stimulation (TMS) studies of motor function have revealed a variety of types of inhibition and these likely arise from these different inhibitory connections. These types of inhibition are generally recognized as clinical neurophysiological phenomena. Their functional role in movement generation is less well understood.

A principle for function of the motor system may be "surround inhibition". Surround inhibition is a concept well accepted in sensory physiology (Angelucci et al., 2002). For example, receptive fields in the visual cortex are organized such that light in the center of field will activate a cell, while light in the periphery will inhibit it. Such a pattern helps to sharpen borders and is an important step in the formation of patterns and objects. Surround inhibition is not so well known in the motor system, but it is a logical concept. When making a movement, the brain must activate the motor system. It is possible that the brain just activates the specific movement. On the other hand, it is more likely that the one specific movement is generated, and, simultaneously, other possible movements are suppressed. The suppression of unwanted movements would be surround inhibition. This should produce a more precise movement, just as surround inhibition in sensory systems produces more precise perceptions.

2. A brief review of types of inhibition revealed by TMS

Short intracortical inhibition (SICI) is obtained with paired pulse methods and reflects interneuron influences in the cortex (Ziemann et al., 1996). In such studies, an initial conditioning stimulus is given, enough to activate cortical neurons, but small enough that no descending influence on the spinal cord can be detected. A second test stimulus, at suprathreshold level, follows at short interval. Intracortical influences

* *Correspondence to*: Dr. Mark Hallett, M.D., Chief, Human Motor Control Section, NINDS, NIH, Building 10, Room 5N226, 10 Center Drive, MSC 1428, Bethesda, MD 20892-1428, USA.
Tel: 301-496-9526; Fax: 301-480-2286;
E-mail: hallettm@ninds.nih.gov

initiated by the conditioning stimulus modulate the amplitude of the motor evoked potential (MEP) produced by the test stimulus. At short intervals, less than 5 ms, there is inhibition that is likely largely a GABAergic effect, specifically GABA-A (Di Lazzaro et al., 2000a) (at intervals between 8 and 30 ms, there is facilitation, called intracortical facilitation, ICF).

The silent period (SP) is a pause in ongoing voluntary EMG activity produced by TMS. While the first part of the SP is due in part to spinal cord refractoriness, the latter part is entirely due to cortical inhibition (Fuhr et al., 1991). This type of inhibition is likely mediated by GABA-B receptors (Werhahn et al., 1999). SICI and the SP show different modulation in different circumstances and clearly reflect different aspects of cortical inhibition.

Intracortical inhibition can also be assessed with paired suprathreshold TMS pulses at intervals from 50 to 200 ms (Valls-Solé et al., 1992). This is called long intracortical inhibition, or LICI, to differentiate it from SICI as noted above. LICI and SICI differ as demonstrated by the facts that with increasing test pulse strength, LICI decreases but SICI tends to increase, and that there is no correlation between the degree of SICI and LICI in different individuals (Sanger et al., 2001). Interestingly, but not surprisingly from what is known about the anatomy of cortical GABAergic cells, one type of inhibition can affect another. Specifically, LICI inhibits SICI (Sanger et al., 2001). The mechanisms of LICI and the SP may be similar in that both seem to depend on GABA-B receptors.

There are two phases of inhibition of the MEP produced by somatosensory stimulation of nerves in the hand, 25–30 ms and 150–200 ms, which can be called short and long peripheral nerve inhibition, SPNI and LPNI (Classen et al., 2000). SPNI appears to depend on muscarinic receptors as demonstrated by its selective blockage by scopolamine (Di Lazzaro et al., 2000b).

Transcallosal inhibition (TCI) is produced by conditioning a test MEP with subthreshold stimulation of the motor cortex in the contralateral hemisphere at an interval of about 10 ms (Netz et al., 1995). Some of this ipsilateral effect on the MEP is likely mediated subcortically (Gerloff et al., 1998). There is also a transcallosal influence of shortening of the silent period, suggesting inhibition of the inhibitory neurons that produce it (Schnitzler et al., 1996).

Cerebellar inhibition is produced by conditioning a test MEP with strong stimulation of the ipsilateral cerebellum at an interval between 5 and 7 ms (Ugawa et al., 1995).

As noted earlier, these different phenomena reflect different central nervous system pathways for inhibition, but how they function in operations of the motor system is not, in general, known.

3. Anatomical and physiological background for functional surround inhibition

The cortex has anatomical and functional connections that allow for surround inhibition. Activation of a region gives rise to activity in short inhibitory interneurons that inhibit nearby neurons. This pattern has been well characterized in models of focal epilepsy where neurons surrounding a focus are inhibited (Collins, 1978).

The basal ganglia can influence inhibition and are anatomically organized to work in a center-surround mechanism. This idea of center-surround organization was one of the possible functions of the basal ganglia circuitry suggested by Alexander and Crutcher (1990). Subsequently, Mink detailed the possible anatomy (Mink, 1996). The direct pathway has a focused inhibition in the globus pallidus while the subthalamic nucleus has divergent excitation. The direct pathway (with two inhibitory synapses) is a net excitatory pathway and the indirect pathway (with three inhibitory synapses) is a net inhibitory pathway. Hence the direct pathway can be the center and the indirect pathway the surround of a center-surround mechanism.

Tremblay and Filion (1989) studied the reactions of single cells in the globus pallidus to stimulation in the striatum. The great majority of responses consisted of an initial inhibition, at a mean latency of 14 ms, followed by excitation, at a mean latency of 35 ms. The early inhibition was always displayed by neurons located in the center of the pallidal zone of influence of each striatal stimulation site, and was ended and often curtailed by excitation. At the periphery of the zone, excitation occurred alone or as the initial component of responses. The authors state that "this topological arrangement suggests that excitation is used, temporally, to control the magnitude of the central striatopallidal inhibitory signal and, spatially, to focus and contrast it onto a restricted number of pallidal neurons". In interpreting this data, it is important to remember that the output of the globus pallidus is inhibitory, so that inhibition would be the "center" signal and excitation the "surround" signal.

14. Evidence for surround inhibition in human motor systems

The concepts that the motor system makes a movement by activating one pattern and inhibiting others, and that the basal ganglia play a role in this process have been discussed for many years. The idea might have been original to Denny-Brown (Denny-Brown and Yanagisawa, 1976), but was emphasized in my own work as well (Hallett and Khoshbin, 1980). There is now explicit evidence that inhibition of unselected tasks actually occurs.

Leocani et al. evaluated corticospinal excitability of both hemispheres during the auditory reaction time (RT) tasks using TMS (Leocani et al., 2000). Subjects performed right and left thumb extensions in simple (SRT), choice (CRT) and go/no-go auditory RT paradigms. TMS, which induced MEPs simultaneously in the extensor pollicis brevis muscles bilaterally, was applied at different latencies from the tone. For all paradigms, MEP amplitudes on the side of movement increased progressively in the 80–120 ms before EMG onset, while the resting side showed inhibition. The inhibition was significantly more pronounced for right than for left thumb movements. After no-go tones, bilateral inhibition occurred at a time corresponding to the mean RT to go tones. Corticospinal inhibition on the side not to be moved suggests that suppression of movement is an active process. Proof that this is active rather than passive comes from studies of no-go trials by Waldvogel et al. (2000) and Sohn et al. (2002). During the period of MEP suppression, intracortical inhibition was determined to be increased using the paired-pulse TMS method. Further evidence for this effect to be cortical comes from the observation of Liepert et al. (2001) who showed that the inhibition of the contralateral hand, while demonstrable with TMS, could not be demonstrated with transcranial electrical stimulation.

Sohn et al. have shown that with movement of one finger there is widespread inhibition of muscles in the contralateral limb (Sohn et al., 2003). Significant suppression of MEP amplitudes was observed when TMS was applied between 35 and 70 ms after EMG onset (Fig. 1). This inhibition affected "adjacent" muscles (those near the homologous muscle in the same extremity) as well as homologous muscles, but more inhibition was observed in adjacent and distal muscles than homologous and proximal muscles. Paired-pulse TMS (at 2- and 10-ms interstimulus intervals) showed a significant increase in intracortical facilitation (ICF) selectively in the homologous muscle when triggered by self-paced movement of the opposite hand, but no change was observed in intracortical inhibition. At the same time, the silent period of the homologous muscle was significantly shortened, but the F-wave and compound muscle action potential were unchanged. The findings demonstrated that voluntary hand movement exerts an inhibitory influence on a diffuse area of the ipsilateral motor cortex. The inhibitory influence is nonselective, while the facilitatory influence (enhancing ICF) appears to act selectively on the homologous muscle. Thus, there is some center-surround character to this transcallosal inhibitory effect.

Sohn et al. have also shown that there is some inhibition of muscles in the ipsilateral limb when those muscles are not involved in any way in the movement (Sohn and Hallett, 2002). Subjects made self-paced movements of the right index finger. TMS was delivered to the left motor cortex from 3 ms to 1000 ms after EMG onset in the flexor digitorum superficialis muscle. MEPs from abductor digiti minimi were unchanged during the movement of the index finger in the face of increased F-wave

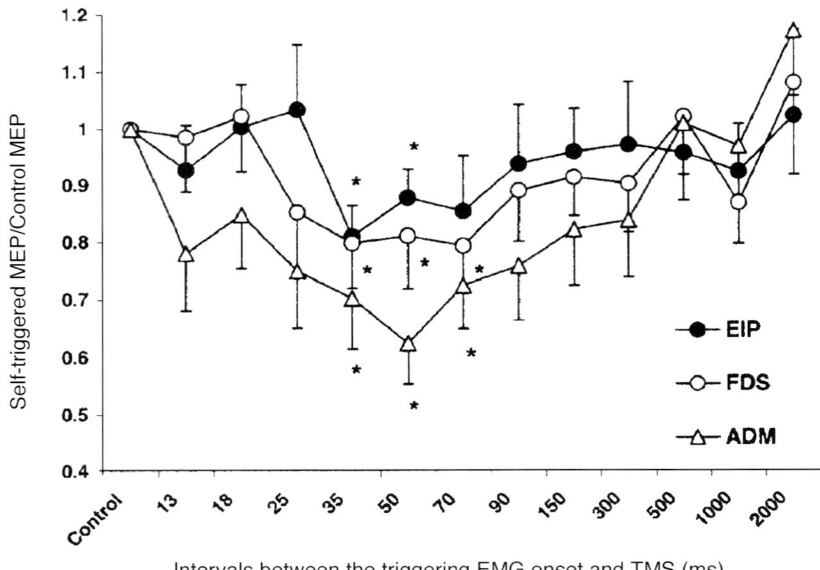

Fig. 1. Time course changes in motor evoked potential (MEP), amplitude of left extensor indicis proprius (EIP, solid circles), flexor digitorum superficialis (FDS, open circles) and abductor digiti minimi (ADM, open triangles) from the EMG onset of right EIP activation. TMS was triggered by right EIP activation at a stimulation intensity of 140% resting motor threshold for left EIP. Data are shown as the ratio (means ± SEM) of the self-triggered MEP amplitude to the control MEP amplitude ($n = 12$; *different from control, $P < 0.05$). There was significant suppression at intervals of 35 and 50 ms in all three muscles, and of 70 ms in FDS and ADM. Non-significant MEP suppression was observed until 300 ms. The MEP suppression was more prominent in ADM than other muscles. From Sohn et al. (Sohn et al., 2003) with permission.

amplitude and persistence, suggesting that the cortical excitability is actually reduced.

In another experiment, Liepert et al. (1998) studied changes in intracortical inhibition associated with two motor tasks requiring a different selectivity in fine motor control of small hand muscles (abductor pollicis brevis muscle, APB, and fourth dorsal interosseous muscle, 4DIO). In experiment 1, subjects completed four sets (5 min duration each) of repetitive thumb movements at 1 Hz. In experiment 2, the subjects produced the same number of thumb movements, but complete relaxation of 4DIO was demanded. Following free thumb movements, amplitudes of MEPs in response to both single and paired TMS showed a trend to increase with the number of exercise sets in both APB and 4DIO. By contrast, more focal, selective thumb movements involving APB with relaxation of 4DIO caused an increase in MEP amplitudes after single and paired pulses only in APB, while there was a marked decrease in MEPs after paired pulses, but not after single TMS, in the actively relaxed 4DIO. Intracortical inhibition within the hand representation appears to vary according to the selective requirements of the motor program. Performance of more focal tasks may be associated with a decrease in intracortical inhibition in muscles engaged in the repetitive action, while at the same time intracortical inhibition may be increased in an actively relaxed muscle.

5. Focal dystonia may result from a failure of surround inhibition

Dystonia is characterized by excessive movement. The excessive movement leads to involuntary movements, distorted voluntary movements and abnormal postures. While it can be present at rest, it is brought out more by attempted voluntary movement. EMG studies have revealed that there is excessive co-contraction of antagonist muscles and there is overflow activation of extraneous muscles (Cohen and Hallett, 1988). With phasic movements, there are prolonged EMG bursts. Given that the central nervous system operates as a balance between excitation and inhibition, excessive movement could arise from increased excitability or reduced inhibition. Evidence has been accumulating that dystonia is generated by a loss of inhibition. If surround inhibition in the motor system is lacking, it would not be surprising that a disorder like dystonia would emerge.

The evidence for loss of inhibition in dystonia comes from studies of spinal and brainstem reflexes and cortical mechanisms. Examples of such data are the loss of reciprocal inhibition in the arm in patient with focal hand dystonia (Rothwell et al., 1983; Nakashima et al., 1989; Panizza et al., 1989, 1990), abnormalities of blink reflex recovery in blepharospasm (Berardelli et al., 1985), and loss of intracortical inhibition in patients with focal hand dystonia (Ridding et al., 1995). A more recent finding is there is also loss of inhibition produced by cutaneous stimulation. Stimulation of the median nerve or index finger, leads to inhibition of MEPs in hand and forearm muscles at various intervals becoming maximal at 200 ms (called LPNI earlier). Patients with focal hand dystonia show facilitation instead (Abbruzzese et al., 2001).

It should be noted that loss of cortical inhibition in motor cortex can give rise to dystonic-like movements in primates. Matsumura et al. showed that local application of bicuculline, a GABA antagonist, onto the motor cortex led to disordered movement and changed the movement pattern from reciprocal inhibition of antagonist muscles to co-contraction (Matsumura et al., 1991). In a second study, they showed that bicuculline caused cells to loose their crisp directionality, converted unidirectional cells to bidirectional cells, and increased firing rates of most cells including making silent cells into active ones (Matsumura et al., 1992). There is preliminary evidence from magnetic resonance spectroscopy that GABA is diminished in the motor cortex region in patients with hand dystonia (Levy and Hallett, 2002).

Bütefisch et al. (2000). have tested whether task-dependent modulation of inhibition within the motor cortex is impaired in dystonia using an experimental design similar to that of Liepert et al. (1998) described above. Paired pulse TMS at short inter-stimulus time intervals was used to measure cortical inhibition in muscles that acted as agonist (abductor pollicis brevis, APB) and synergist (fourth dorsal interosseus muscle, 4DIO) in a selective and non-selective task. The synergistic muscle was activated in the non-selective task but not in the selective task. Following the selective task, the conditioned MEP of the synergist decreased in normal subjects while the conditioned MEP of the agonist increased. In contrast, conditioned MEP of both synergistic and agonist muscles increased in the dystonic subjects. In the non-selective task the conditioned amplitudes of both muscles increased in normal and dystonic subjects. These results suggest that task dependent cortical inhibition is disturbed in patients with dystonia.

As noted earlier, Sohn and Hallett (2002) have shown that there is probable cortical inhibition of the ADM (an uninvolved muscle in the "surround") when the FDS of the index finger is activated. This effect is less in patients with focal hand dystonia. Molloy et al. have shown the same phenomenon in the preparatory period before movement onset (Molloy et al., 2002).

References

Abbruzzese, G., Marchese, R., Buccolieri, A., Gasparetto, B. and Trompetto, C. Abnormalities of sensorimotor integration in focal dystonia: a transcranial magnetic stimulation study. *Brain*, 2001, 124: 537–545.

Alexander, G.E. and Crutcher, M.D. Functional achitecture of basal ganglia circuits: neural substrates of parallel processing. *Trends in Neuroscience*, 1990, 13: 266–271.

Angelucci, A., Levitt, J.B. and Lund, J.S. Anatomical origins of the classical receptive field and modulatory surround field of single neurons in macaque visual cortical area V1. *Prog. Brain Res.*, 2002, 136: 373–388.

Berardelli, A., Rothwell, J.C., Day, B.L. and Marsden, C.D. Pathophysiology of blepharospasm and oromandibular dystonia. *Brain*, 1985, 108: 593–608.

Bütefisch, C.M., Boroojerdi, B., Battaglia, F., Chen, R. and Hallett, M. Task dependent intracortical inhibition is impaired in patients with task specific dystonia. *Movement Disorders*, 2000, 15(Suppl. 3): 153.

Classen, J., Steinfelder, B., Liepert, J., Stefan, K., Celnik, P., Cohen, L.G., et al. Cutaneomotor integration in humans is somatotopically organized at various levels of the nervous system and is task dependent. *Exp. Brain Res.*, 2000, 130: 48–59.

Cohen, L.G. and Hallett, M. Hand cramps: clinical features and electromyographic patterns in a focal dystonia. *Neurology*, 1988, 38: 1005–1012.

Collins, R.C. Use of cortical circuits during focal penicillin seizures: an autoradiographic study with [14C]deoxyglucose. *Brain Res.*, 1978, 150: 487–501.

Denny-Brown, D. and Yanagisawa, N. The role of the basal ganglia in the initiation of movement. In: M.D. Yahr (Ed.), *The Basal Ganglia*. Raven Press, New York, 1976: 115–119.

Di Lazzaro, V., Oliviero, A., Meglio, M., Cioni, B., Tamburrini, G., Tonali, P., et al. Direct demonstration of the effect of lorazepam on the excitability of the human motor cortex. *Clin. Neurophysiol.*, 2000a, 111: 794–749.

Di Lazzaro, V., Oliviero, A., Profice, P., Pennisi, M.A., Di Giovanni, S., Zito, G., et al. Muscarinic receptor blockade has differential effects on the excitability of intracortical circuits in the human motor cortex. *Exp. Brain Res.*, 2000b, 135: 455–461.

Fuhr, P., Agostino, R. and Hallett, M. Spinal motor neuron excitability during the silent period after cortical stimulation. *Electroenceph. Clin. Neurophysiol.*, 1991, 81: 257–262.

Gerloff, C., Cohen, L.G., Floeter, M.K., Chen, R., Corwell, B. and Hallett, M. Inhibitory influence of the ipsilateral motor cortex on responses to stimulation of the human cortex and pyramidal tract. *J. Physiol.*, 1998, 510: 249–259.

Hallett, M., Khoshbin, S. A physiological mechanism of bradykinesia. *Brain*, 1980, 103: 301–314.

Leocani, L., Cohen. L.G., Wassermann, E.M., Ikoma, K. and Hallett, M. Human corticospinal excitability evaluated with transcranial magnetic stimulation during different reaction time paradigms. *Brain*, 2000, 123: 1161–1173.

Levy, L.M. and Hallett, M. Impaired brain GABA in focal dystonia. *Ann. Neurol.*, 2002, 51: 93–101.

Liepert, J., Classen, J., Cohen, L.G. and Hallett, M. Task-dependent changes of intracortical inhibition. *Exp. Brain Res.*, 1998, 118: 421–426.

Liepert, J., Dettmers, C., Terborg, C. and Weiller, C. Inhibition of ipsilateral motor cortex during phasic generation of low force. *Clin. Neurophysiol.*, 2001, 112: 114–121.

Matsumura, M., Sawaguchi, T., Oishi, T., Ueki, K. and Kubota, K. Behavioral deficits induced by local injection of bicuculline and muscimol into the primate motor and premotor cortex. *J. Neurophysiol.*, 1991, 65: 1542–1553.

Matsumura, M., Sawaguchi, T. and Kubota, K. GABAergic inhibition of neuronal activity in the primate motor and premotor cortex during voluntary movement. *J. Neurophysiol.*, 1992, 68: 692–702.

Mink, J.W. The basal ganglia: focused selection and inhibition of competing motor programs. *Prog. Neurobiol.*, 1996, 50: 381–425.

Molloy, F., Sohn, Y.H. and Hallett, M. Surround inhibition is impaired in patients with focal hand dystonia during movement preparation. *Movement Disorders*, 2002, 17 (Suppl 5): S304–S305.

Nakashima, K., Rothwell, J.C., Day, B.L., Thompson, P.D., Shannon, K. and Marsden, C.D. Reciprocal inhibition in writer's and other occupational cramps and hemiparesis due to stroke. *Brain*, 1989, 112: 681–697.

Netz, J., Ziemann, U. and Homberg, V. Hemispheric asymmetry of transcallosal inhibition in man. *Exp. Brain Res.*, 1995, 104: 527–533.

Panizza, M.E., Hallett, M. and Nilsson, J. Reciprocal inhibition in patients with hand cramps. *Neurology*, 1989, 39: 85–89.

Panizza, M., Lelli, S., Nilsson, J. and Hallett, M. H-reflex recovery curve and reciprocal inhibition of H-reflex in different kinds of dystonia. *Neurology*, 1990, 40: 824–828.

Ridding, M.C., Sheean, G., Rothwell, J.C., Inzelberg, R. and Kujirai, T. Changes in the balance between motor cortical excitation and inhibition in focal, task specific dystonia. *J. Neurol., Neurosurg., Psych.*, 1995, 59: 493–498.

Rothwell, J.C., Obeso, J.A., Day, B.L. and Marsden, C.D. Pathophysiology of dystonias. *Adv. Neurol.*, 1983, 39: 851–863.

Sanger, T.D., Garg, R.R. and Chen, R. Interactions between two different inhibitory systems in the human motor cortex. *J. Physiol.*, 2001, 530: 307–317.

Schnitzler, A., Kessler, K.R. and Benecke, R. Transcallosally mediated inhibition of interneurons within human primary motor cortex. *Exp. Brain Res.*, 1996, 112: 381–391.

Sohn, Y.H. and Hallett, M. Impaired surround inhibition in focal hand dystonia during voluntary movement. *Movement Disorders*, 2002, 17 (Suppl 5): S290–S291.

Sohn, Y.H., Wiltz, K. and Hallett, M. Effect of volitional inhibition on cortical inhibitory mechanisms. *J. Neurophysiol.*, 2002, 88: 333–338.

Sohn, Y.H., Jung, H.Y., Kaelin-Lang, A. and Hallett, M. Excitability of the ipsilateral motor cortex during phasic voluntary hand movement. *Exp. Brain Res.*, 2003, 148: 176–185.

Somogyi, P., Tamas, G., Lujan, R. and Buhl, E.H. Salient features of synaptic organisation in the cerebral cortex. *Brain Res. Rev.*, 1998, 26: 113–135.

Tremblay, L. and Filion, M. Responses of pallidal neurons to striatal stimulation in intact waking monkeys. *Brain Res.*, 1989, 498: 1–16.

Ugawa, Y., Uesaka, Y., Terao, Y., Hanajima, R. and Kanazawa, I. Magnetic stimulation over the cerebellum in humans. *Ann. Neurol.*, 1995, 37: 703–713.

Valls-Solé, J., Pascual-Leone, A., Wassermann, E.M. and Hallett, M. Human motor evoked responses to paired transcranial magnetic stimuli. *Electroenceph. Clin. Neurophysiol.*, 1992, 85: 355–364.

Waldvogel, D., van Gelderen, P., Muellbacher, W., Ziemann, U., Immisch, I. and Hallett, M. The relative metabolic demand of inhibition and excitation. *Nature*, 2000, 406: 995–998.

Werhahn, K.J., Kunesch, E., Noachtar, S., Benecke, R. and Classen, J. Differential effects on motorcortical inhibition induced by blockade of GABA uptake in humans. *J. Physiol.* (Lond), 1999, 517: 591–597.

Ziemann, U., Rothwell, J.C. and Ridding, M.C. Interaction between intracortical inhibition and facilitation in human motor cortex. *J. Physiol.* (*Lond.*), 1996. 496: 873–881.

Transcranial Magnetic Stimulation and Transcranial Direct Current Stimulation (Supplements to Clinical Neurophysiology, Vol. 56)
Editors: W. Paulus, F. Tergau, M.A. Nitsche, J.C. Rothwell, U. Ziemann, M. Hallett

Chapter 14

Functional connectivity of the human premotor and motor cortex explored with TMS

T. Bäumer[a], J.C. Rothwell[b] and A. Münchau[a,*]

[a]*Neurology Department, Hamburg University, Martinistrasse 52, D-20246 Hamburg (Germany)*
[b]*Sobell Department of Neurophysiology, Institute of Neurology, Queen Square, London WC1N 3BG (UK)*

1. Background

The dorsolateral premotor cortex (Broca area F4) is located on the crown of the precentral gyrus anterior to the primary motor cortex, that lies in the anterior bank of the central sulcus (Foerster, 1936; Preuss et al., 1996). The close proximity of the premotor and the motor cortex and their similar somatotopic organization (Godschalk et al., 1995; Raos et al., 2003) imply that they are also anatomically and functionally interconnected. Anatomical studies in animals have established that apart from direct connections to the spinal cord large areas of the premotor cortex have dense connections to the motor cortex (Dum and Strick, 1991; Morecraft and Van Hoesen, 1993; Stepniewska et al., 1993; Tokuno and Nambu, 2000). A recent human fMRI study suggests that such cortico-cortical organisation between premotor and motor cortex is somatotopically organised also in human subjects (Buccino et al., 2001). In addition to their connections to the motor cortex different sub-areas of the premotor cortex receive inputs also from the frontal cortex and information on external stimuli via the inferior and superior parietal sulcus (Wise et al., 1997; Battaglia Mayer et al., 1998; Rizzolatti et al., 1998; Marconi et al., 2001). Apart from its importance for the performance of complex skilled movements (Dum and Strick, 1991; Cisek et al., 2003) the premotor cortex has therefore been considered to be involved in externally referenced movements, especially visually guided movements (Wise, 1985). It seems to integrate visual response selection and timing adjustments for the responses, i.e. what to do and when to do it (Sakai et al., 2000).

A number of studies have looked more closely at the neurophysiology of the premotor-motor circuitry in primates and in human subjects (Ghosh and Porter, 1988; Godschalk et al., 1995; Ashby et al., 1999; Tokuno and Nambu, 2000; Civardi et al., 2001; Gerschlager et al., 2001; Münchau et al., 2002a). For instance, microstimulation of premotor cortex neurons in primates can produce excitatory or inhibitory effects in the motor cortex (Ghosh and Porter, 1988; Tokuno and Nambu, 2000). Stimulation of the premotor cortex results predominantly in short latency inhibition of pyramidal tract neurons that may involve excitatory inputs to superficial inhibitory

* *Correspondence to*: Dr. A. Münchau, Neurology Department, Hamburg University, Martinistrasse 52, D-20246 Hamburg, Germany.
Tel.: +49 (40) 42803 3770; Fax: +49 (40) 42803 5086;
E-mail: muenchau@uke.uni-hamburg.de

interneurons in the motor cortex (Tokuno and Nambu, 2000).

The aim of this chapter is to give an overview over neurophysiological, particularly TMS/rTMS studies, that have examined the premotor-motor circuitry in human subjects. We will start with studies on focal electrical stimulation of the premotor and motor area and will then focus on TMS.

2. Subdural electrical stimulation of motor areas

To localise the area from which inhibition and facilitation of corticospinal excitability occur Ashby et al. (1999) performed a paired pulse experiment using electrical stimulation applied over an 8 × 8 cm grid of subdural electrodes implanted for diagnostic purposes in a young, otherwise healthy epileptic woman. Each of the 64 electrodes had a diameter of 5 mm with a centre-to-centre separation of 1 cm. After identifying the "hot spot" of the target muscle (i.e. abductor pollicis brevis muscle) they applied sub motor threshold conditioning pulses through adjacent electrodes at different distances between 1 and 50 ms before suprathreshold electrical test pulses given over the motor "hot spot". They found that when conditioning stimuli were given through a pair of neighbouring electrodes within the hand area of the motor cortex inhibition was obtained at interstimulus intervals (ISIs) of 2 ms and between 30 and 50 ms, and facilitation between 5 and 15 ms. When applying conditioning pulses through more distant electrodes including two that were located anteriorly close to or within the premotor area they showed that facilitation was only induced within a distance of 1 cm from the site where test pulses were given. In contrast, inhibition occurred up to a distance of 1–2 cm anterior and anterior-medial of the motor "hot spot". At distances of more than 2 cm away from the "hot spot" no changes of the motor evoked potential could be evoked by conditioning pulses.

A possible interpretation of these data is that there is a balance of inhibitory and facilitatory inputs, presumably through intracortical interneurons, close to a given motor "hot spot", whereas projections from more distant sites including the premotor area are predominantly inhibitory. Alternatively, the activation threshold of more distant inhibitory interneurons could be lower than that for facilitatory neurons.

3. TMS studies

3.1. Methodological considerations

TMS is an established non-invasive method to chart the functional connectivity of the human motor system, e.g. the corticospinal connection from motor cortex to spinal cord and the transcallosal connection between the two motor cortices (Rothwell et al., 1991; Ferbert et al., 1992; Netz et al., 1995). Several recent TMS/rTMS and combined TMS/EEG or TMS/imaging studies have also explored the connectivity between the motor cortex and non-primary motor areas including the premotor cortex (Praamstra et al., 1999; Civardi et al., 2001; Gerschlager et al., 2001; Siebner et al., 2001; Münchau et al., 2002a, 2002b; Oliviero et al., 2003). Here we focus on TMS and rTMS/TMS studies.

A principal problem of TMS/rTMS experiments where TMS pulses are applied outside the motor cortex in the premotor area is that the effects of premotor stimulation cannot be determined directly but only indirectly through measurements of motor cortex excitability using single or paired pulse TMS over the motor cortex.

An inherent shortcoming of TMS/rTMS is poor spatial accuracy. This is particularly problematic in experiments that aim at identifying differential effects of TMS/rTMS over adjacent brain areas like the motor and premotor cortex. rTMS application over a particular brain area may lead to inadvertent co-activation of adjacent brain areas through physical spread of the stimulus. To avoid such physical spread of TMS pulses from motor to premotor cortex during motor cortex stimulation and vice versa low or very low TMS/rTMS stimulation intensities can be used as was indeed done in the TMS/rTMS studies discussed below. A drawback of low intensity stimulation may, of course, be reduced effectiveness. In addition to physical spread focal rTMS may also lead to physiological spread via synaptic connections.

In fact, this is a prerequisite of TMS/rTMS studies on cortico-cortical connectivity.

Intensities of TMS or rTMS application to the premotor area are traditionally referenced to the motor cortex threshold for TMS pulses, although it is unknown whether the TMS responsiveness of the premotor cortex is similar to that of the motor cortex. For instance, in animal studies it was shown that the threshold for electrical stimulation was lower in the premotor cortex (Preuss et al., 1996). Moreover, it is conceivable that due to its location at the top of the precentral gyrus the premotor cortex is more "accessible" to external stimulation and has thus lower TMS stimulation thresholds.

Conventional coil placement where brain regions other than the motor cortex are stimulated is referenced to the position of the motor "hot spot". However, this does not account for individual variations in the distance between motor areas and the target brain regions and thus leads to variable effective brain stimulation (Herwig et al., 2001). Therefore, to target relevant brain regions accurately neuronavigation systems that guide coil placement on the basis of individual anatomical and functional MRI scans should be used in future studies.

These methodological limitations have to be borne in mind when interpreting data of the following experiments.

3.2. TMS study using single conditioning TMS pulses applied over the premotor area

Previously, it was shown that subthreshold conditioning pulses given over the primary motor cortex (M1) can modulate the size of the ipsilateral test MEP depending on the interstimulus intervals (ISI) with conditioning pulses at short intervals (2–5 ms) producing inhibition and those at longer intervals (6–20 ms) producing facilitation (Kujirai et al., 1993). Ferbert and colleagues demonstrated that conditioning pulses applied to M1 contralaterally also lead to an inhibition of the test MEP, presumably via transcalloasal fibres (Ferbert et al., 1992). Recently, Civardi and colleagues studied the effects of conditioning TMS pulse at different positions anterior to M1 in the premotor and prefrontal area on M1 excitability as determined by the size of supratheshold TMS pulse given over the M1 hand area (Civardi et al., 2001). Two small figure-of-eight coils with an inner diameter of 4 cm were used for the conditioning and the test pulse, respectively. They tested the effects at ISIs of 4, 6 and 8 ms at 13 different positions in a 1×1 cm grid anterior to the interauricular line. At an intensity of the conditioning pulse of 90% active motor threshold (AMT) they found inhibitory effects at an ISI of 6 ms which were most pronounced at two distinct positions. One was located 5 cm anterior to the "hot spot" and 6 cm lateral to the midline (A) and the other in the midline 6 cm anterior to the interauricular line (B) corresponding to the premotor cortex and the pre SMA, respectively.

At point A inhibition of the test pulse at an ISI of 6 ms was only induced with an intensity of the conditioning pulses of 90% AMT, but not with 80%, and a coil position leading to an anterior-posterior (AP) current flow in the brain, whereas a reverse posterior-anterior (PA) current flow produced no significant effects. Facilitation of the test pulse was produced with an intensity of 90% AMT at an ISI of 15 ms and 120% at an ISI of 6 ms, respectively.

This implies that there are both inhibitory and facilitatory inputs from the premotor to the motor cortex that can be activated by low intensity stimulation over the premotor area. At higher intensities facilitatory effects prevail which could be due to current spread to the motor cortex with activation of facilitatory motor cortex interneurons. Alternatively, facilitatory premotor interneurons could have higher activation thresholds.

3.2.1. rTMS studies

rTMS can influence the excitability of human motor cortex when applied directly over the motor cortex area. MEPs are suppressed after low frequency (1 Hz or less) motor rTMS applied for five minutes or more (Chen et al., 1997; Wassermann et al., 1998; Maeda et al., 2000; Muellbacher et al., 2000). In contrast, an increase of the size of EMG responses occurs if higher frequencies, and higher intensities are used (Pascual-Leone et al., 1994; Wu et al., 2000). Moreover motor cortex rTMS trains also affect intrinsic motor cortex excitability as determined with the Kujirai paired pulse paradigm (Kujirai et al., 1993). Thus, high frequency rTMS decreases intracortical inhibition (ICI) in the stimulated hemisphere (Peinemann et al., 2000; Wu et al., 2000). Gerschlager et al. (2001) investigated the effect of subthreshold (90% AMT) 1 Hz rTMS applied to the left lateral premotor, left lateral frontal, left anterior parietal cortex and the hand area of the left M1 on net corticospinal excitability as reflected in the MEP size to suprathreshold TMS pulses applied over left M1. They stimulated at different points on a line parallel to the midline, i.e. directly over M1, 2.5 and 5 cm anterior and 2.5 cm posterior to the M1 "hot spot". Five trains of 300 pulses were given in each condition. MEPs were measured before and following application of 900 and 1500 rTMS pulses. MEP amplitudes were significantly reduced after rTMS over the premotor area, but not at any other stimulation site. This effect occurred after 900 pulses and outlasted the rTMS session for at least 15 min. To examine whether this effect was dependent on the effective current flow during rTMS the authors tested two additional coil orientations for premotor rTMS by rotating the coil by 90° and 180° from the customary coil orientation (handle pointing 45° postero-laterally). MEP suppression of similar magnitude was present after premotor rTMS with the coil handle pointing in the antero-medial direction (rotation by 180°) but not in the lateral-medial direction (rotation by 90°).

The magnetic stimulus had a biphasic waveform with the first phase of the stimulus inducing a PA current flow in the brain when the coil is held in the customary position. According to recent single pulse studies the more effective stimulation occurs during the second phase of the biphasic pulse which thus induces an AP current (Corthout et al., 2001; Kammer et al., 2001). Apparently, premotor-motor projections mediating MEP depression following biphasic 1 Hz premotor rTMS at 90% AMT can be activated both by AP and PA current flow.

To investigate the effects of left premotor rTMS on intrinsic left motor cortex excitability, Münchau et al. (2002a) used 1 Hz premotor rTMS at intensities of 70, 80 and 90% AMT and measured motor thresholds, the MEP size, ICI and intracortical facilitation (ICF) using the Kujirai paired pulse paradigm at ISI between 2 and 7, 10 and 15 ms and the silent period. The coil was always positioned with the handle pointing 45° postero-laterally with the most effective current thus flowing in the AP direction. The rTMS stimulation point over the premotor area was defined as lying 8% of the distance between nasion and inion (typically about 3 cm) anterior to the motor cortex hand area "hot spot", i.e. approximately 0.5 cm more anterior than the stimulation site chosen by Gerschlager et al. (2001). In control experiments they used identical rTMS trains directly over the motor cortex and 3 cm posteriorly of the motor "hot spot", i.e. over the area of the somatosensory cortex. Following premotor rTMS there was a significant increase in intracortical excitability at ISIs of 6 and 7 ms in the paired pulse experiment outlasting the rTMS train by about an hour (Fig. 1). The question arises of whether this effect was caused by effective stimulation of the premotor area under the centre of

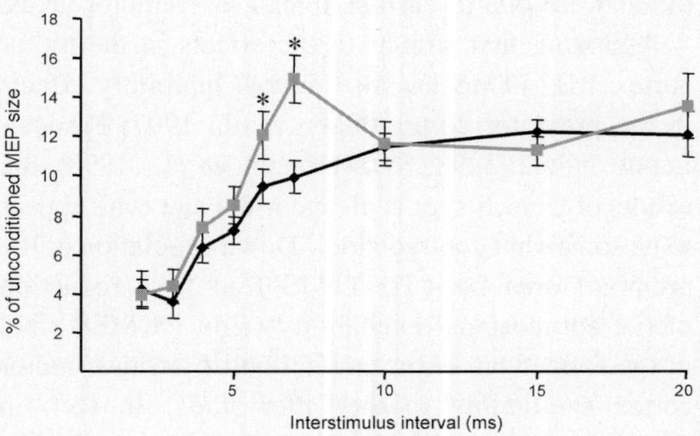

Fig. 1. Intracortical inhibition/facilitation (ICI/ICF) curves before and after 80% AMT rTMS over the premotor area in 13 subjects. Mean (± S.E.M.) time course of the conditioned test motor evoked potential (MEP) after rTMS is superimposed on the time course at baseline. The size of the conditioned test response is expressed as a percentage of the unconditioned test size. After premotor rTMS facilitation was significantly increased at an ISI of 6 and 7 ms. * = $p < 0.05$.

the rTMS coil or in the motor cortex directly because of physical current spread away from the coil. This seems unlikely as after moving the rTMS coil, so that its centre was over the motor hand area, or more posterior, over the sensory cortex, there was no effect on ICI/ICF. Since the intensity of rTMS was the same as the intensity of the first pulse in the ICI/ICF paradigm (80% AMT), and rTMS over motor cortex had no effect on ICI/ICF, we can presume that premotor rTMS was not having a direct effect on the intracortical elements activated in the ICI/ICF paradigm. The conclusion is that premotor rTMS was influencing interneurons in the motor cortex through cortico-cortical premotor-motor connections.

In addition to specific changes of intracortical excitability and corroborating these findings there was also a shortening of the cortical silent period after premotor rTMS but not after motor or sensory rTMS.

In previous studies probing the effect of rTMS on ICI/ICF (Ziemann et al., 1998; Siebner et al., 1999; Peinemann et al., 2000; Wu et al., 2000), rTMS was applied over the motor cortex directly, and at a higher intensity and/or frequency than used in the premotor study by Münchau et al. (2002a) (between 90–120% resting motor threshold). It is therefore possible that some of the effects on intracortical inhibition were due to current spread to premotor areas.

Assuming that similar to the effects in the motor cortex 1 Hz rTMS has also overall inhibitory effects in the premotor cortex (Chen et al., 1997; Pascual-Leone et al., 1998; Wassermann et al., 1998) the results of Gerschlager et al. and Münchau et al. appear to be somewhat contradictory. Down-regulation of the premotor area by 1 Hz rTMS lead to a reduction of net corticospinal excitability (reduced MEP size) in the former but extra facilitation of intrinsic motor cortex excitability in the latter study. In fact, in contrast to the results of Gerschlager et al. (2001), Münchau et al. (2002a) did not find a significant reduction of the MEP amplitudes after 1 Hz premotor rTMS.

The most reasonable explanation for this discrepancy is that lower rTMS stimulation intensities used in the study by Münchau et al. (2002a) (80% AMT) induced changes in different sets of interneuronal projections from the premotor to the motor cortex. Such stimulation may have been sufficient to act on low threshold inhibitory premotor-motor interneurons without activating facilitatory ones. On the other hand, slightly higher intensities in the Gerschlager study (Gerschlager et al., 2001) (90% AMT) may have activated both projections with stronger effects on facilitatory inputs.

Alternatively, the slightly more anterior coil placement in the study by Münchau et al., could have lead to more anterior effective stimulation. On the basis of the work of Ashby et al. (1999) (see above) it is conceivable that under the experimental conditions used down-regulation of the premotor area closer to the motor cortex (Gerschlager et al., 2001) predominantly affected facilitatory premotor-motor projections resulting in net inhibitory effects in the motor cortex (MEP size reduction) whereas "inhibitory" 1 Hz rTMS at a slightly greater distance from the motor cortex (Münchau et al., 2002a) mainly acted on inhibitory pathways from the premotor to the motor cortex causing specific extra facilitation (increase of ICF at an ISI of 6 and 7 ms).

Finally, which premotor-motor projections are predominantly activated or deactivated by TMS may depend on the direction of the current flow. Deactivation of inhibitory premotor-motor projections by premotor conditioning TMS or 1 Hz rTMS was induced by an effective AP current flow in the studies by Civardi et al. (2001) and Münchau et al. (2002), whereas a PA current flow did not produce inhibition, at least in the Civardi study (Civardi et al., 2001) (it was not tested in the study by Münchau et al.). In contrast, net inhibitory effects onto the motor cortex, presumably due to deactivation of facilitatory premotor-motor connection, by 1 Hz premotor rTMS in the study by Gerschlager et al. (2001) could be induced both with an effective AP and PA current flow while only a latero-medial flow did not lead to a change of MEP size.

Taken together, in line with studies in primates (Ghosh and Porter, 1988; Tokuno and Nambu, 2000) these data imply a complex neurophysiological interaction between premotor and motor cortex that can be inhibitory or facilitatory.

The specificity of the extra facilitation only at certain ISI in the study by Münchau et al. (2002a) is noteworthy. It has been argued that ICI occurring at ISI between 2 and 6 ms and ICF at longer ISIs (7–20 ms) are caused by separate mechanisms as the threshold of a conditioning pulse to produce inhibition is lower than that to produce facilitation (Kujirai et al., 1993; Ziemann et al., 1996). Also, ICF depends on the orientation of the stimulation coil whereas ICI does not (Ziemann et al., 1996) and ICI and ICF can be modulated independently by drugs acting on the CNS or are altered independently in a number of neurological conditions (Ziemann et al., 1999). Moreover, closer inspection of the results of other studies using the paired pulse paradigm implies that the paired pulse curve reflects the balance of inhibition and facilitation in a number of different classes of interneurons. For instance, intake of haloperidol leads to an increase in ICF at specific ISI (12 and 15), but not at others (10, 20 or 30 ms) in healthy subjects (Ziemann et al., 1997). In patients with Parkinson's disease Ridding et al. (1995a) found a significant decrease in ICI at 2, 4 and 5 ms, but not at 3 or 7 ms. It is therefore probably more appropriate to consider the motor cortex paired pulse curve as a composite of many interneuronal circuits each of which have certain time constants rather than a curve reflecting the activity in one set of inhibitory and another of facilitatory interneurons. These various sets of interneurons may represent modifiable "excitability modules" (Fig. 2) that can be "accessed" and modulated separately. Apparently, there are projections from the premotor to the motor cortex that modulate those "modules" that shape the paired pulse curve at certain intervals (in this case 6 and 7 ms) but not at others.

It has to be borne in mind that on the basis of the data discussed above it cannot be decided whether the consequences of premotor rTMS on motor cortex excitability are due to lasting effects on ongoing levels of activity in a connection from premotor to motor cortex (as suggested in Fig. 2) or due to rTMS activation of a connection from premotor to motor cortex which then results in an after effect on the activity of neurons in the motor cortex. Thus, it could be that following rTMS activity in the premotor area normalizes quickly and that the after effects are caused by altered motor cortex activity only.

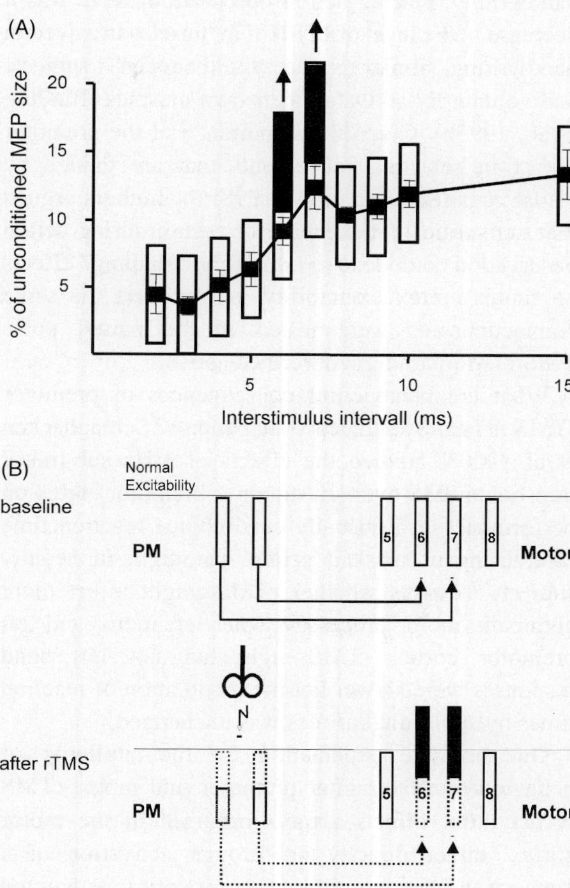

Fig. 2. (A) Schematic drawing of the paired pulse curve with premotor rTMS induced effects. Changes occur at certain ISI (6 and 7 ms) but do not affect the whole "inhibitory" or "facilitatory" part of the curve. The paired pulse curve probably represents a composite of many interneuronal circuits, each of which may correspond to modifiable "excitability modules". These are symbolized by open or filled rectangles. The latter represent those modules that receive premotor inputs. (B) The premotor cortex apparently acts on some modules, e.g. those that determine the level of excitability at an ISI of 6 and 7 ms, but not on others. Under the experimental conditions used in the study by Münchau et al. (2002) this action is inhibitory. "Inhibitory" 1 Hz rTMS then reduces premotor activity thus "releasing" dependent motor cortex interneuronal modules which leads to extra facilitation in the motor cortex.

In a behavioural test of the premotor-motor connection, Strafella and Paus (2000) instructed resting healthy subjects to observe other people during handwriting. During action observation, there was a decrease in the level of ICI/ICF in muscles involved in handwriting, similar to what would happen if subjects had voluntarily activated their own muscles (Ridding et al., 1995b). Given the importance of the premotor cortex in selecting movements that are guided by visual cues (Schluter et al., 1998) the authors argued that activation of the premotor cortex during action observation could lead to inhibitory, "shaping" effects on motor cortex excitability, perhaps via the same connections as were tested in the paired pulse TMS/rTMS paradigm described above.

What are behavioural consequences of premotor rTMS in healthy subjects or in patients? Schlaghecken et al. (2003) studied the effects of 1 Hz sub-motor threshold rTMS over left motor or premotor cortex on performance in a visually cued choice reaction time task, using a 'masked prime' paradigm in healthy subjects to asses whether rTMS might affect more automatic motor processes. After left motor and left premotor cortex rTMS right but not left hand responses were slower but the modulation of reaction times by subliminal primes was unchanged.

One possible explanation for the similarity of behavioural effects after premotor and motor rTMS is that after effects always occurred in the motor cortex, either directly or through activation of a connection from premotor to motor cortex, as pointed out above. Alternatively, as premotor and motor cortex are topographically and functionally closely connected, particularly concerning processing of visuomotor information (Schluter et al., 1998), changes in motor behaviour might ensue whenever activity in either motor or premotor cortex is altered, implying conjoint or parallel rather then sequential processing in these areas.

Given the role of the premotor cortex in visuomotor integration the finding that priming effects were not influenced by rTMS is surprising. It might indicate that priming effects are generated at earlier stages of visuo-motor processing, e.g. at the level of the basal ganglia. Indeed, a recent behavioural and fMRI study of patients with Huntington's disease and healthy subjects using the same 'masked prime' paradigm demonstrated abnormal processing of the subliminal prime stimulus in patients and significant modulation of activity of both the caudate and thalamus during the response inhibition process in healthy subjects (Aron et al., 2003).

As various symptoms suggest that premotor areas are overactive in patients with tic-dominant Gilles de la Tourette syndrome (GTS) (Eidelberg et al., 1997; Peterson et al., 1998; Stern et al., 2000) we studied the effects of 1 Hz motor and premotor rTMS on symptoms in GTS patients. In a single-blinded, placebo-controlled, crossover trial 16 GTS patients received in random sequence 1 Hz motor, premotor (80% AMT) and sham rTMS which each consisted of two 20 min rTMS sessions applied on 2 consecutive days. There was no significant improvement of symptoms after any of the rTMS conditions as assessed with an established rating scale (the MOVES survey) (Münchau et al., 2002b). A possible explanation is that abnormal premotor cortex activity in patients with GTS is compensatory rather than primary. Alternatively, rTMS might have been ineffective to treat symptoms of GTS patients because the rTMS stimulation intensity was too low. Also, as no neuronavigation guidance system was used the negative response may have been caused by inaccurate coil placement.

Clearly, further TMS/rTMS studies, preferably combined with neuronavigation systems, are needed to delineate behaviourally relevant effects of premotor rTMS both in healthy subjects and in patients.

4. Future directions

The premotor-motor TMS/rTMS studies discussed above show that TMS is a useful method to map the functional connectivity in motor networks. The time course and specificity of premotor-motor interactions as demonstrated in the paired pulse TMS/rTMS paradigms render these an attractive technique not only for studies of premotor-motor connectivity but also plasticity.

For instance, we recently examined whether the conditioning effect of premotor 1 Hz rTMS on ipsilateral motor cortex would differ if premotor 1 Hz rTMS was given on 2 consecutive days (Bäumer et al., 2003). We hypothesised that two premotor rTMS sessions applied on 2 consecutive days would increase the magnitude and/or duration of excitability changes in the motor cortex compared to the effects of a single rTMS train. Motor cortex excitability was determined at baseline, immediately after, 30, 60, 120 min and 24 h after each premotor rTMS session. Similar to our previous work (Münchau et al., 2002a) there was a selective increase of paired pulse facilitation at an ISI of 7 ms after premotor rTMS lasting for less than 30 min on day one. This effect was also present after rTMS on day two and had the same magnitude. However, in contrast to day one it persisted for at least 2 h. These data could indicate that 1 Hz premotor rTMS can lead to cumulative plastic changes of intrinsic motor cortex excitability when repeated within 24 h implying the formation of memory after the first rTMS train lasting for at least 1 day. Such a memory effect may represent the basis of long-term rTMS effects observed in patients after repeated rTMS applications. More work needs to be done to delineate the time course, behavioural correlates and also neuropharmacology of these plastic changes.

5. Conclusions

In spite of some methodological shortcomings single and paired pulse TMS and rTMS represent effective, non-invasive tools to study the neurophysiology of premotor-motor connections. TMS studies so far indicate that there are both inhibitory and facilitatory premotor-motor projections, the activation/deactivation of which depends on the TMS intensity, frequency, coil placement and effective current flow. What emerges is a delicate finely tuned motor network consistent with the concept that the premotor area has a "shaping" or "focussing" role in the execution of movements.

Acknowledgement

A. Münchau is supported by the Volkswagenstiftung.

References

Aron, A.R., Schlaghecken, F., Fletcher, P.C., Bullmore, E.T., Eimer, M., Barker, R., Sahakian, B.J. and Robbins, T.W. Inhibition of subliminally primed responses is mediated by the caudate and thalamus: evidence from functional MRI and Huntington's disease. *Brain*, 2003, 126: 713–723.

Ashby, P., Reynolds, C., Wennberg, R., Lozano, A.M. and Rothwell. J. On the focal nature of inhibition and facilitation in the human motor cortex. *Clin. Neurophysiol.*, 1999, 110: 550–555.

Battaglia Mayer, A., Ferraina, S., Marconi, B., Bullis, J.B., Lacquaniti, F., Burnod, Y., Baraduc, P. and Caminiti, R. Early motor influences on visuomotor transformations for reaching: a positive image of optic ataxia. *Exp. Brain Res.*, 1998, 123: 172–189.

Bäumer, T., Lange, R., Liepert, J., Weiller, C., Siebner, H., Rothwell, J.C. and Münchau, A. Repeated premotor rTMS leads to cumulative plastic changes of motor cortex excitability in humans. *Neuroimage* (in press).

Buccino, G., Binkofski, F., Fink, G.R., Fadiga, L., Fogassi, L., Gallese, V., Seitz, R.J., Zilles, K., Rizzolatti, G. and Freund, H.J. Action observation activates premotor and parietal areas in a somatotopic manner: an fMRI study. *Eur. J. Neurosci.*, 2001, 13: 400–404.

Chen, R., Classen, J., Gerloff, C., Celnik, P., Wassermann, E.M., Hallett, M. and Cohen L.G. Depression of motor cortex excitability by low-frequency transcranial magnetic stimulation. *Neurology*, 1997, 48: 1398–1403.

Cisek, P., Crammond, D.J. and Kalaska, J.F. Neural activity in primary motor and dorsal premotor cortex in reaching tasks with the contralateral vs. ipsilateral arm. *J. Neurophysiol.*, 2003, 89: 922–942.

Civardi, C., Cantello, R., Asselman, P. and Rothwell, J.C. Transcranial magnetic stimulation can be used to test connections to primary motor areas from frontal and medial cortex in humans. *Neuroimage*, 2001, 14: 1444–1453.

Corthout, E., Barker, A.T. and Cowey, A. Transcranial magnetic stimulation. Which part of the current waveform causes the stimulation? *Exp. Brain Res.*, 2001, 141: 128–132.

Dum, R.P. and Strick, P.L. The origin of corticospinal projections from the premotor areas in the frontal lobe. *J. Neurosci.*, 1991, 11: 667–689.

Eidelberg, D., Moeller, J.R., Antonini, A., Kazumata, K., Dhawan, V., Budman, C. and Feigin, A. The metabolic anatomy of Tourette's syndrome. *Neurology*, 1997, 48: 927–934.

Ferbert, A., Priori, A., Rothwell, J.C., Day, B.L., Colebatch, J.G. and Marsden, C.D. Interhemispheric inhibition of the human motor cortex. *J. Physiol.* (Lond), 1992, 453: 525–546.

Foerster, O. Motorische Felder und Bahnen. Sensible cortical Felder. In: O. Bumke and O. Foerster (Eds.), *Handbuch der Neurologie*, Vol. 6, Springer, Berlin, 1936: 1–357.

Gerschlager, W., Siebner, H.R. and Rothwell, J.C. Decreased corticospinal excitability after subthreshold 1 Hz rTMS over lateral premotor cortex. *Neurology*, 2001, 57: 449–455.

Ghosh, S. and Porter, R. Corticocortical synaptic influences on morphologically identified pyramidal neurones in the motor cortex of the monkey. *J. Physiol.*, 1988, 400: 617–629.

Godschalk, M., Mitz, A.R., van Duin, B. and van der, B.H. Somatotopy of monkey premotor cortex examined with microstimulation. *Neurosci. Res.*, 1995, 23: 269–279.

Herwig, U., Padberg, F., Unger, J., Spitzer, M. and Schonfeldt-Lecuona, C. Transcranial magnetic stimulation in therapy studies: examination of the reliability of "standard" coil positioning by neuronavigation. *Biol. Psychiatry*, 2001, 50: 58–61.

Kammer, T., Beck, S., Erb, M. and Grodd, W. The influence of current direction on phosphene thresholds evoked by transcranial magnetic stimulation. *Clin. Neurophysiol.*, 2001, 112: 2015–2021.

Kujirai, T., Caramia, M.D., Rothwell, J.C., Day, B.L., Thompson, P.D., Ferbert, A., Wroe, S., Asselman, P. and Marsden, C.D. Corticocortical inhibition in human motor cortex. *J. Physiol. (Lond.)*, 1993, 471: 501–519.

Maeda, F., Keenan, J.P., Tormos, J.M., Topka, H. and Pascual-Leone, A. Modulation of corticospinal excitability by repetitive transcranial magnetic stimulation. *Clin. Neurophysiol.*, 2000, 111: 800–805.

Marconi, B., Genovesio, A., Battaglia-Mayer, A., Ferraina, S., Squatrito, S., Molinari, M., Lacquaniti, F. and Caminiti, R. Eye-hand coordination during reaching. I. Anatomical relationships between parietal and frontal cortex. *Cereb. Cortex*, 2001, 11: 513–527.

Morecraft, R.J. and Van Hoesen, G.W. Frontal granular cortex input to the cingulate (M3), supplementary (M2) and primary (M1) motor cortices in the rhesus monkey. *J. Comp. Neurol.*, 1993, 337: 669–689.

Muellbacher, W., Ziemann, U., Boroojerdi, B. and Hallett, M. Effects of low-frequency transcranial magnetic stimulation on motor excitability and basic motor behavior. *Clin. Neurophysiol.*, 2000, 111: 1002–1007.

Münchau, A., Bloem, B.R., Irlbacher, K., Trimble, M.R. and Rothwell, J.C. Functional connectivity of human premotor and motor cortex explored with repetitive transcranial magnetic stimulation. *J. Neurosci.*, 2002a, 22: 554–561.

Münchau, A., Bloem, B.R., Thilo, K.V., Trimble, M.R., Rothwell, J.C. and Robertson, M.M. Repetitive transcranial magnetic stimulation for Tourette syndrome. *Neurology*, 2002b, 59: 1789–1791.

Netz, J., Ziemann, U. and Homberg, V. Hemispheric asymmetry of transcallosal inhibition in man. *Exp. Brain Res.*, 1995, 104: 527–533.

Oliviero, A., Strens, L.H., Di Lazzaro, V., Tonali, P.A. and Brown, P. Persistent effects of high frequency repetitive TMS on the coupling between motor areas in the human. *Exp. Brain Res.*, 2003, 149: 107–113.

Pascual-Leone, A., Valls-Solé, J., Wassermann, E.M. and Hallett, M. Responses to rapid-rate transcranial magnetic stimulation of the human motor cortex. *Brain*, 1994, 117 (Part 4): 847–858.

Pascual-Leone, A., Tormos, J.M., Keenan, J., Tarazona, F., Canete, C. and Catala, M.D. Study and modulation of human cortical excitability with transcranial magnetic stimulation. *J. Clin. Neurophysiol.*, 1998, 15: 333–343.

Peinemann, A., Lehner, C., Mentschel, C., Münchau, A., Conrad, B. and Siebner, H.R. Subthreshold 5-Hz repetitive transcranial magnetic stimulation of the human primary motor cortex reduces intracortical paired-pulse inhibition. *Neurosci. Lett.*, 2000, 296: 21–24.

Peterson, B.S., Skudlarski, P., Anderson, A.W., Zhang, H., Gatenby, J.C., Lacadie, C.M., Leckman, J.F. and Gore, J.C. A functional magnetic resonance imaging study of tic suppression in Tourette syndrome. *Arch. Gen. Psychiatry*, 1998, 55: 326–333.

Praamstra, P., Kleine, B.U. and Schnitzler, A. Magnetic stimulation of the dorsal premotor cortex modulates the Simon effect. *NeuroReport*, 1999, 10: 3671–3674.

Preuss, T.M., Stepniewska, I. and Kaas, J.H. Movement representation in the dorsal and ventral premotor areas of owl monkeys: a microstimulation study [published erratum appears in *J. Comp. Neurol.*, 1997, Jan 27, 377(4): 611]. *J. Comp. Neurol.*, 1996, 371: 649–676.

Raos, V., Franchi, G., Gallese, V. and Fogassi, L. Somatotopic Organization of the Lateral Part of Area F2 (Dorsal Premotor Cortex) of the Macaque Monkey. *J. Neurophysiol.*, 2003, 89: 1503–1518.

Ridding, M.C., Inzelberg, R. and Rothwell, J.C. Changes in excitability of motor cortical circuitry in patients with Parkinson's disease. *Ann. Neurol.*, 1995a, 37: 181–188.

Ridding, M.C., Taylor, J.L. and Rothwell, J.C. The effect of voluntary contraction on cortico-cortical inhibition in human motor cortex. *J. Physiol. (Lond.)*, 1995b, 487(Part 2): 541–548.

Rizzolatti, G., Luppino, G. and Matelli, M. The organization of the cortical motor system: new concepts. *Electroencephalogr. Clin. Neurophysiol.*, 1998, 106: 283–296.

Rothwell, J.C., Thompson, P.D., Day, B.L., Boyd, S. and Marsden, C.D. Stimulation of the human motor cortex through the scalp. *Exp. Physiol.*, 1991, 76: 159–200.

Sakai, K., Hikosaka, O., Takino, R., Miyauchi, S., Nielsen, M. and Tamada, T. What and when: parallel and convergent processing in motor control. *J. Neurosci.*, 2000, 20: 2691–2700.

Schlaghecken, F., Münchau, A., Bloem, B.R., Rothwell, J.C. and Eimer, M. Slow frequency repetitive transcranial magnetic stimulation over motor and premotor cortex affects reaction times, but not priming effects, in a masked prime task. *Clin. Neurophysiol.*, 2003, 114: 1272–1277.

Schluter, N.D., Rushworth, M.F., Passingham, R.E. and Mills, K.R. Temporary interference in human lateral premotor cortex suggests dominance for the selection of movements. A study using transcranial magnetic stimulation. *Brain*, 1998, 121 (Part 5): 785–799.

Siebner, H.R., Tormos, J.M., Ceballos-Baumann, A.O., Auer, C., Catala, M.D., Conrad, B. and Pascual-Leone, A. Low-frequency repetitive transcranial magnetic stimulation of the motor cortex in writer's cramp. *Neurology*, 1999, 52: 529–537.

Siebner, H., Peller, M., Bartenstein, P., Willoch, F., Rossmeier, C., Schwaiger, M. and Conrad, B. Activation of frontal premotor areas during suprathreshold transcranial magnetic stimulation of the left primary sensorimotor cortex: a glucose metabolic PET study. *Hum. Brain Mapp.*, 2001, 12: 157–167.

Stepniewska, I., Preuss, T.M. and Kaas, J.H. Architectonics, somatotopic organization, and ipsilateral cortical connections of the primary motor area (M1) of owl monkeys. *J. Comp. Neurol.*, 1993, 330: 238–271.

Stern, E., Silbersweig, D.A., Chee, K.Y., Holmes, A., Robertson, M.M., Trimble, M., Frith, C.D., Frackowiak, R.S. and Dolan, R.J. A functional neuroanatomy of tics in Tourette syndrome. *Arch. Gen. Psychiatry*, 2000, 57: 741–748.

Strafella, A.P. and Paus, T. Modulation of cortical excitability during action observation: a transcranial magnetic stimulation study. *NeuroReport*, 2000, 11: 2289–2292.

Tokuno, H. and Nambu, A. Organization of nonprimary motor cortical inputs on pyramidal and nonpyramidal tract neurons of primary motor cortex: An electrophysiological study in the macaque monkey. *Cereb. Cortex*, 2000, 10: 58–68.

Wassermann, E.M., Wedegaertner, F.R., Ziemann, U., George, M.S. and Chen, R. Crossed reduction of human motor cortex excitability by 1-Hz transcranial magnetic stimulation. *Neurosci. Lett.*, 1998, 250: 141–144.

Wise, S.P. The primate premotor cortex: past, present, and preparatory. *Ann. Rev. Neurosci.*, 1985, 8: 1–19.

Wise, S.P., Boussaoud, D., Johnson, P.B. and Caminiti, R. Premotor and parietal cortex: corticocortical connectivity and combinatorial computations. *Ann. Rev. Neurosci.*, 1997, 20: 25–42.

Wu, T., Sommer, M., Tergau, F. and Paulus, W. Lasting influence of repetitive transcranial magnetic stimulation on intracortical excitability in human subjects. *Neurosci. Lett.*, 2000, 287: 37–40.

Ziemann, U., Rothwell, J.C. and Ridding, M.C. Interaction between intracortical inhibition and facilitation in human motor cortex. *J. Physiol.* (*Lond.*), 1996, 496(Part 3): 873–881.

Ziemann, U., Tergau, F., Bruns, D., Baudewig, J. and Paulus, W. Changes in human motor cortex excitability induced by dopaminergic and anti-dopaminergic drugs. *Electroencephalogr. Clin. Neurophysiol.*, 1997, 105: 430–437.

Ziemann, U., Corwell, B. and Cohen, L.G. Modulation of plasticity in human motor cortex after forearm ischemic nerve block. *J. Neurosci.*, 1998, 18: 1115–1123.

Ziemann, U., Lonnecker, S., Steinhoff, B.J. and Paulus, W. Motor excitability changes under antiepileptic drugs. *Adv. Neurol.*, 1999, 81: 291–298.

Transcranial Magnetic Stimulation and Transcranial Direct Current Stimulation (Supplements to Clinical Neurophysiology, Vol. 56)
Editors: W. Paulus, F. Tergau, M.A. Nitsche, J.C. Rothwell, U. Ziemann, M. Hallett

Chapter 15

Inhibitory control of acquired motor programs in the human brain

Christian Gerloff* and Friedhelm Hummel

Cortical Physiology Research Group, Department of Neurology, Eberhard-Karls University Tübingen, Hoppe-Seyler-Str. 3, D-72076 Tübingen (Germany)

Transcranial magnetic stimulation (TMS) can be used to assess inhibitory modulation of neuronal function (e.g. reduction of motor evoked potential (MEP) amplitudes compared with baseline) (Ziemann et al., 1996; Chen et al., 1998; Gerloff et al., 1998). This makes TMS unique, because with other neuroimaging techniques (e.g. regional cerebral blood flow (rCBF), BOLD, oscillatory electrocortical activity) it is largely unclear how inhibitory neuronal activity affects parameters used for the measurement of neuronal function. The present set of experiments was geared at advancing our knowledge on the neuroimaging of inhibitory neuronal processes in the human brain. Why is this relevant? Because an important basis of human behavior is the appropriate retrieval of acquired and memorized behavioral programmes. Appropriate retrieval is warranted if behavioral programs are only activated if necessary and are, probably more often, inhibited if required by the context of a given situation. The best 'real-life' example for this concept might be a car waiting in front of a red traffic light. As the light turns green, the normal driver's behavior is to accelerate (= retrieval of the learned motor program). Non-retrieval (= inhibition) would correspond to the same situation with the signal of an ambulance approaching so that acceleration would be fatal and the normal motor program must be inhibited (Fig. 1). Under physiological conditions, acquired motor programs are readily retrieved and are thus the substrate of effective motor learning. We hypothesized that, rather than being '*activated or disregarded*', these programs are '*activated or actively inhibited*' and that the neuronal correlates of this context-dependent inhibition can be demonstrated by the combined use of TMS and other neuroimaging methods. In the present set of experiments, we combined TMS and EEG. In ongoing follow-up experiments, we have now extended the concept of context-dependent inhibition to metabolic measures (i.e. BOLD, fMRI).

Eighteen volunteers were studied. Cortical function was assessed with transcranial magnetic stimulation over the motor cortex (M1) and with task-related analysis of oscillatory EEG activity. A retrieval (= activation, ACT) and non-retrieval (= inhibition, INH) condition were compared. In both, visual cues were presented at 1/s. In ACT, subjects had to respond to these cues with individual finger movements as learned in a preceding training session. In

* *Correspondence to*: Dr. Christian Gerloff, Cortical Physiology Research Group, Department of Neurology, Eberhard-Karls University Tübingen, Hoppe-Seyler-Str. 3, D-72076 Tübingen, Germany.
E-mail: christian.gerloff@uni-tuebingen.de

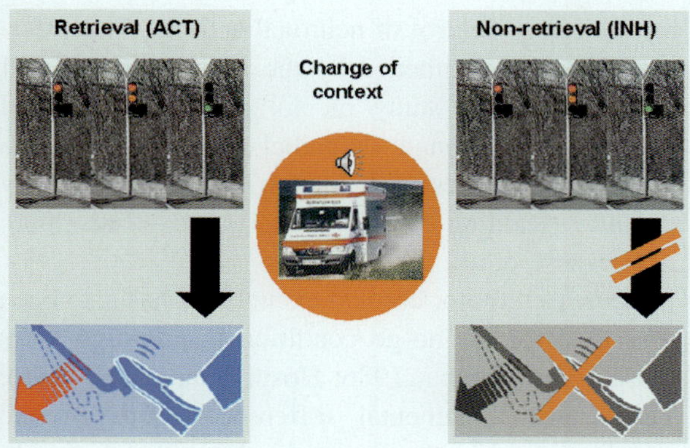

Fig. 1. Illustration of the paradigm. Left, a learned behavioral program must be retrieved in order to follow the instructions given by the green traffic light ('accelerate' = activation, ACT). Middle, in this example 'change of context' corresponds to the approaching ambulance. Right, after the context has changed, the appropriate response to the traffic light turning green is 'non-retrieval', i.e. inhibition of the learned motor program (INH). In the actual experiment, visual cues were presented on a computer screen and finger movements were used as learned motor programs.

INH, subjects had to observe the cues without retrieval of motor responses.

Single-pulse TMS (Magstim Company Ltd, Whitland, Wales, UK) was carried out with the subjects at complete rest. An 8-shaped magnetic coil was used with the handle pointing backwards and laterally at a ~45° angle to the sagittal plane. The optimal scalp position (OP) for activation of the first dorsal interosseus (FDI) muscle was identified. Motor threshold (MT) was defined as the minimal intensity of stimulation capable of inducing 5 MEPs of more than 50 μV out of 10 pulses in the relaxed FDI. Stimulation intensity was adjusted so as to obtain stable baseline MEPs of 1–2 mV (119.0% ± 2.7% MT).

Continuous EEG was recorded from 28 (Ag/AgCl) surface electrodes (Electro-Cap International, Inc., Eaton, Ohio, USA). Impedance was kept below 5 kΩ (Synamp amplifiers and software by NeuroScan Inc., Herndon, VA, USA). Linked earlobe electrodes served as reference. Key presses and visual trigger stimuli (symbols or numbers) were automatically documented with markers in the continuous EEG file and were used for stimulus-locked averaging. For digitization of head shape and electrode positions a magnetic field digitizer (3Space Fastrak®, Polhemus, Colchester, VT, USA) was used. EEG was segmented into artifact-free epochs of 1024 ms duration (± 512 ms visual cue onset). For spectral power analysis, a discrete Fourier transformation was computed for each 1024 ms epoch and all electrodes. In order to account for inter-subject variability, TRPow was expressed as the percentage of spectral power during activation ($Pow_{activation}$) compared to the spectral power during the rest condition (Pow_{rest}). This normalization was computed according to: $\%TRPow = [(Pow_{rest} - Pow_{activation})/Pow_{rest}] \times 100$. Therefore, task-related power decreases (TRPD) are expressed as positive values (color coding, red), task-related power increases (TRPI) as negative values (color coding, blue). Further analysis of the power spectra was focused on the alpha (7–13 Hz) band because the most prominent task-related power changes were observed in this frequency range.

The first main result was a significant MEP reduction in the inhibition condition, i.e. when visual cues were presented on the screen, but no movement was required (Kruskal–Willis, $P < 0.05$). The MEP amplitudes (mean ± SD) evoked by single TMS pulses over the M1 were 0.8 ± 0.7 mV in INH, 1.4 ± 1.1 mV during unconstrained rest, and 3.4 ± 2.1 mV during ACT.

The second main finding was a topographically distinct task-related alpha power increase (α-TRPI) in the EEG over sensorimotor areas in the inhibition condition (left sensorimotor region, α-TRPI –21.7%; ANOVA, inhibition vs. rest $P < 0.05$). This α-TRPI occurred in the upper alpha band (11–13 Hz, maximum at 12 and 13 Hz), was prominent over fronto-central, central, and parietal areas bilaterally, and slightly less pronounced over the midline.

Figure 2 summarizes these results by providing TMS and EEG data of a representative subject for all relevant conditions.

Several control experiments confirmed that, α-TRPI associated with MEP reduction was specifically related to the successful suppression of learned motor programs acquired the day before the electrophysiological measurements. The present findings go beyond the concept of locally increased oscillatory activity as a correlate of idling (Pfurtscheller, 1992) or a 'nil-working' state (Mulholland, 1995).

The main significance of the present study is the demonstration of electrophysiological correlates of appropriate, context-dependent inhibitory control of previously acquired motor programmes. Enhanced oscillatory alpha activity (α-TRPI) over cortical sensorimotor areas was paralleled by a decrease of MEP amplitudes below baseline. In terms of mechanisms, we favor the interpretation that increases of local oscillatory activity (α-TRPI) are instrumental for inhibitory control of neuronal activity. This interpretation is strengthened by the absence of α-TRPI in a preliminary study on six patients with focal dystonia of the hand (Hummel et al., 2002), as a model for diseases with known deficient inhibitory circuitry (Ridding et al., 1995; Tinazzi et al., 2000; Abbruzzese et al., 2001).

Decreased motor cortical excitability has also been described for the no-go condition in go/no-go tasks (Sasaki and Gemba, 1986; Hoshiyama et al., 1996). There are fundamental differences between the paradigm used in the present study and such a task: (i) in a go/no-go task, the S1 stimulus prompts the subjects to prepare the motor act as fast as possible,

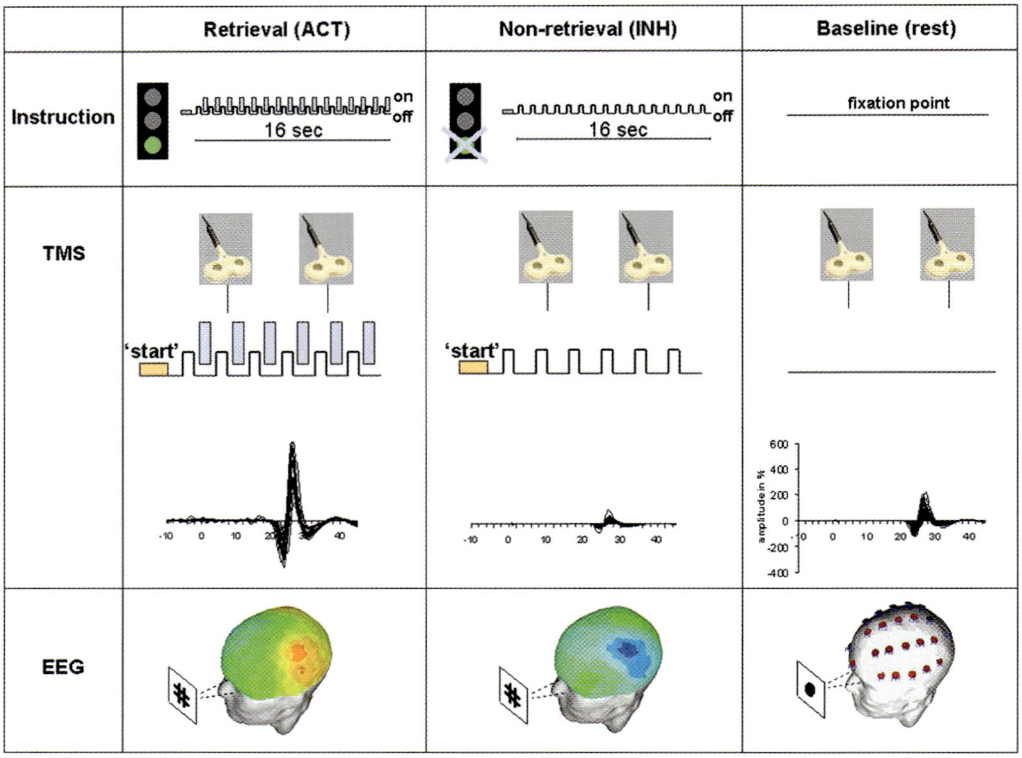

	Retrieval (ACT)	Non-retrieval (INH)	Baseline (rest)
Instruction	on off 16 sec	on off 16 sec	fixation point
TMS	'start'	'start'	600 400 200 0 -200 -400 amplitude in % -10 0 10 20 30 40
EEG			

Fig. 2. Left, in ACT subjects retrieved the previously learned motor program consisting in a finger movement sequence of 16 key presses following visual cues. MEP amplitudes were facilitated and the EEG showed task-related power decreases in the alpha band (red color coding). Middle, after change of context, the previously learned programs were not retrieved but inhibited. This was accompanied by reduced MEP amplitudes (below baseline) and task-related power increases in the EEG (α-TRPI, blue color coding) over the left sensorimotor region. Right, illustration of rest condition (TMS, EEG) and electrode montage (EEG).

and the no-go S2 signal cancels this dynamic, volitional preparation process (Naito and Matsumura, 1996; Grafton et al., 1998). Our subjects did not have to produce any fast voluntary inhibition of volitional motor actions. Whenever an inhibition sequence had been initiated, they were informed in advance that for the upcoming 16 visual cues no motor output was required. Voluntary rapid initiation and inhibition of responses as in go/no-go paradigms can therefore not play a major role in the present experiments; and (ii) go/no-go tasks are reaction time paradigms in which speed of performance is critical (Shibata et al., 1997). In the present study precision of the sequential finger movements was the critical factor and the movement rate was slow (1/s). Hence, results from go/no-go paradigms are not directly comparable with our data.

There is converging evidence that, depending on the context, cortical motor networks integrate facilitatory and inhibitory activity. The importance of 'context' for neuronal activity in premotor and motor areas has recently also been emphasized by Hepp-Reymond et al. (1999) who demonstrated context-dependent modifications of the discharge rates in a grip force task in monkeys. The present results extend these data by demonstrating context-dependent sustained inhibitory and excitatory changes in human cortical activity.

In particular, the present data emphasize the important role of inhibition in the implementation of motor behavior. The critical impact of proper inhibitory capacities of the sensorimotor cortices has been substantiated in various studies, e.g. by Jacobs and Donoghue (1991). They blocked cortical inhibition pharmacologically in adult rats, and found that reduction of inhibition can temporarily change the proper relation patterns between different limb representations in M1 areas.

Preliminary data from ongoing fMRI experiments in our laboratory suggests that MEP reduction and α-TRPI over the left sensorimotor region might be linked to a reduction of the BOLD response below baseline during inhibition. If this can be verified in a larger sample of subjects, the combined use of TMS and EEG, TMS and fMRI, or the combination of all three modalities could provide a new window into understanding inhibitory neuronal processes in the human brain at the level of systems physiology.

References

Abbruzzese, G., Marchese, R., Buccolieri, A., Gasparetto, B. and Trompetto, C. Abnormalities of sensorimotor integration in focal dystonia: A transcranial magnetic stimulation study. *Brain*, 2001, 124: 537–545.

Chen, R., Tam, A., Butefisch, C., Corwell, B., Ziemann, U., Rothwell, J.C., et al. Intracortical inhibition and facilitation in different representations of the human motor cortex. *J. Neurophysiol.*, 1998, 80: 2870–2881.

Gerloff, C., Cohen, L.G., Floeter, M.K., Chen, R., Corwell, B. and Hallett, M. Inhibitory influence of the ipsilateral motor cortex on responses to stimulation of the human cortex and pyramidal tract. *J. Physiol. (Lond.)*, 1998, 510: 249–259.

Grafton, S.T., Hazeltine, E. and Ivry, R.B. Abstract and effector-specific representations of motor sequences identified with PET. *J. Neurosci.*, 1998, 18: 9420–9428.

Hepp-Reymond, M., Kirkpatrick-Tanner, M., Gabernet, L., Qi, H. and Weber, B. Context-dependent force coding in motor and premotor cortical areas. *Exp. Brain Res.*, 1999, 128: 123–133.

Hoshiyama, M., Koyama, S., Kitamura, Y., Shimojo, M., Watanabe, S. and Kakigi, R. Effects of judgement process on motor evoked potentials in Go/No-go hand movement task. *Neurosci. Res.*, 1996, 24: 427–430.

Jacobs, K.M. and Donoghue, J.P. Reshaping the cortical motor map by unmasking latent intracortical connections. *Science*, 1991, 251: 944–947.

Mulholland, T. Human EEG, behavioral stillness and biofeedback. *Int. J. Psychophysiol.*, 1995, 19: 263–279.

Naito, E. and Matsumura, M. Movement-related potentials associated with motor inhibition under different preparatory states during performance of two visual stop signal paradigms in humans. *Neuropsychologia*, 1996; 34: 565–573.

Pfurtscheller, G. Event-related synchronization (ERS): an electrophysiological correlate of cortical areas at rest. *Electroencephalogr. Clin, Neurophysiol.*, 1992, 83: 62–69.

Ridding, M.C., Sheean, G., Rothwell, J.C., Inzelberg, R. and Kujirai, T. Changes in the balance between motor cortical excitation and inhibition in focal, task specific dystonia. *J. Neurol. Neurosurg. Psychiatry*, 1995, 59: 493–498.

Sasaki, K. and Gemba, H. Electrical activity in the prefrontal cortex specific to no-go reaction of conditioned hand movement with colour discrimination in the monkey. *Exp. Brain Res.*, 1986, 64: 603–606.

Shibata, T., Shimoyama, I., Ito, T., Abla, D., Iwasa, H., Koseki, K., et al. The time course of interhemispheric EEG coherence during a GO/NO-GO task in humans. *Neurosci. Lett.*, 1997, 233: 117–120.

Tinazzi, M., Priori, A., Bertolasi, L., Frasson, E., Mauguiere, F. and Fiaschi, A. Abnormal central integration of a dual somatosensory input in dystonia. Evidence for sensory overflow. *Brain*, 2000, 123: 42–50.

Ziemann, U., Rothwell, J.C. and Ridding, M.C. Interaction between intracortical inhibition and facilitation in human motor cortex. *J. Physiol.* (*Lond.*), 1996, 496: 873–881.

Transcranial Magnetic Stimulation and Transcranial Direct Current Stimulation (Supplements to Clinical Neurophysiology, Vol. 56)
Editors: W. Paulus, F. Tergau, M.A. Nitsche, J.C. Rothwell, U. Ziemann, M. Hallett

Chapter 16

Motor control in mirror movements: studies with transcranial magnetic stimulation

M. Cincotta[a,*], A. Borgheresi[a], A. Ragazzoni[a], P. Vanni[a], F. Balestrieri[a], F. Benvenuti[b], G. Zaccara[a] and U. Ziemann[c]

[a] *Unità Operativa di Neurologia, Azienda Sanitaria di Firenze, Florence (Italy)*
[b] *Ospedale INRCA 'I Fraticini', Florence (Italy)*
[c] *Neurologische Klinik, J.W. Goethe-Universität, Frankfurt/Main (Germany)*

1. Introduction

Mirror movements (MM) are unintended movements on one side of the body which occur as mirror reversals of the contralateral voluntary ones; they mainly involve the distal upper limb muscles (Schott and Wyke, 1981; Cohen et al., 1991). MM can be seen in normal children up to 10 years of age but their prevalence and intensity decreases with age (Reitz and Muller, 1998; Mayston et al., 1999). Significant MM are pathological in adulthood (Schott and Wyke, 1981; Cohen et al., 1991), although subtle mirroring can be observed in normal adults performing complex and effortful tasks (Armatas et al., 1994; Mayston et al., 1999).

MM are etiologically heterogeneous. Persistent congenital MM have been described in different conditions, ranging from the absence of other neurological abnormalities to severe hemiparesis (Schott and Wyke, 1981; Carr et al., 1993; Rasmussen et al., 1993). MM can also be observed in association with several acquired conditions, such as Parkinson's disease (PD) (Van den Berg et al., 2000), stroke (Weiller et al., 1993; Netz et al., 1997), focal lesions involving the supplementary motor area (SMA) (Chan and Ross, 1988), and behavioral disorders (Woods and Eby, 1982).

The neurophysiological hallmark of persistent congenital MM is the presence of fast-conducting corticospinal pathways connecting abnormally the hand area of one primary motor cortex (M1) with both sides of the spinal cord. This was demonstrated more than 10 years ago by transcranial electrical stimulation (Farmer et al., 1990; Cohen et al., 1991) and confirmed by close to 20 transcranial magnetic stimulation (TMS) studies, showing that focal stimulation of one M1 elicits bilateral motor evoked potentials (MEP) of normal latency in the resting hand muscles. In patients with congenital MM not associated with other relevant motor abnormalities, ipsilateral MEP are seen after stimulation of either hemisphere (Danek et al., 1992; Cincotta et al., 1994), whereas in patients with severe congenital hemiparesis (CH), they can be seen only after stimulation of the unaffected M1 (Carr et al., 1993; Cincotta et al., 2000). In healthy children and adults,

* *Correspondence to*: Dr. Massimo Cincotta, U.O. di Neurologia, Azienda Sanitaria di Firenze, Ospedale S. Maria Nuova, Piazza S. Maria Nuova 1, 50122 Florence, Italy.
Tel: 39-055-2758894; Fax: 39-055-2758291;
E-mail: cincotta@unifi.it

neurophysiological investigations suggest that 'physiological' mirroring may be merely due to simultaneous activation of crossed corticospinal tracts originating from both M1 (Mayston et al., 1999).

As non-invasive investigations have shed some light on the anatomical and physiological mechanisms that govern MM, several pathophysiological aspects are still debated. In patients with congenital MM not associated with severe hemispheric lesions, one question is whether the existence of the uncrossed corticospinal tracts is the unique abnormality or the M1 ipsilateral to the voluntary movement also contributes to MM in the sense of a 'mirror' cortex. In addition, the origin of the ipsilateral corticofugal pathways is uncertain. One possibility is abnormal branching of crossed corticospinal fibers (Farmer et al., 1990). Another hypothesis favors a separate ipsilateral projection (Mayston et al., 1997). Finally, the neural mechanisms underlying MM in patients with acquired diseases are largely unexplored. We report various novel ways how TMS can be used to address these issues, with particular regard to our experience.

2. Persistent congenital mirror movements

2.1. Congenital mirror movements not associated with severe hemispheric lesions

In otherwise normal patients with congenital MM (Cohen et al., 1991) and in MM patients with X-linked Kallmann's syndrome (Krams et al., 1997), positron emission tomography studies showed abnormal bilateral activation of the M1 during intended unimanual movements. However, activation of the M1 ipsilateral to the 'voluntary' hand was similar to that during passive movements of the 'mirror' hand (Krams et al., 1997). This raises the possibility that the activation of the 'mirror cortex' was not motor activity but caused by the sensory feedback from the mirror hand. In congenital MM, bilateral M1 activation was also suggested by functional magnetic resonance imaging (Leinsinger et al., 1997). However, a control experiment using passive movements was not done. Finally, movement-related cortical potential recordings showed an abnormal bilateral distribution of the pre-movement negativity in MM patients (Shibasaki and Nagae, 1984; Cohen et al., 1991; Mayer et al., 1995). As sensory feedback does not confound this measure, it suggests that both M1 contributed to the preparation of unimanual movements. However, this does not necessarily indicate that the 'mirror M1' produced actual motor output. In order to clarify this, we used focal TMS to interfere with the function of either M1 during intended unilateral isometric contraction of the abductor pollicis brevis (APB) muscle. In normal subjects, stimulation of the M1 contralateral to the target muscle produces a long-lasting silent period (SP) in ongoing voluntary EMG (for review, see Hallett, 1995), whereas ipsilateral stimulation produces a short-lasting SP, which mainly reflects transcallosal inhibition (TI) of the 'active' M1 of the opposite hemisphere (Meyer et al., 1995). If the ipsilateral corticospinal pathways were the unique abnormality in patients with congenital MM, then during intended unimanual contraction, stimulation of the contralateral M1 would evoke a normal SP in both APB. In contrast, when the ipsilateral M1 was also 'active', the SP would be shortened because the motor output from the non-stimulated M1 would produce an early partial recovery of the ongoing EMG, coinciding with the offset of TI. We studied a 15-year-old girl (patient 1) and a 40-year-old woman (patient 2), both right-handed, with congenital MM affecting both hands and forearms. MM were strong and sustained, although less pronounced than the voluntary ones (grade 3 according to the criteria of Wood and Tauber, 1978). The family history of patient 1 was negative, whereas the mother and brother of patient 2 also showed MM. In both patients, the general and neurological examinations were normal except for MM. Representative SP recordings from patient 1 are shown in Fig. 1. In both patients, unilateral focal TMS of either M1 during intended unilateral contraction of either APB resulted in a clearly shorter SP in both muscles when compared to the contralateral SP of normal control subjects (Fig. 1A–B) (Cincotta et al., 1996, 2002). Balbi et al. (2000) reported similar findings in a MM patient suffering from mild perinatal

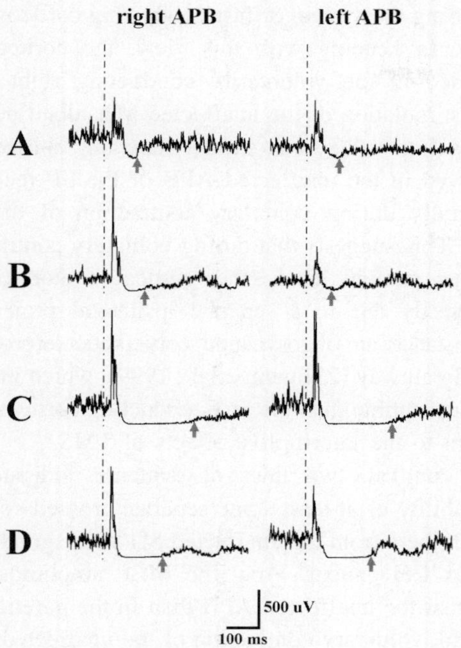

Fig. 1. SP following focal TMS of either the left (A) or right (B) M1 (20% above the resting motor threshold) or bilateral simultaneous stimulation of both M1 (C, 20% or D, 10% above the resting motor threshold to match MEP size with the MEP size in the unilateral TMS conditions) delivered during an intended unilateral isometric contraction of the right APB in patient 1. Each trace is the average of 10 rectified EMG responses. The vertical dotted lines indicate the time of TMS. The SP duration was calculated from the stimulus to the point when the mean post-MEP EMG reached again 20% of the mean pre-stimulus EMG. Arrows indicate the end of the SP. Unilateral stimulation of either M1 produced a shortened contralateral SP in both APB, whereas the duration of the SP following bilateral stimulation was normal.

ischemic damage. Furthermore, in our patients, simultaneous bilateral M1 stimulation produced a normal, long-lasting SP in both APB (Fig. 1C–D) (Cincotta et al., 2002). This experiment indicated that the short SP observed with unilateral stimulation of the M1 contralateral to the voluntarily contracted APB was really due to a contribution of the 'mirror' cortex to the EMG activity.

To investigate the origin of the ipsilateral corticospinal pathways, we tested task-related modulation of short-interval intracortical inhibition (SICI) using the conventional paired-pulse TMS paradigm at 3 ms interstimulus interval (Kujirai et al., 1993). SICI is regulated by cortical circuits projecting onto the corticospinal fibers (Di Lazzaro et al., 1998). In normals, voluntary contraction of the target muscle strongly reduces SICI compared with the rest condition (Ridding et al., 1995). If ipsilateral MEP in patients with congenital MM were exclusively due to branching of crossed corticospinal neurons, then intended unilateral APB contraction would produce the same effects in the 'task' and 'mirror' APB. This was not the case. In patients 1 and 2, when focal TMS of one M1 was delivered during intended unilateral contraction of either APB, SICI decreased markedly in the 'task' APB, but remained unchanged in the 'mirror' one, compared with the rest condition (Cincotta et al., 2001). The dissociation of task-related SICI modulation indicates the existence of a separate, strictly ipsilateral corticospinal projection.

Taken together, these results may have relevant functional implications. Assuming the existence of separate contralateral and ipsilateral corticospinal projections from either hemisphere and bilateral motor output with intended unimanual movements, Mayer et al. (1995) hypothesized that MM patients may reduce the amount of mirroring by preferentially activating the crossed projection from the M1 contralateral to the voluntary movement and the uncrossed projection from the ipsilateral M1. Our TMS findings strongly support this view (Cincotta et al., 1996, 2001, 2002). This model (Fig. 2) could account for the ability of some patients to exert some degree of voluntary control over the MM and provides a rationale for rehabilitation.

2.2. *Mirror movements associated with severe congenital hemiparesis*

A complex pattern of cortical reorganization was documented in a 39-year-old man with severe right CH due to a large porencephalic cavitation in the left hemisphere mainly involving the frontal and parietal lobes (Cincotta et al., 2000; Ragazzoni et al., 2002).

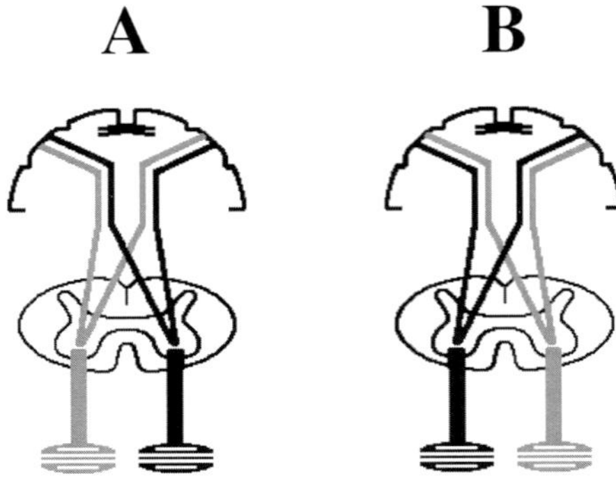

Fig. 2. Schematic drawing representing separate crossed and uncrossed corticospinal fibers and bilateral motor output with intended unimanual movements in otherwise normal patients with congenital MM. Black and grey lines indicate the preferentially and non-preferentially activated pathways, respectively. Patients could reduce the amount of mirror activity by preferentially activating the crossed corticospinal neurons from the right hemisphere and the ipsilateral tract from the left hemisphere during intended unilateral movements of the left hand (A), and vice versa during intended unilateral movements of the right hand (B).

He showed strong and sustained MM affecting both hands and forearms. During intended unilateral phasic movements of either upper limb, MM were less pronounced than the voluntary ones (grade 3 according to the criteria of Wood and Tauber, 1978). Accordingly, during isometric APB contractions, the level of voluntary EMG was above the mirror one. This indicates that the patient was to some extent capable of lateralizing voluntary motor activity. Focal TMS of the right M1 elicited bilateral MEP of normal latency in the resting APB, whereas no motor response was obtained after stimulation of the affected hemisphere.

When paired-pulse TMS of the unaffected M1 was delivered during unilateral contraction of the paretic hand, SICI was not down-regulated in either the 'task' or 'mirror' APB, compared with the rest condition. This finding provides no evidence for a separate ipsilateral corticospinal projection (see also sub-section 2.1) and suggests that, in our CH patient with MM, partial lateralization of motor activity with voluntary movements of the affected hand depended on a different corticofugal pathway, bypassing the system of fast-conducting corticospinal fibers. In keeping with this view, the cortical SP recorded in the voluntarily contracting right APB after stimulation of the unaffected M1, albeit normal in absolute value, was shorter than the 'mirror' SP observed in the unaffected APB or the SP recorded bilaterally during voluntary contraction of the left APB. This suggests that during voluntary contraction of the paretic hand, the cortical motor output was partly due to a separate ipsilateral projection, for instance an oligosynaptic corticoreticulo(proprio)-spinal pathway (Ziemann et al., 1999), which may be less susceptible than the fast-conducting corticospinal system to the interruptive effects of TMS.

In contrast, two lines of evidence indicate the availability of at least some separate crossed corticospinal fibers from the unaffected M1 to the good hand in this CH patient. First, the MEP amplitude was larger in the unaffected APB than in the paretic one. Second, voluntary contraction of the unaffected APB revealed a suppression of SICI in the good hand, but not in the paretic one. This SICI dissociation indicates a selective disinhibition of strictly crossed corticospinal fibers.

3. Mirror movements in Parkinson's disease

We studied an 82-year-old man with tremor-dominant idiopathic PD, mainly affecting the right upper limb. He was treated with levodopa (300 mg/day). MM were bilaterally present with intended unilateral finger movements, although more pronounced during voluntary movements of the right hand.

Focal TMS of either M1 elicited normal MEP in the contralateral APB, whereas no MEP was seen in the ipsilateral hand muscles, either at rest or during voluntary contraction. Focal TMS of one M1 produced a normal, long-lasting SP in the contralateral APB during either voluntary or 'mirror' contraction. Accordingly, stimulation of one M1 produced a normal, short-lasting ipsilateral SP, either during voluntary or 'mirror' contraction of the ipsilateral APB. This indicates that, in our PD patient, MM were not due to unmasking of ipsilateral projections but are best explained by motor output along strictly crossed corticospinal projections from bilateral M1.

These preliminary findings suggest that MM associated with PD may represent an abnormal enhancement of the 'physiological' mechanisms underlying the subtle mirroring sporadically observed in healthy adults (Mayston et al., 1999). Data in lesioned monkeys (Brinkman, 1984) and human patients (Chan and Ross, 1988) suggest that non-mirror transformation of motor programs is orchestrated by a cortical network mainly involving the SMA (for detailed discussion, see Van den Berg et al., 2000). Non-mirror transformation of movement could be a dynamic phenomenon, with a 'breaking point' related to the complexity of the task. In PD, bradykinesia is thought to be due to a failure of basal ganglia output to reinforce the cortical mechanisms that prepare and execute the movements (Berardelli et al., 2001). Likewise, one could hypothesize that enhanced mirroring associated with PD may be due to a failure of basal ganglia output to support the cortical mechanisms responsible for non-mirror transformation of motor programs. Further studies are needed to clarify this intriguing issue.

References

Armatas, C.A., Summers, J.J. and Bradshaw, J.L. Mirror movements in normal adult subjects. *J. Clin. Exp. Neuropsychol.*, 1994, 16: 405–413.

Balbi, P., Trojano, L., Ragno, M., Perretti, A. and Santoro, L. Patterns of motor control reorganization in a patient with mirror movements. *Clin. Neurophysiol.*, 2000, 111: 318–325.

Berardelli, A., Rothwell, J.C., Thompson, P.D. and Hallett, M. Pathophysiology of bradykinesia in Parkinson's disease. *Brain*, 2001, 124: 2131–2146.

Brinkman, C. Supplementary motor area of the monkey's cerebral cortex: short- and long-term deficits after unilateral ablation and the effects of subsequent callosal section. *J. Neurosci.*, 1984, 4: 918–929.

Carr, L.J., Harrison, L.M., Evans, A.L. and Stephens, J.A. Patterns of central motor reorganization in hemiplegic cerebral palsy. *Brain*, 1993, 116: 1223–1247.

Chan, J.L. and Ross, E.D. Left-handed mirror writing following right anterior cerebral artery infarction: evidence for nonmirror transformation of motor programs by right supplementary motor area. *Neurology*, 1988, 38: 59–63.

Cincotta, M., Ragazzoni, A., De Scisciolo, G., Pinto, F., Maurri, S. and Barontini, F. Abnormal projection of corticospinal tracts in a patient with congenital mirror movements. *Neurophysiol. Clin.*, 1994, 24: 427–434.

Cincotta, M., Lori, S., Gangemi, P.F., Barontini, F. and Ragazzoni, A. Hand motor cortex activation in a patient with congenital mirror movements: a study of the silent period following focal transcranial magnetic stimulation. *Electroenceph. Clin. Neurophysiol.*, 1996, 101: 240–246.

Cincotta, M., Borgheresi, A., Liotta, P., Montigiani, A., Marin, E., Zaccara, G. and Ziemann, U. Reorganization of the motor cortex in a patient with congenital hemiparesis and mirror movements. *Neurology*, 2000, 55: 129–131.

Cincotta, M., Borgheresi, A., Boffi, P., Vigliano, P., Benvenuti, F., Ragazzoni, A., Zaccara, G. and Ziemann, U. Modulation of the motor cortical output in congenital mirror movements. *Clin. Neurophysiol.*, 2001, 112 (Suppl. 1): S5.

Cincotta, M., Borgheresi, A., Boffi, P., Vigliano, P., Ragazzoni, A., Zaccara, G. and Ziemann, U. Bilateral motor cortex output with intended unimanual contraction in congenital mirror movements. *Neurology*, 2002, 58: 1290–1293.

Cohen, L.G., Meer, J., Tarkka, I., Bierner, S., Leiderman, D.B., Dubinsky, R.M., Sanes, J.N., Jabbari, B., Branscum, B. and Hallett, M. Congenital mirror movements. Abnormal organization of motor pathways in two patients. *Brain*, 1991, 114: 381–403.

Danek, A., Heye, B. and Schroedter, R. Cortically evoked motor responses in patients with Xp22.3-linked Kallmann's syndrome and in female gene carriers. *Ann. Neurol.*, 1992, 31: 299–304.

Di Lazzaro, V., Restuccia, D., Oliviero, A., Profice, P., Ferrara, L., Insola, A., Mazzone, P., Tonali, P. and Rothwell, J.C. Magnetic transcranial stimulation at intensities below active motor threshold activates intracortical inhibitory circuits. *Exp. Brain Res.*, 1998, 119: 265–268.

Farmer, S.F., Ingram, D.A. and Stephens, J.A. Mirror movements studied in a patient with Klippel-Feil syndrome. *J. Physiol. (Lond.)*, 1990, 428: 467–484.

Hallett, M. Transcranial magnetic stimulation. Negative effects. *Adv. Neurol.*, 1995, 67: 107–113.

Krams, M., Quinton, R., Mayston, M.J., Harrison, L.M., Dolan, R.J., Bouloux, P.M., Stephens, J.A., Frackowiak, R.S. and Passingham, R.E. Mirror movements in X-linked Kallmann's syndrome. II. A PET study. *Brain*, 1997, 120: 1217–1228.

Kujirai, T., Caramia, M.D., Rothwell, J.C., Day, B.L., Thompson, P.D., Ferbert, A., Wroe, S., Asselman, P. and Marsden, C.D. Corticocortical inhibition in human motor cortex. *J. Physiol. (Lond.)*, 1993, 471: 501–519.

Leinsinger, G.L., Heiss, D.T., Jassoy, A.G., Pfluger, T., Hahn, K. and Danek, A. Persistent mirror movements: functional MR imaging of the hand motor cortex. *Radiology*, 1997, 203: 545–552.

Mayer, M., Botzel, K., Paulus, W., Plendl, H., Prockl, D. and Danek, A. Movement-related cortical potentials in persistent mirror movements. *Electroenceph. Clin. Neurophysiol.*, 1995, 95: 350–358.

Mayston, M.J., Harrison, L.M., Quinton, R., Stephens, J.A., Krams, M. and Bouloux, P.M. Mirror movements in X-linked Kallmann's syndrome. I. A neurophysiological study. *Brain*, 1997, 120: 1199–1216.

Mayston, M.J., Harrison, L.M. and Stephens, J.A. A neurophysiological study of mirror movements in adults and children. *Ann. Neurol.*, 1999, 45: 583–594.

Meyer, B.U., Röricht, S., Gräfin von Einsiedel, H., Kruggel. F. and Weindl, A. Inhibitory and excitatory interhemispheric transfers between motor cortical areas in normal humans and patients with abnormalities of the corpus callosum. *Brain*, 1995, 118: 429–440.

Netz, J., Lammers, T. and Homberg, V. Reorganization of motor output in the non-affected hemisphere after stroke. *Brain*, 1997, 120: 1579–1586.

Ragazzoni, A., Cincotta, M., Borgheresi, A., Zaccara, G. and Ziemann, U. Congenital hemiparesis: different functional reorganization of somatosensory and motor pathways. *Clin. Neurophysiol.*, 2002, 113: 1273–1278.

Rasmussen, P. Persistent mirror movements: a clinical study of 17 children, adolescents and young adults. *Dev. Med. Child Neurol.*, 1993, 35: 699–707.

Reitz, M. and Muller, K. Differences between 'congenital mirror movements' and 'associated movements' in normal children: a neurophysiological case study. *Neurosci. Lett.*, 1998, 256: 69–72.

Ridding, M.C., Taylor, J.L. and Rothwell, J.C. The effect of voluntary contraction on cortico-cortical inhibition in human motor cortex. *J. Physiol. (Lond.)*, 1995, 487: 541–548.

Schott, G.D. and Wyke, M.A. Congenital mirror movements. *J. Neurol. Neurosurg. Psychiatry*, 1981, 44: 586–599.

Shibasaki, H. and Nagae, K. Mirror movements: application of movement-related cortical potentials. *Ann. Neurol.*, 1984, 15: 299–302.

Van den Berg, C., Beek, P.J., Wagenaar, R.C. and Van Wieringen, P.C. Coordination disorders in patients with Parkinson's disease: a study of paced rhythmic forearm movements. *Exp. Brain Res.*, 2000, 134: 174–186.

Weiller, C., Ramsay, S.C., Wise, R.J., Friston, K.J. and Frackowiak, R.S. Individual patterns of functional reorganization in the human cerebral cortex after capsular infarction. *Ann. Neurol.*, 1993, 33: 181–189.

Woods, B.T. and Eby, M.D. Excessive mirror movements and aggression. *Biol. Psychiatry*, 1982, 17: 23–32.

Woods, B.T. and Teuber, H.L. Mirror movements after childhood hemiparesis. Neurology, 1978, 28: 1152–1157.

Ziemann, U., Ishii, K., Borgheresi, A., Yaseen, Z., Battaglia, F., Hallett, M., Cincotta, M. and Wassermann, E.M. Dissociation of the pathways mediating ipsilateral and contralateral motor evoked potentials in human hand and arm muscles. *J. Physiol.* (Lond.), 1999, 518: 895–906.

Transcranial Magnetic Stimulation and Transcranial Direct Current Stimulation (Supplements to Clinical Neurophysiology, Vol. 56)
Editors: W. Paulus, F. Tergau, M.A. Nitsche, J.C. Rothwell, U. Ziemann, M. Hallett

Chapter 17

Impact of interhemispheric inhibition on excitability of the non-lesioned motor cortex after acute stroke

Ludwig Niehaus[a,*], Malek Bajbouj[b] and Bernd-Ulrich Meyer[†]

[a] *Department of Neurology, Charité, Campus Virchow-Klinikum, D-13353 Berlin (Germany)*
[b] *Department of Psychiatry, Charité, Campus Benjamin Franklin, Berlin (Germany)*

1. Introduction

The adult human brain is capable of major functional reorganisation in response to ischemic injury. Neuroimaging and neurophysiological studies in patients with stroke have described a number of changes in cortical function in brain areas remote from the ischemic lesion (Feeney and Baron, 1986; Weiller et al., 1993; Cramer et al., 1997; Juhasz et al., 1997; Weiller, 1998). Using paired-pulse transcranial magnetic stimulation (TMS) it has recently been demonstrated that unilateral stroke may alter motor cortex excitability in the unaffected hemisphere (Liepert et al., 2000; Manganotti et al., 2002; Shimizu et al., 2002; Bütefisch et al., 2003). The underlying mechanisms are not yet fully understood. One hypothesis about lesion-induced changes in contralateral cortical function is based on the observation that neuronal activity in the hand-associated motor cortex is modulated by transcallosally mediated inhibitory influences from the homotopic contralateral motor cortex (Ferbert et al., 1992; Meyer et al., 1995; Di Lazzaro, 1999). In large infarctions, changes in excitability of the unaffected motor cortex might result from a loss of interhemispheric inhibition due to damaged intercortical connections.

The aim of the present study was to clarify the possible role of interhemispheric inhibition on motor cortex reorganisation in the nonstroke hemisphere. To address this problem we investigated excitatory and inhibitory effects of focal TMS over the motor cortex in patients with differently localised monohemispheric stroke. Ischemic cortical and subcortical lesions were used as a model for studying the effects of impaired interhemispheric inhibition on neuronal function in the opposite, intact motor cortex (Fig. 1). Functional integrity of the interhemispheric connections was assessed by transcallosal inhibition (TI) of voluntary tonic electromyographic activity elicited by TMS.

2. Methods

2.1. Patients and subjects

With ethics committee approval and informed consent, we studied 25 patients with an acute stroke (8 women, 17 men), aged from 39 to 81 years (mean, 60 years) and 25 normal control subjects (12 women, 13 men;

[†] deceased November 24, 2001.

* *Correspondence to*: PD Dr. L. Niehaus, Neurologische Klinik der Charité, Campus Virchow-Klinikum, Hochschulmedizin Berlin, Augustenburger Platz 1, D-13353 Berlin, Germany.
Tel: +49-030 4505 60011; Fax: +49-30 4505 60901.
E-mail: ludwig.niehaus@charite.de

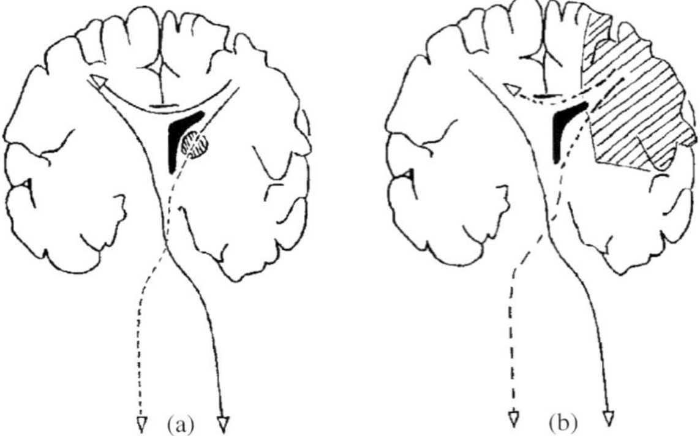

Fig. 1. Simplified model for studying the effects of interhemispheric inhibition on the nonlesioned motor cortex in stroke patients. In case of large hemispheric stroke (a), there was a loss of interhemispheric interaction, while interhemispheric inhibition would keep unaffected in ischemic lesions caudal the corpus callosum (b).

mean age 51 years, range 30–78 years). All patients showed hemiplegia or severe hemiparesis (strength of hand and finger movements ranged from 0 to 2, MRC-scale (Medical Research Council, 1975) at the time of examination. The mean interval between disease onset and examination was 8 ± 5 days. According to the CT and MRI findings patients were divided in two subgroups: 13 patients suffered from a subcortical stroke with a lesion located caudal the corpus callosum ("subcortical group"). Eight of them showed a striatocapsular infarction and five had a lacunar stroke affecting the internal capsule or corona radiata. The other subgroup consisted of 12 patients who showed a large infarction in the territory of the middle cerebral artery ("cortical group"). In all patients the ischemic lesion involved the motor cortex and the adjacent white matter and callosal fibres.

2.2. *Magnetic stimulation and recording*

Focal TMS of the motor cortex was performed with a figure-of-8-shaped coil (o.d. of half coil, 8.5 cm) of the Magstim 200 stimulator (Magstim Company, Dyfed, Wales) with the coil centre placed over the hand representation area. For each subject, the stimulation site for eliciting maximal hand motor responses was determined individually. To determine peripheral conduction times, magnetic stimulation was performed over the cervical nerve roots with a standard round coil (o.d. 11.6 cm).

The elicited surface compound EMG responses were recorded bilaterally from the first dorsal interosseus muscle (FID). Data were collected using a CED 1401 interface and a data collection program (SIGAVG, sampling frequency of 5000/s per channel). To control relaxation or tonic EMG activity, visual and acoustic feedback of the EMG signals was given to the subjects.

2.2.1. *Parameters of cortically elicited motor effects*

Response threshold was determined for the relaxed contralateral hand and defined as the stimulus intensity that evoked small EMG responses (> 0.1 mV) in at least five of 10 trials. Cortex stimulation was then performed during maximal tonic hand muscle contraction. The stimuli were applied over each hemisphere at an intensity of 80% of the maximum stimulator output, since for such intensities inhibitory stimulation effects had previously been found to regularly occur in healthy subjects (Meyer et al., 1995). To assess the excitatory and inhibitory effects 20 consecutive EMG signals elicited by stimulation over each hemisphere were rectified and then averaged. Amplitudes of the contralateral EMG responses were determined baseline-to-peak. In muscles contralateral to the side stimulated, the duration of the postexcitatory inhibition (PI) was measured as the interval between the onset of the excitatory EMG response and the end of the inhibition of tonic EMG activity.

In muscles ipsilateral to stimulation, the onset latency and degree of transcallosally mediated suppression of the tonic EMG activity were determined (transcallosal inhibition, TI). When focal TMS was applied over the affected hemisphere in patients, the coil was centered over the presumed motor cortex which was expected to be located in symmetrical site to the opposite unaffected motor cortex.

2.2.2. *Intracortical inhibition and facilitation*

Intracortical inhibition (ICI) and intracortical facilitation (ICF) were investigated with the previously described paired-pulse technique (Kujirai et al., 1993). Interstimulus intervals (ISI) were set at 1, 2, 3, 4, 5, 6, 7, 10, and 15 ms. The intensity of the conditioning stimulus was adjusted to 95% of the active motor threshold, and the intensity of the test stimulus was set so that the test stimulus alone produced a response of about 1 mV peak-to-peak amplitude. The peak-to-peak amplitude of the conditioned response was expressed as a percentage of the test response amplitude. In stroke patients measurements of ICI and ICF were restricted to the nonlesioned motor cortex.

3. Results

3.1. Corticospinally mediated excitatory and inhibitory effects

On the hemiplegic side hand motor responses were absent in all patients with large hemispheric stroke (cortical group) and in eight of 13 patients with subcortical stroke, while they were significantly reduced in amplitude in the other five patients. On the unaffected side all parameters of excitatory and inhibitory EMG responses were found to be normal (Table 1). Motor thresholds at rest, the response amplitudes and latencies during maximal contraction and the duration of postexcitatory inhibition did not differ between patients and normal subjects.

3.2. Transcallosal inhibition

In all patients with subcortical stroke, TMS applied to the motor cortex of the affected hemisphere were found to suppress ongoing voluntary EMG activity in ipsilateral hand muscles. An example of this finding is illustrated in Fig. 2. Latency and degree of transcallosal inhibition did not differ between normal subjects and patients in the subcortical group (Table 1). In all patients with large hemispheric infarction (cortical group), transcallosal inhibition was absent.

3.3. Intracortical inhibition and facilitation

In normal subjects and patients with subcortical stroke (nonlesioned hemisphere) inhibition of test motor responses occurred at interstimulus intervals (ISIs) of 1–5 ms (values < 100%), whereas facilitation occurred at ISIs of 7, 10, and 15 ms (values > 100%). There was no significant difference in the mean value of ICI (2–4 ms) and ICF (7–15 ms) between controls and patients with subcortical stroke ($P > 0.2$; Mann–Whitney *U*-test) (Fig. 3). In patients with large infarctions (cortical group), ICI was significantly diminished in comparison to healthy controls. This was true when comparing all ISIs at 2–4 ms ($P = 0.028$) and at 5–6 ms ($P = 0.009$, Mann–Whitney *U*-test). There was no significant difference for the

TABLE 1

EXCITATORY AND INHIBITORY EFFECTS OF SINGLE-PULSE TMS OVER BOTH MOTOR CORTICES IN 25 NORMAL SUBJECTS (= 50 HANDS) AND THE UNAFFECTED MOTOR CORTEX IN 25 PATIENTS WITH STROKE ($N = 25$ HANDS). (PI POSTEXCITATORY INHIBITION, TI TRANSCALLOSAL INHIBITION).

	Normal subjects	Patients	
		Subcortical group	Cortical group
Response thresholds (%)	40 ± 6	39 ± 8	39 ± 10
Response amplitude (mV)	4.4 ± 1.1	4.1 ± 0.8	4.5 ± 0.6
Central motor latency (ms)	6.7 ± 1.0	6.9 ± 1.2	7.1 ± 1.2
Duration of PI (ms)	195 ± 38	201 ± 46	171 ± 61
Latency of TI (ms)	37 ± 3	37 ± 4	–
Degree of TI (%)	67 ± 11	65 ± 15	–

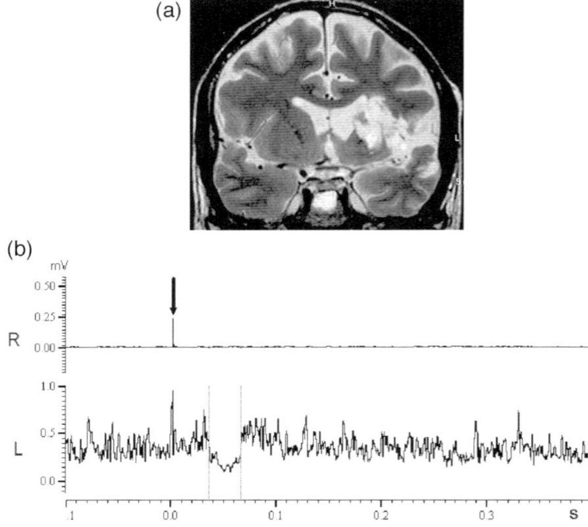

Fig. 2. Interhemispheric inhibition in a patient with striatocapsular infarction. Top: Coronal T2-weighted MRI demonstrated a left-sided subcortical lesion caudal the corpus callosum. Bottom: Traces of averaged and rectified EMG signals from the first dorsal interosseus muscles (FDI). Focal TMS over the left hand-associated motor cortex failed to evoke a contralateral hand motor response, while transcallosally mediated inhibition of tonic EMG activity in the ipsilateral FDI occured with normal onset latency and duration.

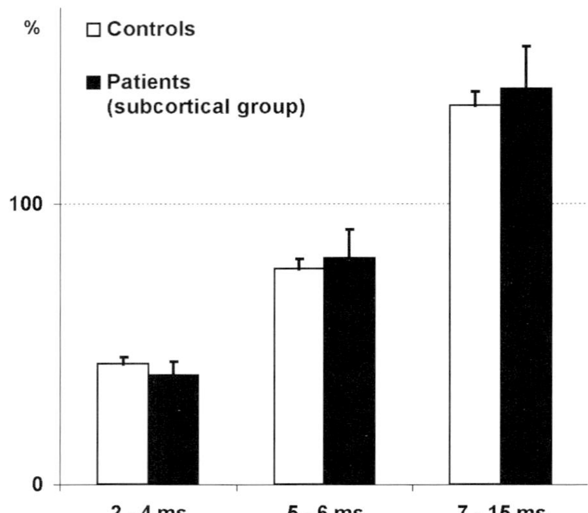

Fig. 3. Intracortical inhibition and facilitation in patients with subcortical stroke and normal subjects expressed as of the mean MEP amplitude of the test pulse alone. Comparison of group means at different ISIs. Error bars represent 1 SEM.

facilitatory ISIs of 7–15 ms between patients and healthy controls (Fig. 4).

4. Discussion

Using single and paired pulse TMS we investigated the function of excitatory and inhibitory neuronal structures in the motor cortex of the nonlesioned hemisphere in acute stroke. Consistent with recent studies (Liepert et al., 2000; Shimizu et al., 2002; Bütefisch et al., 2003) excitability of the corticospinal system was found to be normal. This was true for thresholds and amplitudes of cortically elicited excitatory responses. Furthermore, there was no abnormality in postexcitatory inhibition, i.e. the transcranially elicited inhibition of tonic EMG activity in contralateral hand muscles. The main finding of our study is that ICI is significantly reduced in the undamaged motor cortex in patients with cortical stroke in whom TI is lacking. In contrast, stroke patients with intact TI exhibit normal ICI and ICF in the undamaged hemisphere. These findings indicate a strong relationship between interhemispheric inhibition and motor cortex excitability. In acute stroke, loss of transcallosally mediated inhibition is associated with a decrease in motor cortical inhibition ("disinhibition") over the undamaged hemisphere. As demonstrated by Shimizu et al. (2002) this may also be the case in subacute and chronic stages of stroke.

The findings described above, are similar to observations in animal experiments. In rats, extended cortical and subcortical lesions may induce hyperexcitability of contralateral brain areas which result from downregulation of GABAergic receptor function and enhancement of glutamatergic activity (Buchkremer-Ratzmann et al., 1996; Reinecke et al., 1999; Neumann-Haefelin and Witte, 2000). It is possible that such changes in neurotransmitter systems contribute to

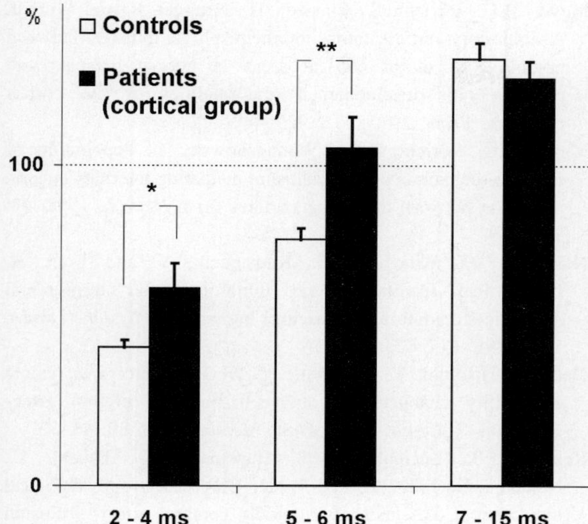

Fig. 4. Intracortical inhibition and facilitation in patients with large hemispheric infarction and normal subjects expressed as of the mean MEP amplitude of the test pulse alone. Comparison of group means at different ISIs. Error bars represent 1 SEM. Asterisks indicate level of significance (* $P < 0.05$, ** $P < 0.01$; Mann–Whitney *U*-test).

the disinhibition in unaffected motor cortex observed in patients with large hemispheric stroke.

In contrast to the resting motor threshold which represents membrane-related neuronal excitability (Ziemann et al., 1996), ICI determined by paired-pulse TMS, reflects the integrity and excitability of inhibitory intraneuronal circuits upstream from corticospinal neurons (Kujirai et al., 1993). Several lines of evidence suggest that ICI is predominantly mediated by GABAergic interneurons within the primary motor cortex (Nakamura et al., 1997; Di Lazzaro et al., 1998; Ziemann et al., 1998). At first glance it seems to be inconsistent that PI which is also attributed to an activation of GABA-mediated inhibitory neuronal circuits (Hallett, 1995) did not change while ICI was abnormally reduced. However, neurophysiological and pharmacological studies indicated that both inhibitory processes are related to different subtypes of GABAergic receptors and may show different thresholds for activation (Ziemann et al., 1996; Siebner et al., 1998; Werhahn et al., 1999; Sanger et al., 2001). Thus, changes in ICI may occur independently from changes in PI even in case of impaired interhemispheric inhibition.

Interhemispheric inhibition as measured by TI is considered to result from an activation of transcallosally projecting neurones which in the other motor cortex activates interneurones with inhibitory influence on corticospinal outputs (Ferbert et al., 1992; Meyer et al., 1998). It is currently unknown which subsets of cortical inhibitory neurons and mechanisms are activated by TI and which are affected by a loss of interhemispheric interactions. The findings of the present study suggest that TI and ICI may share common inhibitory mechanisms and subsets of inhibitory interneurons. However, further experiments are needed to determine the underlying mechanisms of both inhibitory phenomena.

As previously reported by Liepert et al. (1998) ICI can be modulated in a task- and use-dependent matter. It might be argued that enhanced use of the unaffected limb may induce motor cortex hyperexcitability. However, it must be kept in mind that the two groups of patients presented showed similar degrees of paresis in the upper limb. Therefore it is unlikely that there were group differences in the use of the intact hand.

In patients with stroke, both poor and good motor recovery associated with an abnormal excitability over the unaffected hemisphere has been previously reported (Manganotti et al., 2002; Bütefisch et al., 2003). The clinical relevance of motor cortex disinhibition in the undamaged hemisphere need to be elucidated.

In conclusion, our findings document that in acute stroke a loss of interhemispheric inhibition may induce motor cortex disinhibition in the undamaged hemisphere. It remains to be clarified whether this process plays a relevant role in recovery after stroke.

Acknowledgements

This work was supported in part by Deutsche Forschungsgemeinschaft (EI 207/2-1). The authors are grateful to K. Shin-Nolte for her technical assistance and to Dr. M. Gerwig for helpful discussions.

References

Buchkremer-Ratzmann, I., August, M., Hagemann, G. and Witte, O.W. Electrophysiological transcortical diaschisis after cortical photothrombosis in rat brain. *Stroke*, 1998, 27: 1105–1109.

Bütefisch, C.M., Netz, J., Wessling, M., Seitz, R.J. and Hömberg, V. Remote changes in cortical excitability after stroke. *Brain*, 2003, 126: 470–481.

Cramer, S.C., Nelles, G., Benson, R.R., Kaplan, J.D., Parker, R.A., Kwong, K.K., Kennedy, D.N., Finklestein, S.P. and Rosen, B.R. A functional MRI study of subjects recovered from hemiparetic stroke. *Stroke*, 1997, 28: 2518–2527.

Di Lazzaro, V., Restuccia, D., Oliviero, A., Profice, P., Ferrara, L., Insola, A., Mazzone Tonali, P. and Rothwell, J.C. Magnetic transcranial stimulation at intensities below active motor threshold activates intracortical inhibitory circuits. *Exp. Brain Res.*, 1998, 119: 265–268.

Di Lazzaro, V., Insola, A., Mazzone, P., Tonali, P. and Rothwell, J.C. Direct demonstration of interhemispheric inhibition of the human motor cortex produced by transcranial magnetic stimulation. *Exp. Brain Res.*, 1999, 124: 520–524.

Feeney, D.M. and Baron, J.C. Diaschisis. *Stroke*, 1986, 17: 817–830.

Ferbert, A., Priori, A., Rothwell, J.C., Colebatch, J.G., Day, B.L. and Marsden C.D. Interhemispheric inhibition of the human motor cortex. *J. Physiol.* (*Lond.*), 1992, 453: 525–546.

Hallett, M. Transcranial magnetic stimulation. Negative effects. In: M. Hallett, L.O. Lüders and C.D. Marsden (Eds.), Negative motor phenomena. *Advances in Neurology*, Vol. 67. Lippincot-Raven Publishers, Philadelphia. 1995: 107–113.

Juhasz, C., Kamondi, A. and Szirmai, I. Spectral EEG analysis following hemispheric stroke: evidences of transhemispheric diaschisis. *Acta Neurol. Scand.*, 1997, 96: 397–400.

Kujirai, T., Caramia, M.D., Rothwell, J.C., Day, B.L., Thompson, P.D., Ferbert, A., Wroe, S., Asselman, P. and Marsden, C.D. Corticocortical inhibition in human motor cortex. *J. Physiol.*, 1993, 471: 501–519.

Liepert, J., Classen, J., Cohen, L.G. and Hallett, M. Task-dependent changes of intracortical inhibition. *Exp Brain Res.*, 1998, 118: 421–426.

Liepert, J., Hamzei, F. and Weiller, C. Motor cortex disinhibition of the unaffected hemisphere after acute stroke. *Muscle Nerve*, 2000, 23: 1761–1763.

Manganotti, P., Patuzzo, S., Cortese, F., Palermo, A., Smania, N. and Fiaschi, A. Motor disinhibition in affected and unaffected hemisphere in the early period of recovery after stroke. *Clin. Neurophysiol.*, 2002, 113: 936–943.

Meyer, B.U., Röricht, S., Einsiedl, H., Kruggel, F. and Weindl, A. Inhibitory and excitatory interhemispheric transfers between homologeous motor cortical areas in normal subjects and patients with developmental abnormalities of the corpus callosum. *Brain*, 1995, 118: 429–440.

Meyer, B.U., Röricht, S. and Woiciechowsky, C. Topography of fibres in the human corpus callosum mediating interhemispheric inhibition between the motor cortices. *Ann. Neurol.*, 1998, 43: 360–369.

Nakamura, H., Kitagawa, H., Kawaguchi, Y. and Tsuji, H. Intracortical facilitation and inhibition after transcranial magnetic stimulation in conscious humans. *J. Physiol.* (*Lond.*), 1997, 498: 817–823.

Neumann-Haefelin, T. and Witte, O.W. Periinfarct and remote excitability changes after transient middle cerebral artery occlusion. *J. Cereb. Blood Flow. Metab.*, 2000, 20: 45–52.

Reinecke, S., Lutzenburg, M., Hagemann, G., Bruehl, C., Neumann-Haefelin, T. and Witte, O.W. Electrophysiological transcortical diaschisis after middle cerebral artery occlusion (MCAO) in rats. *Neurosci. Lett.*, 1999, 261: 85–88

Sanger, T.D., Garg, R.R. and Chen, R. Interactions between two different inhibitory systems in the human motor cortex. *J. Physiol.*, 2001, 530: 307–317.

Shimizu, T., Hosaki, A., Hino, T., Sato, M., Komori, T., Hirai, S. and Rossini, P.M. Motor cortical disinhibition in the unaffected hemisphere after unilateral cortical stroke. *Brain*, 2002, 125: 1896–1907.

Siebner, H.R., Dressnandt, J., Auer, C. and Conrad, B. Continuous intrathecal baclofen infusions induced a marked increase of the transcranially evoked silent period in a patient with generalized dystonia. *Muscle Nerve*, 1998, 21: 1209–1215.

Weiller, C. Imaging recovery from stroke. *Exp. Brain Res.*, 1998, 123: 13–17.

Weiller, C., Ramsay, S., Wise, R.S.J., Friston, K.J. and Frackowiak, R.S.J. Individual patterns of functional reorganisation in the human cerebral cortex after capsular infarction. *Ann. Neurol.*, 1993, 33: 181–189.

Werhahn, K.J., Kunesch, E., Noachtar, S., Benecke, R. and Classen, J. Differential effects on motorcortical inhibition induced by blockade of GABA-uptake in humans. *J. Physiol.*, 1999, 517: 591–597.

Ziemann, U., Lönnecker, S., Steinhof, B.J. and Paulus, W. Effects of antepileptic drugs on motor cortex excitability in humans: a transcranial magnetic stimulation study. *Ann. Neurol.*, 1996, 40: 367–378.

Ziemann, U., Steinhoff, B.J., Tergau, F. and Paulus, W. Transcranial magnetic stimulation: its current role in epilepsy research. *Epilepsy Res.*, 1998, 30: 11–30.

Transcranial Magnetic Stimulation and Transcranial Direct
Current Stimulation (Supplements to Clinical Neurophysiology, Vol. 56)
Editors: W. Paulus, F. Tergau, M.A. Nitsche, J.C. Rothwell, U. Ziemann, M. Hallett

Chapter 18

Disruption of the neural correlates of working memory using high- and low-frequency repetitive transcranial magnetic stimulation: a negative study

Eva A. Feredoes[a], Perminder S. Sachdev[a,b] and Wei Wen[b]

[a] *School of Psychiatry, Faculty of Medicine, University of New South Wales, Sydney (Australia)*
[b] *Neuropsychiatric Institute, Prince of Wales Hospital, Sydney (Australia)*

1. Introduction

Working memory (WM) is the system which allows for the short-term storage and processing of information (Baddeley, 1986) and is essential for the performance of complex cognitive processes, such as language comprehension, counting and mental arithmetic, syllogistic reasoning and dynamic perceptuomotor control (Baddeley and Logie, 1999). The most widely applied model of WM (Baddeley, 1986) posits a modality-independent central executive (CE) which acts upon information stored in the 'slave systems', more specifically, the phonologic loop and visuospatial scratchpad (Baddeley, 1986). Earlier studies into WM focussed more on the slave systems than the CE, as they were simpler to study (Baddeley, 1986). As knowledge of the WM system has grown, the importance of the CE has become apparent.

The CE has multiple roles in processing information and co-ordinating the slave systems. The so-called executive processes performed by the CE are not rigidly defined, but are thought to include attention and inhibition, task management, planning, monitoring and coding (Smith and Jonides, 1999). The CE, not having a storage capacity of its own, performs these operations upon the information held 'on-line' by the slave systems (Baddeley and Logie, 1999).

There is currently much focus on the anatomical organisation of the CE. Evidence of the possible location(s) of the CE comes from a variety of sources, including human lesion studies (Owen et al., 1996b; Della Salla et al., 1998), animal investigations (Goldman-Rakic, 1971; Marshuetz et al., 2000), neuroimaging (Courtney et al., 1998; D'Esposito et al., 1998; Stern et al., 2000), and transcranial magnetic stimulation (TMS) (Hong et al., 2000; Mottaghy et al., 2000, 2002, 2003; Mull and Seyal, 2001; Oliveri et al., 2001). The prefrontal cortex (PFC) has been implicated in all these studies, but further subdivisions within the PFC is a matter of debate. According to the domain-specific model, the dorsolateral prefrontal cortex (DLPFC) mediates the storage and processing of spatial WM information (Levy and Goldman-Rakic, 2000). On the other hand, the process-specific model argues that the PFC is

* *Correspondence to*: Eva Feredoes, NPI, Euroa Centre, Prince of Wales Hospital, Sydney, NSW 2031, Australia. Tel: +61 2 9382 3809; Fax: + 61 2 9382 3774; E-mail: eva.feredoes@student.unsw.edu.au

segregated according to the nature of the executive process involved (Owen, 1997). There are further variations on these models, exemplifying some of the basic arguments that exist within the field of WM.

The disagreement between WM models has been, in part, due to WM research techniques being unable to establish a causal connection between the activity of a brain area and its specific role in a behavioural output (Pascual-Leone et al., 2000). Transcranial magnetic stimulation (TMS) can address this problem, as it has the unique ability to create 'virtual lesions', transiently disrupting the functioning of a targeted area during the performance of a specific task (Pascual-Leone et al., 1999). Thus, in the manner of traditional lesion studies, the functional link between an activity and disrupted brain area can be made with the advantage of being performed in a controlled experimental environment using healthy, normal human subjects (Pascual-Leone et al., 1999).

Already, a number of studies have reported the impact of single-pulse or repetitive TMS (rTMS) on brain regions previously reported to be involved in executive processing and storage demonstrating disruption of task performance (Hong et al., 2000; Kessels et al., 2000; Mottaghy et al., 2000, 2003; Mull and Seyal, 2001; Oliveri et al., 2001). Mottaghy et al. (2000, 2003) used rTMS over the DLPFCs and combined it with PET scanning to show the underlying neuronal network involved in WM processing. Oliveri et al. (2001) used single-pulse TMS over various PFC areas, including the left and right DLPFC to disrupt visuospatial WM processing.

The present study used both high- and low-frequency rTMS over the DLPFC to disrupt 3-back task performance. Conceptually, rTMS introduces 'random noise' into the organised neuronal functioning during a given behaviour, where the pattern of activity occurring at the time of stimulation is disrupted (Walsh and Rushworth, 1999; Jahanshahi and Rothwell, 2000) but the mechanisms by which high- and low-frequency stimulation act is unclear (Jahanshahi et al., 1998). High-frequency rTMS causes excitation, followed by a period of cortical inhibition (Pascual-Leone et al., 1999), resulting from a GABAergic inhibitory post synaptic potential (Jahanshahi and Rothwell, 2000). Multiple pulses are thought to summate so that the effect of repeated stimuli is more than that produced by a single pulse, and the affected area is also increased (Jahanshahi and Rothwell, 2000). Low frequency stimulation, working in a different but uncertain manner, has been shown to produce effects that last beyond the trains of stimulation, with sub-threshold, low-frequency rTMS most likely causing changes in neuronal excitability (Chen et al., 1997; Fitzgerald et al., 2002; Mottaghy et al., 2002). Our investigations employed a 3-back task during stimulation of the DLPFC. The n-back task is considered a paradigm test of WM (Owen et al., 1999), where it involves an updating, and matching of stimuli to those presented previously in the continuous sequence. The DLPFC is the proposed site of the monitoring and manipulation component of the task (Owen et al., 1996a, b; Smith and Jonides, 1999).

2. Methods

2.1. Subjects

Subjects were healthy volunteers with a mean age of 23 years (range 18–29 years), all right-handed. They were recruited through advertisement, from the student body of the University of New South Wales and provided written consent to participate in the study, which had been approved by the local ethics committee. They were naïve to TMS and were not aware of the specific hypotheses of the studies.

2.2. Stimulation

Stimulation was delivered from a MagStim Rapid stimulator (Magstim Company Ltd, Whitland, UK) using a 70 mm figure-of-eight coil which was positioned tangential to the scalp. All subjects had motor threshold (MT) determination using the method-of-limits procedure (Pascual-Leone et al., 1999). The coil was positioned with the handle in a postero-lateral position, (between 90 and 180° from the midline). Sham stimulation was performed using the one-wing tilt method, where the coil was placed perpendicular to the point of stimulation, at 30% machine intensity.

Stimulation was given over the left and right DLPFC, as well as bilaterally using two machines discharging simultaneously. The DLPFC was defined as the site 5 cm anterior, in the same sagittal plane, to the motor cortex, this being the site of optimal production of evoked potentials in the first dorsal interossus muscle. The vertex (Cz) was used as the site of control stimulation. The correspondence between the site of stimulation and the targeted cortical region was verified in three subjects from 3-D reconstructed MRI of the head that had been scanned after placing vitamin E capsules on the scalp corresponding to the 10–20 international EEG system. The order and site of stimulation were randomised for each subject.

2.3. Tasks

The verbal and visuospatial 3-back tasks were used. For the verbal task (Study 1 only), one of eight letters was presented in the centre of a monitor for 200 ms at intervals of 1800 ms, and subjects were required to press one of two buttons with each hand to indicate if the on-screen stimulus matched or did not match the one presented three stimuli previously. There were an approximately equal number of match and non-match stimuli. Each 'run' comprised 75 stimuli and lasted for 150 s. For the visuospatial task (Studies 1 and 2), a star appeared for 200 ms in one of eight positions around the circumference of an imaginary circle, followed by a blank screen with a fixation cross in the centre for 1800 ms (Study 1) or 1200 ms (Study 2) in which time the position 3-back was required to be matched. Each run lasted for 150 s (Study 1) or 105 s (Study 2). The response was recorded on a Cedrus RB-610 response box placed in a comfortable position selected by the subject. To obviate laterality of response arm, a match was indicated by pressing both index fingers and a non-match by pressing both middle fingers.

2.4. General procedure

Subjects were seated in a reclining chair with a head-rest for stabilisation of the head. The computer screen used for display of the stimuli was at eye-level at a distance of 80 cm from the subject's head. Prior to the test phase, subjects were required to practice on the task for 5–10 trials until they achieved consistency in performance as judged by three runs with scores differing by $< 5\%$. These were averaged to give a baseline score.

Two studies were performed, the first using high-frequency rTMS and the second low-frequency rTMS while the subjects were performing the task. Study 1 used both the verbal and visuospatial tasks whilst Study 2 used the visuospatial task only.

2.5. Study 1: high frequency rTMS during a verbal and visuospatial 3-back task

Ten healthy right-handed individuals (five male, five female) took part in this study. The design of the study is graphically presented in Fig. 1. After having completed the practice trials and reached a satisfactory level of performance ($> 70\%$ accuracy that was consistent over three trials), the subject was seated comfortably as described and the study begun. The subject began the task at the onset of stimulation and continued it for 30 s after stimulation had ceased. For both verbal and visuospatial parts, the subject had eight episodes (four verum and four sham) of stimulation: two each (one verum and one sham) on left DLPFC, right DLPFC, bilateral DLPFC and vertex. Each episode of real stimulation was at 5 Hz, 110% MT, in trains of 151 pulses, an inter-train interval of 2.1 s and an overall stimulation session of 132 s (120 s of rTMS).

2.6. Study 2: low-frequency rTMS during a visuospatial 3-back task

Fourteen healthy right-handed individuals (two male, 12 female) took part in this study. The design of the study is graphically presented in Figs. 1 and 2. After the practice phase 10 min of stimulation was started.

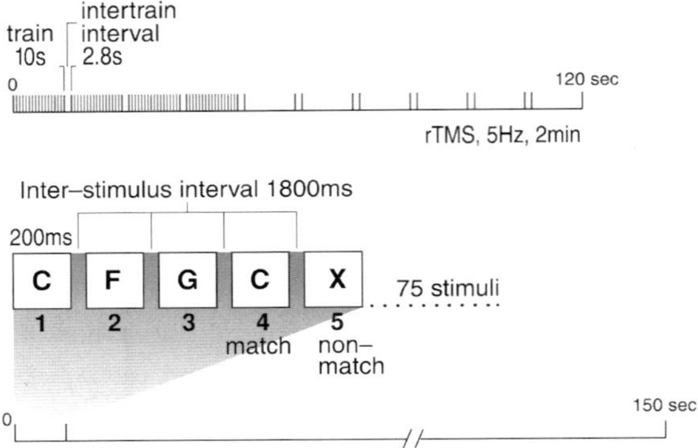

Fig. 1. The design for Study 1 using high-frequency rTMS during verbal and visuospatial 3-back tasks. At the start of the task, stimulation commences (5 Hz, 110% MT). Subjects responded with the index fingers of both hands for a letter matching another 3-back in the sequence of 75 stimuli (200 ms each with an ISI of 1,800 ms). Subjects pressed both middle fingers if the stimulus on-screen was a non- match. Stimulation stopped after 130 s; the task continued until 150 s.

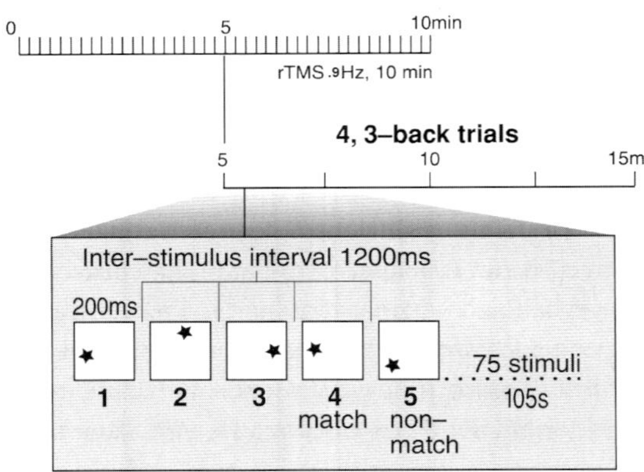

Fig. 2. Study 2 employed a low-frequency stimulation paradigm (0.9 Hz, 90% MT) over 10 min. Five minutes after commencement of stimulation, a visuospatial 3-back task began (75 stimuli, 200 ms each with an ISI of 1,200 ms). Two trials were completed during stimulation. Stimulation stopped after 10 min and a further two trials were completed.

After 5 min of stimulation, two runs of the visuospatial task were performed. Once the stimulation had ceased, two more task runs were performed.

The subject had six episodes (three verum and one sham) of stimulation: one each (one verum) on left DLPFC, right DLPFC and vertex. Sham stimulation was randomly applied once to either the left of right DLPFC. Each episode of real stimualtion was at 0.9 Hz, 90% MT.

2.7. Analysis

The outcome measures for each trial were *percent accuracy and mean reaction time* (RT). An overall analysis of variance (ANOVA) was performed to detect any main effect of stimulation on accuracy or RT or an interaction between them. Follow-up comparisons of conditions were carried out where appropriate.

The 3-D reconstructed MRIs, with vitamin E scalp markers denoting the stimulation sites were analysed using SPM software, to locate the markers to the cortical surface. The corresponding Talairach coordinates were acquired and the Brodmann Areas were determined using the Talairach Daemon Database (v1.1. University of Texas Health Science Centre, San Antonio).

3. Results

The Talairach coordinates and corresponding Brodmann areas underlying the sites of stimulation for three subjects of Study 1 are shown in Table 1, and case 1 shown in Fig. 3. These MRI scans confirmed that stimulation was delivered close to the DLPFC.

3.1. Study 1: high frequency rTMS during a verbal and visuospatial 3-back

3.1.1. Verbal 3-back task

The results for accuracy of performance and RT for different episodes of stimulation are presented in Figs. 4 and 5.

An ANOVA with Stimulation (two levels: active rTMS, sham rTMS) and Site (four levels: left, right, vertex, bilateral) revealed a significant effect of TMS [$F(1,9) = 8.322$; $p = 0.018$], but not for Site

TABLE 1

TALAIRACH COORDINATES OF STIMULATED SITES AND CORRESPONDING BORDMANN AREAS FOR THREE SUBJECTS.

Subject	Talairach coordinates							
	Left			Right			Brodmann area	
	X	Y	Z	X	Y	Z	Left	Right
1	–42.57	20.80	50.71	45.54	25.68	43.39	BA8	BA8
2	–49.40	31.10	33.64	49.70	27.45	28.29	BA8	BA9
3	–43.46	38.90	30.11	43.66	39.29	34.05	BA9	BA9

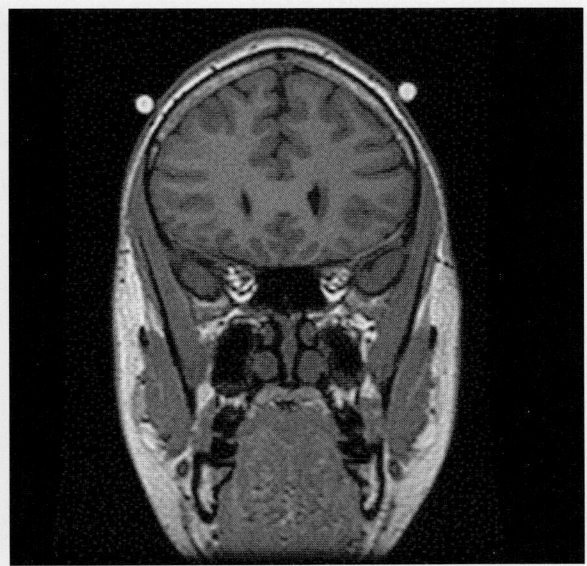

Fig. 3. 3-D reconstructed MRI with vitamin E capsule scalp markers denoting the position of the coil over the left and right mid-DLPFC.

[$F(3,9)$] = 1.345; $p = 0.335$]. There was no interaction between stimulation and the brain region to which it was applied [$F(5,9) = 0.308$; $p = 0.819$).

Subsequent paired t-test comparisons showed that for the verbal task, rTMS over the left and right DLPFC had no significant effect [left: $t(9) = -1.024$; $p = 0.332$]; right: $t(9) = -0.1.294$; $p = 0.228$]. Bilateral rTMS also produced no effect of significance when compared to sham stimulation [$t(9) = -1.705$; $p = 0.122$]. We failed to find any significant effect of active stimulation on RTs [$F(1,9) = 449$; $p = 0.522$] or an effect of stimulation site on RTs [$F(3.9) = 0.420$; $p = 0.745$] and no interaction between TMS and Site [$F = 0.574$; $p = 0.653$] was evident.

3.1.2. *Visuospatial 3-back task*

An ANOVA with TMS and Site revealed a significant effect of TMS on visuospatial task accuracy [$F(1,9) = 5.252$; $p = 0.048$]. There was no effect of Site [$F(3,9) = 0.281$; $p = 0.838$] nor any significant interaction between TMS and Site [$F(5,9) = 0.286$; $p = 0.843$].

Paired t-test comparisons did not show any significant effects of left, right and bilateral active stimulation compared to sham stimulation (left: [$t(9) = 0.326$; $p = 0.752$]; right: [$t(9) = 0.634$; $p = 0.542$]; bilateral: [$t(9) = 1.978$; $p = 0.079$]. RTs were not significantly affected by stimulation (all $p > 0.05$).

3.2. *Study 2: low-frequency rTMS during a visuospatial 3-back task*

The results for accuracy of performance for different episodes of stimulation are presented in Fig. 5.

Four trials were performed under stimulation at each site. The accuracy from each of these trials was collapsed to an overall accuracy at each site and compared to sham stimulation accuracy. Post hoc

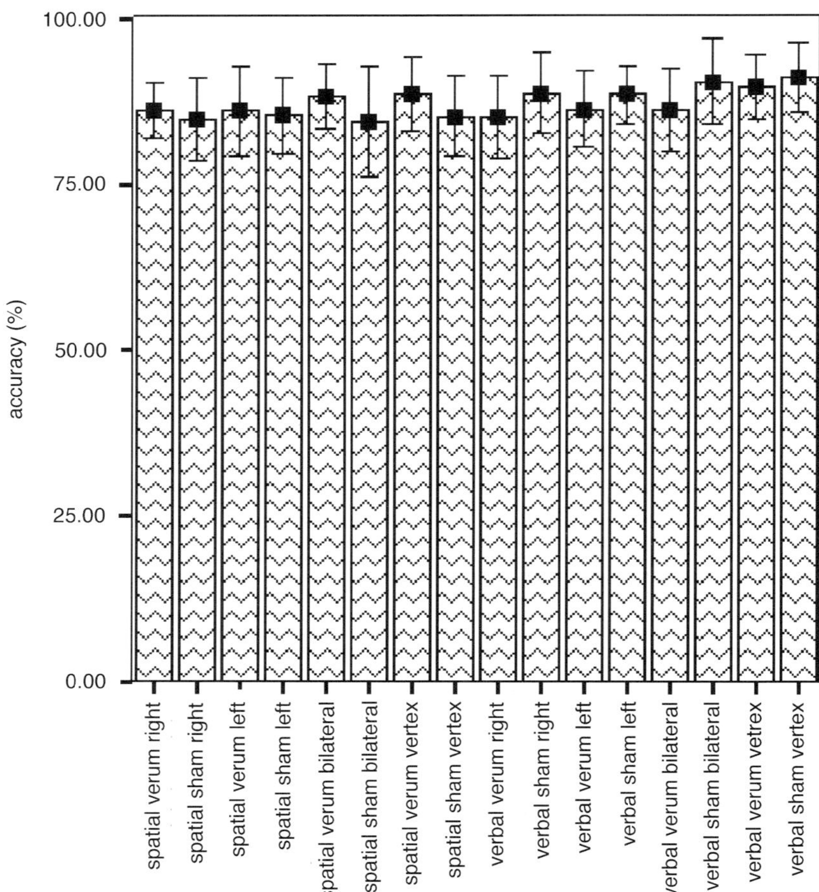

Fig. 4. Study 1. Mean verbal and visuospatial 3-back task accuracy under high-frequency stimulation for both verum and sham stimulation.

analysis compared the two trials after stimulation, combined into an overall post-stimulation accuracy, to the corresponding sham condition.

3.2.1. Visuospatial 3-back task

A repeated measures ANOVA did not reveal a significant difference between the accuracy at the different stimulation sites [$F(14) = 1.282$; $p = 0.329$]. RTs were not significantly affected by rTMS (all $p > 0.05$). For post-stimulation accuracy, we compared the means of stimulation to the left and right DLPFC, vertex and prefrontal sham stimulation. No significant differences were evident between the groups [$F(13) = 0.016$; $p = 0.984$]. Reaction times were not significantly affected by stimulation (all $p > 0.05$).

4. Discussion

We found that healthy subjects performed equally well under conditions of verum and sham stimulation over the DLPFC, with either high- or low-frequency, and irrespective of whether it was unilateral or bilateral stimulation. This was contrary to our expectations of seeing a decrement in performance with

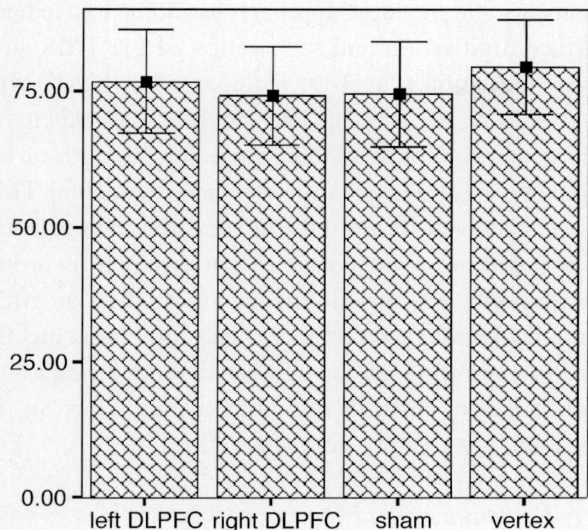

Fig. 5. Study 2. Mean visuospatial 3-back task accuracy under low-frequency stimulation showing real stimualtion of the left and right DLPFC and vertex, and sham stimulation of the PFC.

stimulation over the DLPFC. It is also at variance with a previous study (Mottaghy et al., 2000), which demonstrated a significant reduction in performance accuracy on a verbal 2-back task during high-frequency stimulation. There have been other reports in the literature in which rTMS has been used to disrupt WM tasks (Hong et al., 2000; Mull and Seyal, 2001). In explaining our negative results, we must consider a number of methodological and neurobiological issues. The methodological issues include sample size, differences in stimulation parameters, focality of repetitive stimulation, the nature of the 3-back task and practice effects. The neurobiological aspects that are important include the neuroanatomical basis of WM, and redundancy and compensation within neural systems.

4.1. Sample characteristics

In Study 1, we had power to detect a moderate to high effect size at $\alpha = 0.05$. As no trends were seen, we did not think the result was a Type I error that a larger sample size would have overcome. Nevertheless, the sample size was increased for Study 2 with no difference. Our subjects were highly intelligent university students, and whether this fact contributed to the lack of observable effect is unknown. They were performing at a high level but not at the ceiling, and the presence of a ceiling effect is unlikely.

4.2. Stimulation parameters

Both high- and low-frequency stimulation has been shown to disrupt task performance in previous studies, but there are a number of variables within these stimulation parameters that can produce a different outcome. Our magnetic pulses were not time-locked to task stimuli. It is possible that the individual stimuli did not coincide with the time period when the targeted cortical area was performing its specific aspect of overall task performance (Walsh and Rushworth, 1999). The temporal characteristics of the cortical effects of TMS are incompletely understood. Suprathreshold TMS can delay movements for up to 150 ms, not all of which is due to the pulse's effect on the cortex (Day et al., 1989). At threshold, effects of single pulses on scalp EEG last 20–30 ms (Ilmoniemi et al., 1997). If the disrupting effect of a single stimulus is expected to last a conservative 100 ms, it is likely that in Study 1 a proportion of the task stimuli were presented at a time cortical processing had been disrupted, and a decrement should have been seen. The work of Amassian et al. (1993) has shown that, in fact, frequencies of 4–5 Hz may be sufficient to disrupt cortical functioning continuously. On the other hand, according to Mottaghy et al. (2002), the effect of high-frequency rTMS is seen only for the duration of the pulse train, so the additional 30 s of task without stimulation may have been enough to mask the significant effect caused by stimulation during the first 60 s of the task.

In Study 2 which used low-frequency stimulation, the WM task was started after 5 min of stimulation and continued beyond the 10 min of total stimulation. Recent work has shown that the motor cortex shows sustained inhibition after 5 min of stimulation, and this reaches a peak at about 9 min of stimulation (Gerschlager et al., 2001). It is therefore likely that subjects were performing the task while their DLPFC was continuously inhibited. We examined the performance during the first and second halves of the 10 min task duration, and found no differences between the two, suggesting that early release from inhibition was unlikely to account for the negative effects. It is possible that a larger number of pulses were necessary. Maeda et al. (2002) suggest that the overall number of pulses to produce an effect on motor-evoked potential output should be greater than 1000. Our low-frequency train consisted of only 540 pulses, which may have lowered the size of the TMS effect to below significant.

The threshold of stimulation is another parameter that could have influenced our results. Much of the work on the neurophysiology of TMS has been carried out on the motor cortex. The degree of correspondence between the motor and prefrontal cortices is unknown. We used 110% MT in Study 1 and 90% MT in Study 2. The lower intensity was used in Study 2 to reduce any discomfort in the subjects owing to the prolonged duration of stimulation. It is possible that higher intensity of stimulation might produce different results, although other authors (Mottaghy et al., 2002) have demonstrated decremental effects at similar levels of stimulation.

We also consider coil orientation as another variable that may have contributed to the result. A recent study examining the effects of various coil angles on the results of a cognitive task performance showed that rotating the coil had a significant effect (Hill et al., 2000). With respect to cognitive tasks during TMS, it is difficult to ascertain the optimal coil angle for task disruption, as the behavioural output is not as easily measurable as motor-evoked potentials. Under the circumstances, holding the coil in the postero-lateral position, as shown by Hill et al. (2000), is an acceptable option at present.

4.3. Site of stimulation

The structural MRI scans showed that we were stimulating an area directly overlying the mid-DLPFC (Pascual-Leone et al., 1999). However, there is considerable inter-individual variation in brain anatomy, and the ideal approach would be to use head surface digitisation and registration of the TMS sites onto the subject's 3-D reconstructed head MRI (Miranda et al., 1997). This approach is expensive and generally not available. Since the strength of the magnetic field decays with distance, the actual TMS 'dose' received by the DLPFC and the area affected is not certain. It is possible that a larger neuronal population needs to be influenced to produce an effect on 3-back task performance, therefore reducing the size of the rTMS effect. Higher magnetic fields will recruit large cortical regions, but this has to be balanced with safety and tolerability.

4.4. Redundancy and compensation

Whilst the parameters of rTMS contain a number of variables affecting the outcome of stimulation, the WM network should also be considered an important factor when an rTMS effect is desired. Neuroimaging investigations have shown the distribution of executive processing across the PFC (Courtney et al., 1998; Braver and Bongiolatti, 2002; Cabeza et al., 2002; Collette and Van der Linden, 2002). The high memory load of 3-back recruits a larger number of brain areas compared to the lower WM load of 1- and 2-back tasks (Braver et al., 1997).

Electrophysiological recordings in rats show prefrontal neurons 'tuning' to both spatial and object stimuli depending on task requirements (Rao et al., 1997). A framework is emerging to suggest the multi-role capability of regions where networks span many cortical sites resulting in the overlap of roles (Carpenter et al., 2000). This provides a basis for redundancy or compensation in response to the stimulation of a network component. Redundancy, for example, can occur when the processing of a WM task can still be carried out during stimulation, where another area in the functional network can also perform the required processing. One would conclude that the DLPFC may be an important area involved in WM tasks, but may not be essential for their execution. Alternatively, the processes may involve large cortical regions such that 'noise' in a proportion of the involved cortex would permit the processes to proceed unhindered. Compensation within the WM network was demonstrated by a recent rTMS study investigating the modulation of the brain response to stimulation, during a verbal 2-back task (Mottaghy et al., 2003). A PET scan taken during task performance without rTMS showed a decrease in rCBF in the left DLPFC, probably due to better task performance requiring less recruitment of the DLPFC. rTMS to the left and right DLPFC caused blood flow changes in contralateral homologuous brain regions and posterior regions, most likely in an effort to compensate for the disruptive effects of stimulation. This short-term plasticity has also been observed in experiments that involve cooling the cerebral cortex of cats (Payne et al., 1996), where functionally connected regions can replace the disrupted area/s to maintain a desired behavioural output.

4.5. Task-related issues

An important difference between our experiment and that of Mottaghy et al. (2000) was that we used a 3-back rather than the 2-back used by the other group. The 3-back task is very demanding on WM, and the performance of the subjects suggests that neither ceiling nor floor effects could account for the results. It is possible that the difficulty of the 3-back relative to the 2-back task results in a much wider cortical involvement in the former, such that disruption of a relatively small area does not lead to task disruption. We hope to repeat the experiments using the 2-back task.

The influence of practice on task performance should also be considered. The amount of practice on a task may determine the level of CE involvement. It has been suggested that when a task has been performed more than once, it becomes automatic and is no longer an effective test of executive functioning (Collette and Van der Linden, 2002). The embedded-processes model of WM of Cowan (1999) and the attention scheduling mechanism of Norman and Shallice (1986) both state that a well-rehearsed task no longer fully elicits the CE, compared to a novel task. A well-learned or rehearsed action could mean that the control operates at a lower level when compared to a novel action (Badagaiyan, 2000) and therefore only a novel task is a true test of executive functions (Rabbitt, 1997). Functional neuroimaging has shown that as a visuospatial WM task became more practiced, a number of areas decreased in activation, including prefrontal areas (Garavan et al., 2000). TMS studies have also shown an effect of TMS on a visual search task disappears once the task had been learned. Upon presentation of a novel task, stimulation once again disrupted task performance (Walsh et al., 1998). The nature of the 3-back task, however, makes it likely that demands on WM remain high even after repeat trials. Subjects tended to reach a plateau after a few trials, after which increments in performance was very slow. Practice is therefore unlikely to invalidate the results of this study.

5. Conclusion

We believe that an effect of TMS was not seen on a demanding WM task due to the many factors involved in rTMS itself and the nature of the WM network, acting together. It is possible that the brain region stimulated is not essential in the performance of a WM task such as the 3-back task. The optimal parameters of rTMS, however, that are required to produce a significant 'virtual lesion' are unclear and we highlight the importance of stimulus intensity and frequency, coil placement and pulse timing in any experiment. Our study also brings to focus the plasticity of the neocortex, permitting the brain to adapt quickly to changing cortical excitability. Further work is needed in this field to disentangle the various factors that underlie the performance on WM tasks, and thereby understand the functional neuroanatomy of WM.

References

Amassian, V.E., Maccabee, P.J., Cracco, R.Q., Cracco, J.B., Rudell, A.P. and Eberle, L. Measurement of information processing delays in human visual cortex with repetitve magnetic coil stimulation. *Brain Res.*, 1993, 602: 317–321.

Badagaiyan, R.D. Executive control, willed actions and nonconscious processing. *Hum. Brain Mapp.*, 2000, 9: 38–41.

Baddeley, A.D. *Working Memory* Clarendon Press, Oxford, 1986.

Baddeley, A.D. and Logie, R.H. Working memory: the multiple-component model. In: A. Miyake and P. Shah (Eds), *Models of Working Memory: Mechanisms of Active Maintenance and Executive Control.* Cambridge University Press, Cambridge, 1998: 28–61.

Braver, T.S. and Bongiolatti, S.R. The role of frontopolar cortex in subgoal processing during working memory. *Neuroimage*, 2002, 15: 523–536.

Braver, T.S., Cohen, J.D., Nystrom, L.E., Jonides, J., Smith, E.E. and Noll, D.C. A parametric study of prefrontal cortex involvement in human working memory. *Neuroimage*, 1997, 5: 49–62.

Cabeza, R., Dolcos, F., Graham, R. and Nyberg, L. Similarities and differences in the neural correlates of episodic memory retrieval and working memory. *Neuroimage*, 2002, 16: 317–330.

Carpenter, P.A., Just, M.A. and Reichle, E.D. Working memory and executive function: evidence from neuroimaging. *Curr. Opin. Neurobiol.*, 2000, 10: 195–199.

Chen, R., Classen, J., Gerloff, C., Celnik, P., Wasserman, E.M., Hallett, M. and Cohen, L.G. Depression of motor cortex excitability by low-frequency transcranial magnetic stimulation. *Neurology*, 1997, 48: 1398–1403.

Collette, F. and Van der Linden, M. Brain imaging of the central executive component of working memory. *Neurosci. Biobehav. Rev.*, 2002, 26: 105–125.

Courtney, S.M., Petit, L., Haxby, J.V. and Ungerleider, L.G. The role of prefrontal cortex in working memory: examining the contents of consciousness. *Philos. Trans. R. Soc. Lond. B. Biol. Sci.*, 1998, 353: 1819–1828.

Cowan, N. An embedded-processes model of working memory. In: P. Shah and A. Miyake (Eds.), *Models of Working Memory: Mechanisms of Active Maintenance and Executive Control.* Cambridge University Press, Cambridge, 1999: 62–102.

Day, B.L., Rothwell, J.C., Thompson, P.D., Maertens De Noordhout, A., Nakashima, K., Shannon, K. and Marsden, C.D. Delay in the execution of voluntary movement by electrical or magnetic brain stimulation in intact man. Evidence for the storage of motor programs in the brain. *Brain*, 1989, 112: 649–663.

D'Esposito, M., Aguirre, G.K., Zarahn, E., Ballard, D., Shin, R.K. and Lease, J. Functional MRI studies of spatial and nonspatial working memory. *Cog. Brain Res.*, 1998, 7: 1–13.

Fitzgerald, P.B., Brown, T.L., Daskalakis, Z.J., Chen, R. and Kulkarni, J. Intensity-dependent effects of 1 Hz rTMS on human corticospinal excitability. *Clin. Neurophysiol.*, 2002, 113: 1136–1141.

Garavan, H., Kelley, D., Rosen, A., Rao, S.M. and Stein, E.A. Practice-related functional activation changes in a working memory task. *Microsc. Res. Tech.*, 2000, 51: 54–63.

Gerschlager, W., Siebner, H.R. and Rothwell, J.C. Decreased corticospinal excitability after subthreshold 1Hz rTMS over lateral premotor cotex. *Neurology*, 2001, 57: 449–455.

Goldman-Rakic, P.S., Rosvold, H.E., Vest, B. and Galkin, T.W. Analysis of the delayed-alternation defecit produced by dorsolateral prefrontal lesions in the rhesus monkey. *J. Comp. Physiol. Psychol.*, 1971, 77: 212–220.

Hill, A.C., Davey, N.J. and Kennard, C. Current orientation induced by magnetic stimulation influences a cognitive task. *NeuroReport*, 2000, 11: 3257–3259.

Hong, K., Lee S.K., Kim, J., Kim, K. and Nam, H. Visual working memory revealed by repetitive transcranial magnetic stimulation. *J. Neurolog. Sci.*, 2000, 181: 50–55.

Ilmoniemi, R.J., Virtanen, J., Ruohonen, J., Karhu, J., Aronen, H.J., Naatanen, R. and Katila, T. Neuronal responses to magnetic stimulation reveal cortical reactivity and connectivity. *NeuroReport*, 1997, 8: 3537–3540.

Jahanshahi, M. and Rothwell, J. Transcranial magnetic stimulation studies of cognition: an emerging field. *Exp. Brain Res.*, 2000, 131: 1–9.

Jahanshahi, M., Profice, P., Brown, R.G., Ridding, M.C., Dirnberger, G. and Rothwell, J. The effects of transcranial magnetic stimulation over the dorsolateral prefrontal cortex on suppression of habitual counting during random number generation. *Brain*, 1998, 121: 1533–1544.

Kessels, R.P., D'Alfonso, A.A., Postma, A. and De Haan, E.H. Spatial working memory performance after high-frequency repetitive transcranial magnetic stimulation of the left and right posterior parietal cortex in humans. *Neurosci. Lett.*, 2000, 287: 68–70.

Levy, R. and Goldman-Rakic, P.S. Segregation of working memory within the dorsolateral prefrontal cortex. *Exp. Brain Res.*, 2000, 133: 23–32.

Maeda, F., Gangitano, M., Thall, M. and Pascual-Leone, A. Inter- and intra-individual variability of paired-pulse curves with transcranial magnetic stimulation (TMS). *Clin. Neurophysiol.*, 2002, 113: 376–382.

Marshuetz, C., Smith, E.E., Jonides, J., DeGutis, J. and Chenevert, T.L. Order information in working memory: fMRI evidence for parietal and prefrontal mechanisms. *J. Cogn. Neurosci.*, 2000, 12: 130–144.

Miranda, P.C., de Carvalho, M., Conceicao, T., Luis, M.C. and Ducla-Soares, E. A new method for reproducible coil positioning in transcranial magnetic stimulation mapping. *Electroenceph. Clin. Neurophysiol.*, 1997, 105: 116–123.

Mottaghy, F.M., Krause, B.J., Kemna, L.J., Topper, R., Tellmann, L., Beu, M., Pascual-Leone, A. and Muller-Gartner, H.W. Modulation of the neuronal circuitry subserving working memory in healthy human subjects by repetitive transcranial magnetic stimulation. *Neurosci. Lett.*, 2000, 280: 167–170.

Mottaghy, F.M., Gangitano, M., Sparing, R., Krause, B.J. and Pascual-Leone, A. Segregation of areas related to visual working memory in the prefrontal cortex revealed by rTMS. *Cereb. Cortex*, 2002, 12: 369–375.

Mottaghy, F.M., Pascual-Leone, A., Kemna, L.J., Topper, R., Herzog, H., Muller-Gartner, H.W. and Krause, B.J. Modulation of a brain-behavior relationship in verbal working memory by rTMS. *Cog. Brain Res.*, 2003, 15: 241–249.

Mull, B.R. and Seyal, M. Transcranial magnetic stimulation of left prefrontal cortex impairs working memory. *Clin. Neurophysiol.*, 2001, 112: 1672–1675.

Norman, D. and Shallice, T. Attention to action: willed and automatic control of behaviour. In: R.J. Davidson, G.E. Schwartz and D.E. Shapiro (Eds), *Consciousness and Self-Regulation: Advances in Research and Theory*, Vol. 4. Plenum, New York, 1986: 1–18.

Oliveri, M., Turriziani, P., Carlesimo, G.A., Koch, G., Tomaiuolo, F., Panella, M. and Caltagirone, C. Parieto-frontal interactions in visual-object and visual-spatial working memory: evidence from transcranial magnetic stimulation. *Cereb. Cortex*, 2001, 11: 606–618.

Owen, A.M. Cognitive planning in humans: neuropsychological, neuroanatomical and neuropharmacological perspectives. *Prog. Neurobiol.*, 1997, 53: 431–450.

Owen, A.M., Evans, A.C. and Petrides, M. Evidence for a two-stage model of spatial working memory processing within the lateral frontal cortex: a positron emission tomography study. *Cereb. Cortex*, 1996a, 6: 31–38.

Owen, A.M., Morris, R.G., Sahakian, B.J., Polkey, C.E. and Robbins, T.W. Double dissociations of memory and executive functions in working memory tasks following frontal lobe excisions, temporal lobe excisions or amygdalo-hippocampectomy in man. *Brain*, 1996b, 119: 1597–1615.

Owen, A.M., Herrod, N.J., Menon, D.K., Clark, J.C., Downey, S.P., Carpenter, T.A., Minhas, P.S., Turkheimer, F.E., Williams, E.J., Robbins, T.W., Sahakian, B.J., Petrides, M. and Pickard, J.D. Redefining the functional organization of working memory processes within human lateral prefrontal cortex. *Eur. J. Neurosci.*, 1999, 11: 567–574.

Pascual-Leone, A., Bartres-Faz, D. and Keenan, J.P. Transcranial magnetic stimulation: studying the brain-behaviour relationship by induction of 'virtual lesions'. *Philos. Trans. R. Soc. Lond. B. Biol. Sci.*, 1999, 354: 1229–1238.

Pascual-Leone, A., Walsh, V. and Rothwell, J. Transcranial magnetic stimulation in cognitive neuroscience – virtual lesion, chronometry, and functional connectivity. *Curr. Opin. Neurobiol.*, 2000, 10: 232–237.

Payne, B.R., Lomber, S.G., Villa, A.E. and Bullier, J. Reversible deactivation of cerebral network components. *Trends Neurosci.*, 1996, 19: 535–542.

Rabbitt, P. Introduction: Methodologies and models in the study of executive function. In: P. Rabbitt (Ed.), *Methodology of Frontal and Executive Function*. Psychology Press Ltd, East Sussex. 1999: 1–36.

Rao, S.G., Rainer, G. and Miller, E.K. Integration of the what and where in the primate prefrontal cortex. *Science*, 1997, 276: 821–824.

Smith, E.E. and Jonides, J. Storage and executive processes in the frontal lobes. *Science*, 1999, 283: 1657–1661.

Stern, C.E., Owen, A.M., Tracey, I., Look, R.B., Rosen, B.R. and Petrides, M. Activity in Ventrolateral and Mid-Dorsolateral Prefrontal Cortex during Nonspatial Visual Working Memory Processing: Evidence from Functional Magnetic Resonance Imaging. *Neuroimage*, 2000, 11: 392–399.

Walsh, V. and Rushworth, M. A primer of magnetic stimulation as a tool for neuropsychology. *Neuropsychologia*, 1999, 37: 125–135.

Walsh, V., Ashbridge, E. and Cowey, A. Cortical plasticity in perceptual learning demonstrated by transcranial magnetic stimulation. *Neuropsychologia*, 1998, 36: 363–367.

Transcranial Magnetic Stimulation and Transcranial Direct Current Stimulation (Supplements to Clinical Neurophysiology, Vol. 56)
Editors: W. Paulus, F. Tergau, M.A. Nitsche, J.C. Rothwell, U. Ziemann, M. Hallett

Chapter 19

Motor and phosphene thresholds: consequences of cortical anisotropy

Thomas Kammer[a,b,*], Sandra Beck[a], Klaas Puls[a], Claire Roether[a] and Axel Thielscher[c]

[a] *Department of Neurobiology, Max Planck Institute for Biological Cybernetics, Tübingen (Germany)*
[b] *Department of Neurology, University of Tübingen, Tübingen (Germany)*
[c] *Department Psychiatry III, University of Ulm, Ulm (Germany)*

1. Introduction

Excitability of cortical areas assessed by TMS depends on the induced current direction. This has been extensively demonstrated for the motor cortex. In case of monophasic pulses currents passing the precentral gyrus from back to front are more efficient than currents in the reverse direction (Brasil-Neto et al., 1992; Mills et al., 1992; Niehaus et al., 2000; Di Lazzaro et al., 2001; Kammer et al., 2001b). The optimal current orientation is perpendicular to the central sulcus (Brasil-Neto et al., 1992; Mills et al., 1992; Nithi and Mills, 2000). In recent years, it was found that other cortical areas also show this anisotropic response behavior when stimulated with TMS. In the visual system, early reports suggested a preferential current direction from lateral to medial, both in the induction of phosphenes (Meyer et al., 1991) and for the visual extinction effect (Amassian et al., 1994). Our group confirmed this anisotropy with the first phosphene threshold study systematically varying current directions (Kammer et al., 2001a). Lowest phosphene thresholds were obtained with latero-medial currents in both hemispheres, highest threshold with medio-lateral currents. Vertical oriented currents yielded threshold values between both extremes. For a third region, the prefrontal cortex, a current direction preference has been demonstrated using a behavioral task (Hill et al., 2000).

In the present study we directly compare the current direction effect of monophasic pulses on thresholds in the visual and motor system using two different stimulator types. With a frameless stereotactic positioning system, we further demonstrate a dependency of phosphene maps from the visual cortex on current direction.

2. Methods

Six healthy subjects (age 21 to 37 years, 4 males, 2 females) participated in the study after giving their written informed consent. The study was approved by the local internal review board of the Medical Faculty, University of Tübingen.

* *Correspondence to*: Dr. Thomas Kammer, Department of Neurology, University Hospital of Tübingen, Hoppe-Seyler-Str. 3, D-72076 Tübingen, Germany.
Tel: +49 7071 29 80469; Fax: +49 7071 29 5326;
E-mail: thomas.kammer@uni-tuebingen.de

Two stimulators were used: the Medtronic-Dantec Magpro (Skovlunde, Denmark) in the monophasic mode (maximal rate 0.33 Hz) and the Magstim 200 (Whitland, Dyfed, Wales, maximal rate 0.2 Hz). Both stimulators were fitted with their standard figure-of-8 coil. Coil position in relation to the head was monitored and registered continuously in all six degrees of freedom – three translational and three rotational – with a custom-made positioning system (Kammer et al., 2001b).

Data of phosphene thresholds presented here were taken from Kammer et al. (2001a), left hemisphere. They have been measured with the method of constant stimuli. Subjects had to report the presence or absence of a phosphene at stimulation with 10 different intensities (step size 2%) tested 10 times in a randomized order. Threshold was then calculated using a sigmoidal Boltzmann fit to the data. Three independent measurements with 100 stimuli each were averaged. For more details, *see* Kammer et al. (2001a).

Resting motor thresholds were measured in the right abductor pollicis brevis muscle as described in Kammer et al. (2001b). The threshold criterion was 50 μV peak-to-peak amplitude. Ten trials were performed at each stimulator intensity, varied in steps of 1%. Thresholds were calculated using a sigmoidal Boltzmann fit.

In order to compare threshold data from both stimulators, they were normalized with respect to $\sqrt{E_{max}}$, the maximal energy stored in the stimulator (cf. Barker et al., 1991; Kammer et al., 2001b). E_{max} of Medtronic-Dantec is 300 J, E_{max} of Magstim 200 is 720 J.

For phosphene mapping, subjects looked at a fixation point in the middle of the screen with a background intensity of 0.3 cd/m^2. They observed phosphenes induced by a single TMS pulse and drew the contours of the observed phosphene directly on the screen using a mechanical digitizing arm programmed as a drawing device. Traces of the drawing appeared as white lines on the screen. Subjects could freely release stimulation pulses in order to compare the drawings with the perceived phosphene and if necessary correct the drawing. Finally the drawing was saved on the computer together with the exact stimulation site of the coil as measured by the positioning system. The drawings were off-line classified according to the visual hemifield the phosphenes appeared in right (coded in red), left (blue) or bilateral (yellow). A 3D mesh of the cortical surface was obtained with the software BrainVoyager (Brain Innovation, Maastricht, The Netherlands) based on a segmentation of the white matter in a T1-weighted anatomical scan of the subject. Stored coil positions (midpoint of the figure-of-8 coil, peak electric field) were projected on the 3D mesh of the individual subject's cortical surface. They were colored according to the phosphene hemifield classification.

3. Results

Mean normalized threshold values from the left visual and motor cortex are shown in Fig. 1. They were subjected to a three-way analysis of variance (ANOVA) with factors of *threshold type* (phosphene vs. motor), *stimulator type* (Medtronic-Dantec vs. Magstim), and *current direction* (latero-medial vs. medio-lateral for phosphene threshold, antero-posterior vs. postero-anterior for motor threshold). Significant main effects of *stimulator type* ($F(1,5) = 144.6$; $p < 0.0001$) and *current direction* ($F(1,5) = 113.7$; $p < 0.0002$) were obtained. No significant difference was found for the factor *threshold type* ($F(1,5) = 1.54$; $p = 0.27$), as well as no significant interaction. Medtronic-Dantec was more efficient compared to Magstim. The ratio of Magstim/Medtronic-Dantec thresholds in the visual system was 1.26; in the motor system the ratio was 1.32. The mean threshold ratio for the different current directions was 1.19 in the visual system (medio-lateral/latero-medial) and 1.32 in the motor system (antero-posterior/postero-anterior).

Correlation of phosphene and motor thresholds for the individual subjects is depicted in Fig. 2 for each of the four measurement types (two stimulators, two current directions). Linear regressions revealed no systematic dependency of phosphene and motor thresholds in the individual subjects.

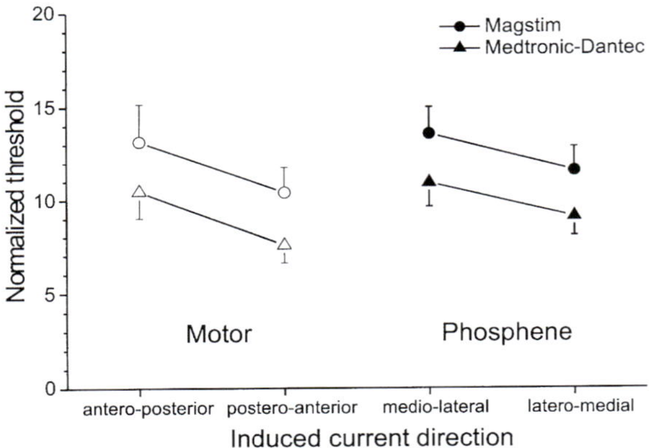

Fig. 1. Comparison of motor and phosphene thresholds (mean ± SD) measured in the left hemisphere in six subjects. Motor thresholds in the right abductor policis brevis muscle were measured with the coil over the left motor hot spot. The coil handle was oriented perpendicular to the central sulcus. Phosphene thresholds were measured over the left occipital pole with the coil handle oriented horizontally. Notice that thresholds were normalized with respect to the maximal energy stored in the stimulator. For ANOVA, see text.

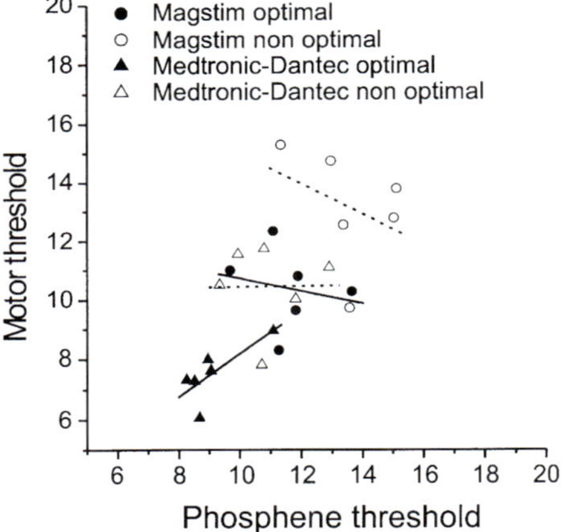

Fig. 2. Correlation of threshold values between motor and visual cortex. The normalized individual values of six subjects × four conditions are plotted. The two different stimulator types are coded as dots (Magstim) and triangles (Medtronic-Dantec). Induced current directions are indicated by filled (optimal direction, latero-medial or postero-anterior) and open (non optimal direction: medio-lateral or antero-posterior) symbols. Linear regression lines are solid (optimal direction) or stippled (non optimal direction). None of the linear regressions was statistically significant.

In Fig. 3 a map of perceived phosphenes in dependence of the coil position is shown. Horizontally oriented stimulation pulses at a constant stimulus intensity were applied at several sites of the occipital cortex. The pins indicate the midpoint of the coil inducing a certain phosphene coded by the color of the pin. At the lateral stimulation sites over one hemisphere the evoked phosphenes appeared in the contralateral visual hemifield (red or blue pins). More medial stimulation sites resulted in the perception of phosphenes in both visual hemifields (yellow pins) indicating the supra-threshold stimulation of both hemispheres. The borders between unilateral and bilateral stimulation depend on the induced current direction which is indicated by the arrows. They were not found in symmetry to the interhemispheric cleft but were shifted in the direction of the induced current. In the depicted example the amount of shift was 12 mm. The shift could be observed with both stimulators, Magstim 200 as well as Medtronic-Dantec in the monophasic mode. It was confirmed in four subjects investigated, ranging from 7–15 mm

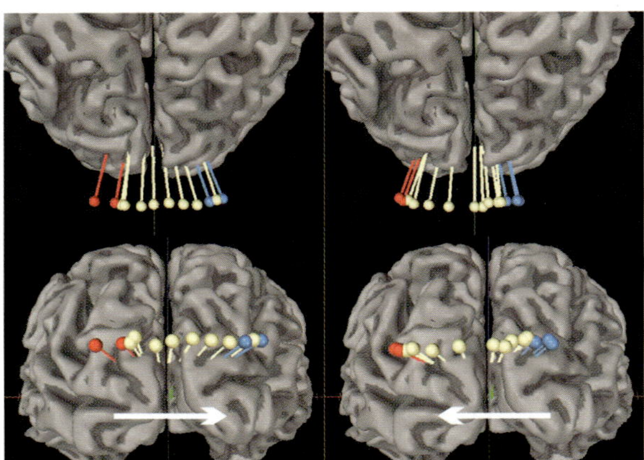

Fig. 3. Phosphene map in dependence of induced current direction. The upper and lower images are two different views on the occipital pole of subject KP, showing the same measurement. Coil positions (midpoint of the figure-of-8 coil) are depicted as colored pins. The color indicates the visual hemifield where the subject perceived a phosphene. Red: right hemifield, blue: left hemifield, yellow: both visual hemifields. The induced current direction is indicated by the large arrows. Stimulation parameters: Medtronic-Dantec, monophasic, 80% intensity.

(data not shown). It did neither depend on the stimulation strength nor on the horizontal position of the coil but could be observed within a large area over the occipital pole.

4. Discussion

Excitability of the visual cortex depends on current direction, similar to excitability of the motor cortex. In case of monophasic pulses in both hemispheres at the occipital pole latero-medial currents are more efficient compared to medio-lateral currents (Kammer et al., 2001a). The data presented here extend our previous results by direct comparison of phosphene thresholds and motor thresholds in the same subjects. The mean of motor thresholds in six subjects confirms the pattern reported in a previous study (Kammer et al., 2001b), i.e. lower thresholds for postero-anterior oriented currents compared to antero-posterior currents. Furthermore, normalization of threshold values with respect to the maximal stored energy (Barker et al., 1991; Kammer et al., 2001b) reveals that the Medtronic-Dantec stimulator transfers stimulation energy more efficient to the brain compared to the Magstim stimulator. The main reason for this difference is the coil geometry of the two figure-of-8 coils, as shown in a modeling approach (Thielscher, 2002). In case of Medtronic-Dantec the two circular windings are bent to each other forming an angle of 140°, whereas in case of Magstim the two windings are placed in a plane thus forming an angle of 180.

In our sample of six subjects we did not observe a significant correlation between motor and visual thresholds. This finding confirms previous observations (Stewart et al., 2001; Boroojerdi et al., 2002) that excitability of the two areas differ within a subject. However, we cannot exclude that these results are based on variations of the coil-cortex distance within a subject (Kozel et al., 2000; McConnell et al., 2001). Further studies combining careful threshold measurement and a model of field strength in dependence of the coil-cortex distance (Thielscher and Kammer, 2002) are required to clarify this important question.

Phosphene mapping revealed that stimulation sites evoking phosphenes bilaterally in the left and right visual field depend on the induced current direction. Under the assumption that the generator of an unilateral phosphene sits in the contralateral hemisphere bilateral phosphenes require a suprathreshold stimulation of both occipital lobes. The shift of the border from bilateral to unilateral stimulation can be directly explained as a consequence of threshold differences. The suprathreshold stimulation of the hemisphere stimulated in the preferred current direction still works with a coil position shifted over the non-preferred hemisphere. This explanation assumes, in addition, that the stimulus site under the coil depends on the electric field strength with its maximum at the midpoint of the coil (Amassian et al., 1992; Ilmoniemi et al., 1999), an assumption that has recently been proved for the motor cortex (Thielscher and Kammer, 2002).

Our data demonstrate that a preference in current direction does exist in the visual cortex, comparable to the motor cortex preference. It seems to be a general feature of cortical networks to have a preferred current direction since it has been demonstrated in prefrontal cortex, too (Hill et al., 2000). Studies in the motor system have demonstrated that a change in the current direction changes the response pattern of the cortical network (Day et al., 1989; Sakai et al., 1997; Di Lazzaro et al., 2001). It is still unclear whether different sites of the same population are stimulated or whether different cell populations respond with reversing current direction. Why do we find differences in the cortical responses in dependence of induced current orientation? Neurons are optimal stimulated with extracellular currents oriented in parallel to longitudinal structures, i.e. the axons of the cells (Rushton, 1927). The striking dependency on current orientation indicates an orientation preference of axons in the cortex. In an histological study of the human motor cortex, Marin-Padilla (1970) described a preferential orientation of dendritic and axonal fields of large basket cells perpendicular to the main axis of the central gyrus thus corresponding to the preferential current direction in TMS. However, using systematic sections alternatively parallel and perpendicular to the main axis of the human precentral gyrus, Meyer (1987) failed to confirm the preferential orientation perpendicular but rather found an orientation dominance in parallel to the main gyrus' axis. We are not aware of histological studies of other cortical areas revealing a general orientation preference in relation of the gyral architecture.

In order to explain threshold differences with polarity reversion of the currents the anatomical orientation preference has to be accomplished by a functional anisotropy implementing a diode-like rectifying response behavior. A hypothesis could be derived from the concept of virtual anodes surrounding a stimulating cathode (Rattay, 1987). It has been shown that certain geometric arrangements of electrodes lead to depolarization of axons with unidirectional propagation. (Ranck, 1975; Van den Honert and Mortimer, 1979; Ungar et al., 1986). It remains to be clarified whether the geometry of electromagnetically induced currents can mimic such a behavior.

Acknowledgements

We thank Kuno Kirschfeld, and Hans-Günther Nusseck for support and for many fruitful discussions. Michael Erb and Wolfgang Grodd provided us with anatomical MR scans of the subjects.

References

Amassian, V.E., Eberle, L., Maccabee, P.J. and Cracco, R.Q. Modelling magnetic coil excitation of human cerebral cortex with a peripheral nerve immersed in a brain-shaped volume conductor: the significance of fiber bending in excitation. *Electroenceph. Clin. Neurophysiol.*, 1992, 85: 291–301.

Amassian, V.E., Maccabee, P.J., Cracco, R.Q., Cracco, J.B., Somasundaram, M., Rothwell, J.C., Eberle, L., Henry, K. and Rudell, A.P. The polarity of the induced electric field influences magnetic coil inhibition of human visual cortex: implications for the site of excitation. *Electroenceph. Clin. Neurophysiol.*, 1994, 93: 21–26.

Barker, A.T., Garnham, C.W. and Freeston, I.L. Magnetic nerve stimulation: the effect of waveform on efficiency, determination of neural membrane time constants and the measurement of stimulator output. *Electroenceph. Clin. Neurophysiol.*, 1991, (Suppl.) 43: 227–237.

Boroojerdi, B., Meister, I.G., Foltys, H., Sparing, R., Cohen, L. G. and Töpper, R. Visual and motor cortex excitability: a transcranial magnetic stimulation study. *Clin. Neurophysiol.*, 2002, 113: 1501–1504.

Brasil-Neto, J.P., Cohen, L.G., Panizza, M., Nilsson, J., Roth, B.J. and Hallett, M. Optimal focal transcranial magnetic activation of the human motor cortex: effects of coil orientation, shape of induced current pulse, and stimulus intensity. *J. Clin. Neurophysiol.*, 1992, 9: 132–136.

Day, B.L., Dressler, D., Maertens de Noordhout, A., Marsden, C. D., Nakashima, K., Rothwell, J.C. and Thompson, P.D. Electric and magnetic stimulation of human motor cortex: surface EMG and single motor unit responses. *J. Physiol. (Lond.)*, 1989, 412: 449–473.

Di Lazzaro, V., Oliviero, A., Saturno, E., Pilato, F., Insola, A., Mazzone, P., Profice, P., Tonali, P. and Rothwell, J.C. The effect on corticospinal volleys of reversing the direction of current induced in the motor cortex by transcranial magnetic stimulation. *Exp. Brain Res.*, 2001, 138: 268–273.

Hill, A.C., Davey, N.J. and Kennard, C. Current orientation induced by magnetic stimulation influences a cognitive task. *Neuroreport*, 2000, 11: 3257–3259.

Ilmoniemi, R.J., Ruohonen, J. and Karhu, J. Transcranial magnetic stimulation – a new tool for functional imaging of the brain. *Crit. Rev. Biomed. Eng.*, 1999, 27: 241–284.

Kammer, T., Beck, S., Erb, M. and Grodd, W. The influence of current direction on phosphene thresholds evoked by transcranial magnetic stimulation. *Clin. Neurophysiol.*, 2001a, 112: 2015–2021.

Kammer, T., Beck, S., Thielscher, A., Laubis-Herrmann, U. and Topka, H. Motor thresholds in humans. A transcranial magnetic stimulation study comparing different pulseforms, current directions and stimulator types. *Clin. Neurophysiol.*, 2001b, 112: 250–258.

Kozel, F.A., Nahas, Z., deBrux, C., Molloy, M., Lorberbaum, J. P., Bohning, D., Risch, S.C. and George, M.S. How coil-cortex distance relates to age, motor threshold, and antidepressant response to repetitive transcranial magnetic stimulation. *J. Neuropsychiatry Clin. Neurosci.*, 2000, 12: 376–384.

Marin-Padilla, M. Prenatal and early postnatal ontogenesis of the human motor cortex: a Golgi study. II The basked-pyramidal system. Brain Res. 23, 185–191.

McConnell, K. A., Nahas, Z., Shastri, A., Lorberbaum, J. P., Kozel, F. A., Bohning, D. E. and George, M. S. (2001) The transcranial magnetic stimulation motor threshold depends on the distance from coil to underlying cortex: A replication in healthy adults comparing two methods of assessing the distance to cortex. *Biol. Psychiatry*, 1970, 49: 454–459.

Meyer, B.U., Diehl, R.R., Steinmetz, H., Britton, T.C. and Benecke, R. Magnetic stimuli applied over motor cortex and visual cortex: Influence of coil position and field polarity on motor responses, phosphenes, and eye movements. *Electroenceph. Clin. Neurophysiol.*, 1991, (Suppl.) 43: 121–134.

Meyer, G. Forms and Spatial Arrangement of Neurons in the Primary Motor Cortex of Man. *J. Comparative Neurology*, 1987, 262: 402–428.

Mills, K.R., Boniface, S.J. and Schubert, M. Magnetic brain stimulation with a double coil: the importance of coil orientation. *Electroenceph. Clin. Neurophysiol.*, 1992, 85, 17–21.

Niehaus, L., Meyer, B.U. and Weyh, T. Influence of pulse configuration and direction of coil current on excitatory effects of magnetic motor cortex and nerve stimulation. *Clin. Neurophysiol.*, 2000, 111: 75–80.

Nithi, K.A. and Mills, K.R. Mapping motor cortex projections to single motor units in humans with transcranial magnetic stimulation. *Muscle Nerve*, 2000, 23: 1542–1548.

Ranck, J.B. Which elements are excited in electrical stimulation of mammalian central nervous system: a review. *Brain Res.*, 1975, 98: 417–440.

Rattay, F. Ways to approximate current-distance relations for electrically stimulated fibers. *J. Theor. Biol.*, 1987, 125: 339–349.

Rushton, W.A.H. The effect upon the threshold for nervous excitation of the length of nerve exposed, and the angle between current and nerve. *J. Physiol.* (*Lond.*), 1927, 63: 357–377.

Sakai, K., Ugawa, Y., Terao, Y., Hanajima, R., Furubayashi, T. and Kanazawa, I. Preferential activation of different I wave by transcranial magnetic stimulation with a figure-of-eight-shaped coil. *Exp. Brain. Res.*, 1997, 113: 24–32.

Stewart, L.M., Walsh, V. and Rothwell, J.C. Motor and phosphene thresholds: a transcranial magnetic stimulation correlation study. *Neuropsychologia*, 2001, 39: 415–419.

Thielscher, A. Abschätzung zum Ort der Nervenstimulation durch Magnetfelder – Ein Beitrag zu den biophysikalischen Grundlagen der Transkraniellen Magnetstimulation. Dissertation, Abteilung Psychiatrie III, Universität Ulm, 2002.

Thielscher, A. and Kammer, T. Linking Physics with Physiology in TMS: A sphere field model to determine the cortical stimulation site in TMS. *Neuroimage*, 2002, 17: 1117–1130.

Ungar, I.J., Mortimer, J.T. and Sweeney, J.D. Generation of unidirectional propagating action potentials using a monopolar electrode cuff. *Ann. Biomed. Engineer.*, 1986, 14: 437–450.

Van den Honert, C. and Mortimer, J.T. Generation of unidirectionally propagated action potentials in a peripheral nerve by brief stimuli. *Science*, 1979, 206: 1311–1312.

Transcranial Magnetic Stimulation and Transcranial Direct Current Stimulation (Supplements to Clinical Neurophysiology, Vol. 56)
Editors: W. Paulus, F. Tergau, M.A. Nitsche, J.C. Rothwell, U. Ziemann, M. Hallett

Chapter 20

The organisation and re-organisation of human swallowing motor cortex

Shaheen Hamdy*

Clinical Sciences Building, Department of GI Sciences, Hope Hospital, Eccles Old Road, Salford M6 8HD (UK)

1. Overview

Swallowing problems can affect as many as one in three patients in the period immediately after a stroke. In some cases this can lead to serious morbidity, in particular malnutrition and pulmonary aspiration. Despite this, swallowing usually recovers to a safe level in the majority of patients within weeks. This propensity for recovery is likely to relate to how swallowing motor cortex is organised and then reorganised after cerebral injury. A better understanding of these processes may therefore help in developing therapeutic interventions that can drive plasticity and so encourage the recovery process. In this chapter, I will examine present knowledge about the cortical control of swallowing in man particularly from investigations with TMS, and explore what aspects of its organisation are important for compensating for recovery after damage. In addition, I will describe approaches, which may be useful in speeding up the process of recovery.

2. CNS control of swallowing

It is now well established that the cerebral cortex plays an important functional role in the regulation of swallowing (Martin and Sessle, 1993). While the reflexive component of swallowing depends on swallowing centres in the brainstem, the initiation of swallowing is a voluntary action that involves the integrity of motor areas of the cerebral cortex (Miller, 1982). In anaesthetised animals, electrical stimulation of either hemisphere can induce swallowing (Sumi, 1969). This might be interpreted as indicating that both hemispheres have an equal role in controlling the swallowing process (Martin and Sessle, 1993). Analogous neurosurgical studies of the motor cortex in humans (Penfield and Boldery, 1937; Woolsey et al., 1979) have usually been confined to one hemisphere, so that a direct comparison with animal data has not been possible. However, these human data show that the locus of cortical control of swallowing lies within and antero-caudal to the face area of primary motor cortex (Penfield and Boldery, 1937).

3. The problem of dysphagia after stroke

Injury to swallowing areas of motor cortex and/or their connections to the brainstem will usually result in problems with swallowing (dysphagia). The

* *Correspondence to*: Dr. Shaheen Hamdy, MD, Clinical Sciences Building, Department of GI Sciences, Hope Hospital, Eccles Old Road, Salford M6 8HD, UK.
Tel: +161-787-4414; Fax: +161-787-1495;
E-mail: shamdy@fs1.ho.man.ac.uk

commonest reason for dysphagia in the U.K. is now stroke (Gordon et al., 1987). Up to half of all stroke patients experience dysphagia, which is associated with the life threatening complications of pulmonary aspiration and malnutrition (Gordon et al., 1987; Barer, 1989). Dysphagia leads to increased length of stay in hospital, and greater demands on health service resources, estimated to be an extra £400 M per year in the U.K. (Smithard et al., 1996). Diagnosing dysphagia in stroke (and other neurological diseases) can be difficult, and therefore, requires a high level of clinical suspicion. The pattern of disordered swallowing in stroke is usually a combination of oral and pharyngeal abnormalities (Gordon et al., 1987), typically delayed swallowing reflex with pooling or stasis of residue, reduced pharyngeal peristalsis and weak tongue control, but occasionally oesophageal abnormalities may be apparent. Clinical suspicion of swallowing difficulty should be followed up by a thorough bedside swallowing assessment and where appropriate, videofluoroscopy. The bedside examination incorporates a number of clinical measures including assessment consisting of the patients' feeding status, posture, breathing and co-operation levels before examining the patients' oral musculature, oral reflexes, pharyngeal swallow and a trial feed with a 5–10 ml water bolus. While the bedside assessment is cheap, easy to perform and involves no radiation exposure, it does not give detailed information of the pharyngeal stage of swallowing, making it prone to missing significant aspiration, especially silent aspiration. By comparison, videofluoroscopy gives a detailed anatomical assessment of the pharyngeal swallow, but is expensive, involves radiation, and uses a non-physiological medium, i.e. barium, which may not give a true picture of the patients swallowing performance.

The management of dysphagia after stroke is therefore critical. With severe dysphagia the risk of aspiration is high, and the patient is therefore kept nil by mouth, with early commencement of parental fluids. With less severe dysphagia, based upon videofluoroscopic and bedside swallowing assessment outcomes, therapeutic interventions may be tried. These interventions often include changes in diet, posture and food placement adjustments, as well as methods for sensitising, or desensitising the oropharynx to alter the swallow reflex, although their efficacy is a matter of some controversy. At present there are no randomised controlled trials of these interventions to show proven efficacy in improving swallowing after stroke (Kerr et al., 1999), consequently patients require nasogastic tube or gastrostomy feeding until swallowing improves spontaneously (Finucane and Bynum, 1996).

4. Studies of dysphagia after stroke and cerebral injury

Despite inferential animal evidence for bilateral control, studies after brain damage tend to suggest that at least in man, one or other hemisphere may be dominant (Bastian, 1898; Tuch and Nielson, 1941; Meadows, 1973; Robbins and Levine, 1988; Daniels and Foundas, 1997). Indeed, one of the earliest observations of a unilateral cerebral lesion producing dysphagia was in 1898 when Bastian reported on the case of a man who had been admitted to hospital with a hemiplegia and aphasia, but who also had transient "difficulty in deglutition". Later necropsy revealed that apart from two limited lesions in the left hemisphere, the brain was healthy. More recently, Meadows (1973) reported on six cases of dysphagia. All of them had confirmed unilateral lesions of the cerebral cortex, five of which affected the right hemisphere. Since then a number of studies (Veis and Logemann, 1985; Robbins and Levine, 1988; Robbins et al., 1993; Kidd et al., 1995; Daniels and Foundas, 1997) have confirmed that perhaps 40% or more of patients with unilateral hemispheric stroke may have swallowing difficulties. There was an increased tendency for the pharynx to be involved if the damage was limited to the cortex, and was on the right hemisphere (Robbins and Levine, 1988).

5. The organisation of human swallowing motor cortex

The missing piece of data in these studies has been lack of information about the normal pattern of cortical projections to swallowing muscles in normal humans. Recently, the technique of transcranial magnetic stimulation (TMS) has been able to fill the gaps in our knowledge. This technique uses a very short, rapidly changing magnetic field to induce electric current in the brain beneath the stimulator (Barker et al., 1985; Rothwell, 1997). The site of stimulation is less well localised compared to an electrode applied directly to the surface of the brain, so that the effective area of stimulation is larger than that obtained in acute experiments on anaesthetised subjects or animals. However, the centre of the most effective site for stimulation is very similar to that seen during neurosurgery, being slightly anterior to the best points for obtaining responses in muscles of the hand or arm (Wassermann et al., 1992; Metman et al., 1993). One important difference between the techniques is that in previous work, the brain has been stimulated with a train of several hundred stimuli at a rate of 50–60 Hz. Such stimuli can induce a full swallowing cycle visible to the experimenter (Penfield and Boldery, 1937). However, because of the risk of inducing epileptic seizures in awake subjects, TMS studies usually employ only single shocks given several seconds apart. The consequence is that a full swallow is never evoked. Instead the response has to be monitored by recording the EMG of pharynx and oesophagus from an intraluminal catheter inserted into the oesophagus (Aziz et al, 1995; Hamdy et al, 1996). A single stimulus evokes a simple EMG potential that has a latency of about 8–10 ms, compatible with a fairly direct and rapidly conducting pathway from cortex via brainstem to the muscle. Mapping these projections demonstrates that the various swallowing muscles are arranged somatotopically, with the oral muscles (mylohyoid) lateral and the pharynx and oesophagus more medial. However, the most important finding from a large group of subjects (Hamdy et al., 1996) was that in the majority of individuals, the projection from one or other hemisphere tended to be larger than the other, i.e. asymmetric representation for swallowing between the two hemispheres, independent of handedness. It was also observed to be discordant in a pair of identical right-handed twins, suggesting little genetic contribution to its development.

6. The functional neuroanatomy of human swallowing

Whilst information gathered from TMS has helped delineate in greater detail the organisation of projections from motor cortex to swallowing muscles, this approach does not allow an assessment of cerebral activity associated with functional swallowing. The recent technological advances in functional imaging of human brain have revolutionised our understanding of how the cerebral cortex operates in processing sensory and motor information. In particular, positron emission tomography (PET) and functional magnetic resonance imaging (fMRI) have become established as useful methods for exploring the spatial localisation of changes in neuronal activity during tasks, within both cortical and subcortical structures. Both techniques have been applied to the study of human swallowing (Hamdy et al., 1999a, b; Zald and Pardo, 1999), and broadly speaking, the results have been similar. A number of brain regions with increased activation were detected with PET (Hamdy et al., 1999b). These loci included: right orbito-frontal cortex; left mesial premotor cortex and cingulate; right caudo-lateral sensorimotor cortex; left caudo-lateral sensorimotor cortex; right anterior insula; left temporopolar cortex merging with left amygdala; right temporopolar cortex; left medial cerebellum, which merged across the mid-line with the right medial cerebellum; and dorsal brainstem. Strongest activations were found to be in the sensorimotor cortices, insula and cerebellum. Therefore, swallowing recruits multiple cerebral regions, often in an asymmetric manner, particularly in the insula, which was predominantly on the right and in the cerebellum, being mainly on the left. These latter observations would be in keeping with the earlier observations with TMS, that motor cortex representation for swallowing musculature displays degrees of asymmetry.

7. Mechanisms of dysphagia after unilateral cerebral stroke

The results from patients with dysphagia also tend to confirm this idea of inter-hemispheric asymmetry in the cortical representation of swallowing. In a TMS study (Hamdy et al., 1997a) the projections from both hemispheres to the swallowing muscles were examined in a large series of pure unilateral stroke patients. Half of the patients had dysphagia, whereas the other half did not. The authors of this study reasoned that if there were a true asymmetry of swallowing representation in normal subjects, then perhaps dysphagia would occur if the damage had affected the side of the brain with the largest ("most dominant") projection. The results showed that although stimulation of the damaged hemisphere produced little or no response in either group of patients, stimulation of the undamaged hemisphere tended to evoke a much larger response in the non-dysphagic than in the dysphagic subjects. Thus, the size of the hemispheric projection to swallowing muscles may have determined the presence or absence of dysphagia.

8. Cortical re-organisation and swallowing recovery after stroke

Given sufficient time, many dysphagic stroke patients eventually recover their ability to swallow. However, the mechanism for this recovery, seen in as many as 90% of initially dysphagic stroke patients (Barer, 1989), has remained controversial. In a detailed study of stroke using TMS, both dysphagic and non-dysphagic patients were serially mapped over several months while swallowing recovered (Hamdy et al., 1998a). The findings of the study showed that the area of pharyngeal representation in the undamaged hemisphere increased markedly in patients who recovered, whilst there was no change in patients who had persistent dysphagia or in patients who were non-dysphagic. No changes were seen in the damaged hemisphere in any of the groups. These observations imply that over a period of weeks, the recovery of swallowing after stroke depends on compensatory re-organisation in the undamaged hemisphere. The situation appears to differ from that in the limb muscles where some TMS studies have indicated that limb recovery after hemiparesis is more likely to result from an increase in the activity of remaining viable cortex in the damaged hemisphere (Turton et al., 1996). In such cases, the scope for expansion of a normal connection from the undamaged part of the brain may be a limiting factor in recovery.

9. Driving re-organisation in human swallowing motor cortex

Given that the intact hemisphere plays an important role in the recovery of swallowing after stroke, then we are provided with an interesting opportunity for studying plasticity of an intact (normal) pathway. Indeed, it could be suggested that any future therapies aimed at enhancing swallowing recovery should be targeted towards manipulating re-organisation on the intact side. One potential candidate for such a therapy might be the manipulation of sensory input to the cortex. Sensory input from the gut not only has a major influence on the activity of brainstem swallowing centres, but also converges onto cortical sensory and motor areas (Miller, 1982). Furthermore, it has been shown that the excitability of the cortical projection to swallowing muscles can be influenced by stimulation of afferent fibres in the vagal and trigeminal nerves (Hamdy et al., 1997b). Single stimuli, used in those studies, had a very short lasting effect, but recent work has shown that prolonged electrical stimulation of the pharynx can induce changes in cortical excitability that outlast the stimulus by up to 30 min (Hamdy et al., 1998b).

In this study, at 10 min train of electrical stimuli was applied to the pharynx at a just perceived intensity using a pair of intra-luminal electrodes. Motor cortex projections to pharynx were measured before and after this conditioning input using TMS. The authors found that following the pharyngeal input, cortico-pharyngeal evoked responses were increased for 30 min after pharyngeal stimulation, without changes in brainstem reflexes, or in responses evoked to transcranial electrical stimulation. The implication was that short-term (sensory) stimuli could induce longer term changes in motor cortical excitability, providing evidence for a driven "cross-system" effect to increased input. More recent work has suggested that the direction of these changes in swallowing motor cortex is highly dependent on the stimulus frequency, intensity and duration used. Fraser et al. (2002), showed that whilst medium to low frequency stimulation (≤ 10 Hz) was excitatory, high frequency pharyngeal stimulation (> 10 Hz) resulted in long-lasting cortical inhibition and a reduction in the pharyngeal motor map. In addition, the stronger the stimulation the more pronounced the effect, however 20 min of stimulation appeared no better than 10 min.

9.1. Sensory-induced plasticity and changes in swallowing behaviour

Whilst evidence from the swallowing model appears to show a clear effect of sensory stimulation on motor cortex organisation, the critical question remains: can sensory induced plasticity alter function, as a prelude to formulating stimulation-therapies to promote functional recovery after injury? Fraser et al. (2002) used functional magnetic resonance imaging to demonstrate that those patterns of pharyngeal input associated with enhanced motor cortical excitability, could alter the recruitment pattern of cortical activations associated with the task of swallowing. The group was able to show that pharyngeal stimulation resulted in functionally stronger, bilateral, cortical (sensorimotor) activation in areas related to swallowing.

Despite this finding, there has been no direct demonstration in man that any form of plasticity inducing stimuli produces a measurable improvement in function after cerebral injury. Of relevance, however, the effects of pharyngeal stimulation on swallowing have been recently investigated in acute dysphagic stroke patients (Fraser et al., 2002). The application of 10 min of 5 Hz of pharyngeal electrical stimulation at 75% of that maximally tolerated by the patient was used. The stimulation resulted in a long-term (60 min) increase in swallowing cortico-bulbar excitability predominantly within the undamaged, but not the damaged hemisphere. Critically, this was strongly associated with an improvement in swallowing using videofluoroscopy, the standard marker of swallowing performance during the same time frame. The exciting implication from these results is that that sensory input to the human adult brain can be programmed to promote beneficial changes in plasticity that result in an improvement of function after cerebral injury. Whilst the more long-term (days to weeks) effects of this approach still need to be established, the observations hold great promise for future neuro-rehabilitative strategies.

9.2. Direct cortical stimulation and swallowing motor cortex plasticity

Given the possibility of inducing lasting cortical change and the premise that swallowing recovery from dysphagic stroke relates to cortical re-organisation in the unaffected hemisphere, we sort to evaluate repetitive TMS (rTMS) as a potential tool for influencing this process. We proceeded to examine the effects of limited trains of fast rate rTMS (5 Hz) on the dominant swallowing motor cortex. In assessing the "dose" of rTMS to be administered, we chose 5 Hz frequency since that was optimal for up-regulating cortical excitability following afferent stimulation.

Given the possible underlying mechanism of how rTMS might induce change in the motor cortex, we decided to look at changes in excitability as measured by TMS over a period of 2 h post intervention. In healthy individuals the effect of active 5 Hz rTMS to the dominant pharyngeal motor cortex was compared with a sham procedure, which utilised an anterior coil tilt. Active stimulation resulted in a significant increase in cortical excitability lasting for more than one-hour post stimulation. This effect was not noted in the sham. The magnitude of this effect is not as great as that produced by pharyngeal electrical stimulation which is probably related to the fact that the sensory projection provides a more directed input to motor cortex than rTMS at the scalp. Although the rTMS data is only available in healthy subjects there is sufficient promise to proceed to investigate the effect in dysphagic stroke patients. There may be a role for combining rTMS with sensory stimulation to optimise the "up-regulation" of the pharyngeal motor representation in dysphagic subjects.

10. Conclusions

The application of transcranial magnetic stimulation and other functional neuroimaging techniques to study the control of swallowing has provided unique information about how midline musculature is organised and reorganised within the motor cortex after stroke. The observations with sensory manipulation and direct cortical stimulation give new insights both for the mechanisms of plasticity within cortical swallowing circuitry and for potential therapies for rehabilitation. These studies contribute new understanding our knowledge of the neurophysiology of human swallowing both in health and disease.

References

Aziz, Q., Rothwell, J.C., Barlow, J. and Thompson D.G. Modulation of esophageal responses to magnetic stimulation of the human brain by swallowing and by vagal stimulation. *Gastroenterology*, 1995, 109: 1437–1445.

Barer, D.H. The natural history and functional consequences of dysphagia after hemispheric stroke. *J. Neurol. Neurosurg. Psychiatry*, 1989, 52: 236–224.

Barker, A.T., Jalinous, R. and Freestone, I.L. Non-invasive magnetic stimulation of the human motor cortex. *Lancet*, 1985, 1: 1106–1107.

Bastian, H.C. A treatise on aphasia and other speech defects, Lewis, London, 1898.

Daniels, S.K. and Foundas, A.L. The role of the insular cortex in dysphagia. *Dysphagia*, 1997, 12: 146–156.

Finucane, T.E. and Bynum, J.P.W. Use of tube feeding to prevent aspiration pneumonia. *Lancet*, 1996, 348: 1421–1424.

Fraser, C., Power, M., Hamdy, S., Rothwell, J., Hobday, D., Hollander, I., Tyrell, P., Hobson, A., Williams, S. and Thompson, D. Driving plasticity in human adult motor cortex is associated with improved motor function after brain injury. *Neuron*, 2002, 34(5): 831–840.

Gordon, C., Langton Hewer, R. and Wade, D.T. Dysphagia in acute stroke. *Br. Med. J.*, 1987, 295: 411–414.

Hamdy, S., Aziz, Q., Rothwell, J.C., Singh, K., Barlow, J., Hughes, D., Tallis, R.C. and Thompson, D.G. The cortical topography of human swallowing musculature in health and disease. *Nat. Med.*, 1996, 2(11): 1217–1224.

Hamdy, S., Aziz, Q., Rothwell, J.C., Crone, R., Hughes, D.G, Tallis, R.C. and Thompson, D.G. Explaining oropharyngeal dysphagia after unilateral hemispheric stroke. *Lancet*, 1997a, 350: 686–692.

Hamdy, S., Aziz, Q., Rothwell, J.C., Hobson, A., Barlow, J. and Thompson, D.G. Cranial nerve modulation of human cortical swallowing motor pathways. *Am. J. Physiol.*, 1997b, 272: G802–808.

Hamdy, S., Aziz, Q., Rothwell, J.C., Power, M., Singh, K., Nicholson, D.A., Tallis, R.C. and Thompson, D.G. Recovery of swallowing after dysphagic stroke relates to functional reorganisation in intact motor cortex. *Gastroenterology*, 1998a, 115: 1104–1112.

Hamdy, S., Rothwell, J. C., Aziz, Q., Singh, K.D. and Thompson, D.G. Long-term reorganisation of human motor cortex driven by short-term sensory stimulation. *Nat. Neurosci.*, 1998b, 1(1): 64–68.

Hamdy, S., Mikulis, D.J, Crawley, A., Xue, S., Lau, H., Henry, S. and Diamant N.E. Cortical activation during human volitional swallowing: an event related fMRI study. *Am. J. Physiol.*, 1999a, 277: G219–G225.

Hamdy, S., Rothwell, J.C., Brooks, D.J., Bailey, D.L., Aziz, Q. and Thompson, D.G. Identification of the cerebral loci processing human swallowing with H2O15 PET activation. *J. Neurophysiol.*, 1999b, 81: 1917–1926.

Kerr, J.E., Bath, M.J. and Bath, P.M.W. Interventions for dysphagia in acute stroke (protocols). In Cochrane Library, Update Software, Oxford, 1999.

Kidd, D., Lawson, J., Nesbitt, R. and MacMahon, J. The natural history and clinical consequences of aspiration in acute stroke. *Q. J. Med.*, 1995, 88: 409–413.

Martin, R.E. and Sessle, B.J. The role of the cerebral cortex in swallowing. *Dysphagia*, 1993, 8: 195–202.

Meadows, J. Dysphagia in unilateral cerebral lesions. *J. Neurol. Neurosurg. Psychiatry*, 1973, 36: 853–860.

Metman, L.V., Bellevich, J.S., Jones, S.M., Barber, M.D. and Streletz, L.J. Topographic mapping of human motor cortex with transcranial magnetic stimulation: Homunculus revisited. *Brain Topogr.*, 1993, 6: 13–19.

Miller, A.J. Deglutition. *Physiol. Rev.*, 1982, 62: 129–184.

Penfield, W. and Boldery, E. Somatic motor and sensory representation in the cerebral cortex of man as studied by electrical stimulation. *Brain*, 1937, 60: 389–443.

Robbins, J. and Levine, R.L. Swallowing after unilateral stroke of the cerebral cortex: preliminary experience. *Dysphagia*, 1988, 3: 11–14.

Robbins, J., Levine, R.L., Maser, A., Rosenbek, J.C. and Kempster, G.B. Swallowing after unilateral stroke of the cerebral cortex. *Arch. Phys. Med. Rehabil.*, 1993, 74: 1295–1300.

Rothwell, J.C. Techniques and mechanisms of action of transcranial stimulation of the human motor cortex. *J. Neurosci. Methods*, 1997, 74: 113–122.

Smithard, D.G., O'Neill, P.A., Park, C., Morris, J., Wyatt, R., England, R. and Martin, D.F. Complication and outcome after acute stroke. Does dysphagia matter? *Stroke*, 1996, 27: 1200–(1204).

Sumi, T. Some properties of cortically evoked swallowing in rabbits. *Brain Res.*, 1969, 15: 107–120.

Tuch, B.E. and Nielson, J.M. Apraxia of swallowing. *Bull. LA Neurol. Seminar*, 1941, 6: 52–54.

Turton, A., Wroe, S., Trepte, N., Fraser, C. and Lemon, R.N. Contralateral and ipsilateral EMG responses to transcranial magnetic stimulation during recovery of arm and hand function after stroke. *Electroenceph. Clin. Neurophysiol.*, 1996, 101(4): 316–328.

Veis, S.L. and Logemann, J.A. Swallowing disorders in persons with cerebrovascular accident. *Arch. Phys. Med. Rehabil.*, 1985, 66: 372–375.

Wassermann, E.M., McShane, L.M., Hallet, M. and Cohen, L.G. Non-invasive mapping of muscle representation in the human motor cortex. *Electroenceph. Clin. Neurophysiol.*, 1992, 85: 1–8.

Woolsey, C.N., Erikson, T.C. and Gilson, W.E. Localization in somatic sensory and motor areas of human cerebral cortex as determined by direct recording of evoked potentials and electrical stimulation. *J. Neursurg.*, 1979, 51: 476–506.

Zald, D.H., and Pardo, J.V. The functional neuroanatomy of voluntary swallowing. *Ann. Neurol.*, 1999, 46: 281–286.

Transcranial Magnetic Stimulation and Transcranial Direct Current Stimulation (Supplements to Clinical Neurophysiology, Vol. 56)
Editors: W. Paulus, F. Tergau, M.A. Nitsche, J.C. Rothwell, U. Ziemann, M. Hallett

Chapter 21

Exploring paradoxical functional facilitation with TMS

Hugo Théoret, Masahito Kobayashi, Antoni Valero-Cabré and Alvaro Pascual-Leone*

Laboratory for Magnetic Brain Stimulation, Beth Israel Deaconess Medical Center, Harvard Medical School, 330 Brookline Avenue, Boston, MA 02215 (USA)

1. Introduction

Current theories about the representation of function in the brain are increasingly dominated by the notion of distributed neural networks, a series of assemblies of neurons that might be widely dispersed anatomically but are structurally interconnected and can be functionally integrated to serve a specific behavioral role (Mesulam, 1990, 2000). Certain distributed networks subserving specific functional domains can be identified. For example, spatial attention appears to be supported by the parietal lobes connected by callosal fibers and via the inferior colliculus, the prefrontal cortex (particularly on the right) and cingulate gyrus, along with connections via the superior occipito-frontal fasciculus and the cingulum. Another common example is language, subserved by Broca's and Wernicke's areas in the dominant hemisphere and connections along the arcuate fasciculus and the extreme capsule. However, it is important to recognize that depending on behavioral demands, neuronal assemblies can be integrated into *different* functional networks by shifts in weighting of connections (functional and effective connectivity). Indeed, *timing* of interactions between elements of a network, beyond integrity of structural connections, might be a critical binding principle for the functional establishment of given network action and behavioral output (Engel and Singer, 2001). Such notions of dedicated, but multifocal, networks, which can dynamically shift depending on demands for a given behavioral output, provide a current resolution to the long-standing dispute between localizionists and equipotential theorists. Function comes to be identified with a certain pattern of activation of specific, spatially distributed but interconnected neuronal assemblies in a specific time window and temporal order. In such distributed networks, specific nodes may be critical for a given behavioral outcome. Knowledge of such instances is clinically useful to explain findings in patients and localize their lesions, but provides an oversimplified conceptualization of brain–behavior relations. We may be better served realizing that behavior is never the result of the lesion, but rather the consequence of how the rest of the brain is capable of sustaining

* *Correspondence to*: Dr. Alvaro Pascual-Leone, Department of Neurology, Beth Israel Deaconess Medical Center, 330 Brookline Avenue, KS-454, Boston, MA 02215, USA
Tel: 617-667-0203; Fax: 617-975-5322;
E-mail: apleone@bidmc.harvard.edu

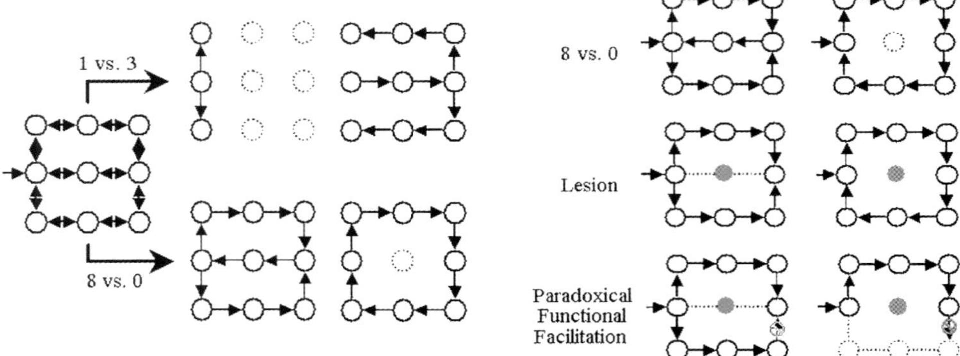

Fig. 1. Schematic representation of the hypothesized effects of a lesion in a distributed network. After the first lesion state, 0 and 8 are no longer distinguishable because they share the same activational pattern caused by the the modified spread of activation due to the lesion, whereas the second leasion re-establishes different activation patterns, and only the difference, not the exact pattern itself, is important for the distinction of the states.

function following a given lesion. This provides a conceptual framework to explain instances of paradoxical functional facilitation (Kapur, 1996), when a second lesion can restore behavioral integrity (e.g. Villeumier et al., 1996).

Imagine, for example, a distributed neural network made up of nine assemblies of neurons (nodes) and their connections (Fig. 1). A given behavior might be to differentiate between a state '1' and a state '3'. A different behavior, supported by some of the same neuronal assemblies but engaged into a different network might be to differentiate '0' from '8'. In the later case, a lesion to one, and only one neuronal assembly will cause a failure of the behavior and we might be tempted to conclude that '8' is localized in that one node, a conclusion that would certainly be incorrect despite the reality of the behavioral impact of the focal, single 'lesion'. In this dysfunctional state, a second 'lesion' may restore the ability to differentiate '0' from '8', hence paradoxically restoring function, even though the new expression of '0' and '8' may well be different.

In this chapter, we wish to first briefly describe experiments conducted in cats to underscore the local and distant effects exerted by repetitive TMS. The better understanding of the modulatory effects of rTMS can then lead to the experimental testing of specific hypotheses relating to the paradoxical effects of TMS-induced 'virtual lesions'. We will then describe studies on attention and motor performance that highlight the potential of TMS as a tool to reveal functional facilitations and ultimately offer the possibility to use such an approach for therapeutic purposes. Kapur had predicted this potential of TMS for the systematic exploration and therapeutic utilization of paradoxical facilitations in the human brain (Kapur, 1996; Ovsiew, 1997). We believe that we are now at a stage where such work ought to be conducted.

2. Repetitive stimulation and the creation of 'virtual lesions': animal evidence

Transcranial magnetic stimulation (TMS) provides a means of interfering with the activity in a specific cortical area and probing the functional changes that may result. The effects can be transient or extend beyond the duration of a train of stimuli, depending on the parameters of stimulation. Applied as trains of repetitive stimuli at appropriate frequency and intensity, TMS can be used to transiently disrupt the function of a given cortical target thus creating a temporary, "virtual brain lesion" (Pascual-Leone et al., 1999). The use of repetitive TMS (rTMS) to disrupt brain function stems from studies of the motor cortex, where it has been shown that applied to the primary motor area, a train of TMS pulses at a frequency of 1 Hz induces a transient reduction of cortical excitability in most subjects that outlasts the stimulation itself (Chen et al., 1997; Maeda et al., 2000). The notion that cortical excitability can be reduced in the motor cortex following low-frequency rTMS suggested that it could also modulate behavioral output when applied to non-motor areas. This idea was first applied to the visual cortex, where it was shown that a 1 Hz, 10 min rTMS train to the occipital pole could impair performance in a visual perception and imagery task (Kosslyn et al., 1999). This rationale has since then been applied to a variety of cortical areas, including parietal (Hilgetag et al., 2001; Lewald et al., 2002; Sack et al., 2002; Brighina et al., 2003), somatosensory (Satow et al., 2003), visual (Thut et al., 2003) and prefrontal (Mottaghy et al., 2001; Robertson et al., 2001; Shapiro et al., 2002) cortices, as well as to the cerebellum (Théoret et al., 2001).

This approach, which is devoid of the usual caveats associated with lesion studies (size of lesion, general cognitive impairments, plastic brain reorganization, etc.) (Robertson et al., in press) should also allow the investigation of paradoxical functional facilitations. However, regardless of the frequent and extensive use of rTMS for the study of cognitive functions in the human cortex, not much is yet known about its effects on networks of neural cells active during the development of a cognitive task. Animal studies should be used to answer questions that cannot be easily addressed in human subjects because of methodological or safety limitations.

Confirming that certain regions of the animal brain, such as the motor cortex, respond in a similar way as the human when targeted with (r)TMS is a critical first step to validate the model. The development of such an animal model is not a straightforward project. Four important aspects need to be taken into account to be able to generate information that can be extrapolated from animals to humans. First, the ratio of the size of the TMS coil over the size of the head and brain of the animal needs to allow specific stimulation of areas with differential contributions to a task. This question poses technical limitations since smaller coils have less penetration power and may thus activate the brain differently. Second, the animal species chosen should be able to be kept and manipulated in relatively large numbers in order to control for the impact of interindividual variability of the TMS effects. Animals have to tolerate single and repetitive TMS at low and high frequencies in an awake state or, if anesthesia is needed, at anesthesia levels that do not significantly interfere with the cortical function of the area of interest. Training to get the animal accustomed to the TMS at different intensities and frequencies is needed to avoid confounding aspects such as stress, particularly when dealing with cognitive functions. Third, it has to be possible to record the effect of TMS by means of neurohistological, electrophysiological (motor evoked potentials, evoked neuronal field potentials) and imaging techniques (2-deoxyglucose (2-DG) uptake, optical imaging intrinsic signal). Ideally, it should be possible to induce similar behavioral disruptions as those shown in equivalent tasks in humans so as to be able to establish a detailed correlate between behavioral and neurobiological effects. Finally, an extensive knowledge of the anatomy and function of cortical and subcortical networks involved in a task in that particular animal species is fundamental in order to interpret the impact of TMS. Obviously, previous anatomical, functional and behavioral data of the metabolic and behavioral impact of the same areas by irreversible (lesions) or reversible (pharmacological studies, cooling probes) deactivation techniques will help enormously in the interpretation of TMS results.

We have developed an animal model that meets these criteria and allows the study of TMS-induced behavioral, metabolic, and electrophysiological disruption in an awake preparation (Valero-Cabré et al., 2002). Motor evoked potentials (MEPs) can be easily and consistently recorded after TMS of the primary motor cortex (Fig. 2a). The MEPs have amplitudes and latencies consistent with those observed in humans (Figs. 2c, 2d). Moreover, low frequency rTMS but not sham stimulation of the

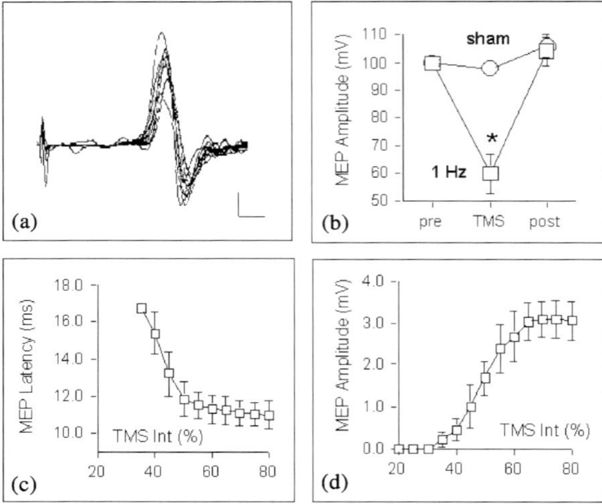

Fig. 2. (a) Overlapped motor evoked potentials recorded in the right flexor radialis muscle of the awake cat by consecutive TMS pulses delivered in the left primary motor cortex. Horizontal bar: 3 ms, vertical bar: 1 mV. (b) Average modulation of the MEP amplitude in three awake cats prior (pre), immediately after (TMS) and 20 min after (post) two conditions: 1 Hz stimulation during 15 min (900 pulses) or sham stimulation at identical parameters, both over the left primary motor cortex; * $p < 0.05$ vs. pre- and post-MEP amplitudes. (c) Changes in onset latency of the MEP at increasing levels of intensity of stimulation (% vs. maximal TMS machine output). (d) Recruitment of MEP amplitudes at increasing levels of TMS intensity.

primary motor cortex is able to inhibit contralateral MEP responses (Fig. 2b), much as is the case in humans (Chen et al., 1997; Maeda et al., 2000). Neuroimaging data in humans, using PET or fMRI, are limited by methodological constraints and artifacts that affect the detailed spatial and temporal resolution of the TMS impact. Overcoming these limitations, the feline model has been used successfully to examine the metabolic impact of on-line rTMS. Valero-Cabré et al. (2002) stimulated two cats with real 20 Hz rTMS and one cat with sham rTMS for 28 min in the visuo-parietal (VP) cortex area implicated in visual attention. We found a decrease in the uptake of ^{14}C-radiolabeled glucose in the targeted cortical area (Fig. 3a) compared to analogous structures in the contralateral hemisphere. Moreover, a transsynaptic deactivation of several targets receiving strong afferent connections and located far away from the reach of the direct effect of the magnetic field was found in the superior colliculus (SC) (Fig. 3b) and the splenial visual area (SVA) (Fig. 3c). It is worth mentioning that the direct impact on cortical areas was significantly greater than the transsynaptic impact and that the transsynaptic effect was highly specific along known anatomical connections, proportional in its magnitude with the strength of those connections, and in all cases led to a suppression of activity in the distant structures. Control structures with less or no connections to the directly stimulated area VP, such as the inferior colliculus (IC), medial geniculate (MGN) and lateral geniculate (LGN) nuclei showed no change in the 2-DG uptake (Fig. 3d). These results, match cooling deactivation experiments of the same areas in the cat (Vanduffel et al., 1997), and demonstrate a remarkably precise spatial resolution of TMS. Furthemore, in agreement with the function attributed to the VP area in cooling deactivation experiments, slow frequency stimulation (1 Hz) for 15 min in the awake cat induces a reversible neglect in the contralateral visual field, in agreement with studies in normal humans (Hilgetag et al., 2001) (Fig. 3e).

3. Dirsupting the brain with TMS to improve behavior

3.1. Attention

Brain plasticity following a brain lesion may not lead to recovery but rather provide the substrate for deficits to become chronically established. In such instances, focal disruption of brain activity may lead to behavioral improvement. For example, some patients with unilateral right brain damage suffer from extinction, a condition in which stimuli delivered to the contralesional side are not perceived when a simultaneous ipsilesional stimulus is presented (Vallar, 1998). It has been hypothesized that this phenomenon of "extinction to double simultaneous stimulation" and "neglect" is related to an imbalance between the hemispheres resulting from the release

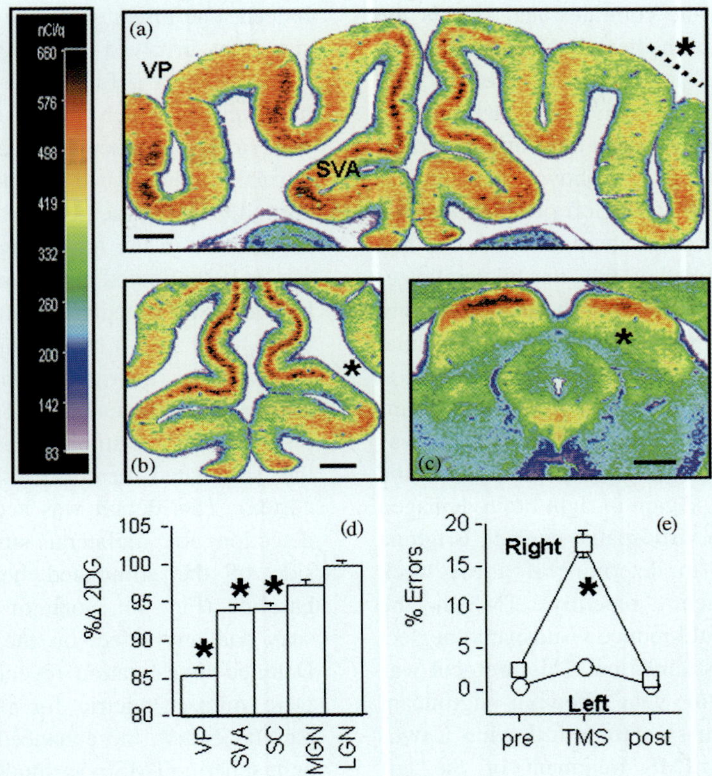

Fig. 3. (a) ^{14}C-2-deoxyglucose (^{14}C-2-DG) autoradiography from a cat brain submitted to 20 Hz rTMS of the left visuo-parietal cortex (*). Note differences between the stimulated (left *) and the non-stimulated (right) hemisphere. (b) Detail of the transynaptical impact of rTMS on the left splenial visual area (SVA) (*). (c) Detail of the rTMS effect on the left superior colliculus (SC) (*). (d) Average percentage of change with respect to the analogous area in the contralateral hemisphere of the ^{14}C-2-DG levels in visuo-parietal cortex (VP), splenial visual area (SVA), superior colliculus (SC), medial geniculate (MGN) and lateral geniculate (LGN) nuclei. * $p < 0.01$ vs. contralateral hemisphere. (e) Number of errors in the detection of visual stimuli presented randomly to the right and left visual hemifields before (pre), during the 15 min following 1 Hz rTMS stimulation at 40% on the VP cortex (TMS) and 60 min after the end of the stimulation. Note the increase in the number of mistakes in detecting visual stimuli in the right but not the left visual hemifield. (*) stimulated hemisphere. Scales bars = 2 mm.

of reciprocal inhibitory influences (Kinsbourne, 1977). Lesion of one hemisphere results in trans-hemispheric release of inhibition onto the healthy hemisphere that becomes "hyperactive", creating "hyper-attention" to the ipsilesional side. In humans, support for this hypothesis first came from the report of a patient who suffered from severe spatial neglect (the failure to explore contralesional space) following a right parietal lesion (Vuilleumier et al., 1996). Following a second lesion to the left frontal cortex, the neglect symptoms completely and abruptly disappeared, lending creedence to the notion of a dynamic balance between the two hemispheres for the allocation of attentional resources. Animal studies by Sprague and later Payne and Lomber (Sprague, 1966; Payne et al., 1996) have provided critical insights into the underlying physiology.

Oliveri et al. (1999) took advantage of the non-invasive nature of single pulse TMS to re-visit the famous case described by Vuilleumier et al. (1996).

If failure to orient to the contralesional side is the result of hyperactivity of the healthy hemisphere, then transient disruption of left cortical areas in right parietal-damaged patients may also temporarily alleviate extinction symptoms. In a group of 14 right brain-damaged patients, it was shown that application of single-pulse TMS to the left prefrontal cortex significantly reduced contralateral extinction when the TMS pulse was applied 40 ms after bilateral electrical stimulation of the fingers. These results were later replicated by the same group in a visuospatial task using high-frequency repetitive TMS (Oliveri et al., 2001). The performance of five right brain-damaged patients in a line bisection task was significantly improved following parietal rTMS of the unaffected hemisphere. Again in right brain-damaged patients suffering from visuospatial neglect, Brighina et al. (2003) set out to determine if a two-week regimen of low-frequency repetitive TMS to the healthy hemisphere could reduce visuospatial neglect beyond the period of stimulation. This protocol was based on experimental data showing significant reduction of depressive symptoms following a two-week low-frequency rTMS treatment of the left prefrontal cortex in medication resistant depressed individuals (see Wassermann and Lisanby, 2001). One Hz rTMS was applied to the left parietal cortex in three patients with a right parieto-temporal lesion every other day for 14 days. Visuospatial performance (clock drawing and line bisection tasks) was significantly improved immediately after treatment and for at least 15 days. The authors interpreted these results as additional evidence for the idea that hyperexcitability of the unlesioned hemisphere may underlie neglect syndromes and that inhibition of these overactive areas, whether transiently with single-pulse TMS, for a few days with repetitive TMS or permanently with a second lesion, may restore function.

The concept of reciprocal inter-hemispheric inhibition and its link to attentional performance was further investigated with rTMS in normal subjects (Hilgetag et al., 2001). Here, it was hypothesized that visual spatial attention could be improved following transient cortical impairment in healthy subjects. Indeed, one might speculate that the disinhibition of structures involved in inter-hemispheric competition might lead to a functional release in the opposite hemisphere, which could result in a measurable behavioral enhancement. To verify this hypothesis, normal subjects had to detect small rectangular stimuli briefly presented on a computer monitor either unilaterally in the left or right periphery, or bilaterally in both. Spatial detection performance was tested before and immediately after a ten minute, 1 Hz rTMS train to: (a) right parietal cortex; (b) left parietal cortex; (c) right primary motor cortex; and (d) sham stimulation. We observed a clear extinction phenomenon for stimuli presented contralaterally to the stimulated hemisphere (right or left parietal cortex). This deficit was accompanied by increased detection for unilateral stimuli presented on the side of the stimulated hemisphere compared to baseline (Fig. 4). None of the control stimulation sites had any effect on the detection performance. Detailed investigation revealed that although trends were mirror-symetric for rTMS of left and right parietal cortex, the enhancement produced by right-hemispheric rTMS was significantly greater than that after left hemisphere and only right hemispheric stimulation produced a significant ipsilateral detection enhancement. These data suggest that in normal subjects, decreasing left parietal cortex excitability with rTMS disinhibits the contralateral cortex leading to improvements in performance.

3.2. *Motor performance*

The paradoxical effects of rTMS-induced 'virtual lesions' are not limited to studies of attention. For example, we have recently showed a motor cortex effect similar to that observed in parietal areas. Patients with strokes involving the primary motor cortex (M1) often display increased excitability of the contralateral M1 and intracortical inhibition is generally suppressed, presumably through impaired transcallosal inhibition (Traversa et al., 1997; Shimuzu et al., 2002). Single-pulse TMS studies have revealed mainly inhibitory interactions between both primary motor cortices (Ferbert et al., 1992; Gerloff

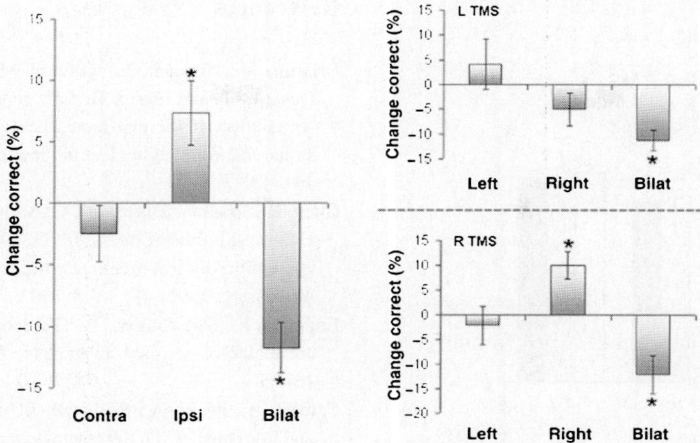

Fig. 4. Modified from Hilgetag et al. (2001) with permission. Changes in correct stimulus detection after parietal rTMS. The diagrams are based on changes in the number of correctly detected stimuli (relative to the total number of presented stimuli) averaged for both stimulus sizes and all subjects. (a) The pooled data show a significant increase in performance ipsilateral to the parietal rTMS location (increase in relative percentage points: 7.3% SEM: 2.6%), and a trend to decreased contralateral performance (reduction by 2.5%, SEM: 2.3%). In addition, detection of bilateral stimuli decreased significantly (–11.7%, SEM: 2.0%). These trends are also apparent after separating data for (b) left parietal TMS and (c) right parietal rTMS. Significant trends (as determined by z-tests, are marked by stars.

et al., 1998) and we thus hypothesized that low-frequency rTMS over M1 might lead to the disinhibition of the contralateral M1, and the subsequent improvement in motor performance. Indeed, it was shown that following 10 mins of 1 Hz rTMS, execution times in a well-learned key-pressing task were significantly shortened for the hand ipsilateral to the magnetic stimulation compared to baseline performance (Fig. 5a). Performance in the contralateral hand remained unchanged and we observed increased intracortical excitability in the un-stimulated M1 (Fig. 5b). It does appear that a phenomenon of interhemispheric rivalry, as postulated for attentional processes, is also at play between motor cortices, whereby suppression of the excitability of one motor cortex can enhance motor performance with the ipsilateral hand through, presumably, suppression of transcallosal inhibition.

4. Conclusion

Taken together, these results underscore the potential of TMS as a tool to probe the paradoxical functional facilitations that may occur following lesions to a particular node of a complex and distributed neural network. Work in cats has shown the robust metabolic effects of rTMS on local and distant cortical and subcortical sites. This has important implications for the study of paradoxical functional facilitations in human subjects since improvements in performance following a cortical lesion are often believed to result from plastic changes occuring in parts of a distributed network functionally related to the lesioned area (Kapur, 1996). TMS work on attention and motor performance in human subjects has highlighted the mechanisms that may underlie functional facilitations by providing experimental support for the hypothesis that some brain functions operate in a state of dynamic hemispheric competition. Manipulation of the hemispheric balance with single or repetitive TMS affords the investigation of the neural mechanisms underlying plasticity following brain lesions and can provide valuable knowledge on the inner workings of the normal brain. One can hope that these ideas will result in the development of meaningful therapeutic approaches, such as the

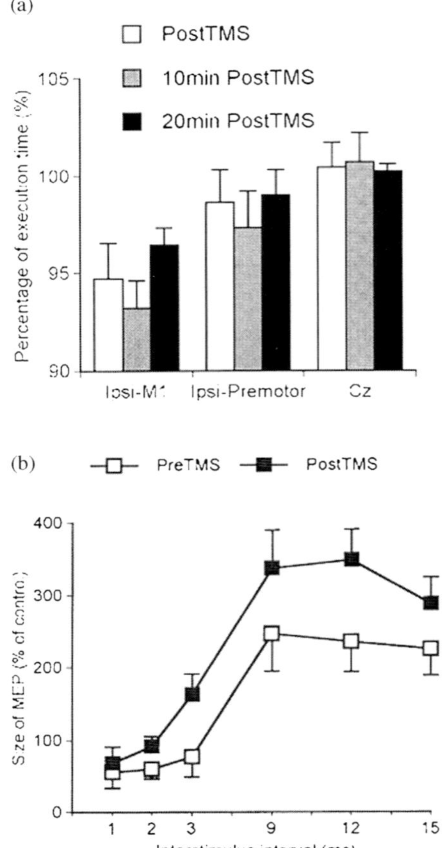

Fig. 5. (a) Ratio of execution times following rTMS at three different sites (ipsilateral M1, ipsilateral premotor cortex and Cz). Reaction times were significantly shorter after ipsilateral rTMS over primary motor cortex. (b) Changes in MEP sizes of the left first dorsal interosseus muscle with various interstimulus intervals.

treatment of motor, attentional and language impairments associated with strokes.

Acknowledgements

Some of the work described was supported by grants from the Canadian Institutes of Health Research and the National Alliance for Autism Research (HT) and the National Institutes of Health (APL).

References

Brighina, F., Bisiach, E., Oliveri, M., Piazza, A., La Bua, V., Daniele, O. and Fierro, B. 1 Hz repetitive transcranial magnetic stimulation of the unaffected hemisphere ameliorates contralesional visuospatial neglect in humans. *Neurosci. Lett.*, 2003, 16: 131–133.

Chen, R., Classen, J., Gerloff, C., Celnik, P., Wassermann, E. M., Hallett, M. and Cohen, L. G. Depression of motor cortex excitability by low-frequency transcranial magnetic stimulation. *Neurology*, 1997, 48: 1398–1403.

Engel, A.K. and Singer, W. Temporal binding and the neural correlates of sensory awareness. *Trends Cogn. Sci.*, 2001, 5: 16–25.

Ferbert, A., Priori, A., Rothwell, J.C., Day, B.L., Colebatch, J.G. and Marsden, C.D. Interhemispheric inhibition of the human motor cortex. *J Physiol.*, 1992, 453: 525–546.

Gerloff, C., Cohen, L.G., Floeter, M.K., Chen, R., Corwell, B. and Hallett, M. Inhibitory influence of the ipsilateral motor cortex on responses to stimulation of the human cortex and pyramidal tract. *J. Physiol.*, 1998, 510: 249–259.

Hilgetag, C.C., Theoret, H. and Pascual-Leone, A. Enhanced visual spatial attention ipsilateral to rTMS-induced 'virtual lesions' of human parietal cortex. *Nat. Neurosci.*, 2001, 4: 953–957.

Kapur, N. Paradoxical functional facilitation in brain-behaviour research. A critical review. *Brain*, 1996, 119: 1775–1790.

Kinsbourne, M. Hemi-neglect and hemisphere rivalry. In: E.A. Weinstein and R.P. Friedland (Eds.), Hemi-inattention and hemisphere specialization. *Advances in Neurology*, Vol. 18. Raven Press, New-York, 41–49.

Lewald, J., Foltys, H. and Töpper, R. Role of the posterior parietal cortex in spatial hearing. *J. Neurosci.*, 2002: 22, RC207.

Maeda, F., Keenan, J.P., Tormos, J.M., Topka, H. and Pascual-Leone, A. Modulation of corticospinal excitability by repetitive transcranial magnetic stimulation. *Clin. Neurophysiol.*, 2000, 111: 800–805.

Mesulam, M.M. Large-scale neurocognitive networks and distributed processing for attention, language, and memory. *Ann. Neurol.*, 1990, 28: 597–613.

Mesulam, M.M. Behavioral neuroanatomy. Large-scale neural networks, association cortex, frontal systems, the limbic system, and hemispheric specializations. In: M.M. Mesulam (Ed.), *Principles of Behavioral and Cognitive Neurology*, 2nd ed. Oxford University Press, New York, 2000: 1–120.

Mottaghy F.M., Hungs, M., Brugmann, M., Sparing, R., Boroojerdi, B., Foltys, H., Huber W. and Topper, R. Facilitation of picture naming after repetitive transcranial magnetic stimulation. *Neurology*, 1999, 53: 1806–1812.

Oliveri, M., Rossini, P.M., Traversa, R., Cicinelli, P., Filippi, M. M., Pasqualetti, P., Tomaiuolo, F. and Caltagirone C. Left frontal transcranial magnetic stimulation reduces contralesional extinction in patients with unilateral right brain damage. *Brain*, 1999, 122: 1731–1739.

Oliveri, M., Bisiach, E., Brighina, F., Piazza, A., La Bua, V., Buffa, D. and Fierro B. rTMS of the unaffected hemisphere transiently reduces contralesional visuospatial hemineglect. *Neurology*, 2001, 57: 1338–1340.

Ovsiew, F. Paradoxical functional facilitation in brain-behavior research: a critical review. *Brain*, 1997, 120: 1261–1264.

Pascual-Leone, A., Bartres-Faz, D. and Keenan, J.P. Transcranial magnetic stimulation: studying the brain-behaviour relationship by induction of 'virtual lesions'. *Philos. Trans. R. Soc. Lond. B. Biol. Sci.*, 1999, 354: 1229–1238.

Paus, T. Imaging the brain before, during, and after transcranial magnetic stimulation. *Neuropsychologia*, 1999, 37: 219–224.

Payne, B.R., Lomber, S.G., Geeraerts, S., van der Gucht, E. and Vandenbussche, E. Reversible visual hemineglect. *Proc. Natl. Acad. Sci. USA*, 1996, 93: 290–294.

Robertson, E.M., Tormos, J.M., Maeda, F. and Pascual-Leone, A. The role of the dorsolateral prefrontal cortex during sequence learning is specific for spatial information. *Cereb. Cortex*, 2001, 11: 628–635.

Robertson, E., Théoret, H. and Pascual-Leone, A. Studies in Cognition: The problems solved and created by Transcranial Magnetic Stimulation. *J. Cogn. Neurosci.*, in press.

Sack, A.T., Sperling, J.M., Prvulovic, D., Formisano, E., Goebel, R., Di Salle, F., Dierks, T. and Linden, D.E. Tracking the mind's image in the brain II: transcranial magnetic stimulation reveals parietal asymmetry in visuospatial imagery. *Neuron*, 2002, 35: 195–204.

Satow, T., Mima, T., Yamamoto, J., Oga, T., Begum, T., Aso, T., Hashimoto, N., Rothwell, J.C. and Shibasaki, H. Short-lasting impairment of tactile perception by 0.9Hz-rTMS of the sensorimotor cortex. *Neurology*, 2003, 60: 1045–1047.

Shapiro, K.A., Pascual-Leone, A., Mottaghy, F.M., Gangitano, M. and Caramazza, A. Grammatical distinctions in the left frontal cortex. *J. Cogn. Neurosci.*, 2001, 13: 713–720.

Shimizu, T., Hosaki, A., Hino, T., Sato, M., Komori, T., Hirai, S. and Rossini, P.M. Motor cortical disinhibition in the unaffected hemisphere after unilateral cortical stroke. *Brain*, 2002, 125: 1896–1907.

Sprague, J.M. Interaction of cortex and superior colliculus in mediation of visually guided behavior in the cat. *Science*, 1966, 153: 1544–1547.

Thut, G., Théoret, H., Pfennig, A., Ives, J., Kampmann, F., Northoff, G. and Pascual-Leone A. Differential effects of low-frequency rTMS at the occipital pole on visual-induced alpha desynchronization and visual-evoked potentials. *Neuroimage*, 2003, 18: 334–347.

Traversa, R., Cicinelli, P., Bassi, A., Rossini, P.M. and Bernardi, G. Mapping of motor cortical reorganization after stroke. A brain stimulation study with focal magnetic pulses. *Stroke*, 1997, 28: 110–117.

Valero-Cabré, A., Rushmore, J., Pascual-Leone, A., Lomber, S and Payne, B. High frequency repetitive TMS decreases the cortical uptake of glucose. 32nd Society for Neuroscience 2002, Orlando, 2–7 2002. SFN Abstract Viewer and Itinerary Planner, 208.6

Vallar, G. Spatial hemineglect in humans. *Trends Cogn. Sci.*, 1999, 2: 87–97.

Vanduffel, W., Payne, B.R., Lomber, S.G. and Orban, G.A. Functional impact of cerebral connections. *Proc. Natl. Acad. Sci. USA*, 1997, 94: 7617–7620.

Vuilleumier, P., Hester, D., Assal, G. and Regli, F. Unilateral spatial neglect recovery after sequential strokes. *Neurology*, 1996, 46: 184–189.

Wassermann, E.M. and Lisanby, S.H. Therapeutic application of repetitive transcranial magnetic stimulation: a review. *Clin. Neurophysiol.*, 2001, 112: 1367–1377.

Transcranial Magnetic Stimulation and Transcranial Direct Current Stimulation (Supplements to Clinical Neurophysiology, Vol. 56)
Editors: W. Paulus, F. Tergau, M.A. Nitsche, J.C. Rothwell, U. Ziemann, M. Hallett

Chapter 22

Repetitive magnetic and functional electrical stimulation reduce spastic tone increase in patients with spinal cord injury

Phillip Krause* and Andreas Straube

Department of Neurology, University of Munich, Klinikum Grosshadern, D-81377 Munich (Germany)

1. Introduction

A complete or incomplete spinal cord injury (SCI) often leads to a spastic tone increase (STI) in muscles distal to the lesion. STI is a characteristic feature of spastic paresis, one component of the upper motoneuron syndrome (Lance, 1980). While STI can have positive effects on rest mobility, it can also pose problems during the rehabilitation process and in daily life (Greenwood, 1998). Physiotherapy remains the best and most important treatment (Dietz, 2000; Mauritz, 2002; Paci, 2003); however, it is often insufficient. Drug treatment is frequently accompanied by negative side effects (Abbruzzese, 2002).

Thus, alternative methods for treating STI are needed. Transcutaneous electrical nerve stimulation (TENS) and functional electrical muscle stimulation (fES) have been shown to have long-term effects in reducing STI (Bajd et al., 1985; Katz et al., 1987; Franek et al., 1988; Granat et al., 1993). The application of repetitive magnetic stimulation (rMS) at peripheral nerves and the spinal cord was also found to reduce STI (Nielsen et al., 1995; Struppler et al., 1997).

The aim of our study was to determine whether individual fES of lower limb muscles or rMS of lumbar nerve roots innervating the lower limbs can have a positive influence on STI in SCI patients.

2. Methods

2.1. Patients

Six SCI patients participated. Three had complete SCI and no clinical STI at the time of investigation, whereas the other three had incomplete SCI with severe spastic tone of the lower limbs. The mean age was 36 (range from 32 to 47 years); mean time since injury was 5 years (range from 2 to 12 years); no pharmacological treatment was administered. All patients gave their informed consent, and the study was approved by the local ethics committee.

2.2 Measurements

The STI was assessed in two ways: (1) clinically with the modified Ashworth scale (MAS) (Bohannon et al., 1987) and (2) technically with a modified form (Bajd et al., 1984) of Wartenbergs' (1951) pendulum test of spasticity. The MAS assigns a grade to the

* *Correspondence to*: Dr. Phillip Krause, Department of Neurology, Klinikum Grosshadern, Marchioninistrasse 15, D-81377 Munich, Germany.
Tel: 0049-(0)89-7095-4818; Fax: 0049-(0)89-7095-4805;
E-mail: pkrause@nefo.med.uni-muenchen.de

spastic tone by measuring passive movements of the lower leg against the upper leg on a scale of 0 (no spastic tone) to 4 (most severe tone, in which no movements are possible).

The pendulum test measures freely damped pendular swinging movements of the lower leg against the upper leg by an electrical goniometer placed on the knee. Optimal relaxation is an important prerequisite for valid results. A pendulum test of a healthy subject and of a patient are shown in Fig. 1. The analogous output of the goniometer data was later analyzed with a customized program using Matlab®. This program allowed a semiautomatic analysis of the knee angles over time (Bajd et al., 1984). For further evaluation the peak velocity of the first swing was calculated, from a stretched position to a position of maximum flexion. The peak velocity depends on muscle resistance during the passive stretching phase and is measured in deg/s. The mean of 10 completed pendulum tests per subject was calculated.

To monitor the extent of muscle relaxation during the pendulum test, we used a surface EMG of the quadriceps muscle with acoustic monitoring of voluntary muscle contraction. The surface EMG was constantly recorded during leg swing.

2.3. Magnetic stimulation

The rMS was applied with a Magstim® Rapid (MAGSTIM® Company, UK) that had a maximum output of 1.275 Tesla. A circular coil with a diameter of 90 mm was positioned at the level of vertebrae L3 and L4 about 2 cm paravertebrally. Because the stimulator switched the coil off when it became too warm, two magnetic coils were used alternately. Before rMS was begun, the best position on the back was determined by applying single stimuli with certain suprathreshold intensities. The location at which the largest motor response could be detected was then marked. This point was used to define the resting motor threshold, the lowest intensity at which at least five of ten single stimuli led to responses in the surface EMG larger than 50 μV. EMG recordings were done in both quadriceps muscles. The motor threshold was determined for the more affected leg. There were no recorded stimuli for the other side. For this reason, the terms "stimulated and not-stimulated side" were not used, but rather "ipsilateral and contralateral" stimulation side. The single magnetic stimuli did not cause any visible muscle responses, whereas the rMS induced visible muscle contractions in some patients.

The stimulation intensity of the rMS was about 120% of resting motor threshold. Ten series of rMS at 20 Hz were applied to each subject, each series lasting for 10 s, the inter series-interval was 50 s. Altogether 2000 single magnetic stimuli were given. The side stimulated was always the clinically more affected leg.

Certain subthreshold stimulation intensities (10% of maximum stimulator output) were used for sham

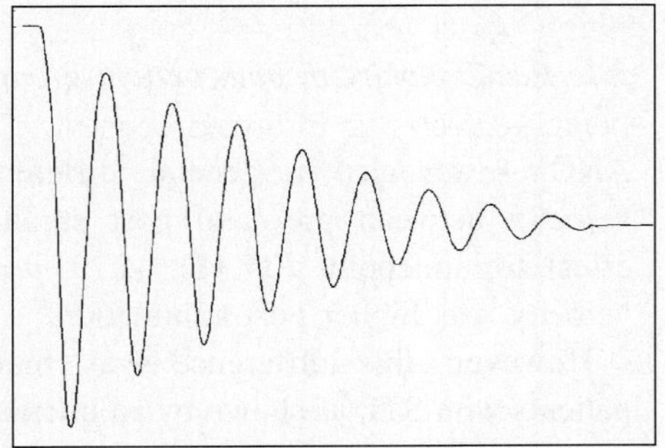
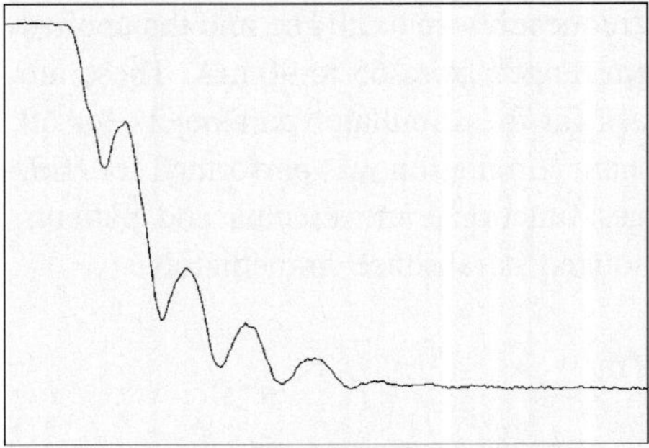

Fig. 1. Examples of a typical pendulum test of a healthy subject (left) and a patient with a MAS of about 3 (severe spastic tone; right). The range of motion (deg/sec), starting from a stretched position, is shown and recorded over time.

rMS. Patients were not informed if they were being treated with rMS or sham rMS. During the sham rMS session patients were told that a different magnetic coil (having the same intensity) was being used in order to explain the difference in stimulation that they were certain to notice. Our aim was to change the real stimulation setting as little as possible and not to apply any strong stimuli. In this way we wanted to minimize subjective effects felt by the patients even when the magnetic coil was held behind the back.

2.4. Functional electrical muscle stimulation

The fES was applied using common programmable electrical stimulators, type microstim 8 (Krauth + Timmermann®, Germany) with biphasic rectangular impulses, tunable in 10–500 μs width, and frequencies from 0.1 to 50 Hz. Reusable commercial surface electrodes of different sizes were used (5×9, 5×13 cm rectangular and 4×6 cm oval formed, Krauth + Timmermann®, Germany). Since all patients had been affiliated with our spinal cord outpatient clinic for fES training for many years, individual stimulation programs were applied. These programs contained the stimulator parameters needed to achieve the desired functional movements. For example, three patients used the stimulator program for standing, two for standing and walking, and one for bicycle training. In the fixed stimulator program all training sessions for each patient were always identical. Electrodes were placed over hip and thigh muscles. The mean stimulation periods lasted up to 10 min, with frequencies up to 20 Hz, and the applied current strength ranged from 65 to 90 mA. These are averaged values for the stimulator parameters for all patients. No sham stimulation was performed for fES, since it induces functional movements and patients would have noticed its absence immediately.

2.5. Procedures

The patients sat at a recording desk for evaluation by MAS and the pendulum test before, and after, stimulation. Between these two evaluations, the rMS, sham rMS, or fES was applied. All patients were retested by fES and rMS at least three times. Sham rMS was tested in three patients only once.

2.6. Statistics

The peak velocity of the first leg swing and the MAS were submitted to separate repeated measures ANOVA. For analysis of peak velocity, patient group (with and without STI) was entered as a between-subjects factor. Analysis of the MAS was performed for patients with STI only, because this measure was always 0 for patients without STI, and consequently, the variances would have been inhomogeneous. Timepoint (pre- and post stimulation), stimulation method (fES, rMS), and stimulated side (ipsi- and contralateral) were entered as within-subject factors. Data from sham rMS were available for only three patients; for each only one measurement, not three like with rMS and fES. Since this would have considerably reduced the number of valid cells for the ANOVA, sham rMS was not included in the above analysis, but submitted to statistics separately.

Differences between pre- and post stimulation values for the three stimulation methods were calculated. These differences were analyzed using the Wilcoxon test for related samples.

3. Results

The data for the following results are also shown graphically in Fig. 2.

3.1. Peak velocity in both patient groups

ANOVA revealed a general difference in peak velocity between pre- and post stimulation (main effect for timepoint $F(1,11) = 4.79$, $p = 0.05$): peak velocity was higher post stimulation.

However, this difference was mainly due to patients with STI, as shown by an interaction of timepoint and patient group ($F(1,11) = 5.33$, $p < 0.05$). Peak velocity was the same pre and post stimulation for patients without STI.

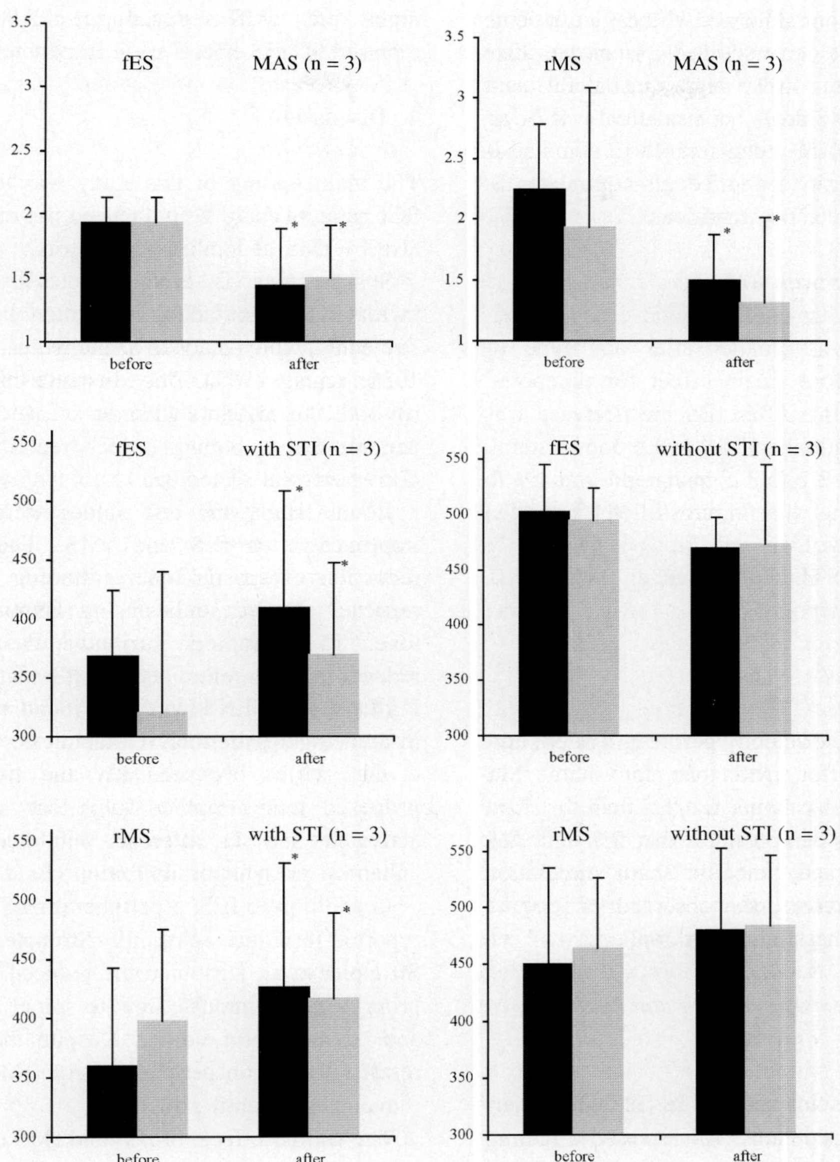

Fig. 2. Top: patient MAS values before and after fES (left) and rMS (right). Middle: peak velocity (deg/s) before and after fES in patients with (left) and without (right) clinical STI. Bottom: peak velocity (deg/s) before and after rMS in patients with (left) and without (right) clinical STI. Mean and standard deviation for the ipsilateral (black) and the contralateral (gray) sides are always shown. Columns marked with (*) show statistically significant changes. The MAS value within the group of patients without spastic tone was always 0 and is therefore not shown here.

Independently of timepoint and stimulation method, patients with STI generally had a lower peak velocity than patients without STI (main effect for patient group, $F(1,11) = 8.77$, $p < 0.05$).

In patients with STI, the peak velocity of the first swing increased after fES (368.2 deg/s to 409.2 deg/s ipsilateral and 320 deg/s to 369.5 deg/s contralateral) and rMS (360.5 deg/s to 426.8 deg/s ipsilateral and

398 deg/s to 415.9 contralateral), whereas in patients without STI peak velocity showed a decrease after fES (502.5 deg/s to 469.6 deg/s ipsilateral and 495.1 deg/s to 473.3 deg/s contralateral) and an increase after rMS (450.1 deg/s to 480.2 deg/s ipsilateral and 464.5 deg/s to 484.3 deg/s contralateral). These differences were not significant.

3.2. *MAS in patients with STI*

The MAS value was smaller after any type of stimulation than before (main effect for timepoint, $F(1,7) = 5.3$; $p < 0.01$). After fES the decrease was from 1.9 to 1.4 ipsilateral and 1.9 to 1.5 contralateral, and after rMS from 2.2 to 1.5 ipsilateral and 1.9 to 1.3 contralateral. Thus, the findings of MAS parallel those for peak velocity.

Patients without STI always had an MAS of 0, independently of timepoint.

3.3. *Sham rMS*

The difference in peak velocity before and after stimulation was larger for rMS than for sham rMS ($p = < 0.05$). It was also larger for fES than for sham rMS ($p = 0.01$). This demonstrates that fES and rMS positively affected peak velocity; sham stimulation had no effect. Therefore, the observed effects are most likely due to the stimulation applied.

3.4. *Subjective assessment of both stimulation methods*

As the patients were adapted to the fES, they tolerated it without any problems. All reported a feeling of increased relaxation in the muscles after fES, but noted also the diurnal occurrence of the spastic tone.

The rMS was also well tolerated. No patient complained of any unpleasant feeling during or after stimulation. On the contrary, after repeated rMS, patients reported having a pleasant feeling of relaxed legs, which at night allowed them to sleep better. Furthermore, some reported that it was easier to move, for example, from the wheelchair to the bed, a situation in which spastic reactions often occur. At night after rMS reduced spastic reactions were reported. These effects were in part felt for ca. 24 h.

4. Discussion

The main finding of this study was that the STI in SCI patients could be influenced not only by fES but also by rMS at lumbar nerve roots.

Spastic tone is typically characterized by an increased reflex activity during passive muscle stretching, which leads to a sudden resistance (Lance, 1980; Young, 1994). This resistance can be measured by both the MAS (Bohannon et al., 1987) and the pendulum test, both of which record more or less decreased peak velocities.

In our study the test values were significantly improved after fES and rMS. This indicates a reduction of spastic tone, a finding that was also reported in earlier studies using fES to reduce spastic tone. These authors attributed their findings to reduced spastic reflex activity (Granat et al., 1993). Furthermore, TENS was also found to be effective in reducing spastic tone (Goulet et al., 1996; Joodaki et al., 2001). Consequently the hypothesis was proposed that atrophied inhibitory synapses were activated and Ia afferents inhibited due to an enhanced presynaptic inhibition (Bajd et al., 1985).

In addition to fES, a peripheral rMS has also been reported to reduce spasticity (Struppler et al., 1997). Struppler et al. attributed the reduced spasticity to a proprioceptive impulse flow to spinal motor systems and to the motor cortex. Despite these promising results, studies on peripheral nerve rMS in STI have remained rare until now.

The similar effects of fES and rMS on spastic tone in our study and the results of earlier investigations point to similar influences, although fES and rMS are different. The aim of the electrical method is to produce functional movements; it is individually adapted to the patient's needs and is a more active tool. Magnetic stimulation is a more passive stimulation; it causes less muscle activity, and it aims not to elicit functional movements. Thus, the similar effects might result from the stimulation of different structures. The use of different stimulation locations (muscle vs. lumbar nerve roots) and common differences, like painlessness of rMS vs. pain sensations with fES in some cases, further underline this hypothesis. Our results allow us to only describe these effects. Any discussion concerning fiber systems would be too speculative.

Sham rMS did not cause large changes in either the MAS or the pendulum test. Analyzed with the Wilcoxon test and compared pairwise with the rMS and fES, significant differences did not point to any changes after sham rMS. It is clear that these results can only show a tendency and more patient data are necessary.

Interestingly, fES and rMS tended to cause different changes in peak velocity (decrease after fES and increase after rMS) in patients without clinical STI. Since these were relatively small, most probably due to the limited number of patients tested they were not significant. Larger patient groups are required to confirm these effects.

5. Conclusion

Lumbar rMS can reduce spastic tone of the lower limbs as fES does. Since rMS was well tolerated and caused no discomfort, it could perhaps become an additional therapeutic tool or alternative in the rehabilitation process of SCI patients with spastic tone increase. Therefore its role should be evaluated in more detail as well as the possibilities of using it in patients without STI.

References

Abbruzzese, G. The medical management of spasticity. *Eur. J. Neurol.*, 2002, 9 (Suppl. 1): 30–34.

Bajd, T. and Vodovnik, L. Pendulum testing of spasticity. *J. Biomed. Eng.*, 1984, 6(1): 9–16.

Bajd, T., Gregoric, M., Vodovnik, L. and Benko, H. Electrical stimulation in treating spasticity resulting from spinal cord injury. *Arch. Phys. Med. Rehabil.*, 1985, 66(8): 515–517.

Bohannon, R.W. and Smith, M.B. Interrater reliability of a modified Ashworth scale of muscle spasticity. *Phys. Ther.*, 1987, 67(2): 206–207.

Dietz, V. Spastic movement disorder. *Spinal Cord*, 2000, 38(7): 389–393.

Franek, A., Turczynski, B. and Opara, J. Treatment of spinal spasticity by electrical stimulation. *J. Biomed. Eng.*, 1988, 10(3): 266–270.

Goulet, C., Arsenault, A.B., Bourbonnais, D., Laramee, M.T. and Lepage, Y. Effects of transcutaneous electrical nerve stimulation on H-reflex and spinal spasticity. *Scand. J. Rehabil. Med.*, 1996, 28(3): 169–176.

Granat, M.H., Ferguson, A.C., Andrews, B.J. and Delargy, M. The role of functional electrical stimulation in the rehabilitation of patients with incomplete spinal cord injury – observed benefits during gait studies. *Paraplegia*, 1993, 31(4): 207–215.

Greenwood, R. Introduction: spasticity and the upper motor neurone syndrome. In: G. Sheean (Ed.), *Spasticity Rehabilitation*, 1st ed. Churchill Communications Ltd 1998, 1–5.

Joodaki, M.R., Olyaei, G.R. and Bagheri, H. The effects of electrical nerve stimulation of the lower extremity on H-reflex and F-wave parameters. *Electromyogr. Clin. Neurophysiol.*, 2001, 41(1): 23–28.

Katz, R.T., Green, D., Sullivan, T. and Yarkony, G. Functional electric stimulation to enhance systemic fibrinolytic activity in spinal cord injury patients. *Arch. Phys. Med. Rehabil.*, 1987; 68(7): 423–426.

Lance, J.W. Symposium synopsis. In: R.G. Feldman, R.R. Young and W.P. Koella (Eds.), *Spasticity: Disordered Motor Control*. Chicago: Yearbook Medical 1980: 485–494.

Mauritz, K.H. Gait training in hemiplegia. *Eur. J. Neurol.*, 2002, 9 (Suppl. 1): 23–29.

Nielsen, J.F., Klemar, B., Hansen, H.J. and Sinkjaer, T. A new treatment of spasticity with repetitive magnetic stimulation in multiple sclerosis. *J. Neurol. Neurosurg. Psychiatry*, 1995, 58(2): 254–255.

Paci, M. Physiotherapy based on the Bobath concept for adults with post-stroke hemiplegia: a review of effectiveness studies. *J. Rehabil. Med.*, 2003, 35(1): 2–7.

Struppler, A., Havel, P., Müller-Barna, P. and Lorenzen, H.W. A new method for rehabilitation of central palsy of arm and hand by peripheral magnetic stimulation. *Neurol. Rehabil.*, 1997, 3: 145–158.

Wartenberg, R. Pendelousness of the legs as a diagnostic test. *Neurology*, 1951, 1: 18–24.

Young, R.R. Spasticity: a review. *Neurology*, 1994, 44(11, Suppl. 9): S12–S20.

Transcranial Magnetic Stimulation and Transcranial Direct Current Stimulation (Supplements to Clinical Neurophysiology, Vol. 56)
Editors: W. Paulus, F. Tergau, M.A. Nitsche, J.C. Rothwell, U. Ziemann, M. Hallett

Chapter 23

Pharmacology of TMS

Ulf Ziemann

Clinic of Neurology, J.W. Goethe-University Frankfurt, Theodor-Stern-Kai 7, D-60590 Frankfurt am Main (Germany)

1. Introduction

Recent years have witnessed the development of a large array of transcranial magnetic stimulation (TMS) measures to probe motor cortical excitability. One important contribution to our understanding of the physiology underlying these various TMS measures came from pharmacological studies which tested the effects of CNS active drugs on these measures. This chapter will review the currently available data on the pharmacology of TMS. Only studies on healthy subjects will be considered. The most often used experimental approach is to measure motor cortical excitability before (baseline) and at one or more time points after intake of a single dose of the drug under study (post measurements). The post measurements are then compared with the baseline measurements. Another experimental approach is to test drug effects in a blinded placebo-controlled parallel or cross-over design.

* *Correspondence to*: Dr. Ulf Ziemann, Clinic of Neurology, Johann Wolfgang Goethe-University Frankfurt, Schleusenweg 2–16, D-60528 Frankfurt am Main, Germany.
Tel: +49-69-63015739; Fax: +49-69-63016842;
E-mail address: u.ziemann@em.uni-frankfurt.de

2. Effects of CNS active drugs on TMS measures of motor cortical excitability

2.1. Motor threshold

Motor threshold is the minimum intensity that is necessary to elicit a small (usually $> 50\ \mu V$) motor evoked potential (MEP) in the target muscle in at least half of the trials. Motor threshold is lower in the voluntarily contracting muscle (active motor threshold, AMT) compared to the resting muscle (resting motor threshold, RMT), usually by about 10% of stimulator output. Conceptually, motor threshold should depend on the excitability of cortico-cortical and/or thalamo-cortical axons excited by TMS, and the excitability of their excitatory synaptic contacts with the cortico-spinal neurones. Axon excitability is regulated mainly by voltage-gated sodium channels while fast excitatory synaptic neurotransmission is regulated by ionotropic glutamatergic non-NMDA receptors, in particular the AMPA receptor. Accordingly, motor threshold is elevated by drugs which block voltage-gated sodium channels (Mavroudakis et al., 1994; Ziemann et al., 1996c; Chen et al., 1997; Boroojerdi et al., 2001) but decreased by the indirect AMPA receptor agonist ketamine (Di Lazzaro et al., 2003) (Table 1).

TABLE 1

SYNOPSIS OF DRUG EFFECTS ON TMS MEASURES OF MOTOR CORTICAL EXCITABILITY

Drug	Mode of action	MT	MEP	CSP	SICI	ICF	IWF	SLAI
Carbamazepine	Na+	▲○	○	○	○○	○▼	○	
Phenytoin	Na+	▲▲	○○	○○○				
Lamotrigine	Na+	▲▲	▼	○	○	○	○	
Losigamone	? Na+/Ca++	▲		○	○	○		
Valproic acid	Na+ / GABA	○		○	○	○		
Lorazepam	$GABA_A$	○○○	▼▼	▲	▲▲○	▼○	▼	
Diazepam	$GABA_A$	○	▼○	▼	▲○	○		
Thiopental	$GABA_A$	○	▼	○				
Vigabatrin	GABA	○	○○	○○	○	▼	▼	
Tiagabin	GABA	○	○	▲	▼	▲		
Baclofen	$GABA_B$	○○	○○	○○	▲	▼	○	
Gabapentin	? GABA/anti-GLU	○○	○	▲	▲▲	▼▼	○	
Levetiracetam	?	○	▼	○	○	○		
Topiramate	Na+/$GABA_A$/anti-GLU	○		○	▲	▼		
Piracetam	?						▼	
Dextrometorphan	NMDA antagonist	○	○	○	▲	▼		
Memantine	NMDA antagonist	○○	○	○	▲	▼	○	
Riluzole	anti-GLU	○○		○○	▲○	▼▼		
Ketamine	NMDA antagonist ? AMPA	▼	▲					
L-DOPA	DA precursor	○	○	▲	○	○		
Bromocriptine	DA agonist	○			▲	○		
Pergolide	DA agonist	○	○	▲	▲	○		
Cabergoline	DA agonist	○	▼		▲	▼		
Selegiline	MAO-B inhibitor	○			○	○		
Haloperidol	DA antagonist	○	▲		▼	▲		
Sulipiride	DA antagonist	○			○	○		
Methylphenidate	NE agonist	○○	▲	○	▼○	○▲		
d-Amphetamine	NE/DA agonist	○	▲		○	▲		
Reboxetine	NE reuptake inhibitor	○▼	▲		▼○	▲▲		
Yohimbine	α2 antagonist	○○	▲		○	▲		
Prazosin	α1 antagonist	○	○		○	○		
Guanfacine	α2 agonist	○	▼		▲	▼		
Sertraline	SSRI	▲	○	○	○	▼		
Zolmitriptan	5-HT1B/1D agonist	○	○	○	▼	○		
Atropine	M1/M2 antagonist	○	○	○	▼	▲		
Scopolamine	M1 antagonist	▼	▲	○	○	○		▼

Drugs are grouped according to main mode of action. ○, no effect; ▼, reduction; ▲, increase; GLU, glutamate; SSRI, serotonin reuptake inhibitor; M, muscarinic receptor. Data in this table provide a survey of the currently (April 2003) available literature. Important references are in the main text

2.2. MEP size

MEP size increases with stimulus intensity in a sigmoid fashion. At a clearly supra-threshold stimulus intensity late I-waves (I2–I4) contribute significantly to the MEP whereas small MEP just above threshold are produced mainly by the I1-wave (Di Lazzaro et al., 1998). The amplitude of late I-waves can be modified by many processes such as conditioning stimulation of the tested motor cortex, the opposite motor cortex, or a peripheral nerve. Very likely, late I-waves depend on synaptic transmission through a chain of several excitatory interneurones. Therefore, it may be expected that the amplitude of large MEP (> 500 μV) is regulated by inhibitory (GABA) and excitatory neurotransmitters (glutamate), and neuromodulators (dopamine (DA), norepinephrine (NE), serotonin (5-HT), acetylcholin). Neuromodulators are potent modifiers of synaptic neurotransmission. The widespread diffuse innervation of the cortex by neuromodulators arises from various brainstem nuclei and, in contrast to neurotransmitters, appears largely transmitted by volume diffusion, not by activity-dependent synaptic release. It was found that $GABA_A$ receptor agonists (Inghilleri et al., 1996; Di Lazzaro et al., 2000a; Boroojerdi et al., 2001), the DA agonist cabergoline (own unpublished observation) and the NE antagonist guanfacine (Korchounov et al., 2003) decrease MEP size. In contrast, the indirect AMPA receptor agonist ketamine (Di Lazzaro et al., 2003), the DA antagonist haloperidol (own unpublished observation), NE agonists (Boroojerdi et al., 2001; Plewnia et al., 2001; Plewnia et al., 2002; Ilic et al., 2003) and the serotonin reuptake inhibitor sertraline (Ilic et al., 2002a) increase MEP size. Most of these changes in MEP size occur without changes in motor threshold (Table 1). MEP size is a rather sensitive measure to detect changes in neurotransmission and may be the only TMS measure that is affected by the drug under study, as is the case for the novel anticonvulsant levetiracetam (Sohn et al., 2001).

2.3. Cortical silent period (CSP)

The CSP refers to a TMS induced interruption of voluntary activity in the EMG of the target muscle. CSP duration increases linearly with stimulus intensity and may reach 200–300 ms in hand muscles (Cantello et al., 1992). It is currently believed that the CSP reflects a long-lasting cortical inhibition mediated by $GABA_B$ receptors. The experimental evidence in support of this hypothesis is relatively weak, though. In two studies, the $GABA_B$ receptor agonist baclofen did lead to a lengthening of the CSP (Inghilleri et al., 1996; Ziemann et al., 1996c). However, the applied dosages were probably too low to result in effective drug levels in the brain. One patient with generalised dystonia who was treated with incremental doses of intrathecal baclofen showed a significant lengthening of the CSP starting at a dose of 1000 μg/d (Siebner et al., 1998). However, a contribution of changes in spinal excitability to that effect was not ruled out. The $GABA_B$ hypothesis was further supported by a lengthening of the CSP by the GABA reuptake inhibitor tiagabin (Werhahn et al., 1999). Furthermore, neuromodulation by dopaminergic drugs appears to lengthen the CSP (Priori et al., 1994). Other drug effects were inconsistent (Table 1).

2.4. Short-interval intracortical inhibition (SICI).

SICI is determined in a paired-pulse TMS protocol, using a sub-threshold first (conditioning) followed after a short inter-stimulus interval of approximately 2–4 ms by a supra-threshold second (test) pulse (Kujirai et al., 1993). Another short-interval inhibition at very short intervals of ~1 ms is probably distinct from SICI (Fisher et al., 2002) and will not be considered here. It is currently believed that the sub-threshold first pulse produces an IPSP at the corticospinal neurones through activation of a low-threshold inhibitory cortical circuit which inhibits action potential generation by EPSPs coming from the supra-threshold second pulse (Ilic et al., 2002b). Accordingly, $GABA_A$ receptor agonists (Ziemann et al., 1996b; Di Lazzaro et al., 2000a; Reis et al., 2002) and anti-glutamatergic drugs (Ziemann et al., 1998a; Schwenkreis et al., 1999; Schwenkreis et al., 2000) increase SICI. The GABA reuptake inhibitor Tiagabin, however, decreases SICI (Werhahn et al., 1999). This was explained by activation of pre-synaptic $GABA_B$ autoreceptors located on GABAergic nerve terminals which results in auto-inhibition. Neuromodulators also affect SICI: DA agonists (Ziemann et al., 1996a; Ziemann et al., 1997) and the NE antagonist guanfacine (Korchounov et al., 2003) increase SICI. Conversely, the DA antagonist haloperidol (Ziemann et al., 1997) and NE agonists (Herwig et al., 2002; Ilic et al., 2003) decrease SICI (Table 1).

2.5. *Intracortical facilitation (ICF)*

ICF is tested by the same protocol as SICI but longer ISI of 7–20 ms are used (Kujirai et al., 1993; Ziemann et al., 1996d). Compared to SICI, the physiology of ICF is less clear. The leading hypothesis is that ICF probes the excitability of excitatory neuronal circuits in motor cortex. The pharmacological profile of ICF is similar but not identical to SICI (Table 1). $GABA_A$ receptor agonists (Ziemann et al., 1996b; Reis et al., 2002) and anti-glutamatergic drugs (Liepert et al., 1997; Ziemann et al., 1998a; Schwenkreis et al., 1999; Schwenkreis et al., 2000) decrease ICF. Neuromodulators also exert consistent effects on ICF. The DA agonist cabergoline (own unpublished observation), the NE antagonist guanfacine (Korchounov et al., 2003) and sertraline (Ilic et al., 2002a) decrease ICF whereas the DA antagonist haloperidol (Ziemann et al., 1997), NE agonists (Boroojerdi et al., 2001; Plewnia et al., 2001, 2002; Herwig et al., 2002; Moll et al., 2003) and atropine (Liepert et al., 2001) increase ICF (Table 1).

2.6. *I-wave facilitation (IWF)*

IWF is also measured in a paired-pulse TMS protocol, but in contrast to SICI and ICF, the first pulse is supra-threshold and the second pulse is sub-threshold (Ziemann et al., 1998b), or both pulses are of approximately threshold intensity (Tokimura et al., 1996). IWF occurs at discrete ISI of about 1.1–1.5 ms, 2.3–2.9 ms and 4.1–4.4 ms. IWF originates through direct excitation of initial axon segments of excitatory interneurones by the sub-threshold second pulse which were made hyperexcitable through EPSP by the first pulse (Hanajima et al., 2002; Ilic et al., 2002b). IWF is reduced by GABAergic drugs (Ziemann et al., 1998c; Ilic et al., 2002b) and piracetam (Wischer et al., 2001), while all other drugs tested so far had no effect (Table 1). These data suggest that the excitatory interneurones where the facilitatory interaction between the two pulses takes place are controlled by GABAergic circuits.

2.7. *Short latency afferent inhibition (SLAI)*

SLAI is defined as a MEP inhibition produced by a conditioning afferent pulse applied to the median nerve at the wrist contralateral to the test motor cortex approximately 20 ms prior to TMS (Tokimura et al., 2000). Pharmacological experiments revealed that this inhibition is physiologically distinct from SICI because it can be reduced by the anticholinergic scopolamine which does not affect SICI (Di Lazzaro et al., 2000b). The effects of other drugs on SLAI have not been tested yet.

3. Summary and conclusions

Testing the effects of CNS active drugs (neurotransmitters, neuromodulators) on motor cortical excitability by means of TMS has developed into an important field of research. At least two major avenues can be followed up. First, testing a drug with a known singular mode of action may provide information on the physiological properties of a novel TMS measure. For instance, it was shown that the recently discovered short latency afferent inhibition was significantly reduced by the anticholinergic (M1 antagonist) scopolamine (Di Lazzaro et al., 2000b). This opened up the opportunity to use short latency afferent inhibition (SLAI) to detect deficiency of central cholinergic innervation in neurological disease, for instance in Alzheimer's disease (Di Lazzaro et al., 2002). The other avenue is to use an array of well characterised TMS measures to obtain knowledge about the modes of action at the systems level of human cortex of a drug with unknown or multiple modes of action. One example is the novel anticonvulsant topiramate for which multiple modes of action were identified in animal experiments, including blocking effects on voltage-gated sodium channels, positive modulation of the $GABA_A$ receptor, inhibition of the kainate and AMPA subtypes of the glutamate receptor, inhibition of L-type voltage-gated calcium channels, and increase of cerebral GABA levels. Topiramate resulted in a selective increase of SICI and decrease of ICF without affecting motor threshold or CSP (Reis et al., 2002). From these results it was concluded that the main modes of action of topiramate at the level of the human motor cortex are its enhancing action on $GABA_A$ receptors and/or inhibition of glutamate receptors.

TMS offers now a wide array of measures of motor cortical excitability which covers many different forms of excitability, such as axon and inhibitory and excitatory synaptic excitability. Increasing numbers of different forms of cortical inhibition are being discovered, such as SICI ($GABA_A$ dependent), CSP ($GABA_B$ dependent) and SLAI (cholinergic), and it is very likely that more will follow soon.

References

Boroojerdi, B., Battaglia, F., Muellbacher, W. and Cohen, L.G. Mechanisms influencing stimulus-response properties of the human corticospinal system. *Clin. Neurophysiol.*, 2001, 112: 931–937.

Cantello, R., Gianelli, M., Civardi, C. and Mutani, R. Magnetic brain stimulation: the silent period after the motor evoked potential. *Neurology*, 1992, 42: 1951–1959.

Chen, R., Samii, A., Canos, M., Wassermann, E.M. and Hallett, M. Effects of phenytoin on cortical excitability in humans. *Neurology*, 1997, 49: 881–883.

Di Lazzaro, V., Oliviero, A., Profice, P., Saturno, E., Pilato, F., Insola, A., Mazzone, P., Tonali, P. and Rothwell, J.C. Comparison of descending volleys evoked by transcranial magnetic and electric stimulation in conscious humans. *Electroencephalogr. Clin. Neurophysiol.*, 1998, 109: 397–401.

Di Lazzaro, V., Oliviero, A., Meglio, M., Cioni, B., Tamburrini, G., Tonali, P. and Rothwell, J.C. Direct demonstration of the effect of lorazepam on the excitability of the human motor cortex. *Clin. Neurophysiol.*, 2000a, 111: 794–799.

Di Lazzaro, V., Oliviero, A., Profice, P., Pennisi, M.A., Di Giovanni, S., Zito, G., Tonali, P. and Rothwell, J.C. Muscarinic receptor blockade has differential effects on the excitability of intracortical circuits in human motor cortex. *Exp. Brain Res.*, 2000b, 135: 455–461.

Di Lazzaro, V., Oliviero, A., Tonali, P.A., Marra, C., Daniele, A., Profice, P., Saturno, E., Pilato, F., Masullo, C. and Rothwell, J.C. Noninvasive in vivo assessment of cholinergic cortical circuits in AD using transcranial magnetic stimulation. *Neurology*, 2002, 59: 392–397.

Di Lazzaro, V., Oliviero, A., Profice, P., Pennisi, M.A., Pilato, F., Zito, G., Dileone, M., Nicoletti, R., Pasqualetti, P. and Tonali, P.A. Ketamine increases motor cortex excitability to transcranial magnetic stimulation. *J. Physiol.*, 2003.

Fisher, R.J., Nakamura, Y., Bestmann, S., Rothwell, J.C. and Bostock, H. Two phases of intracortical inhibition revealed by transcranial magnetic threshold tracking. *Exp. Brain Res.*, 2002, 143: 240–248.

Hanajima, R., Ugawa, Y., Terao, Y., Enomoto, H., Shiio, Y., Mochizuki, H., Furubayashi, T., Uesugi, H., Iwata, N.K. and Kanazawa, I. Mechanisms of intracortical I-wave facilitation elicited with paired- pulse magnetic stimulation in humans. *J. Physiol.*, 2002, 538: 253–261.

Herwig, U., Bräuer, K., Connemann, B., Spitzer, M. and Schönfeldt-Lecuona, C. Intracortical excitability is modulated by a norepinephrine-reuptake inhibitor as measured with paired-pulse transcranial magnetic stimulation. *Psychopharmacol.*, 2002, 164: 228–232.

Ilic, T.V., Korchounov, A. and Ziemann, U. Complex modulation of human motor cortex excitability by the specific serotonin re-uptake inhibitor sertraline. *Neurosci. Lett.*, 2002a, 319: 116–120.

Ilic, T.V., Meintzschel, F., Cleff, U., Ruge, D., Kessler, K.R. and Ziemann, U. Short-interval paired-pulse inhibition and facilitation of human motor cortex: the dimension of stimulus intensity. *J. Physiol.*, 2002b, 545(1): 153–167.

Ilic, T.V., Korchounov, A. and Ziemann, U. Methylphenydate facilitates and disinhibits the motor cortex in intact humans. *Neuroreport*, 2003, 14: 773–776.

Inghilleri, M., Berardelli, A., Marchetti, P. and Manfredi, M. Effects of diazepam, baclofen and thiopental on the silent period evoked by transcranial magnetic stimulation in humans. *Exp. Brain Res.*, 1996, 109: 467–472.

Korchounov, A., Ilic, T.V. and Ziemann, U. The alpha2-adrenergic agonist guanfacine reduces excitability of human motor cortex through disfacilitation and increase of inhibition. *Clin. Neurophysiol.*, 2003, 114 (in press).

Kujirai, T., Caramia, M.D., Rothwell, J.C., Day, B.L., Thompson, P.D., Ferbert, A., Wroe, S., Asselman, P. and Marsden, C.D. Corticocortical inhibition in human motor cortex. *J. Physiol. (Lond.)*, 1993, 471: 501–519.

Liepert, J., Schwenkreis, P., Tegenthoff, M. and Malin, J.-P. The glutamate antagonist Riluzole suppresses intracortical facilitation. *J. Neural. Transm.*, 1997, 104: 1207–1214.

Liepert, J., Schardt, S. and Weiller, C. Orally administered atropine enhances motor cortex excitability: a transcranial magnetic stimulation study in human subjects. *Neurosci. Lett.*, 2001, 300: 149–152.

Mavroudakis, N., Caroyer, J.M., Brunko, E. and Zegers de Beyl, D. Effects of diphenylhydantoin on motor potentials evoked with magnetic stimulation. *Electroencephalogr. Clin. Neurophysiol.*, 1994, 93: 428–433.

Moll, G.H., Heinrich, H. and Rothenberger, A. Methylphenidate and intracortical excitability: opposite effects in healthy subjects and attention-deficit hyperactivity disorder. *Acta. Psychiatr. Scand.*, 2003, 107: 69–72.

Plewnia, C., Bartels, M., Cohen, L. and Gerloff, C. Noradrenergic modulation of human cortex excitability by the presynaptic alpha(2)-antagonist yohimbine. *Neurosci. Lett.*, 2001, 307: 41–44.

Plewnia, C., Hoppe, J., Hiemke, C., Bartels, M., Cohen, L. and Gerloff, C. Enhancement of human cortico-motoneuronal excitability by the selective norepinephrine reuptake inhibitor reboxetine. *Neurosci. Lett.*, 2002, 330: 231–234.

Priori, A., Berardelli, A., Inghilleri, M., Accornero, N. and Manfredi, M. Motor cortical inhibition and the dopaminergic system. Pharmacological changes in the silent period after transcranial brain stimulation in normal subjects, patients with Parkinson's disease and drug-induced parkinsonism. *Brain*, 1994, 117: 317–323.

Reis, J., Tergau, F., Hamer, H.M., Muller, H.H., Knake, S., Fritsch, B., Oertel, W.H. and Rosenow, F. Topiramate selectively decreases intracortical excitability in human motor cortex. *Epilepsia*, 2002, 43: 1149–1156.

Schwenkreis, P., Witscher, K., Janssen, F., Addo, A., Dertwinkel, R., Zenz, M., Malin, J.-P. and Tegenthoff, M. Influence of the N-methyl-D-aspartate antagonist mementine on human motor cortex excitability. *Neurosci. Lett.*, 1999, 270: 137–140.

Schwenkreis, P., Liepert, J., Witscher, K., Fischer, W., Weiller, C., Malin, J.-P. and Tegenthoff, M. Riluzole suppresses motor cortex facilitation in correlation to its plasma level. *Exp. Brain Res.*, 2000, 135: 293–299.

Siebner, H.R., Dressnandt, J., Auer, C. and Conrad, B. Continuous intrathecal baclofen infusions induced a marked increase of the transcranially evoked silent period in a patient with generalized dystonia. *Muscle Nerve*, 1998, 21: 1209–1212.

Sohn, Y.H., Kaelin-Lang, A., Jung, H.Y. and Hallett, M. Effect of levetiracetam on human corticospinal excitability. *Neurology*, 2001, 57: 858–863.

Tokimura, H., Ridding, M.C., Tokimura, Y., Amassian, V.E. and Rothwell, J.C. Short latency facilitation between pairs of threshold magnetic stimuli applied to human motor cortex. *Electroencephalogr. Clin. Neurophysiol.*, 1996, 101, 263–272.

Tokimura, H., Di Lazzaro, V., Tokimura, Y., Oliviero, A., Profice, P., Insola, A., Mazzone, P., Tonali, P. and Rothwell, J.C. Short latency inhibition of human hand motor cortex by somatosensory input from the hand. *J. Physiol.*, 2000, 523: 503–513.

Werhahn, K.J., Kunesch, E., Noachtar, S., Benecke, R. and Classen, J. Differential effects on motorcortical inhibition induced by blockade of GABA uptake in humans. *J. Physiol. (Lond.)*, 1999, 517: 591–597.

Wischer, S., Paulus, W., Sommer, M. and Tergau, F. Piracetam affects facilitatory I-wave interaction in the human motor cortex. *Clin. Neurophysiol.*, 2001, 112: 275–279.

Ziemann, U., Bruns, D. and Paulus, W. Enhancement of human motor cortex inhibition by the dopamine receptor agonist pergolide: evidence from transcranial magnetic stimulation. *Neurosci. Lett.*, 1996a, 208: 187–190.

Ziemann, U., Lönnecker, S., Steinhoff, B.J. and Paulus, W. The effect of lorazepam on the motor cortical excitability in man. *Exp. Brain Res.*, 1996b, 109: 127–135.

Ziemann, U., Lönnecker, S., Steinhoff, B.J. and Paulus, W. Effects of antiepileptic drugs on motor cortex excitability in humans: a transcranial magnetic stimulation study. *Ann. Neurol.*, 1996c, 40: 367–378.

Ziemann, U., Rothwell, J.C. and Ridding, M.C. Interaction between intracortical inhibition and facilitation in human motor cortex. *J. Physiol. (Lond.)*, 1996d, 496: 873–881.

Ziemann, U., Tergau, F., Bruns, D., Baudewig, J. and Paulus, W. Changes in human motor cortex excitability induced by dopaminergic and anti-dopaminergic drugs. *Electroencephalogr. Clin. Neurophysiol.*, 1997; 105: 430–437.

Ziemann, U., Chen, R., Cohen, L.G. and Hallett, M. Dextromethorphan decreases the excitability of the human motor cortex. *Neurology*, 1998a, 51: 1320–1324.

Ziemann, U., Tergau, F., Wassermann, E.M., Wischer, S., Hildebrandt, J. and Paulus, W. Demonstration of facilitatory I-wave interaction in the human motor cortex by paired transcranial magnetic stimulation. *J. Physiol. (Lond.)*, 1998b, 511: 181–190.

Ziemann, U., Tergau, F., Wischer, S., Hildebrandt, J. and Paulus, W. Pharmacological control of facilitatory I-wave interaction in the human motor cortex. A paired transcranial magnetic stimulation study. *Electroencephalogr. Clin. Neurophysiol.*, 1998c, 109: 321–330.

Transcranial Magnetic Stimulation and Transcranial Direct Current Stimulation (Supplements to Clinical Neurophysiology, Vol. 56)
Editors: W. Paulus, F. Tergau, M.A. Nitsche, J.C. Rothwell, U. Ziemann, M. Hallett

Chapter 24

Bihemispheric plasticity after acute hand deafferentation

Konrad J. Werhahn[a], Jennifer Mortensen[b], Robert W. Van Boven[c] and Leonardo G. Cohen[d]

[a] *Department of Neurology, Johannes Gutenberg University, Rhineland-Palatinate, Mainz (Germany)*
[b] *Brigham Young University, Provo, UT (USA)*
[c] *Laboratory of Brain and Cognition, National Institute of Neurological Disorders and Stroke, Bethesda, MD (USA)*
[d] *Human Cortical Physiology Section, National Institute of Neurological Disorders and Stroke, National Institutes of Health, Bethesda, MD (USA)*

1. Introduction

There is considerable evidence that the adult human cortex maintains the ability to reorganize throughout life and is highly dynamic. This capacity to reorganize may be the basis for recovery following injury. The term "plasticity" is defined as "any enduring change in cortical properties either morphological or functional" (Donoghue et al., in Bloedel et al., 1996). One model to induce cortical plasticity is deprivation of sensory input in non-human animals that results in significant reorganisation of cortical representation (Merzenich and Kaas, 1982; Kaas et al., 1983; Jones, 2000). For example, plastic changes in receptive fields or topography have been observed in somatosensory (Rasmusson, 1982; Pons et al., 1991) auditory (Rajan, 1998) and visual (Kaas et al., 1990; Gilbert and Wiesel, 1992) cortex and these changes become apparent within minutes (Kelahan and Doetsch, 1984; Calford and Tweedale, 1988; Silva et al., 1996). In the motor cortex, various forms of deafferentation including peripheral nerve lesions (Kolarik et al., 1994) and limb amputations (Chen et al., 1998; Qi et al., 2000) result in reorganisation of the motor representation in the deafferented hemisphere (Cohen et al., 1991). In humans, ischemic nerve block (INB) implemented by inflating a tourniquet around the forearm has been used as a model for acute sensory deafferentation. The acute, reversible deprivation of somatosensory input results in well described functional changes in the contralateral motor cortex (Brasil-Neto et al., 1992, 1993; Ridding and Rothwell, 1995; Ziemann et al., 1998a) that are thought to be similar to those observed in animal experiments. Most reports have focused on the effects of deafferentation on contralateral cortical representations. Here we summarize experiments showing that deprivation of somatosensory input could also elicit organisational changes in the hemisphere contralateral to the deafferented one. The

* *Correspondence to*: Dr. K.J. Werhahn, Department of Neurology, University of Mainz, Langenbeckstr. 1, D-55131 Mainz, Germany.
Tel: +49-6131-175275; Fax: +49-6131-173271;
E-mail: Werhahn@uni-mainz.de

existence of interactions between homotopic sites within cortical representations in both hemispheres provides a substrate for such an effect (Asanuma and Okudo, 1962; Ferbert et al., 1992; Di Lazzaro et al., 1999; Hanajima et al., 2001). For example, in primates and flying foxes, acute deafferentation leads to rapid changes of receptive fields in the somatosensory cortex in both hemispheres (Calford and Tweedale, 1990). It has been proposed that chronic deafferentation, in association with long term practice as in blind (Van Boven et al., 2000), deaf (Levänen and Hamdorf, 2001), or individuals with amputation (Haber, 1958) results in compensatory gains in the same and in other sensory modalities. However, the long-term changes described are mild and the question whether blind or deaf people develop enhanced capacities of their remaining senses is still controversial (Rauschecker, 1995). Acute deafferentation leads to rapid changes of contra- and ipsilateral cortical representations (Calford and Tweedale, 1990; Sadato et al., 1995). These immediate changes most likely result from unmasking of existing anatomical connections enforcing competition between afferents within a single modality. Much less is known about the behavioural consequences of acute deafferentation in humans (Ziemann et al., 2001). It is conceivable that there are "built-in" mechanisms by which interruption of sensory input from one region leads to perceptual compensatory enhancements in a different site (MacAvoy et al,, 1987). An immediate behavioural improvement in a different body site or modality following acute deafferentation could reflect the existence of compensatory mechanisms to allow coping with the new deficit (Miller, 1996).

2. Deafferentation induced excitability changes in motor cortex

Temporary removal of somatosensory input by ischaemic nerve block (INB) results in the reduction of inhibition within the motor cortex (Brasil-Neto et al., 1992, 1993). The amplitudes of motor evoked potentials (MEP) to transcranial magnetic stimulation (TMS) from muscles immediately proximal to INB at the forearm increase within minutes after the onset of anaesthesia and return to control values after termination of anaesthesia. Further experiments by the same group showed that the deafferented motor cortex becomes modifiable by inputs that are normally subthreshold for inducing changes in excitability (Ziemann et al., 1998a). Moreover, using repetitive transcranial magnetic stimulation (rTMS) and stimulating the "plastic" cortex these deafferentation-induced plastic changes can be up-regulated and likely via inhibitory projections down-regulated by stimulation of the opposite cortex. This increase in MEP size induced by a combination of INB and rTMS involves rapid removal of GABA-related cortical inhibition and short-term changes in synaptic efficacy dependent on Na^+ or Ca^{2+} channels (Ziemann et al., 1998b). Pharmacological interventions suggested further that some long-lasting (> 60 min) excitatory effects might be related to long-term potentiation-like mechanisms given their duration and the involvement of NMDA receptor activation (Ziemann et al., 1998b).

Based on the knowledge acquired through these experiments and given the previous evidence pointing to interactions between homotopic sites within both motor cortices (Asanuma and Okudo, 1962; Calford and Tweedale, 1990; Ferbert et al., 1992; Di Lazzaro et al., 1999; Hanajima et al., 2001) a series of experiments were performed to look into a possible influence of deafferentation on the motor cortex contralateral to the deafferented one (Werhahn et al., 2002a). In healthy subjects MEP amplitudes were subsequently measured during, 10, 30 and 60 min after INB of the right hand. The latest measurement during INB (around 40 min into INB) was obtained under the condition of a complete motor block and light touch anaesthesia. MEPs were elicited by TMS applied at rest at the optimal stimulation position for small hand, biceps (Bic), tibialis anterior (TA) or pectoralis (Pec) muscles bilaterally using a stimulus intensity well above motor threshold. Tourniquet inflation leading to INB resulted progressively in numbness and paresthesias in the deafferented hand paralled by a gradual decrease of MEP amplitude in small hand muscles distal to INB, consistent with a motor block effect. At the same time, INB led to larger MEP responses (max. by 176% compared to baseline) in the right Bic muscle, immediately proximal to the tourniquet in the absence of changes in RMT (Fig. 1).

In addition to changes in cortical excitability of muscles ipsilateral to INB (right arm), tourniquet inflation resulted in larger MEP amplitudes in the left first dorsal interosseus muscle (FDI) contralateral to the ischemic hand as well. In accord to a focal effect, INB at the right forearm did not elicit significant changes in contralateral Bic, ipsi- and contralateral Pec, and TA muscles suggesting that the increases in right Bic and left FDI were not due to a generalized and hence unspecific change of cortical excitability. Also, INB and anaesthesia of the right foot did not lead to significant changes in MEP amplitudes in hand muscles or biceps relative to baseline arguing against an unspecific effect of INB on alertness causing the site-specific changes. Similar to what has been shown previously for the effect in upper arm muscles on the side of deafferentation (Brasil-Neto et al., 1993) amplitude changes in the left hand during right hand anaesthesia were of cortical origin since they could only be obtained by TMS but not by brainstem electrical stimulation (Ugawa et al., 1991). A single oral dose of lorazepam (LZP) a short-acting benzodiazepine that causes cell hyperpolarisation by enhancing Cl^- currents via $GABA_A$ receptors (Macdonald, 1995) blocked the enhancing effect of right hand INB on left FDI MEP amplitude present

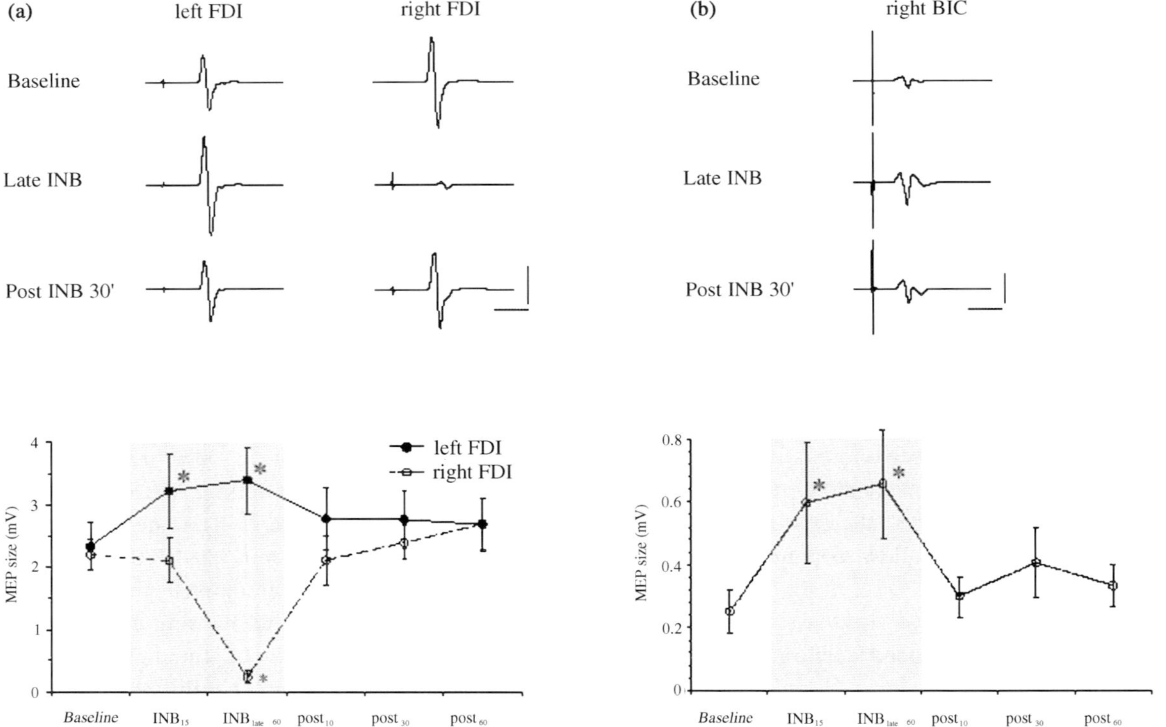

Fig. 1. Effect of deafferentation of the right hand by ischemic nerve block (INB) on MEP amplitudes in small hand muscles bilaterally (a) and in the biceps brachii (Bic) immediately proximal to the tourniquet (b). The upper half shows EMG raw data from the left and right first dorsal interosseus (FDI) and the right Bic muscles of one representative subject. The lower half depicts the time course of the effect, the shaded areas illustrating the period of INB. Data represent group means + SEM. * $p < 0.01$ in post-hoc testing. Calibration bars: 1 mV, 20 ms. Permission for reprint from Werhahn et al., 2002a was granted by Oxford Journals.

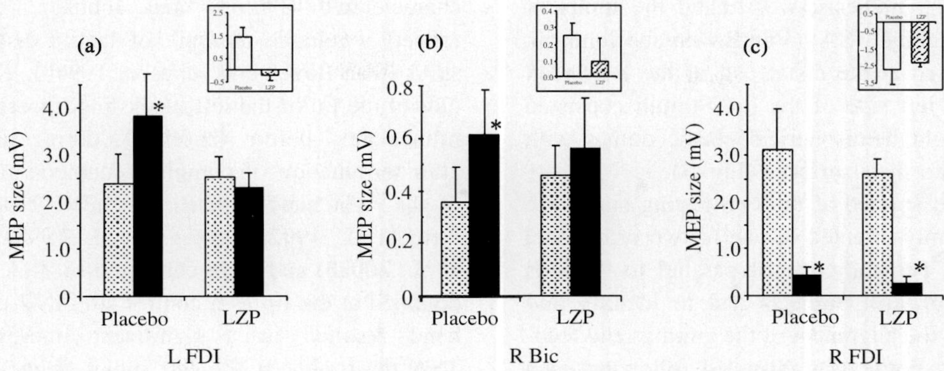

Fig. 2. MEP amplitudes from left FDI (a), right biceps brachii (Bic) (b) and right FDI (c) at baseline (dotted bars) and INBlate (filled bars) in the placebo and lorazepam (LZP) sessions. MEP amplitude changes at INBlate relative to baseline are shown in the insets. Note that LZP did not modify the reduction in right FDI MEP amplitudes secondary to motor block (c). In contrast, LZP blocked and substantially attenuated the increase in left FDI (a) and right Bic (b) MEP amplitudes. Data represent group means + SEM. * $p < 0.05$ in post-hoc testing. Permission for reprint from Werhahn et al., 2002a was granted by Oxford Journals.

in the placebo sessions suggesting that the observed effect was mediated via a reduction of GABAergic neurotransmission (Fig. 2).

3. Deafferentation induced enhancement of perceptual abilities in homotopic body parts

The behavioural consequences of interruption of sensory input are incompletely understood. For example, amputations, may lead to a condition called phantom limb pain, which consists of excruciating painful sensations referred to the missing limb (Ramachandran and Hirstein, 1998). and is thought to represent a form of "maladaptive" cortical reorganization (Flor et al., 1995). On the other hand, deafferentation may lead to compensatory gains in patients with chronic loss of sensory input (Cohen et al., 1997; Van Boven et al., 2000; Levänen and Hamdorf, 2001). However, in these cases, input deprivation was associated with increased use or practice. For example, blind individuals who frequently read Braille experience improvements in tactile perceptual skills (Pascual-Leone et al., 1995). Still, it is not known if acute deafferentation alone, in the absence of increased use, has a behavioural impact which may be consistent with findings of focal increases in motor cortical excitability during acute deafferentation (Brasil-Neto et al., 1992; Ziemann et al., 1998a; Werhahn et al., 2002a).

Acute deafferentation not only results in bihemispheric increases of motor cortical excitability (Brasil-Neto et al., 1992; Ziemann et al., 1998a; Werhahn et al., 2002a) but also causes rapid bilateral cortical reorganisation in the sensory domain (Merzenich et al., 1983; Robertson and Irvine, 1989; Calford and Tweedale, 1990; Gilbert and Wiesel, 1992; Shin et al., 1997). For instance, anaesthesia of a digit results in an immediate bilateral expansion of cortical receptive fields representing nearby fingers (Rasmusson, 1982; Merzenich et al., 1983; Calford and Tweedale, 1990). Similarly, in human amputees, functional changes have been described in both contralateral and ipsilateral cortical body part representations (Kew et al., 1994) and acute hand deafferentation in healthy adults has similar effects in homotopic regions of both sensorimotor cortices (Sadato et al., 1995). These reports led us to explore the hypothesis that acute hand deafferentation could result in enhanced perceptual abilities in the remaining hand (Werhahn et al., 2002b).

To test this hypothesis, we studied the limits of tactile spatial acuity (TSA) (Van Boven and Johnson, 1994b) measured at the distal pad of the left index finger and the left side of the lip. Stimuli consisted of a set of eight hemispherical plastic domes with gratings cut into their surfaces (Fig. 3).

Stimuli were applied at the two testing sites with gratings randomly oriented in one of two orthogonal directions (i.e. perpendicular or parallel to the axis of the finger or lip). Subjects had to identify and verbally report the alignment of the gratings and feedback on the response was provided following each trial. Manual application yields reliable data since cutaneous spatial resolution is relatively insensitive to force (Johnson and Phillips, 1981) and the spatial profile for the neural response to complex surfaces are relatively insensitive to the depth of indentation (Vega-Bermudez and Johnson, 1999). Subjects, naive to the purpose of the experiments were tested before, during and after acute cutaneous anaesthesia of the right hand. TSA thresholds, defined as the groove width yielding a 75% correct performance (Van Boven and Johnson, 1994a; Sathian and Zangaladze, 1998), were determined using a grating orientation test (GOT) that is reproducible (Van Boven and Johnson, 1994a; Sathian and Zangaladze, 1998), well

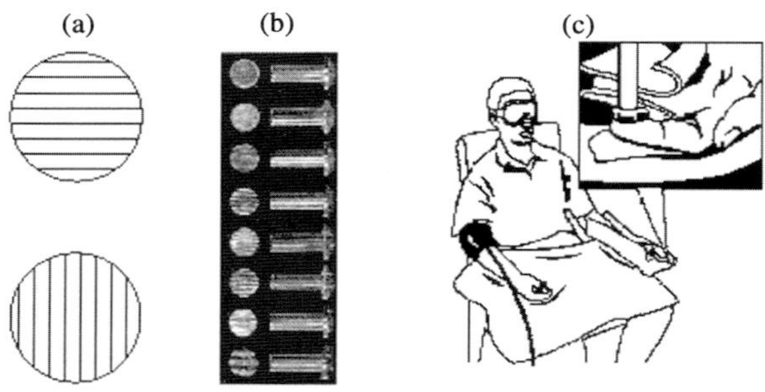

Fig. 3. Experimental set-up for grating orientation task (GOT). (a) Gratings were placed in two orthogonal orientations relative to the long axis of the left index finger and (b) consisted of a set of eight hemispherical plastic domes. Subjects left arm and finger were immobilized by a cast, while a tourniquet was placed around the right forearm (c). Permission for reprint from Werhahn et al., 2002b was obtained by NPG.

characterized (Phillips and Johnson, 1981) and reflects a reliable measure of tactile discriminative skills (Van Boven and Johnson, 1994b). TSA thresholds at the tip of the left index finger were measured immediately before (baseline), during and 15 min after termination of complete cutaneous anaesthesia of the right hand by ischemic nerve block (Brasil-Neto et al., 1992; Ziemann et al., 1998a; Werhahn et al., 2002b) and were compared to TSA thresholds obtained at the lip as a control site. INB of the right hand resulted in a significant improvement in TSA thresholds at the left index finger relative to baseline (from 1.1 + 0.09 mm to 0.89 + 0.07 mm) that returned to baseline levels (1.1 + 0.01 mm) after the end of anaesthesia (Fig. 4).

TSA thresholds at the lip measured during the same procedure did not show significant changes. In a control experiment starting from similar baseline TSA measurements as in the other sessions, anaesthesia of the right foot failed to elicit performance improvements in TSA thresholds at the left index finger suggesting that the improvement in TSA only occurs with deafferentation of the opposite hand. Given that other conflicting variables like the duration of deafferentation and discomfort induced by the intervention were similar between arm and leg sessions, these results are consistent with a topographically selective effect of hand deafferentation on performance in the non-deafferented hand. In an additional experiment, we tested the effects of right hand anaesthesia on TSA thresholds in naïve subjects compared to subjects that practised the GOT task twice the day before. In both groups, with and without practice, right hand anaesthesia resulted in significant improvements in TSA thresholds that did not differ from each other. To investigate whether these behavioural findings are paralleled by neurophysiological changes we also measured amplitudes of the short-latency cortical components of somatosensory evoked potentials (SSEPs) recorded over the right primary sensory cortex during INB of the right hand or right foot. These recordings revealed a significant enlargement of the N1 and N1-P1 components of the SSEP (Fig. 5) during hand but not during right foot deafferentation reflecting an increase

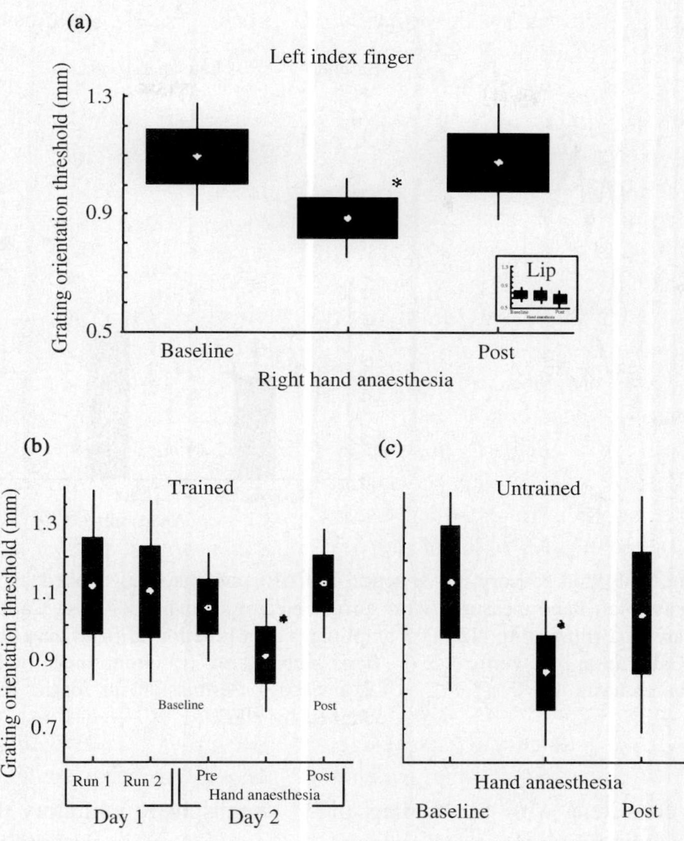

Fig. 4. Effect of cutaneous anaesthesia on tactile spatial acuity. GOT thresholds at the left index finger (a) ($n = 19$; mean $\pm$ 1 and 2 SEM) before, during (* $F_{2,19} = 9.3$, $p < 0.001$), and after anaesthesia of the right hand. The inset illustrates GOT thresholds at the left side of the lower lip ($n = 13$) during right hand anaesthesia. Below, mean GOT thresholds at the left index finger in trained ($n = 9$) (b) and untrained ($n = 10$) (c) individuals (* post-hoc $p < 0.05$). Permission for reprint from Werhahn et al., 2002b was obtained by NPG.

in the excitability of the right primary somatosensory cortex.

These changes were not due to alterations of the input in the peripheral afferent volley between recordings since SSEP were also enlarged when correcting for the size of the sensory nerve actions potentials recorded from the median nerve. On the other hand, subcortical SSEP components were unaffected by INB also pointing to a cortical site of the effect (Allison et al., 1980).

In contrast to situations in which behavioural gains have been ascribed to an increased reliance on the remaining senses like in blind (Van Boven et al., 2000) or deaf subjects (Neville and Lawson, 1987), the gains described in this report did not depend on training. Our findings demonstrate that deafferentation can acutely lead to a rapid improvement in tactile discriminative skills in the absence of increased practice. The increase in tactile spatial acuity was identified shortly after the onset of deafferentation pointing to the involvement of existing cortical or subcortical substrates. The enhancement of the cortical SSEP components originated in S1 (Allison et al., 1989) in the absence of changes in subcortical generators (Allison et al., 1980). This points to changes in processing within the primary somatosensory cortex.

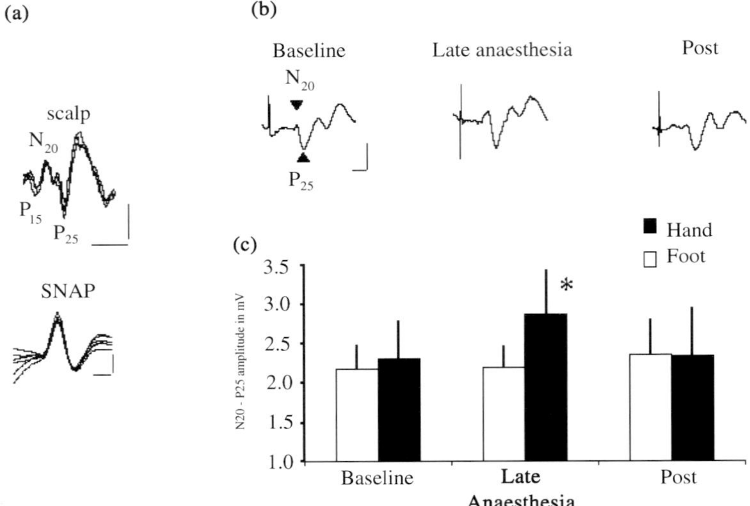

Fig. 5. Components of scalp and sensory nerve action (SNAP) potentials (a) evoked by cutaneous stimulation of digits 2–4 in the non-deafferented left hand measured with surface electrodes over the wrist. Calibration bars vertical: 2 (V, horizontal: 10 ms. In (b), raw data illustrating N20-P25 amplitudes as a function of hand anaesthesia (baseline, late anaesthesia, and post anaesthesia). Calibration bars vertical: 2 (V, horizontal: 10 ms. (c) Group mean (+ SEM) N20-P25 amplitudes with hand ($n = 10$) or foot anaesthesia ($n = 7$) (* $F_{2,10} = 4.2$, $p < 0.01$). Permission for reprint from Werhahn et al., 2002b was obtained by NPG.

Such contention is consistent with the finding of enlarged receptive fields (Calford and Tweedale, 1990) and increased regional cerebral blood flow (rCBF) in the sensorimotor cortex ipsilateral to an acutely deafferented hand (Sadato et al., 1995). It is possible that unmasked intracortical horizontal connections within the somatosensory cortex underlie behavioural gains in a way similar to that shown to mediate behavioural improvements in the visual (Crist et al., 2001) and motor (Rioult-Pedotti et al., 1998) cortex. The precise site within the cortex where this interaction occurs remains to be determined. There are direct interhemispheric connections linking the primary motor cortices and it has been proposed that they could exert inhibitory influences on homotopic sites in the contralateral hemisphere (Asanuma and Okudo, 1962; Ferbert et al., 1992; Di Lazzaro et al., 1999; Hanajima et al., 2001). Such connections could be the substrate for the transfer of INB-induced cortical excitability changes between homologous body part representations. For example, a reduction of the interhemispheric inhibitory drive through deafferentation could lead to disinhibition of contralateral motor areas. However, anatomical commissural connections linking hand representations in both primary motor cortex (Jones and Powell, 1969a; Jenny, 1979) and in the primary somatosensory areas 3b, 1 and 2 (Jones and Powell, 1969a; Jones et al., 1979; Killackey et al., 1983) are sparse. Alternative interhemispheric pathways mediating this effect include those linking the supplementary motor areas, which have denser commissural projections between the hand representations than the primary motor cortex (Jones and Powell, 1969b; Gould et al., 1986) or those linking somatosensory areas 1 and 2 (Jones et al,, 1979; Disbrow et al., 2001). In the latter case, the transferred information could be transmitted to area 4 through point-to-point corticocortical connections (Jones and Powell, 1969b; Jones et al., 1978; Pons and Kaas, 1986). Further experiments need to determine if S1 acts as the single substrate or just as a portal for a corticocortical gating of this effect. Other sites possibly involved include the secondary somatosensory cortex (Disbrow et al., 2001), the parietal association areas (Bodegard et al., 2001) and regions in parieto-occipital junction (Sathian et al., 1997) since all of them are active in association with the tactile perception of a spatial form. Finally, a combination or network of these sensory competent cortical regions could also be responsible for the related improvement of tactile abilities.

In summary, our experiments demonstrate that acute hand deafferentation leads to excitability changes in the ipsilateral human sensorimotor cortex that are influenced by GABA. This transfer of excitability across hemispheric boundaries seems to render the capability of a rapid behavioral compensatory gain through enhanced processing in the opposite representation. Such increase could support the remaining hand's need to tackle increased environmental requirements and is consistent with interhemispheric competition models of sensory processing (Kinsbourne, 1977).

References

Allison, T., Goff, W.R., Williamson, P.D. and VanGilder, J.C. On the neural origin of early components of the human somatosensory evoked potentials. In: J.E. Desmedt (Ed.), *Clinical Uses of Cerebral, Brainstem and Spinal Somatosensory Evoked Potentials,* Vol 7. Basel: Karger, 1980: 51–68.

Allison, T., McCarthy, G., Wood, C.C., Williamson, P.D. and Spencer, D.D. Human cortical evoked potentials by stimulation of the median nerve. I. Cytoarchitectonic areas generating short-latency activity. *J. Neurophysiol.*, 1989, 62: 694–710.

Asanuma, H. and Okudo, O. Effects of transcallosal volleys on pyramidal tract cell activity of the cat. *J. Neurophysiol.*, 1962, 25: 198–208.

Bloedel, J.R., Ebner, T.J. and Wise, S.P. *The acquisition of motor behavior in vertebrates*. Cambridge: MIT Press, 1996.

Bodegard, A., Geyer, S., Grefkes, C., Zilles, K. and Roland, P.E. Hierarchical processing of tactile shape in the human brain. *Neuron*, 2001, 31: 317–328.

Brasil-Neto, J.P., Cohen, L.G., Pascual-Leone, A., Jabir, F.K., Wall, R.T. and Hallett, M. Rapid reversible modulation of human motor outputs after transient deafferentation of the forearm: a study with transcranial magnetic stimulation. *Neurology*, 1992, 42: 1302–1306.

Brasil-Neto, J.P., Valls-Sole, J., Pascual-Leone, A., Cammarota, A., Amassian, V.E., Cracco, R. et al. Rapid modulation of human cortical motor outputs following ischaemic nerve block. *Brain*, 1993, 116: 511–525.

Calford, M.B. and Tweedale, R. Immediate and chronic changes in responses of somatosensory cortex in adult flying-fox after digit amputation. *Nature*, 1988, 332: 446–448.

Calford, M.B. and Tweedale, R. Interhemispheric transfer of plasticity in the cerebral cortex. *Science*, 1990, 249: 805–807.

Chen, R., Corwell, B., Yaseen, Z., Hallett, M. amd Cohen, L.G. Mechanisms of cortical reorganization in lower-limb amputees. *J. Neurosci.*, 1998, 18: 3443–3450.

Cohen, L.G., Bandinelli, S., Findley, T.W. and Hallett, M. Motor reorganization after upper limb amputation in man. Astudy with focal magnetic stimulation. *Brain*, 1991, 114: 615–627.

Cohen, L.G., Celnik, P., Pascual-Leone, A., Corwell, B., Falz, L., Dambrosia, J. et al. Functional relevance of cross-modal plasticity in blind humans. *Nature*, 1997, 389: 180–183.

Crist, R.E., Li, W. and Gilbert, C.D. Learning to see: experience and attention in primary visual cortex. *Nat. Neurosci.*, 2001, 4: 519–525.

Di Lazzaro, V., Oliviero, A., Profice, P., Insola, A., Mazzone, P., Tonali, P. et al. Direct demonstration of interhemispheric inhibition of the human motor cortex produced by transcranial magnetic stimulation. *Exp. Brain Res.*, 1999, 124: 520–524.

Disbrow, E., Roberts, T., Poeppel, D. and Krubitzer, L. Evidence for interhemispheric processing of inputs from the hands in human S2 and PV. *J. Neurophysiol.*, 2001, 85: 2236–2244.

Ferbert, A., Priori, A., Rothwell, J.C., Day, B.L., Colebatch, J.G. and Marsden, C.D. Interhemispheric inhibition of the human motor cortex. *J. Physiol.* (*Lond.*), 1992, 453: 525–546.

Flor, H., Elbert, T., Knecht, S., Wienbruch, C., Pantev, C., Birbaumer, N. et al. Phantom-limb pain as a perceptual correlate of cortical reorganization following arm amputation. *Nature*, 1995, 375: 482–484.

Gilbert, C.D. and Wiesel, T.N. Receptive field dynamics in adult primary visual cortex. *Nature*, 1992, 356: 150–152.

Gould, H.J.I., Cusik, C.G., Pons, T.P. and Kaas, J.H. The relationship of corpus callosum connections to electrical stimulation maps of motor, supplementary motor, and frontal eye fields in owl monkeys. *J. Comp. Neurol.*, 1986, 247: 297–325.

Haber, W.B. Reactions to loss of limb: physiological and psychological aspects. *Ann. NY Acad. Sci.*, 1958, 74: 14–24.

Hanajima, R., Ugawa, Y., Machii, K., Mochizuki, H., Terao, Y., Enomoto, H. et al. Interhemispheric facilitation of the hand motor area in humans. *J. Physiol.* (*Lond.*), 2001, 531: 849–859.

Jenny, A.B. Commissural projections of the cortical hand motor area in monkeys. *J. Comp. Neurol.*, 1979, 188: 137–145.

Johnson, K.O. and Phillips, J.R. Tactile spatial resolution. I. Two-point discrimination, gap detection, grating resolution, and letter recognition. *J. Neurophysiol.*, 1981, 46: 1177–1192.

Jones, E.G. Cortical and subcortical contributions to activity-dependent plasticity in primate somatosensory cortex. *Annu. Rev. Neurosci.*, 2000, 23: 1–37.

Jones, E.G. and Powell, T.P. Connections of the somatic sensory cortex of the rhesus monkey. II. Contralateral cortical connections. *Brain*, 1969a, 92: 717–730.

Jones, E.G. and Powell, T.P. Connexions of the somatic sensory cortex of the rhesus monkey. I. Ipsilateral cortical connexions. *Brain*, 1969b, 92: 477–502.

Jones, E.G., Coulter, J.D. and Hendry, S.H. Intracortical connectivity of architectonic fields in the somatic sensory, motor and parietal cortex of monkeys. *J. Comp. Neurol.*, 1978, 181: 291–347.

Jones, E.G., Coulter, J.D. and Wise, S.P. Commissural columns in the sensory-motor cortex of monkeys. *J. Comp. Neurol.*, 1979, 188: 113–135.

Kaas, J.H., Merzenich, M.M. and Killackey, H.P. The reorganization of somatosensory cortex following peripheral nerve damage in adult and developing mammals. *Annu. Rev. Neurosci.*, 1983, 6: 325–356.

Kaas, J.H., Krubitzer, L.A., Chino, Y.M., Langston, A.L., Polley, E.H. and Blair, N. Reorganization of retinotopic cortical maps in adult mammals after lesions of the retina. *Science*, 1990, 248: 229–231.

Kelahan, A.M. and Doetsch, G.S. Time-dependent changes in the functional organization of somatosensory cerebral cortex following digit amputation in adult raccoons. *Somatosens. Res.*, 1984, 2: 49–81.

Kew, J.J., Ridding, M.C., Rothwell, J.C., Passingham, R.E., Leigh, P.N., Sooriakumaran, S. et al. Reorganization of cortical blood flow and transcranial magnetic stimulation maps in human subjects after upper limb amputation. *J. Neurophysiol.*, 1994, 72: 2517–2524.

Killackey, H.P., Gould, H.J.D., Cusick, C.G., Pons, T.P. and Kaas, J.H. The relation of corpus callosum connections to architectonic fields and body surface maps in sensorimotor cortex of new and old world monkeys. *J. Comp. Neurol.*, 1983, 219: 384–419.

Kinsbourne, M. Hemi-neglect and hemisphere rivalry. *Adv. Neurol.*, 1977, 18: 41–49.

Kolarik, R.C., Rasey, S.K. and Wall, J.T. The consistency, extent, and locations of early-onset changes in cortical nerve dominance aggregates following injury of nerves to primate hands. *J. Neurosci.*, 1994, 14: 4269–4288.

Levänen, S. and Hamdorf, D. Feeling vibrations: enhanced tactile sensitivity in congenitally deaf humans. *Neurosci. Lett.*, 2001, 301: 75–77.

Levänen, S. and Hamdorf, D. Feeling vibrations: enhanced tactile sensitivity in congenitally deaf humans. *Neurosci. Lett.*, 2001, 301: 75–77.

MacAvoy, M.G., Bruce, C.J. and Rakic, P. Effect of prenatal monocular enucleation on vernier hyperacuity in rhesus monkeys. *Soc. Neurosci. Abstr.*, 1987, 13: 1244.

Macdonald, R.L. Benzodiazepines. In: R.H. Levy, R.H. Mattson and B.S. Meldrum (Eds.), *Antiepileptic Drugs*, Vol 4. New York: Raven Press, 1995: 695–703.

Merzenich, M.M. and Kaas, J.H. Reorganization of mammalian somatosensory cortex following peripheral nerve injury. *TINS*, 1982, 434–436.

Merzenich, M.M., Kaas, J.H., Wall, J., Nelson, R.J., Sur, M. and Felleman, D. Topographic reorganization of somatosensory cortical areas 3b and 1 in adult monkeys following restricted deafferentation. *Neuroscience*, 1983, 8: 33–55.

Miller, K.D. Synaptic economics: competition and cooperation in synaptic plasticity. *Neuron*, 1996, 17: 371–374.

Neville, H.J. and Lawson, D. Attention to central and peripheral visual space in a movement detection task: an event-related potential and behavioral study. II. Congenitally deaf adults. *Brain Res.*, 1987, 405: 268–283.

Pascual-Leone, A., Wassermann, E.M., Sadato, N. and Hallett, M. The role of reading activity on the modulation of motor cortical outputs to the reading hand in Braille readers. *Ann. Neurol.*, 1995, 38: 910–915.

Phillips, J.R. and Johnson, K.O. Tactile spatial resolution. II. Neural representation of Bars, edges, and gratings in monkey primary afferents. *J. Neurophysiol.*, 1981, 46: 1192–203.

Pons, T.P. and Kaas, J.H. Corticocortical connections of area 2 of somatosensory cortex in macaque monkeys: a correlative anatomical and electrophysiological study. *J. Comp. Neurol.*, 1986, 248: 313–335.

Pons, T.P., Garraghty, P.E., Ommaya, A.K., Kaas, J.H., Taub, E. and Mishkin, M. Massive cortical reorganization after sensory deafferentation in adult macaques. *Science*, 1991, 252: 1857–1860.

Qi, H.X., Stepniewska, I. and Kaas, J.H. Reorganization of primary motor cortex in adult macaque monkeys with long-standing amputations. *J. Neurophysiol.*, 2000, 84: 2133–2147.

Rajan, R. Receptor organ damage causes loss of cortical surround inhibition without topographic map plasticity. *Nat. Neurosci.*, 1998, 1: 138–143.

Ramachandran, V.S. and Hirstein, W. The perception of phantom limbs. The D. O. Hebb lecture. *Brain*, 1998, 121: 1603–1630.

Rasmusson, D.D. Reorganization of raccoon somatosensory cortex following removal of the fifth digit. *J. Comp. Neurol.*, 1982, 205: 313–326.

Rauschecker, J.P. Compensatory plasticity and sensory substitution in the cerebral cortex. *Trends Neurosci.*, 1995, 18: 36–43.

Ridding, M.C. and Rothwell, J.C. Reorganisation in human motor cortex. *Can. J. Physiol. Pharmacol.*, 1995, 73: 218–222.

Rioult-Pedotti, M.S., Friedman, D., Hess, G. and Donoghue, J.P. Strengthening of horizontal cortical connections following skill learning. *Nat. Neurosci.*, 1998, 1: 230–234.

Robertson, D. and Irvine, D.R. Plasticity of frequency organization in auditory cortex of guinea pigs with partial unilateral deafness. *J. Comp. Neurol.*, 1989, 282: 456–471.

Sadato, N., Zeffiro, T.A., Campbell, G., Konishi, J., Shibasaki, H. and Hallett, M. Regional cerebral blood flow changes in motor cortical areas after transient anesthesia of the forearm. *Ann. Neurol.*, 1995, 37: 74–81.

Sathian, K. and Zangaladze, A. Perceptual learning in tactile hyperacuity: complete intermanual transfer but limited retention. *Exp. Brain Res.*, 1998, 118: 131–134.

Sathian, K., Zangaladze, A., Hoffman, J.M. and Grafton, S.T. Feeling with the mind's eye. *NeuroReport*, 1997, 8: 3877–3881.

Shin, H.C., Won, C.K., Jung, S.C., Oh, S., Park, S. and Sohn, J.H. Interhemispheric modulation of sensory transmission in the primary somatosensory cortex of rats. *Neurosci. Lett.*, 1997, 230: 137–139.

Silva, A.C., Rasey, S.K., Wu, X. and Wall, J.T. Initial cortical reactions to injury of the median and radial nerves to the hands of adult primates. *J. Comp. Neurol.*, 1996, 366: 700–716.

Ugawa, Y., Rothwell, J.C., Day, B.L., Thompson, P.D. and Marsden, C.D. Percutaneous electrical stimulation of corticospinal pathways at the level of the pyramidal decussation in humans. *Ann. Neurol.*, 1991, 29: 418–427.

Van Boven, R.W. and Johnson, K.O. The limit of tactile spatial resolution in humans: grating orientation discrimination at the lip, tongue, and finger. *Neurology*, 1994a, 44: 2361–2366.

Van Boven, R.W. and Johnson, K.O. A psychophysical study of the mechanisms of sensory recovery following nerve injury in humans. *Brain*, 1994b, 117: 149–167.

Van Boven, R.W., Hamilton, R.H., Kauffman, T., Keenan, J.P. and Pascual-Leone, A. Tactile spatial resolution in blind braille readers. *Neurology*, 2000, 54: 2230–2236.

Vega-Bermudez, F. and Johnson, K.O. SA1 and RA receptive fields, response variability, and population responses mapped with a probe array. *J. Neurophysiol.*, 1999, 81: 2701–2710.

Werhahn, K.J., Mortensen, J., Kaelin-Lang, A., Boroojerdi, B. and Cohen, L.G. Cortical excitability changes induced by deafferentation of the contralateral hemisphere. *Brain*, 2002a, 125: 1402–1413.

Werhahn, K.J., Mortensen, J., Van Boven, R.W., Zeuner, K.E. and Cohen, L.G. Enhanced tactile spatial acuity and cortical processing during acute hand deafferentation. *Nat. Neurosci.*, 2002b, 5: 936–938.

Ziemann, U., Corwell, B. and Cohen, L.G. Modulation of plasticity in human motor cortex after forearm ischemic nerve block. *J. Neurosci.*, 1998a, 18: 1115–1123.

Ziemann, U., Hallett, M. and Cohen, L.G. Mechanisms of deafferentation-induced plasticity in human motor cortex. *J. Neurosci.*, 1998b, 18: 7000–7007.

Ziemann, U., Muellbacher, W., Hallett, M. and Cohen, L.G. Modulation of practice-dependent plasticity in human motor cortex. *Brain*, 2001, 124: 1171–1181.

Transcranial Magnetic Stimulation and Transcranial Direct Current Stimulation (Supplements to Clinical Neurophysiology, Vol. 56)
Editors: W. Paulus, F. Tergau, M.A. Nitsche, J.C. Rothwell, U. Ziemann, M. Hallett

Chapter 25

Modulation of use-dependent plasticity by D-amphetamine

Cathrin M. Bütefisch

Neurological Therapeutic Center and Department of Neurology, Heinrich-Heine University, D-40591 Düsseldorf (Germany)

The organization of the primary motor cortex is modified by use (Kaas, 1991; Pascual-Leone et al., 1994; Karni et al., 1995; Donoghue et al., 1996; Nudo et al., 1996; Classen et al., 1998; Kleim et al., 1998; Rioult-Pedotti et al., 1998) a process often referred to as plasticity. Because use-dependent plasticity may play a beneficial role in the functional recovery following injury to the central nervous system (Bütefisch et al., 1995; Nudo et al., 1996) and in motor learning (Donoghue et al., 1996), enhancing this process would be of significant utility. Modulation of use-dependent plasticity by pharmacological agents represents one innovative approach to such an enhancement.

D-amphetamine (AMPH) is a drug that exerts its effect through the pre-synaptic release of the monoamines noradrenaline, dopamine and serotonin and inhibition of their re-uptake from the synaptic cleft (Creese and Iversen, 1975; Boyeson, 1989; Goldstein, 1993; Boyeson et al., 1994). It can enhance the beneficial effects of physical therapy after cortical injury in animal models and in stroke patients (Feeney et al., 1982; Crisostomo et al., 1988; Walker-Batson et al., 1992, 1995). Because AMPH facilitates behaviorally assessed memory storage (Doty and Doty, 1966; Krivanek and McGaugh, 1969; Evangelista and Izquierdo, 1971; Soetens et al., 1993, 1995) through its effect on memory consolidation (Soetens et al., 1993) and may exert a facilitatory effect on long-term potentiation (LTP) (Delanoy et al., 1983; Gold et al., 1984) it is possible that AMPH enhances plastic changes that may be involved in the recovery after injury to the brain.

One paradigm to study use-dependent plasticity in humans exploits the fact that such plasticity can be elicited by motor training (Classen et al., 1998; Bütefisch et al., 2000). Simple, voluntary, repetitive thumb movements in a specific direction elicits reorganization of the cortical representation of the thumb that encodes the kinematic details of the practiced movements (Classen et al., 1998; Bütefisch et al., 2000). More specifically, previous work showed that such training causes changes in the direction of thumb movements and electromyographic responses evoked by transcranial magnetic stimulation (TMS). In addition to the training induced directional changes in TMS-evoked movements, the MEP amplitude of the muscle supporting the training movement (MEP

* *Correspondence to*: Dr. Cathrin Bütefisch, Neurological Therapeutic Center, Institute at the Heinrich-Heine University, Hohensandweg 37, D-40591 Düsseldorf, Germany.
Tel: +49 211 7816193; Fax: +49 211784353.
E-mail: cathrin.buetefisch@uni-duesseldorf.de

training$_{agonist}$) increased and the MEP amplitude of the muscle antagonising the training movement (MEP training$_{antagonist}$) decreased (Classen et al., 1998; Bütefisch et al., 2000). This differential modulation of muscle groups controlling thumb movements points to an increased excitability of the muscle representations mediating movements in the training direction and decreased excitability of the muscle representations antagonistic to the training movement. The mechanisms operating in this form of plasticity share similarities to mechanisms of long-term potentiation (LTP) (Hess et al., 1996), as demonstrated by the involvement of NMDA receptor activation and $GABA_A$ mediated inhibition (Bütefisch et al., 2000).

In the current study (Bütefisch et al., 2002), the effect of AMPH on use-dependent plasticity was studied in healthy volunteers using this paradigm in a placebo controlled, randomized double-blind, counterbalanced experimental design. The end point measure of the study was the magnitude of training-induced changes in TMS-evoked kinematic and electromyographic responses. Under AMPH, the training time required to elicit directional changes in TMS-evoked movement directions was consistently reduced to 5–10 min as compared to 30 min in the placebo condition, indicating that AMPH accelerates the induction of use-dependent plasticity. This conclusion was underscored by the two findings of additional experiments using a similar experimental design (Bütefisch et al., 2002; Sawaki et al., 2002). First, regardless of total training time (10 or 30 min), when premedicated with AMPH, training induced directional changes were long-lasting (more than 30 min). Second, in healthy subjects in whom the training consistently failed to elicit directional changes of TMS evoked movements, when premedicated with AMPH, training induced directional changes of TMS evoked thumb movements in two out of six subjects (Sawaki et al., 2002). One possible explanation is that AMPH reduces the necessary training time in these two subjects to 30 min or less to allow directional changes to occur. In the four other subjects that did not show directional changes with AMPH, the training time may still not be of sufficient length.

Following completion of motor training, directional changes lasted for 10–15 min in the placebo condition but for more than 30 min in the AMPH condition regardless of total training time (30 or 10 min). This result indicates that the longer duration of the training effect under AMPH cannot be explained by a longer training time after the change in TMS-induced movement directions had occurred. Instead, AMPH substantially prolonged the duration of use-dependent plasticity, an effect consistent with the action of this drug on memory processes (Reus et al., 1979; Soetens et al., 1995). Because AMPH-induced shifts in attention (Usher et al., 1999) or vigilance (Spiegel, 1978) or reported side effects had no measurable effect on the training kinematics in these studies, the enhancing effect of AMPH on use-dependent plasticity is not due to differences in the quality of the motor training. Moreover, consistent with other TMS-studies (Boroojerdi et al., 2001; Ziemann et al., 2002) and in vitro studies (Gold, 1984; Bröcher et al., 1992), AMPH did not elicit massive changes in cortico-motoneuronal excitability prior to training, as indicated by the similarity of measures of corticomotoneuronal excitability such as motor thresholds (Mavroudakis et al., 1994; Ziemann et al., 1996), movement thresholds and MEP amplitudes recorded at suprathreshold intensity (Amassian et al., 1987; Ridding and Rothwell, 1997) across conditions.

In contrast to the placebo condition, when premedicated with AMPH, training induced an increase in the MEP amplitudes of muscles supporting and antagonizing the training movement. However, the size of the MEP amplitude of the training agonist still exceeded the size of the antagonist. These results are consistent with the idea that AMPH facilitated activity-dependent plasticity in excitatory neuronal circuits. Changes in cortical and subcortical levels could theoretically underlie use-dependent plasticity described in this model (Classen et al., 1998). While previous experiments suggested the involvement of modifications in synaptic efficacy in the cortical networks representing the thumb (Classen et al., 1998; Bütefisch et al., 2000), subcortical contributions can not be completely ruled out. Similarly, it is conceivable that amphetamine also favored changes in cortical and/or subcortical structures. For example, amphetamine may modulate LTP (Delanoy et al., 1983; Gold, 1984; Bröcher et al., 1992) and if so, enhancement of LTP-like mechanisms might contribute to the facilitation of use-dependent plasticity demonstrated in this study.

In summary, AMPH paired with motor training facilitates the induction and retention of use-dependent plasticity. Use-dependent plasticity is thought to contribute to functional recovery after brain injury (Bütefisch et al., 1995; Nudo et al., 1996). Therefore, it is conceivable that this drug enhances recovery of function after cortical lesions (Feeney et al., 1981; Feeney and Hovda, 1983; Crisostomo et al., 1988; Goldstein and Davis, 1990; Walker-Batson et al., 1992, 1995, 2000) through its effects on use-dependent plasticity. Because studies with AMPH are hampered by the involvement of different monoamines, further studies with drugs that interact specifically with single neurotransmitter systems are needed to address the question of the relative contributions of noradrenaline, dopamine and serotonin to this effect.

References

Amassian, V.E., Quirk, G.L. and Stewart, M. Magnetic coil vs. electrical stimulation of monkey motor cortex (abstract). *J. Physiol. (Lond.)*, 1987, 394: 119P.

Boroojerdi, B., Battaglia, F., Müllbacher, W. and Cohen, L.G. Mechanisms influencing stimulus-response properties of the human corticospinal system. *Clin. Neurophysiol.*, 2001, 112: 931–937.

Boyeson, M.G. Intraventricular Norepinephrine facilitates motor recovery following sensorimotor cortex injury. *Pharmacol. Biochem. Behav.*, 1989, 35: 497–501.

Boyeson, M.G., Jones, J.L. and Harmon, R.L. Sparing of motor function after cortical injury. A new perspective on underlying mechanisms. *Arch. Neurol.*, 1994, 51: 405–414.

Bröcher, S., Artola, A. and Singer, W. Agonists of cholinergic and noradrenergic receptors facilitate synergistically the induction of long-term potentiation in slices of rat visual cortex. *Brain Res.*, 1992, 573: 27–36.

Bütefisch, C.M., Hummelsheim, H., Denzler, P. and Mauritz, K.H. Repetitive training of isolated movements improves the outcome of motor rehabilitation of the centrally paretic hand. *J. Neurol. Sci.*, 1995, 130: 59–68.

Bütefisch, C.M., Davis, B.C., Wise, S.P., Sawaki, L., Kopylev, L., Classen, J. and Cohen, L.G. Mechanisms of use-dependent plasticity in the human motor cortex. *Proc. Natl. Acad. Sci. USA*, 2000, 97: 3661–3665.

Bütefisch, C.M., Davis, B.C., Sawaki, L., Waldvogel, D., Classen, J., Kopylev, L. and Cohen, L.G. Modulation of use-dependent plasticity by d-amphetamine. *Ann. Neurol.*, 2002, 51: 59–68.

Classen, J., Liepert, J., Wise, S.P. Hallett, M. and Cohen, L.G. Rapid plasticity of human cortical movement representation induced by practice. *J. Neurophysiol.*, 1998, 79: 1117–1123.

Creese, I. and Iversen, S.D. The pahrmacological and anatomical substrates of the amphetamine response in the rat. *Brain Res.*, 1975, 83: 419–436.

Crisostomo, E.A., Duncan, P.W., Propst, M. Dawson, D.V. and Davis, J.N. Evidence that amphetamine with physical therapy promotes recovery of motor function in stroke patients. *Ann. Neurol.*, 1988, 23: 94–97.

Delanoy, R.L., Tucci, D.L. and Gold, P.E. Amphetamine effects on long term potentiation in dentate granule cells. *Pharmacol. Biochem. Behav.*, 1983, 18: 137–139.

Donoghue, J.P., Hess, G. and Sanes, J. Substrates and mechanisms for learning in motor cortex. In: J. Boedel (Ed.), *Acquisition and mechanisms for learning in motor cortex*, 1996: 363–386.

Doty, B. A. and Doty, L. A. Facilitative effects of amphetamine on avoidance conditioning in relation to age and problem difficulty. *Psychopharmacologia*, 1966, 9: 234–241.

Evangelista, A.M. and Izquierdo, I. The effect of pre- and post-trial amphetamine injections on avoidance responses of rats. *Psychopharmacologia*, 1971, 20: 42–47.

Feeney, D.M. and Hovda, D.A. Amphetamine and apomorphine restore tactile placing after motor cortex injury in the cat. *Psychopharmacology*, 1983, 79: 67–71.

Feeney, D.M., Gonzales, A. and Law, W.A. Amphetamine restores locomotor function after motor cortex injury in the rat. *Proc. West. Pharmacol. Soc.*, 1981, 24: 15–17.

Feeney, D.M., Gonzales, A. and Law, W.A. Amphetamine, haloperidol, and experience interact to affect rate of recovery after motor cortex injury. *Science*, 1982, 217; 855–857.

Gold, P.E. Modulation of Long-Term Potentiation by peripherally administered amphetamine and epinephrine. *Brain Res.*, 1984, 305: 103–107.

Goldstein, L.B. Basic and clinical studies of pharmacologic effects on recovery from brain injury. *J. Neural. Transplant. Plast.*, 1993, 4: 175–192.

Goldstein, L.B. and Davis J.N. Restorative neurology. Drugs and recovery following stroke. *Stroke*, 1990, 21: 1636–1640.

Hess, G., Aizenman, C. and Donoghue, J.P. Conditions for the induction of long-term potentiation in layer II/III horizontal connections of the rat motor cortex. *J. Neurophysiol.*, 1996, 75: 1765–1778.

Kaas, J.H. Plasticity of sensory and motor maps in adult mammals. *Annu. Rev. Neurosci.*, 1991, 14: 137–167.

Karni, A., Meyer, G., Jezzard, P., Adams, M.M., Turner, R. and Ungerleider, L.G. Functional MRI evidence for adult motor cortex plasticity during motor skill learning. *Nature*, 1995, 377: 155–158.

Kleim, J.A., Barbay, S. and Nudo, J.R. Functional reorganization of the rat motor cortex following motor skill learning. *J. Neurophysiol.*, 1998, 80: 3321–3325.

Krivanek, J.A. and McGaugh, J.L. Facilitating effects of pre- and posttrial amphetamine administration on discrimination learning in mice. *Agents Actions*, 1969, 1: 36–42.

Mavroudakis, N., Caroyer, J.M., Brunko, E. and Beyl, D.Z. Effects of dephenylhydantoin on motor potentials evoked with magnetic stimulation. *Electroencephalogr. Clin. Neurophysiol.*, 1994, 93: 428–433.

Nudo, J.R., Wise, B.M., SiFuentes, F.S. and Milliken, G.W. Neural substrates for the effects of rehabilitative training on motor recovery after ischemic infarct. *Science*, 1996, 272: 1791–1794.

Pascual-Leone, A., Grafmann, J. and Hallett, M. Modulation of cortical motor output maps during development of implicit and explicit knowledge. *Science*, 1994, 263: 1287–1289.

Reus, V., Silberman, E., Post, R. and Weingartner, H. d-Amphetamine: effects on memory in a depressed population. *Biol. Psychiatry*, 1979, 14: 345–356.

Ridding, M.C. and Rothwell, J.C. Stimulus/response curves as a method of measuring motor cortical excitability in man. *Electroencephalogr. Clin. Neurophysiol.*, 1997, 105: 340–344.

Rioult-Pedotti, M.S., Friedman, D., Hess, G. and Donoghue, J.P. Stengthening of horizontal cortical connections following skill learning. *Nature Neurosci.*, 1998, 1: 230–234.

Sawaki, L., Cohen, G., Classen, J., Davis, B.C. and Bütefisch, C.M. Enhancement of use-dependent plasticity by d-amphetamine. *Neurology*, 2002, 59: 1262–1264.

Soetens, E., D'Hooge, R. and Hueting, J. Amphetamine enhances human-memory consolidation. *Neurosci. Lett.*, 1993, 161: 9–12.

Soetens, E., Casaer, S., D'Hooge, R. and Hueting, J.E. Effect of amphetamine on long-term retention of verbal material. *Psychopharmacology (Berl.)*, 1995, 119: 155–162.

Spiegel, R. Effects of amphetamines on performance and on pölygraphic sleep parameters in man. *Adv. Biosci.*, 1978, 21: 189–201.

Usher, M., Cohen, J.D., Servan-Schreiber, D., Rajkowski, J. and Aston-Jones, G. The role of locus coeruleus in the regulation of cognitive performance. *Science*, 1999, 283: 549–554.

Walker-Batson, D. Use of pharmacotherapy in the treatment of aphasia. *Brain Lang.*, 2000, 71: 252–254.

Walker-Batson, D., Unwin, H. and Curtis, S. Use of amphetamine in the treatment of aphasia. *Restor. Neurol. Neurosci.*, 1992, 4: 47–50.

Walker-Batson, D., Smith, P, Curtis, S., Unwin, H. and Greenlee, R. Amphetamine paired with physical therapy accelerates motor recovery after stroke. Further evidence. *Stroke*, 1995, 26: 2254–2259.

Ziemann, U., Lonnecker, S., Steinhoff, B.J. and Paulus, W. Effects of antiepileptic drugs on motor cortex excitability in humans: a transcranial magnetic stimulation study. *Ann. Neurol.*, 1996, 40: 367–378.

Ziemann, U., Tam, A., Bütefisch, C.M. and Cohen, L.G. Dual modulating effects of amphetamine on neuronal excitability and stimulation-induced plasticity in human motor cortex. *Clin. Neurophysiol.*, 2002, 113: 1308–1315.

Section IV

Transcranial Direct Current Stimulation

Transcranial Magnetic Stimulation and Transcranial Direct Current Stimulation (Supplements to Clinical Neurophysiology, Vol. 56)
Editors: W. Paulus, F. Tergau, M.A. Nitsche, J.C. Rothwell, U. Ziemann, M. Hallett

Chapter 26

Transcranial direct current stimulation (tDCS)

W. Paulus

Department of Clinical Neurophysiology, University of Göttingen, Robert-Koch-Strasse 40, D-37075 Göttingen (Germany)

1. Transcranial direct current stimulation (tDCS)

Four years ago, at this Göttingen Neurobiology Conference, the idea of using transcranial direct current stimulation (tDCS) arose in the Department of Clinical Neurophysiology during a theoretical talk on neuronal membrane function. Already attempting to modulate neuronal excitability in man by means of repetitive transcranial magnetic stimulation (rTMS), we began to pursue the idea of manipulating membrane potentials directly by passing weak direct currents through the skull. Michael Nitsche agreed to explore tDCS as a possible alternative to rTMS in order to induce excitability changes non-invasively in the human brain. The first ethics committee proposal was written and permission to start was given in 1999. Peter Wenig, our electronics technician, built the first stimulator. At that time Priori et al. (1998) had already used TMS to evaluate tDCS effects during current stimulation. However, this work did not turn out to be very helpful for us, since the results were quite different from what we found (cf. Nitsche et al., this volume). Since the older literature was not well represented in the PubMed system, it took some time to get an overview, which in the end revealed an astonishing number of animal, as well as human, DC stimulation studies (cf. Nitsche et al., this volume). The main finding, which was demonstrated by Bindman et al. (1964), proved to be that in order to get after-effects, a minimum duration of DC stimulation of at least some minutes seemed to be necessary. With this knowledge, M. Nitsche was able quite quickly to show the first after-effects of tDCS by means of single pulse transcranial magnetic stimulation (TMS). Depending on the direction of current flow, excitability increases or decreases could be induced during stimulation which persisted after the end of stimulation (Nitsche and Paulus, 2000).

The tDCS-induced after-effects developed if the stimulation lasted at least 3 min (Nitsche and Paulus, 2000). Prolongation of stimulation duration proportionally increased after-effect duration (Nitsche and Paulus, 2000, 2001; Nitsche et al., 2003a). Subsequent studies using different methods have added further insight into tDCS-induced excitability changes (cf. Nitsche et al., this volume). An fMRI study with BOLD measurements confirmed that cathodal tDCS lowered cortical activation in interconnected areas significantly, but not in the stimulated motor cortex

* *Correspondence to*: Prof. W. Paulus, Department of Clinical Neurophysiology, University of Göttingen, Robert-Koch-Strasse 40, D-37075 Göttingen, Germany.
Tel: +49 5 51 39-6650; Fax: +49 5 51 39-8126;
E-mail: w.paulus@med.uni-goettingen.de

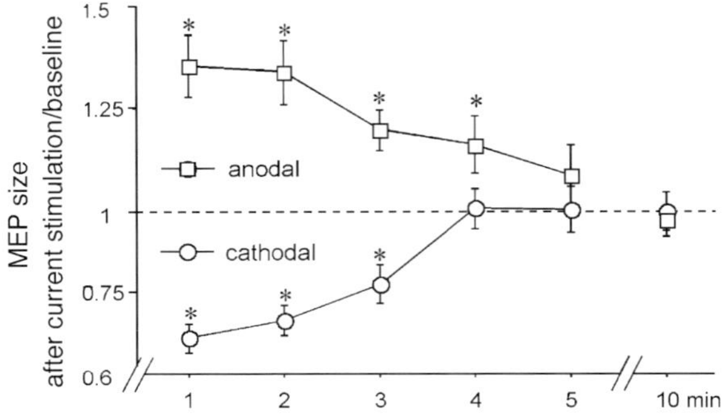

Fig. 1. After-effects of 5 min anodal and cathodal stimulation on the MEP size. (From Nitsche and Paulus, 2000, with permission.)

itself, whereas anodal stimulation tended to raise activation, however insignificantly (Baudewig et al., 2001). Psychophysical measurements (Antal et al., 2001, 2003) in the visual system and behavioural effects (Nitsche et al., 2003b) added confirmatory evidence to the efficacy of tDCS in humans (Lang et al., in preparation).

Does a bridge exist between tDCS and rTMS after-effects? Knowledge about the concept of modulating the neuronal membrane potential may lead to a reconsideration of rTMS-induced after-effects. A first step towards inducing a more direct alteration of the neuronal membrane potential by rTMS could have been made by comparing monophasic and biphasic TMS. It appeared that monophasic TMS pulses produced longer lasting after-effects than biphasic (Antal et al., 2002; Sommer et al., 2002). However, it remains to be proven whether monophasic (or asymmetric) pulses are better suited to induce membrane potential changes than biphasic (or symmetric). Although so far in our lab compared to tDCS rTMS is distinctly less effective in the induction of excitability changes, rTMS still has the advantage that it is restricted to one site and does not bear the possibility of unwanted effects under a second electrode. So far, none have been observed, however stimulation of the cortex at the site of the second electrode with opposite polarity cannot be avoided by tDCS. A possible approach to minimise possible undesired effects could be a relative enlargement of the second electrode.

2. Possible sites of action of transcranial direct current stimulation (tDCS)

In order to gain a better understanding of the underlying mechanisms of tDCS-induced effects, studies should probably focus on neuronal membranes and their behaviour with changing membrane potentials. Since there are no modern membrane studies on DCS effects, much is speculative at the moment. The lipid bi-layer of the plasma membrane of nerve or glial cells is almost impermeable to ions and it serves as an insulator separating cytoplasm and the extracellular fluid. Ions cross the membrane only through specialised pores such as ion channels. Transmembrane crossing of ions is essential for establishing the resting membrane potential as well as for neuronal signaling, which depends on rapid changes in the electrical potential difference across neuronal membranes. Ion channels recognise, select and conduct specific ions, and open and close in response to specific electrical, mechanical or chemical signals. tDCS presumably targets neuronal signaling by manipulating ion channels or by shifting electrical gradients which influence the electrical balance of ions inside and outside of the neuronal membrane, e.g. by changing the membrane potential. It seems unlikely that tDCS distinguishes between those channels responsible for membrane potential changes and those devoted to signal transmission.

Most likely, tDCS affects primarily non-gated or resting channels open in the cell at rest, and voltage-gated channels. Most gated channels are closed when the membrane is at rest, in contrast to resting channels. Gated channels may become involved in tDCS effects after altering the resting membrane potential. Their probability of opening is regulated by changes in membrane potential, ligand binding or membrane stretch. Ligand-gated channels could be affected by tDCS only secondarily, e.g. by modulation of neurotransmission through affecting other cells in a network. Mechanically gated channels will probably not be affected at all. The rate of transmission between the open and closed states of a voltage-gated channel depends strongly on the membrane potential, with time scales varying from several microseconds to a minute. Also, many but not all voltage-gated channels can enter a refractory state after activation. The response of a single neuron to tDCS after having shifted the resting membrane potential is determined by the proportions of different types of voltage-gated channels in the cell's integrative and trigger zones (for an overview: Kundel et al., 2000).

Even if the reaction of a single neuronal membrane to tDCS became clear, within a complex array of nerve cells tDCS responses would be even more difficult to predict. They depend on neuronal geometry, on direction of current flow and on the type of cells stimulated predominantly: some cells respond to a constant excitatory input with only a single action potential, others with a constant-frequency train of action potentials or with accelerating or decelerating trains of action potentials. In order to target other cells, alternating cathodal with anodal stimulation might be sensible, as they are neurons in which a preceding steady hyperpolarizing input makes the cell less responsive to a succeeding excitatory input and vice versa.

Finally, tDCS may also affect signal transmission to adjacent nerve cells at electrical synapses via gap-junction channels. Gap junctions are found between glial cells as well as between neurons. Electrical transmission is particularly rapid and useful for connecting larger groups of neurons or glial cells. In the latter, the gap junctions seem to mediate both intercellular and intracellular communication. However, the role of glial cells in tDCS effects still has to be determined.

3. Role of neuropharmacology in evaluating tDCS effects in man

The hypothesis that membrane potential changes are involved in the effects of tDCS has been tested in a first human experiment by blocking voltage-dependent Na-channels with the antiepileptic drug carbamazepine (Liebetanz et al., 2002). Here we were able to block anodal excitatory after-effects, whereas inhibitory cathode-induced after-effects were left unchanged. Apart from membrane potential changes, chemical neurotransmission, either pre- or postsynaptically, may also play a role in tDCS effects (Liebetanz et al., 2002) (Fig. 3).

We think that pharmacological studies of tDCS should be separated into three groups. Effects *during*: (i) tDCS may behave differently from short-; (ii) and long-lasting; (iii) tDCS after-effects. Longer lasting, but not short-lasting, effects may include the build-up of new synapses (Engert and Bonhoeffer, 1999), and should therefore be looked at separately. Two of the most relevant neuronal functions in the latter context are long-term potentiation (LTP) and long-term depression (LTD), for years well investigated in neuronal slice preparations. LTP and LTD share at least common characteristics with tDCS regarding the duration of after-effects (Nitsche and Paulus, 2000, 2001).[1] LTP requires the activation of NMDA receptors by glutamate. Therefore, the proof that NMDA antagonists cancelled tDCS after-effects would allow to assume an involvement of an LTP-like mechanism. According to this hypothesis, the afore-mentioned pharmacological study by our group also revealed, that the NMDA antagonist Dextromethor-phan, an anti-coughing drug, which has been widely used in the past as an NMDA antagonist in human studies (e.g. Ziemann et al., 1998), abolished tDCS-induced after-effects (Liebetanz et al., 2002). So far, the glutamatergic system, in particular NMDA receptors, seems to be necessary for induction and maintenance of neuroplastic after-effects, excitability enhancement as well as diminution (Liebetanz et al., 2002). Nevertheless, during almost every reviewing process we were cautioned by the reviewers concerning possible links to LTP and LDP, simply due to the fact that both have been defined on the cellular level and not in complex neuronal systems as the intact human.

1 If tDCS effects turn out to be basically interconnected with LTP and LTD effects, the statement by Andersen (2003) "Responses lasting for more than 1 h were not reported until 1973" might turn out not to be true.

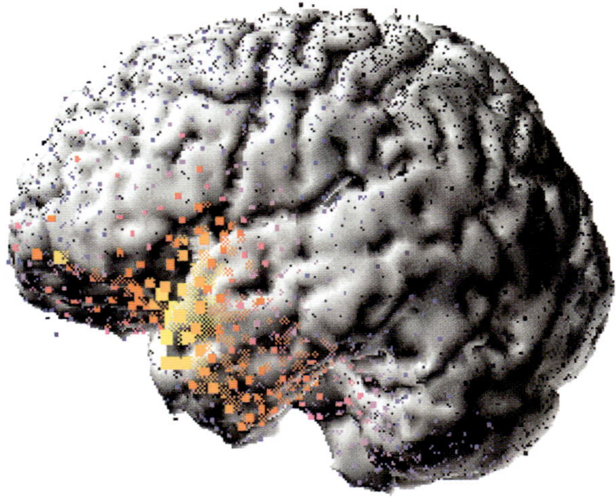

Fig. 2. Recalculated distribution of epileptic activity in a realistic head model by aid of 64 channel recordings. Note that epileptic activity may extend across a somewhat larger region and that in particular opposing walls of a gyrus may be affected. Thus, direct current passing through a gyrus may induce opposite effects on opposing walls.

4. Neuropharmacology and its possible role in overcoming problems due to cortex folding

Apart from the possibility of unraveling receptor and channel effects of tDCS by simultaneous application of specific neuropharmacological drugs, another pharmacological aspect may be of similar importance. This aspect concerns the geometry of the cortex, which will play a distinctive role with regard to the use of tDCS, e.g. in epilepsy (Weiss et al., 1998). Supposing that an epileptic focus extends to both sides of a cortical gyrus, currents passing through this gyrus will elicit a net excitatory effect on one side of the gyrus and an inhibitory one on the opposite wall, or vice versa, depending on the direction of current flow. As has been shown from our very first papers, the direction of current flow plays a critical role with respect to facilitation or inhibition and orientation of neuronal cells.

If an epileptic focus extends to both sides of the wall there will be an unintended effect on at least one site. Thus, a drug which prevents excitatory effects and after-effects in the whole system, might

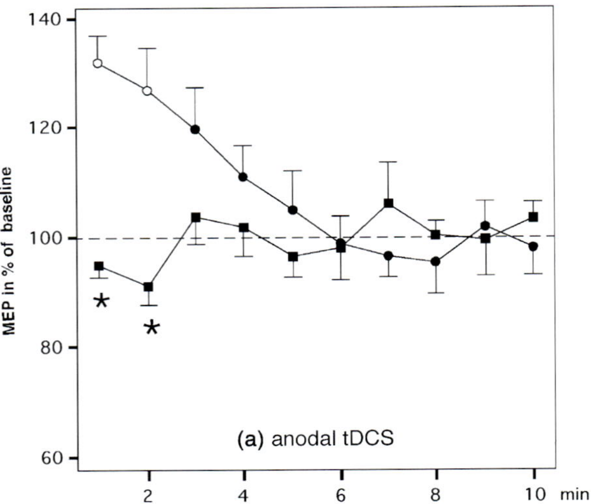

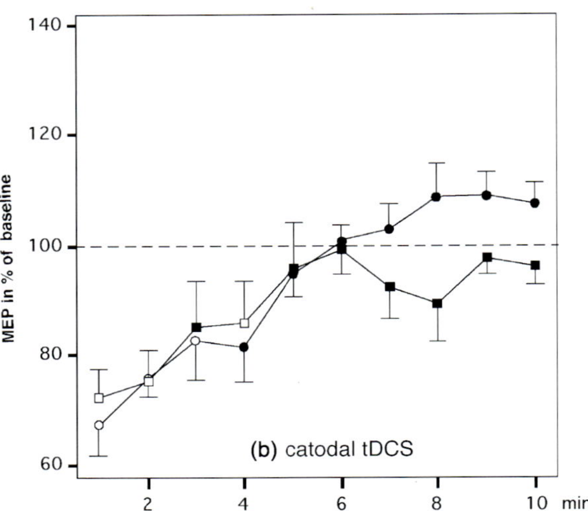

Fig. 3. Carbamazepine eliminates anodal induced tDCS after-effects on the TMS induced MEP, while leaving cathodal effects unchanged. (From Liebetanz et al., 2002, with permission.)

allow epileptic activity to be reduced without the potential of activating it at other sites. As a first approach to this, we showed that all excitatory after-effects were abolished under carbamazepine, probably by blocking voltage-dependent Na^+ channels, whereas the cathodal after-effects remained unchanged (Liebetanz et al., 2002).

This might lead to the (so-far remote) possibility of being able to pass currents in a deliberately chosen

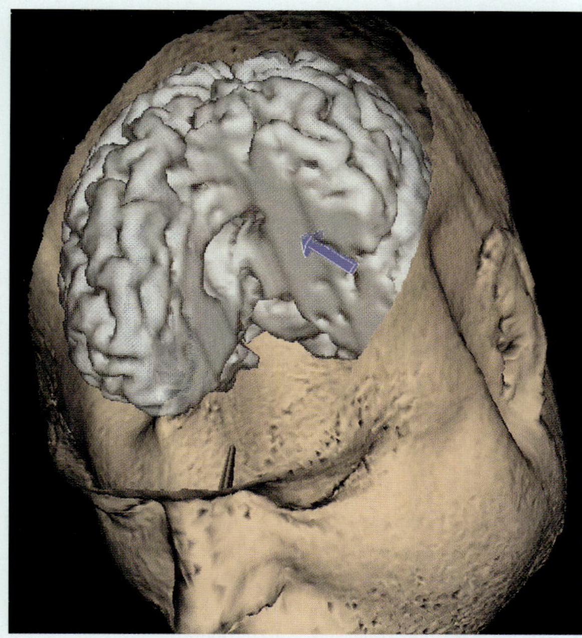

Fig. 4. Dipole orientation (blue arrow) derived from 64 channel surface recordings of epileptic spikes in a realistic head model. Suggested parallel direct current flow (white arrow) for influencing epileptic activity. Passing hyperpolarizing current into an epileptic focus and hereby inhibiting epileptic activity may be a possible future application of tDCS. Nevertheless, although effective in the animal model (Weiss et al., 1998) this idea may turn out to be too simple. Chronic human epilepsies may alter their channel or neurotransmitter characteristics quite dramatically. In carbamazepine-resistant patients the use-dependent block of Na^+ channels by carbamazepine has been shown to be absent (Remy et al., 2003). Also, in human temporal lobe epilepsy GABAergic neurotransmission may be excitatory (Cohen et al., 2002).

direction through the brain in order to induce only inhibitory effects. Nevertheless, it would be most helpful to place the electrodes in such a way that current direction is optimally suited to reduce epileptic activity. A possible approach to this might be to determine the source of epileptic activity, as revealed in Fig. 4 in a realistic, and in Fig. 5 in a spherical, head model. Current flow calculations work in both directions; computer programmes such as BESA® allow optimal electrode positions to be calculated (M. Scherg, personal communication). Back

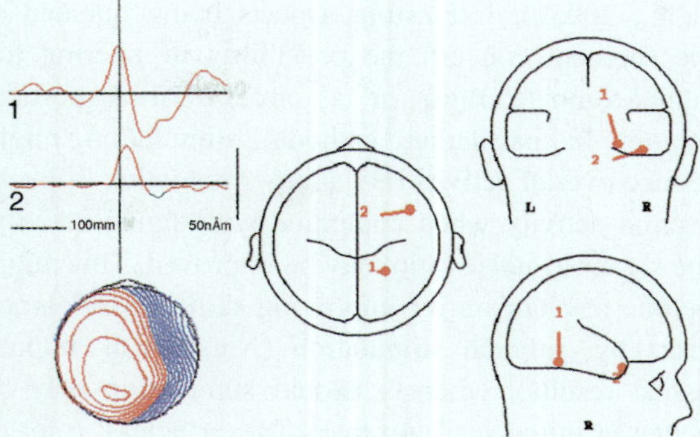

Fig. 5. Dipole modelling of a propagated epileptic spike in a non-realistic head model. Upper right: orientation of two different spike components. Upper left: time course of electric activity in source 1 and 2. Lower left: Projection of electric source activity to the skull surface. The latter method may be used for optimal positioning of electrodes for tDCS.

projection of the equivalent dipole to the surface (Fig. 5, lower left) delineates suggested electrode positions on the skull.

5. tDCS and its possible role in learning

For several reasons motor learning is particularly well suited as a model for studying learning mechanisms in humans: (i) Manipulation of plasticity is possible by a diversity of methods, in many combinations: activity-dependent learning, input manipulation by electrical peripheral nerve stimulation or deafferentation, TMS, neuropharmacological intervention and DC stimulation. In addition, lesions associated with stroke as well as patients with diseases like dystonia, may serve as plasticity models with the motor cortex involved. (ii) Alterations in cortical organisation may be monitored not only by functional imaging, but in addition by movement analysis and by TMS. (iii) The motor cortex provides an easy way to effect evaluation by all available TMS methods.

Here tDCS adds a further tool for manipulating motor cortex function in learning studies. The stable excitability increase or decrease which can so far be achieved for about 1 h allows us to study learning processes during increased or decreased motor cortex excitability (see Lang et al., this volume; Nitsche et al., 2003b). Interesting aspects being pursued at the moment concern the possibility of altering the signal-to-noise ratio in a circumscribed cortical region. In particular, cathodal stimulation might reduce overall activity. By a larger reduction of background activity when compared with signal activity, the signal-to-noise ratio may be improved. This might be one mechanism for improving skill in overlearned tasks by cathodal stimulation (Antal et al, unpublished results), whereas anodal stimulation may be better in initial learning tasks. Nevertheless, a lot of work remains to be done in order to categorise tDCS effects in such areas as homosynaptic or heterosynaptic mechanisms (Bailey et al., 2000) or others.

6. Summary and conclusions

tDCS appears to be a promising tool in neuroplasticity research with some tentative perspectives in clinical neurophysiology. The next steps to be carried out encompass better histological safety data. In order to preclude the possibility of neuronal damage, extending tDCS duration should be limited until more direct safety criteria are available than those derived from Agnew and McCreery (1987) (cf. Nitsche et al, this volume). Safe stimulation protocols have to be developed which allow an extension of the duration of after-effects towards a somewhat permanent state, supposing a beneficial effect can be found in neurological diseases or in neurorehabilitation.

References

Antal, A., Nitsche, M.A. and Paulus, W. External modulation of visual perception in humans. *NeuroReport*, 2001, 12: 3553–3555.

Antal, A., Kincses, T.Z., Nitsche, M.A., Bartfai, O., Demmer, I., Sommer, M. et al. Pulse configuration-dependent effects of repetitive transcranial magnetic stimulation on visual perception. *NeuroReport*, 2002, 13: 2229–2233.

Antal, A., Kincses, T.Z., Nitsche, M.A. and Paulus, W. Manipulation of phosphene thresholds by transcranial direct current stimulation in man. *Exp. Brain Res.*, 2003.

Bailey, C.H., Giustetto, M., Huang, Y.Y., Hawkins, R.D. and Kandel, E.R. Is heterosynaptic modulation essential for stabilizing Hebbian plasticity and memory? *Nat. Rev. Neurosci.*, 2000, 1: 11–20.

Baudewig, J., Nitsche, M.A., Paulus, W. and Frahm, J. Regional modulation of BOLD MRI responses to human sensorimotor activation by transcranial direct current stimulation. *Magn. Reson. Med.*, 2001, 45: 196–201.

Bindman, L.J., Lippold, O.C.J. and Redfearn, J.W.T. Comparison of the effects on electrocortical activity of general body cooling and local cooling of the surface of the brain. *Electroencephalogr. Clin. Neurophysiol.*, 1962a, 15: 238–245.

Bindman, L.J., Lippold, O.C.J. and Redfearn, J.W.T. The prolonged after-action of polarizing currents on the sensory cerebral cortex. *J. Physiol. (Lond.)*, 1962b, 162: 45 P.

Bindmann, L.J., Lippold, O.C. and Redfearn, J.W.T. The action of brief polarizing currents on the cerebral cortex of the rat (1) during current flow and (2) in the production of long-lasting after-effects. *J. Physiology*, 1964, 172: 369–382.

Cohen, I., Navarro, V., Clemenceau, S., Baulac, M. and Miles, R. On the origin of interictal activity in human temporal lobe epilepsy in vitro. *Science*, 2002, 298: 1418–1421.

Engert, F. and Bonhoeffer, T. Dendritic spine changes associated with hippocampal long-term synaptic plasticity. *Nature*, 1999, 399: 66–70.

Kundel, E.R., Schwan, J.H. and Jessell, T.M. *Principles of neural science*. McGraw Hill, New York, 2000.

Liebetanz, D., Nitsche, M.A., Tergau, F. and Paulus, W. Pharmacological approach to the mechanisms of transcranial DC-stimulation-induced after-effects of human motor cortex excitability. *Brain*, 2002, 125: 2238–2247.

Nitsche, M.A. and Paulus, W. Excitability changes induced in the human motor cortex by weak transcranial direct current stimulation. *J. Physiol.*, 2000, 527: 633–639.

Nitsche, M.A. and Paulus, W. Sustained excitability elevations induced by transcranial DC motor cortex stimulation in humans. *Neurology*, 2001, 57: 1899–1901.

Nitsche, M.A., Nitsche, M.S., Klein, C.C., Tergau, F., Rothwell, J.C. and Paulus, W. Level of action of cathodal DC polarisation induced inhibition of the human motor cortex. *Clin. Neurophysiol.*, 2003a, 114: 600–604.

Nitsche, M.A., Schauenburg, A., Lang, N., Liebetanz, D., Exner, C., Paulus, W. et al. Facilitation of implicit motor learning by weak transcranial direct current stimulation of the primary motor cortex in the human. *J. Cog. Neurosci.*, 2003b, 15: 619–626.

Priori, A., Berardelli, A., Rona, S., Accornero, N. and Manfredi, M. Polarization of the human motor cortex through the scalp. *Neuroreport*, 1998, 9: 2257–2260.

Remy, S., Gabriel, S., Urban, B.W., Dietrich, D., Lehmann, T.N., Elger, C. et al. A novel mechanism underlying drug resistance in chronic epilepsy. *Ann. Neurol.*, 2003, 53: 469–479.

Sommer, M., Lang, N., Tergau, F., Paulus, W. Neuronal tissue polarization induced by repetitive transcranial magnetic stimulation? *Neuroreport*, 2002, 13: 809–811.

Weiss, S.R., Eidsath, A., Li, X.L., Heynen, T. and Post, R.M. Quenching revisited: low level direct current inhibits amygdala-kindled seizures. *Exp. Neurol.*, 1998, 154: 185–192.

Transcranial Magnetic Stimulation and Transcranial Direct Current Stimulation (Supplements to Clinical Neurophysiology, Vol. 56)
Editors: W. Paulus, F. Tergau, M.A. Nitsche, J.C. Rothwell, U. Ziemann, M. Hallett

Chapter 27

Modulation of cortical excitability by weak direct current stimulation – technical, safety and functional aspects

Michael A. Nitsche*, David Liebetanz, Andrea Antal, Nicolas Lang, Frithjof Tergau and Walter Paulus

Department of Clinical Neurophysiology, University of Göttingen, Robert Koch Strasse 40, D-37075 Götingen (Germany)

1. Introduction

Achieving short- or even long-term neuroplastic functional modifications of cortical networks through the modulation of activity and excitability of neuronal ensembles has been the focus of many research activities in the past decades (Bennett, 2000). The application of weak direct currents has been shown to elicit cortical excitability and activity shifts during, and after the end of stimulation in animals and humans, and thus could evolve as a promising technique in this field of research. In animals, intracortical or epidural electrodes have been used for DC stimulation. However, even transcranial application of weak direct currents can induce an intracerebral current flow sufficiently large to achieve the intended effects. In monkeys it has been shown that approximately 50% of the transcranially applied currents enter the brain through the skull (Rush and Driscoll, 1968), and these results have been replicated in humans (Dymond et al., 1975). Thus, weak direct currents can be applied to humans non-invasively, transcranially and painlessly to induce focal, prolonged, but yet reversible shifts of cortical excitability, the duration and direction of which depend on stimulation duration and polarity (Nitsche and Paulus, 2000, 2001; Nitsche et al., 2003a). This chapter will first give an overview of the basic and functional effects of weak direct current stimulation in animals and in humans. Then, technical considerations will be discussed and available safety criteria, which are expected to prevent harmful or unwanted effects of the stimulation will be summarised.

2. Basic effects

2.1. Physical parameters

The combination of current strength, size of stimulated area and stimulation duration are thought to be the relevant parameters that describe stimulation

* *Correspondence to*: Dr. Michael A. Nitsche, Department of Clinical Neurophysiology, University of Göttingen, Robert Koch Strasse 40, D-37075 Göttingen, Germany.
Tel: +49-551-396650; Fax: +49-551-3918126;
E-mail: mnitsch1@gwdg.de

strength and thus, control the efficacy of stimulation (Agnew and McCreery, 1987). A formula referring directly to these parameters is total charge ((current strength (A)/area (cm^2)* stimulation duration (s)) (Yuen et al., 1981). This formula was originally developed for suprathreshold electrical stimulation. It seems to be appropriate also for weak subthreshold DC stimulation, because different current intensities per area will result in different amounts of neuronal de- or hyperpolarisation and it has been shown that different stimulation durations result in a different time course of the induced excitability shifts (Bindman et al., 1964; Nitsche and Paulus, 2000). Thus, in the following sections, stimulation strength will be referred to as total charge wherever it is possible to deduce these from the original studies (Tables 1 and 2). Apart from the above-mentioned physiological reasons, this is carried out in order to render stimulation paradigms used in different studies comparable and because for total charge at least preliminary limits for a safe stimulation are available (Yuen et al., 1981). However, it has to be kept in mind that different charges combined with different stimulation durations, which result in an identical total charge, may result in qualitatively quite different effects: a short strong stimulation may induce supra-threshold depolarisation, whereas a weak prolonged stimulation may fail to elicit action potentials of a given neuron, both resulting in identical total charge. Thus, the comparability of different studies in behalf of total charge is limited and should always be qualified by a separate equation of current density and stimulation duration.

Another parameter which seems to be important to achieve the intended stimulation effects – most probably by determing the neuronal population stimulated – is the direction of current flow, which is defined generally by the electrode positions and polarity. As shown for the human motor cortex, only two of six different electrode position combinations tested so far effectively influenced cortical excitability, and the effective combinations may have modulated different neuronal populations (Priori et al., 1998, see below; Nitsche and Paulus, 2000). This has not been tested in animals directly, but it was shown that differently oriented neuronal populations were influenced differently by a constant current flow direction (Creutzfeldt et al., 1964; Purpura and McMurtry, 1965), which strongly suggests that the relation of current flow direction and neuronal orientation is crucial for the efficacy of stimulation and the direction of the current-induced changes of cortical excitability and activity.

2.2. Cortical excitability and activity changes during DC stimulation

For the human motor cortex, it was shown recently that short transcranial direct current stimulation (tDCS) with a total charge of 0.00014 Ci/cm^2 can change motor cortical excitability during stimulation: anodal stimulation *diminished* cortico-spinal excitability, as revealed by single pulse TMS, if it was preceded by cathodal stimulation and a motor cortex-chin electrode montage was used (Priori et al., 1998). By using a different electrode montage (motor cortex-contralateral orbit) under otherwise similar stimulation conditions (Table 1), an excitability *enhancement* by anodal and a respective *diminution* by cathodal stimulation was found by studies of another group (Nitsche and Paulus, 2000). These changes were in the range of 30% compared to baseline. Since electrode position was the only variable which differed substantially between these studies, it most probably caused the discrepant effects.

More detailed knowledge about the origin and effects of cortical DC stimulation has been gained from early animal experiments. For the visual and motor cortex of the cat and rat, it was shown that a DC stimulus between 0.00013–0.3 Ci/cm^2 increased spontaneous neuronal activity if the anode was placed above or within the cortex, whilst cathodal polarity resulted in reduced activity (Creutzfeldt et al., 1962; Bindman et al., 1964; Purpura and McMurtry, 1965). This was due to a subthreshold membrane depolarisation by anodal and a hyperpolarisation by cathodal stimulation (Purpura and McMurtry, 1965; Scholfield, 1990). However, the results were not the same for all neurons studied: Apart from the dominant net shift of cortical activation, some

TABLE 1

OVERVIEW OF STIMULATION PARAMETERS AND FUNCTIONAL EFFECTS OF TDCS IN HUMANS

Authors	Electrode position	Electrode size (cm^2)	Stimulation duration (s)	Current strength (A)	Current density (A/cm^2)	Total charge ($A*s/cm^2$)	Effects
Antal et al., 2001	Oz vs. Cz	35	420	0.001	0.00002857	0.012	Elevated visual perception threshold by cathodal tDCS
Antal et al., 2003	Oz vs. Cz	35	420	0.001	0.00002857	0.012	Phosphene threshold reduced by anodal and increased by cathodal tDCS
Baudewig et al., 2001	C3 vs. contralateral supraorbital	35	300	0.001	0.00002857	0.008571	Reduced BOLD answer after cathodal tDCS (fMRI, finger tapping task)
Bogdanov et al., 1994	Anode frontal right hemisphere, cathode C3 or mastoid left side	6	3,000	0.0002–0.0008	0.000033–0.00013	0.099–0.39	In cerebral palsy clinical severity, muscular hypertonus and reflex answers diminished, enhanced motor learning even after the end of stimulation
Dymond et al., 1975	Frontal vs. mastoid	90 (proposed)	0.001	0.0001–0.0015	0.0000011–0.000016	0.0000000011–0.000000016	Intracerebral voltage linearly correlated to current strength
Elbert et al., 1991	Vertex vs. ear lobe	1.77	5	0.00026	0.00014711	0.00073555	Improved performance in a forced choice reaction time task during anodal stimulation
Jaeger et al., 1987	C3 vs. C4	0.50	2	0.0003	0.00059675	0.0011935	Improved performance in a forced choice reaction time task during anodal stimulation
Korsakov and Matveeva, 1982	Occipital vs. mastoid	0.79	8,000–12,000	0.0002	0.00025461	2.03688–3.05532	Anodal stimulation. VEP-modulations, slow cortical activity changes, less perception sensitivity
Lippold and Redfearn, 1964	Frontal vs. knee	0.5 (proposed)	Up to 14,400	0.0005	0.001	14.4	Anodal stimulation induces elated mood, cathodal withdrawal and silence, but not tiredness

TABLE 1

CONTINUED

Authors	Electrode position	Electrode size (cm^2)	Stimulation duration (s)	Current strength (A)	Current density (A/cm^2)	Total charge ($A*s/cm^2$)	Effects
Nitsche and Paulus, 2000	Primary motor cortex vs. contralateral supraorbital	35	4–300	0.0002–0.001	0.000006–0.00003	0.00012–0.009	Excitability enhancement by anodal and reduction by cathodal stimulation
Nitsche and Paulus, 2001	Primary motor cortex vs. contralateral supraorbital	35	300–780	0.001	0.00003	0.009–0.0234	Long lasting excitability enhancement by anodal stimulation
Nitsche et al., 2003a	Primary motor cortex vs. contralateral supraorbital	35	300–540	0.001	0.00003	0.009–0.0162	Long lasting excitability reduction by cathodal stimulation
Nitsche et al., 2003b	Primary motor cortex vs. contralateral supraorbital	35	540/780	0.001	0.00003	up to 0.0234	Improved implicit motor learning by anodal tDCS
Priori et al., 1998	Primary motor cortex vs. chin	25	7	0.0005	0.00002	0.00014	After cathodal stimulation, anodal tDCS diminishes motor cortical excitability
Pfurtscheller, 1970	Eyes vs. neck or extremities	5.25	4	0.00005–0.0005	0.00001–0.0001	0.00004–0.0004	In regard to evoked potentials diminished 5a/P2 during cathodal, and enhanced during anodal stimulation; EEG: anodal stimulation enhances β- and reduces alpha/theta activity, theta/alpha is enhanced by cathodal stimulation
Shelyakin et al., 1998	Anode frontal right hemisphere, cathode C3 or mastoid left side	1–6	1,200–2,400	0.0003	0.00005–0.0003	0.06–0.72	In cerebral palsy clinical severity diminished. Muscular hypertonus, and reflex answers diminished, enhanced motor learning

TABLE 1

CONTINUED

Authors	Electrode position	Electrode size (cm^2)	Stimulation duration (s)	Current strength (A)	Current density (A/cm^2)	Total charge ($A*s/cm^2$)	Effects
Wieser, 1998	Implanted electrodes amygdala, hippocampus, reference scalp	0.01	120	0.000001–0.00006	0.0001–0.006	0.012–0.72	Anodal stimulation diminished epileptic activity in EEG, one time psychosis because of forced normalisation; cathodal stimulation resulted in seizure

TABLE 2

OVERVIEW OF STIMULATION PARAMETERS AND FUNCTIONAL EFFECTS DC-STIMULATION IN ANIMALS

Authors	Electrode position	Electrode size (cm^2)	Stimulation duration (s)	Current strength (A)	Current density (A/cm^2)	Total charge ($A*s/cm^2$)	Effects
Basics							
Andreasen and Nedergaard, 1996	Electrodes near slices	0.2	0.12	0.00005–0.0045	0.000417–0.0375	0.0000834–0.0075	According to direction of electrical field hyper- or depolarisation; in distal apical dendrites by supra-threshold stimulation (0.05–0.3 mA) Na- and Ca-channel-triggered spiking
Bindman et al., 1964	Epidural sensori-motor cortex	up to 1,200	0.12	0.000003	0.000025	0.03	Anodal stimulation reduces positive evoked potential (EP) wave and increases negative wave, increases spontaneous activity, cathodal stimulation induces reverse changes, effects maximum after minutes, remaining up to hours if stimulation lasts sufficiently long
	Intracortical. sensori-motor cortex	up to 1,200	0.0000000707	0.00000025	3536.0	4342.2	Same effects
Bishop and O'Leary, 1950	Corpus geniculatum laterale	No information available					Anodal stimulation increases threshold and action potential-amplitude, diminishes positive EP wave, and increases negative wave. Cathodal stimulation results in opposite effects. Dendritic amplitudes increased by anodal and diminished by cathodal stimulation
Chan and Nicholson, 1986	Cerebellum in chamber, electrodes at bottom and ceiling of chambers	1–20	2	0.0002–0.005	0.0001–0.0025	0.0001–0.05	Field strength correlates with discharge rate. Purkinje cell somata, primary as well as distal dendrites and most of the stellate cells showing enhanced activity during cathodal stimulation, but other during anodal stimulation; effectivity of stimulation depends on dendritic/neuronal geometry

TABLE 2

CONTINUED

Authors	Electrode position	Electrode size (cm^2)	Stimulation duration (s)	Current strength (A)	Current density (A/cm^2)	Total charge ($A*s/cm^2$)	Effects
Chan et al., 1988	Cerebellum in chamber, electrodes at bottom and ceiling of chambers	10	2	0.002–0.01	0.001–0.005	0.01–0.05	Same polarisation results in different effects in different layers (hyper-, or depolarisation); stronger polarisation elicits spiking
Creutzfeldt et al., 1962	Intracortical, visual and motor cortex	0.001	0.0078525	bis 0.001	0.12735	0.00012735	Most neurons activated by anodal and deactivated by cathodal stimulation; reversed effect in deep layers and in sulci. Linear correlation between current strength and effects from 200 μA on.
Gartside, 1968a	Surface sensorimotor cortex	600	0.12	0.0001–0.0005	0.00083–0.0041	0.498–2.46	Increased spontaneous activity by anodal stimulatiom even after electric decoupling and cooling
Gartside, 1968b	Surface sensorimotor cortex						After-effect following anodal polarisation can be prevented by application of cytostatics
Landau et al., 1964	Motor, visual, somatosensory cortex surface	10–30 (proposed)	0.25	0.0001–0.0025	0.0004–0.01	0.004–0.3	Anodal stimulation increases amplitude of negative and decreases amplitude of positive EP waves, cathodal effect opposite, in surface and deep layers opposite effect; dependent on neuronal orientation; stronger stimulation results in stronger effects
Lukhanina and Litvinova, 1986	Implanted electrodes caudate, thalamus vs. fronto-nasal bone	bis 180	0.000201	0.0003–0.0005	1.4925–2.4875	268.65–447.75	Inhibition at 300 μA by anodal stimulation, after-effects for up to 20 min

TABLE 2

CONTINUED

Authors	Electrode position	Electrode size (cm^2)	Stimulation duration (s)	Current strength (A)	Current density (A/cm^2)	Total charge (A*s/cm^2)	Effects
Morrell, 1961	Implanted electrodes motor cortex	more than 60					In case of anodal stimulation light flash results in motor reaction, even 20 min after cessation of stimulation; increased motor neuron discharges following an acoustic trigger stimulus
Purpura and McMurtry, 1964	Epidural electrodes motor cortex	5–40	0.04–0.2	0.0006–0.0012	0.003–0.008; 0.01–0.04	0.015–0.32; 0.03–1.92	Positive EP-waves diminished and negative increased by anodal stimulation; reversed effect by cathodal stimulation; below 80 μA no effect on PT neurons; above this values depolarisation of PT cell soma by anodal and hyperpolarisation by cathodal stimulation; in non PT cells different effects; long lasting stimulation (40 s and longer) results in long lastig after-effects
Richter et al., 1994	Epidural electrodes	30	0.08	0.000005–0.00002	0.0000625–0.00025	0.001875–0.0075	Spreading depression suppressed by DC stimulation, reoccurs 45–60 min following anodal or cathodal stimulation; cathodal stimulation more effective
Richter et al., 1996	Epidural electrodes	480	0.08	0.00001–0.00003	0.000125–0.000375	0.06–0.18	Spreading depression suppressed by DC stimulation, reoccurs 45–60 min following cathodal stimulation; minimum 30 μA
Scholfield, 1990	Implanted electrodes	4	0.000012564	0.000000025	0.0019898	0.0079592	Anodal stimulation results in depolarisation, cathodal in hyperpolarisation of presynaptical unmyelinated axons
Hattori et al., 1990	Biochemical epidural electrodes sensori-motor cortex	1,800 10,800	0.0078525	0.0000003; 0.000003; 0.00003	0.00003820; 0.0003820; 0.003820	0.06876–41.256	30 min anodal stimulation with 3 μA increases cAMP level. 0.3 μA decreases it. 3 h stimulation duration decreases cAMP under all conditions

TABLE 2

CONTINUED

Authors	Electrode position	Electrode size (cm^2)	Stimulation duration (s)	Current strength (A)	Current density (A/cm^2)	Total charge ($A*s/cm^2$)	Effects
Islam et al., 1995a	Epidural electrodes sensori-motor cortex	1,800	0.0078525	0.000003	0.000382	0.6876	Intraneuronal Ca accumulation and dark neurones until 72 h after the end of anodal stimulation
Islam et al., 1995b	Epidural electrodes sensori-motor cortex	1,800 10,800	0.0078525	0.000003; 0.00003	0.0003820; 0.003820	0.6876–41.256	NMDA-dependent c-Fos expression increased by anodal stimulation
Islam et al., 1997	Epidural electrodes sensori-motor cortex	1,800 10,800	0.0078525	0.0000003; 0.000003; 0.00003	0.00003820; 0.0003820; 0.003820	0.06876–41.256	0.3 mA for 30 min, 3 mA for 30 min and 3 h anodal stimulation are elevating PKCg. All other combinations are not effective; begin 1 h, maximum 3 h after stimulation. Vanished after 72 h
Functional							
Albert, 1966	Medial cortex epidural electrodes	60 repetitively	0.015	0.000012	0.008	0.48	Interhemispheric transfer task; transfer enhanced by anodal, diminished by cathodal stimulation
Hayashi et al., 1990	Implanted electrodes subst. nigra	1,800	0.0003141	0.000003	0.009551	171918,0	During anodal polarisation no effect. After polarisation enhanced contralateral rotation up to 10 days
Hori et al., 1975	Intracranial electrodes (in the bone) over the sensori-motor cortex	1,800 repeated	0.017635–0.17635	0.000001–0.00001	0.00001239–0.0001239	0.023302–0.23302	Enhanced flight-reflex reminding spontaneous movements after anodal polarisation elicited by acoustic or visual cue for hours and days. "dominant focus"
Kupfermann, 1965	Visual cortex, implanted epidural electrodes	400 (proposed)	0.2	0.0002	0.001	0.4	Cathodal stimulation diminishes learning, but not performance; anodal stimulation not effective

TABLE 2

CONTINUED

Authors	Electrode position	Electrode size (cm^2)	Stimulation duration (s)	Current strength (A)	Current density (A/cm^2)	Total charge ($A*s/cm^2$)	Effects
Kyazimova, 1999	tDCS motor cortex	900–2,400					Changing dominance of two dominant foci shows that they are connected
Lu et al., 1994	tDCS, electrodes implanted in the bone over the sensori-motor cortex	1,800 ten times repeated in 3 days	0.0078525	0.0000003; 0.000003; 0.00003	0.00003820; 0.0003820; 0.003820	0.06876–6.876	Between 1–3 μA anodal stimulation increased spontaneous movement of forelimb. decreased forelimb struggle at 10 and 30 μA.
Luchkova, 1979	Implanted electrodes hypothalamus, thalamus	900–1,800					Anodal stimulation prevents conditioning and EEG-synchronisation
Morrell and Naitoh, 1962	Epidural electrodes visual cortex	600 and more	0.05	0.00005	0.001	0.6	Cathodal stimulation impairs performance. anodal improves it the next day with regard to learning
Murik, 1996	Epidural electrodes visual and auditory cortices	600 and more	0.2	0.00014	0.0007	0.42	Anodal stimulation results in less movement in new environment (positive emotion), cathodal in increased (distress, fear)
Proctor et al., 1964	Epidural electrodes visual and auditory cortices	30 (proposed)	0.0706725	0.0000706725	0.001	0.03	Auditory learning disturbed by cathodal stimulation; anodal stimulation not effective
Rosen and Stamm, 1972	Dorsolateral prefrontal, epidural electrodes	Up to 1,920	0.0078525–0.015705	0.00001–0.00004	0.000637–0.00255	1.22304–4.896	Improved learning in delayed reaction task by anodal stimulation, diminished by cathodal stimulation; continuous stimulation acts best

TABLE 2

CONTINUED

Authors	Electrode position	Electrode size (cm^2)	Stimulation duration (s)	Current strength (A)	Current density (A/cm^2)	Total charge ($A*s/cm^2$)	Effects
Rusinova, 1988	Epidural electrodes sensorimotor cortex	No information available					Induction of dominant focus by anodal stimulation; changes in EEG and behavior are detectable even after cessation of stimulation, but extinguishable, it is possible to re-activate them
Rusinova, 1999	Epidural electrodes sensorimotor cortex	No information available					Anodal stimulation results in EEG coherence changes; reduction of alpha and delta-bands and isolation
Rusinova, 1989	Epidural electrodes sensorimotor cortex	No information available					Motor behavior contralateral to stimulation changes, CA3-EEG changes ipsilaterally
Stamm and Rosen, 1971	Dorsolateral prefrontal, epidural electrodes	Up to 1,920	0.0078525–0.015705	0.00001–0.00004	0.000637–0.00255	1.22304–4.896	Improved learning in delayed reaction time task by anodal stimulation, diminished by cathodal stimulation; continuous stimulation acts best
Szeligo, 1976	Epidural electrodes occipital	45			0.0009	0.0405	Increased negative VEP waves by anodal stimulation; more effective with repetitive stimulation, less time to learn needed in visual avoidance task
Vartanyan et al., 1980	Implanted electrodes cortex, Caudate, reticular formation	1,800 repetitively		0.0000004–0.00018	0.00008–0.0003	0.144–0.54	Motor learning and recall can be improved by stimulation of cortex, hippocampus, Ncl. caudatus and mesencephalic reticular formation

TABLE 2

CONTINUED

Authors	Electrode position	Electrode size (cm^2)	Stimulation duration (s)	Current strength (A)	Current density (A/cm^2)	Total charge ($A*s/cm^2$)	Effects
Ward, 1969	Epidural electrodes visual cortex	1,800					Visual discrimination decreased by anodal stimulation during and after stimulation; effect depends on stimulation duration and intensity
Weiss et al., 1998	Implanted electrodes amygdala	300–900 for 7–14 days					Epileptic seizures and after-discharges reduced for 1 month after stimulation
Yamaguchi et al., 1975	Implanted electrodes pre-motor cortex	No information available					Increased spontaneous movement contralaterally for 4–100 days after repeated anodal stimulation; similar to flight-flexes

neurons were modulated conversely. Thus, in the cat motor cortex neurons situated in deep cortical layers were often de-activated by anodal and activated by cathodal stimulation (Creutzfeldt et al., 1962). The same was found for superficially situated motor cortical non-pyramidal tract (PT) neurons (Purpura and McMurtry, 1965). It was argued that these neurons were spatially oriented in a way that reversed current flow direction through the neuron compared to the dominant type of neuron, which would result in an opposite-direction polarisation.

Moreover, the type of neurons modulated by DC stimulation seems to depend on stimulation strength: whereas total charges up to 0.008 μCi/cm^2 modulated predominantly non-PT cells, higher intensities were necessary to change spontaneous activity of PT neurons (Purpura and McMurtry, 1965).

Apart from changes of spontaneous discharge rate, subthreshold DC stimulation modulated the cortical response to thalamic stimulation in the cat: anodal stimulation enhanced the positive and reduced the negative component of the respective electro-cortical potentials, whilst cathodal stimulation resulted in opposite changes (Landau et al., 1965; Purpura and McMurtry, 1965). Conversely, with regard to sensory-evoked potentials in the rat, anodal stimulation decreased the positive waves, while increasing the negative ones; again, cathodal stimulation resulted in reverse effects (Bindman et al., 1964). Because stimulation intensities were similar in both cases and the position of the reference electrode was proved to be unimportant (Bindman et al., 1964; Purpura and McMurtry, 1965), these discrepancies may be due to spatially differently organised cortices of the species.

Taken together, the reported studies show that during cortical DC stimulation, spontaneous neuronal activity and processing of afferent signals are modulated by polarity-specific shifts of resting membrane potential in a de- or hyperpolarising direction. Those effects can be obtained in motor as well as visual cortices. The direction of change depends on an interaction of current flow and neuronal orientation in space, the type of neurons involved and total charge.

2.3. After-effects of DC stimulation on cortical excitability and activity

It was shown recently in humans that tDCS which exceeds a certain threshold of stimulation duration and intensity, results in motor cortical excitability modifications that continue after the end of stimulation: depending on total charge, after-effect durations from a few minutes (0.0087 Ci/cm^2) up to 1 h after the end of stimulation (0.022 Ci/cm^2) were accomplished (Fig. 1a, b; Nitsche and Paulus, 2000, 2001; Nitsche et al., 2003). The respective excitability shifts are in the range of 40–50% compared to baseline. This stimulation paradigm does not only shift cortical excitability but also activity (Baudewig et al., 2001), and the effects are localized intracortically. As shown by a pharmacological study, the evolving after-effects depend on changes of NMDA receptor-efficacy (Liebetanz et al., 2002). The efficacy of tDCS in eliciting after-effects is not restricted to the human motor cortex. Occipital stimulation can modulate visual cortical function (Antal et al., 2001, in press), and the directions of those changes are identical to those in the motor cortex with regard to tDCS polarity.

In animal experiments, the capability of DC stimulation to elicit prolonged cortical excitability and activity changes has been known for some time. Given a total charge of 0.03 Ci/cm^2, anodal stimulation of the rat sensorimotor cortex induced long-lasting increases in the negative wave amplitude of sensory-evoked potentials and spontaneous discharge rates, whilst cathodal stimulation resulted in reverse effects (Fig. 2a, b; Bindman et al., 1964). These shifts were stable at least for some hours after the end of stimulation. Somewhat shorter after-effect durations (about 20 s) were seen in the cat for a total charge of 0.06 Ci/cm^2 (Purpura and McMurtry, 1965). Because stimulation duration differed between the experiments, being much shorter in the second one, it is likely that stimulation duration beyond total charge is an important separate parameter for inducing after-effects. Alternative explanations could be inter-species or anesthetic differences, which might have prevented long-lasting modifications in the latter experiment.

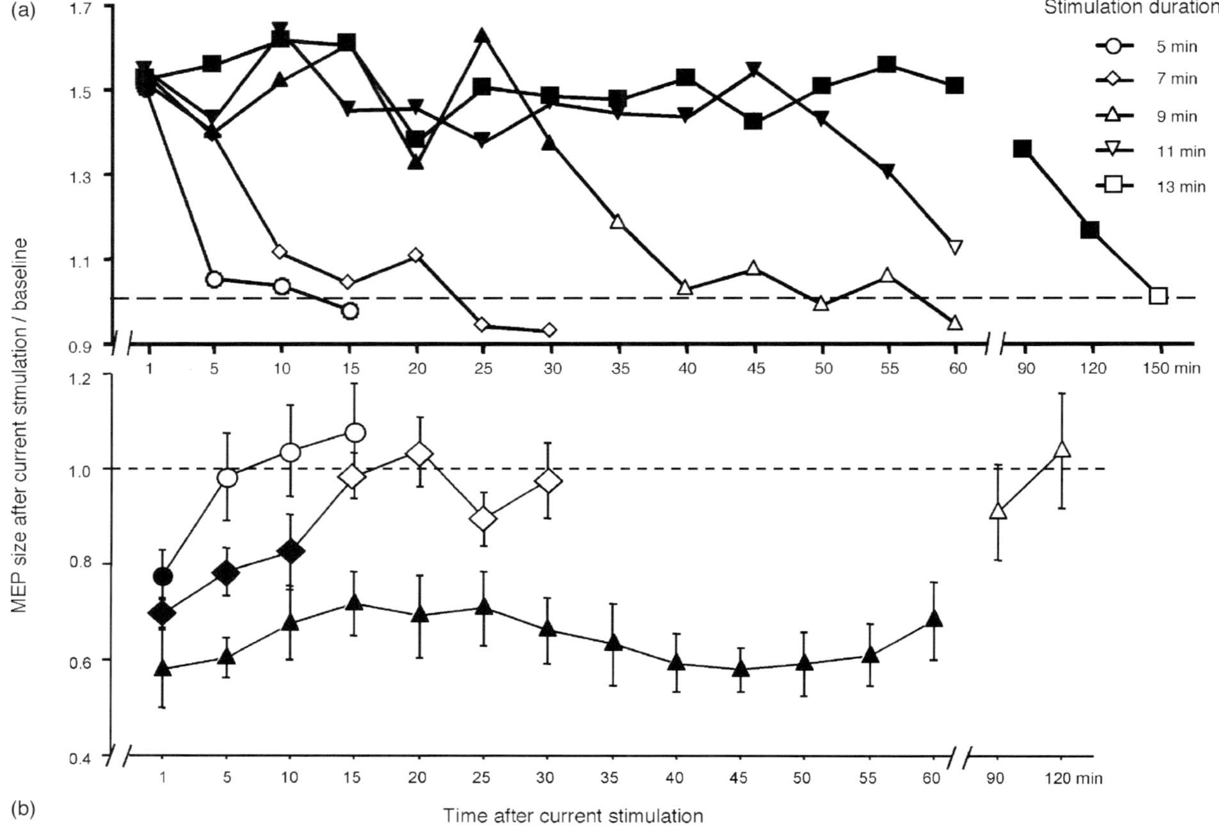

Fig. 1. tDCS of the human motor cortex modulates the MEP-amplitudes after stimulation duration-dependently for up to an hour after tDCS. Anodal stimulation (a) enhances, while cathodal (b) diminishes cortical excitability. Note that 5–7 min stimulation results in short-lasting after-effects, while prolonged tDCS increases the duration of the after-effects over-proportionally (Nitsche and Paulus, 2001; Nitsche et al., 2003a, with permission of *Neurology and Clin. Neurophysiol.*).

Further animal experiments revealed some of the mechanisms that lead to these effects. These are not just electrical phenomena, since intermittent complete cortical inactivation by cooling or application of Kcl did not eliminate them (Gartside, 1968a), but depend on protein-synthesis (Gartside, 1968b). As revealed by histological studies, anodal stimulation modified intracellular cAMP level dependent on noradrenaline and increased the intracellular calcium level as well as early gene expression, the latter was shown to be NMDA receptor-dependent (Hattori et al., 1990; Islam et al., 1995a, b, 1997). These changes were elicited by a total charge between 0.068–0.68 Ci/cm^2, however, lower stimulation intensities were not tested. Remarkably, the modulation of cAMP level dependent on total charge: whereas 0.068 Ci/cm^2 decreased cAMP level, 0.68 Ci/cm^2 increased it.

Thus, in humans, as well as in animals, weak DC stimulation is capable of eliciting long-lasting changes of cortical excitability and activity at similar charge densities. These changes depend on protein synthesis and involve NMDA receptors as well as modifications in intracellular calcium as well as cAMP concentration, and early gene expression.

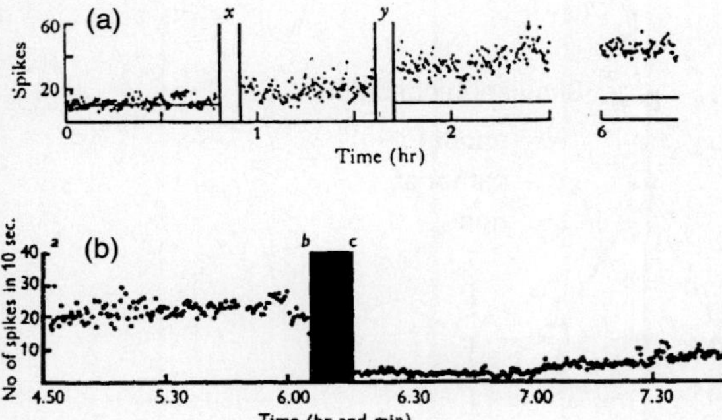

Fig. 2. In vivo weak direct current stimulation of the rat sensori-motor cortex induces prolonged shifts of spontaneous neuronal activity. The time-course of the number of spontaneous discharges before and after stimulation recorded by extracellular field potential measures is depicted. Here, 20 min anodal stimulation (a) results in an prolonged activity enhancement, while 10 min cathodal stimulation (b) reduces it. Vertical bars indicate stimulation phases (Bindman et al., 1964, with permission of *J. Physiol.*).

2.4. *Functional effects of DC stimulation*

2.4.1. *Human experiments*

Human studies exploring a possible functional relevance for DC stimulation can be divided into two categories: those modulating cognitive or neurophysiological functions, and clinical studies.

With regard to the first group, it was shown that anodal stimulation of the motor cortex with a total charge similar to that known to result in cortical excitability changes (Table 1) optimised performance in a choice reaction time task (Jaeger et al., 1987; Elbert et al., 1991) and improved implicit motor *learning* in its aquisition phase (Fig. 3; Nitsche et al., 2003b), most probably due to an excitability enhancement. Moreover, at this total charge tDCS with both polarities reduced *training*-induced changes of motor cortical excitability patterns and re-established the pre-use dominant excitability pattern of a given cortical area (Rosenkranz et al., 2000). The most parsimonous explanation for the latter result is a deactivation of transiently use-dependently activated networks by cathodal and a re-activation of transiently use-dependently inhibited networks by anodal tDCS, thus, both tDCS conditions would shift the focus of excitability back to the pre-use dominant ones. Furthermore, these results imply that the functional effects of tDCS may depend on task characteristics.

For the visual cortex it was shown that relatively strong (up to 3.06 Ci/cm^2) anodal stimulation worsened visual perception in a brightness discrimination task during, and after the end of stimulation (Korsakov and Matveeva, 1982). However, by use of a different electrode montage and much weaker stimulation (0.012 Ci/cm^2), cathodal stimulation, which hyperpolarises the cortex, increased perception threshold, whilst anodal stimulation had no effect (Antal et al., 2001). The surprising difference could be, at first glance, caused by a maximum activation of visual cortical neurons by strong anodal stimulation in the first experiment, which would make it difficult to perceive small differences in brightness due to a ceiling effect, whereas in the weak stimulation condition an inhibition of visual cortical neurons would diminish perception at a given contrast intensity. Because it was shown recently that anodal and cathodal tDCS are able to modulate phosphene threshold stimulation polarity-dependently with a total charge similar to the latter study (Antal et al., 2003), this explanation seems to be plausible. However, it cannot be ruled out that the modulation of different neuronal populations by the respective stimulation protocols caused the effects, since it is known that electrode position and current density are critical for the tDCS-induced excitability modulation of specific neuronal populations.

Clinical studies have so far been largely confined to the treatment of psychiatric diseases, namely depression. Although these earlier experiments included some cortical stimulation, most probably the positioning of the electrodes (supraorbital-knee montage) primarily resulted in predominant brain stem stimulation. However, it was shown by Pfurtscheller (1970) that this kind of stimulation could change EEG patterns and evoked potentials at the cortical level (Table 1) and thus, has to be regarded as effective. Anodal (polarity referring to the frontal electrode) tDCS (14.4 Ci/cm^2) diminished depressive symptomatology (Constain et al., 1964),

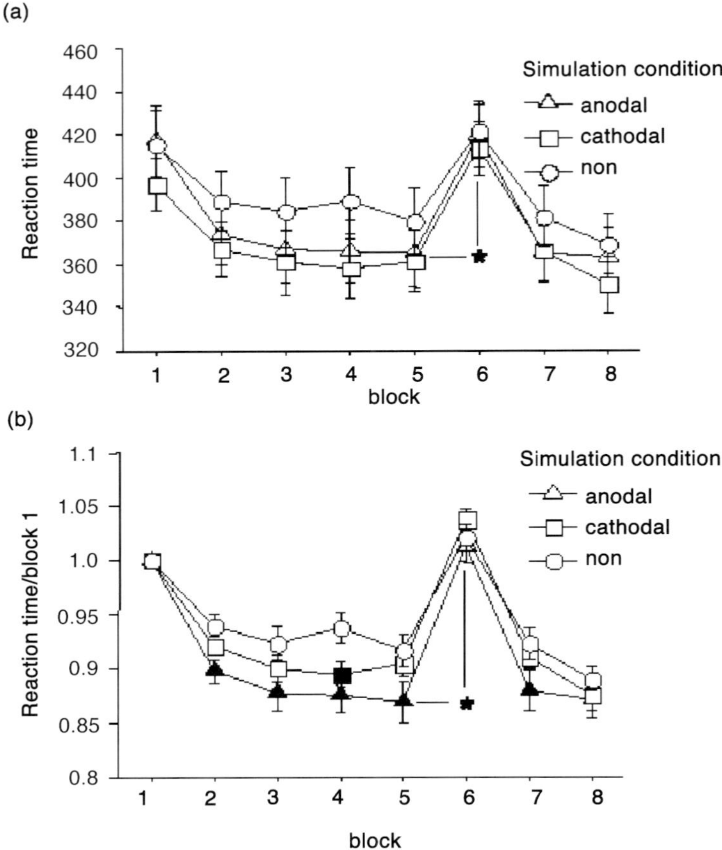

Fig. 3. Anodal tDCS of the primary motor cortex improves performmance in the Serial Reaction Time Task, a standard paradigm to test implicit motor learning. In this task, subjects have to perform a sequential finger movement task without being aware of a rehersal of the sequence. In blocks 2–5 and 7–8 the same sequence is presented 10 times, in block 1 and 6 a random sequence is presented. Reaction time differences between block 5 and 6 are selectively due to implicit motor learning. During anodal stimulation (given during the whole course of the experiment), subjects performed significantly faster during block 5 relative to block 6, as compared by the non-current condition. Figure (a) shows absolute reaction times, Fig. (b) those standardised to block 1 (Nitsche et al., 2003b, with permission of *J. Cog. Neurosci.*).

while cathodal stimulation of the same total charge reduced manic symptoms (Carney, 1969). In healthy subjects, anodal stimulation resulted in increased activity and elated mood, while cathodal stimulation was followed by quietness and apathy (Lippold and Redfearn, 1964). However, these effects could not be replicated by all follow-up studies, maybe because of different patient subgroups, or because measures of changes or other factors that were not controlled systematically (for an overview see Lolas, 1977). In schizophrenic patients, applying direct currents seemed to be without effect in one study (Lifshitz and Harper, 1968). Other studies suggest that anodal stimulation of the frontal cortex (total charge between 0.06 and 0.72 Ci/cm^2) diminished electrophysiological and clinical symptoms of infantile cerebral palsy (Vartayan et al., 1981; Bogdanov et al., 1994), and that anodal DC stimulation of the amygdala with a similar charge density could prevent seizures, whilst cathodal stimulation elicited them (Wieser, 1998).

Although these studies imply that tDCS could be helpful in some neurological and psychiatric diseases, the results are difficult to interpret, because, so far it has not been shown if the excitability changes resulting from tDCS of the frontal cortex or even subcortical stimulation are similar to those induced by motor cortical tDCS. This is not a trivial problem, since neuronal orientation relative to the flow of the current determines the effects of stimulation and it is not improbable that the foldings of the frontal cortex and neuronal orientation in the amygdala result in stimulation effects different from those obtained by stimulation of the primary motor and visual cortices.

2.4.2. Animal experiments

Since learning requires functional changes in cortical architecture that involve excitability modulations, the induction of neuroplastic changes by weak direct current stimulation is an interesting potenital tool to modulate these processes. Indeed, it was shown in some early experiments that learning processes are influenced by DC stimulation: in the monkey, anodal stimulation of the dorsolateral prefrontal cortex improved performance in a delayed reaction time task, while cathodal stimulation of the same region worsened it (Fig. 4, Rosen and Stamm, 1972). The same pattern of results was found by Albert (1966) and Morrell and Naitoh (1962) for a conditioned avoidance task in the rabbit. Total charge varied between 0.48 and 4.8 Ci/cm^2 (Table 2). Thus, an externally induced increase of cortical excitability seems to be beneficial to learning processes, while decreasing it results in a more negative outcome. This is in accordance with current opinions that long-term potentiation, which could be enhanced by an excitability elevation and diminished by a respective reduction of excitability, is the crucial mechanism for the formation of memory traces (Rioult-Pedotti et al., 2000). With regard to visual and auditory cortex stimulation, the results are less conclusive so far: Kupfermann (1965) found decreased learning in a visual categorisation task caused by cathodal occipital lobe stimulation of 0.4 C/cm^2, whilst anodal DC stimulation was not effective. Proctor et al. (1964) describe similar results

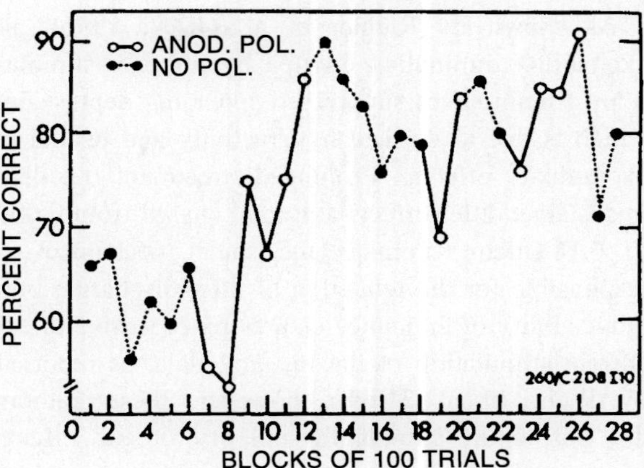

Fig. 4. In vivo anodal weak direct current stimulation of the monkeys dorsolateral prefrontal cortex enhances performance during learning of a delayed reaction time task. Filled symbols represent trials during anodal stimulation, open symbols without stimulation (Rosen and Stamm, 1972, with permission of *Exp. Neurol.*).

for an auditory learning task at a somewhat lower total charge of 0.03 Ci/cm^2. However, Szeligo (1976) describes improved learning by anodal visual cortex stimulation in a visual avoidance task at a total charge of 0.04 Ci/cm^2. Similar to the results achieved in the human motor cortex, most probably task differences or differences of stimulation intensity explain the conflicting results.

Another early branch of research dealt with the induction of a so-called dominant focus in the rabbit motor cortex: it was found that prolonged anodal direct current stimulation resulted in reflex-like motor reactions to sensory stimuli, and that these reactions could not be elicited before the stimulation (Hori et al., 1975; Lu et al., 1994; Rusinova, 1988). It was argued that an externally induced excitability enhancement facilitated the release of flight reflexes which were formerly actively inhibited (Hori et al., 1975). Interestingly, these behavioral modifications remained after the end of stimulation, and the neuronal activity of the stimulated region differed from that of the remaining cortex, which demonstates that neuroplastic changes are induced by this paradigm. Total charges were in the range of the learning experiments, as far as reconstructable (Table 2).

As shown by Richter et al. (1994, 1996), an excitability diminution elicited by cathodal stimulation of brain slices suppressed spreading depression, which is due to cortical hyperactivity and results in excitotoxic effects. Prolonged treatment resulted in sustained after-effects at a total charge from 0.002 to 0.18 Ci/cm^2. Perhaps the same mechanism is responsible for the reduction of after-discharges and inductability of epileptic seizures by repetitive direct current stimulation of the rat amygdala, as reported by Weiss et al. (1998), however, these authors did not report stimulation polarity or the effects of stimulation onto spontaneous cortical activity or excitability. Interestingly, it was shown recently that depending on stimulation polarity direct current stimulation can enhance or diminish epileptic activity in slice preparations (Durant and Bikson, 2001).

2.4.3. Safety aspects

So far, virtually no systematic studies have been performed which are optimally suited to define criteria for safe transcranial direct current stimulation. However, some preliminary statements regarding safety aspects can be derived from available studies. It has to be kept in mind that they were originally developed and studied for relatively strong, long-lasting suprathreshold pulsed stimulation.

Important possible features of electrical brain stimulation, which may cause brain damage, are electrochemically produced toxic brain products and electrode dissolution products on the one hand, caused by the (metallic) electrode-tissue interface (Agnew and McCreery, 1987). As stated by the authors, these factors are not important for transcranial stimulation – as performed by tDCS – with the exception of a possible skin injury, because by transcranial stimulation electrodes and brain tissue are not in direct contact. Since tDCS is performed with water-soaked sponge electrodes by our group, and thus, chemical reactions at the electrode-skin interface are minimised, the only remaining possibility of a damaging effect to the skin will be the heating of the electrode (which has been tested not to happen), if our tDCS protocols are used (Nitsche and Paulus, 2000). On the other hand, electrical stimulation could cause tissue damage by neuronal hyperactivity and brain tissue heating (Agnew and McCreery, 1987). Since the damaging effect due to cortical hyperactivity originally refers to the excitotoxic effect of near-tetanic supra-threshold stimulation and tDCS using our protocols induces only moderate changes of cortical excitability (about 40% as compared to baseline), has been shown in the animal to increase spontaneous firing rate also only to a moderate degree (Bindman et al., 1964), and does not elicit supra-threshold effects, a damaging effect by neuronal hyperactivity is improbable, if these protocols are used. The damaging effect of neuronal tissue heating can be ruled out keeping in mind that this was not the case directly under the electrodes (Nitsche and Paulus, 2000) and that only about 50% of charge/total charge, which could cause those effects, will reach the brain (Rush and Driscoll, 1968). However the situation could be different if the stimulation is applied above foramina, where current flow would be focused and thus, the effective electrode size diminished (Rush and Driscoll, 1968). Consequently, this should be avoided. Given total charge, which is the probably most appropriate parameter – but tested only for suprathreshold electrical stimulation (Yuen et al., 1981) so far – at least approximately comparable to tDCS, the stimulation intensity applied in our protocols (up to 0.03 Ci/cm^2) is much lower than the minimum total charge tested by Yuen et al. (1981) (216 Ci/cm^2), which only in cases of prolonged relatively strong suprathreshold stimulation elicited some damaging effects. Similarly, our stimulation protocols are below the minimum current density (25 mA/cm^2) resulting in brain tissue damage, as described by McCreery et al. (1990). Other parameters studied for suprathreshold electrical stimulation like, charge per phase and, charge density refer to only one pulse within a suprathreshold stimulation session lasting for several hours (Yuen et al., 1981; Agnew and McCreery, 1987) without including the overall applied charge – which determines the damaging effects on neuronal tissue substantially – in the formula. The fact that in regard to these parameters in contrast to suprathreshold electrical stimulation the whole stimulation session will be included in case of tDCS, because tDCS involves only one phase of stimulation, makes them unapplicable for defining safety limits of tDCS. Thus, in regard to the above-mentioned indirect criteria, tDCS should be regarded as safe with the protocols used by our group. Moreover, for these stimulation protocols further direct evidence for the safety of the protocols is available: it was shown that they do not cause heating effects under the electrode (Nitsche and Paulus, 2000), do not elevate serum neurone-specific enolase level (Nitsche and Paulus, 2001; Nitsche et al., 2003), a sensitive marker of neuronal damage (Steinhoff et al., 1999) and do not result in changes of diffusion weighted or contrast-enhanced MRI or pathological EEG changes (unpublished observations). Additionally, the accomplished excitability changes of about 40% compared to baseline should not result in excitotoxic effects, and the restricted duration of the effects seems not to induce stable (in terms of days or weeks) functional or structural cortical modifications, which could be dysfunctional in healthy subjects. This paradigm has been tested in about 500 subjects in our laboratory so far without any side-effects apart from a slight itching under the electrode and a short light flash if the stimulation was switched on or off abruptly. For this reason, and for the prevention of stimulation break effects, which have been shown to diminish the initial effects after the end of stimulation (Bindman et al., 1964), we now prefer ramping for switching the current on or off. Because it seems that current densities above 0.00002857 A/cm^2 (which refers to 1 mA/35 cm^2, it is important to realise that the current strength per area will cause this effect) could be painful (unpublished observations), we suggest that this value should not be exeeded. Nevertheless, for the extension of the after-effects, most probably inducible by a further prolongation of stimulation duration, which is needed for clinical applications, additional systematic safety studies are urgently needed and currently performed in our laboratory.

Some additional precautions should be considered for safe stimulation: electrode montages that could result in brainstem or heart nerve stimulation can be dangerous and should be ommitted. After stimulating the brainstem, Lippold and Redfearn (1964) describe one case of disturbed breathing, speech arrest and psychosis, and it cannot be ruled out completely that a current flow could modulate rhythmogenesis of the heart. Thus, according to currently available knowledge, not only the cortical stimulation electrode, but also the remote one should be positioned at a place preventing current flow through the brainstem. The stimulation device should guarantee a constant current strength, since current strength and not voltage is the relevant parameter for inducing neuronal damage (Agnew and McCreery, 1987) and a constant voltage device could result in unwanted changes of current strength, if resistance is unstable. Stimulation above foramina of the cranial bones should be avoided since this could result in a local excess of total charge and current density due to a focusing effect. Stimulation durations which are likely to result in excitability changes of more than an hour should be applied cautiously in healthy subjects, since excitability changes remaining for such a long time may be consolidated and stabilised (Abraham et al., 1993), and could be dysfunctional. For the same reason, long-term excitability changes should not be induced more than once a week, since repetitive daily stimulation results in excitabiltiy changes stable for weeks or even months in animals (Weiss 1998).

2.4.4. Perspectives

Transcranial direct current stimulation seems to be a promising method to induce acute as well as prolonged cortical excitability and activity modulations could thus evolve as a promising tool in the field of neuroplasticity research.

If safety criteria involving stimulation strength per area, electrode positioning and duration of after-effects are met, the technique should be regarded as safe.

Future studies should evaluate systematically the effect of tDCS onto additional cortices, and should gather information about involved neuronal systems, receptors, ion channels and the dependancy of the effects on stimulation intensity.

For this tool to become relevant, not only for basic research purposes but also for clinical application, it must be shown to induce excitability changes in the human cortex which are stronger, and longer lasting, than those already achieved so far. Before these studies begin, safety studies need to be performed to determine the maximum stimulation intensities and durations that can be applied without causing harmful effects.

References

Abraham, W.C., Mason, S.E., Demmer, J., Williams, J.M., Richardson, C.L., Tate, W.P., Lawlor, P.A. and Dragunow, M. Correlations between immediate early gene induction and the persistence of long-term potentiation. *Neuroscience*, 1993, 56: 717–727.

Agnew, W.F. and McCreery, D.B. Considerations for safety in the use of extracranial stimulation for motor evoked potentials. *Neurosurgery*, 1987, 20: 143–147.

Andreasen, M. and Nedergaard, S. Dendritic electrogenesis in rat hippocampal CA1 pyramidal neurons: functional aspects of Na^+ and $Ca2^+$ currents in apical dendrites. *Hippocampus*, 1996, 6: 79–95.

Antal, A., Nitsche, M.A. and Paulus, W. External modulation of visual perception in humans. *Neuroreport*, 2001, 12: 3553–3555.

Antal, A., Kincses, Z.T., Nitsche, M.A. and Paulus, W. Manipulation of phosphene thresholds by transcranial direct current stimulation in man. *Exp. Brain Res.*, 2003, 150: 375–378.

Baudewig, J., Nitsche, M.A., Fahm, J. and Paulus, W. Regional modulation of BOLD MRI responses to human sensorimotor activation by transcranial direct current stimulation. *Magn. Reson. Med.*, 2001, 45: 196–201.

Bennett, M.R. The concept of long term potentiation of transmission at synapses. *Progr. Neurobiol.*, 2000, 60: 109–137.

Bishop, G.H. and O'Leary, J.L. The effects of polarizing currents on cell potentials and their significance in the interpretation of central nervous system activity. *EEG Clin. Neurophysiol.*, 1950, 2: 389–400.

Bogdanov, O.V., Pinchuk, D.Y., Pisar'kova, E.V., Shelyakin, A.M. and Sirbiladze, K.T. The use of the method of transcranial micropolarization to decrease the severity hyperkineses in patients with infantile cerebral palsy. *Neurosci. Behav. Physiol.*, 1994, 24; 442–445.

Bindman, L.J., Lippold, O.C.J. and Redfearn, J.W.T. The action of brief polarizing currents on the cerebral cortex of the rat (1) during current flow and (2) in the production of long-lasting after-effects. *J. Physiol.*, 1964, 172: 369–382.

Carney, M.W.P. Negative polarisation of the brain in the treatment of manic states. *I. J. Med. Sci.*, 1969, 2: 133–135.

Chan, C.Y. and Nicholson, C. Modulation by applied electric fields of Purkinje and stellate cell activity in the isolated turtle cerebellum. *J. Physiol.*, 1986, 371: 89–114.

Chan, C.Y., Hounsgaard, J. and Nicholson, C. Effects of electric fields on transmembrane potential and excitability of turtle cerebellar Purkinje cells in vitro. *J. Physiol.*, 1988, 402: 751–771.

Costain, R., Redfearn, J.W.T. and Lippold, O.C.J. A controlled trial of the therapeutic effects of polarization of the brain in depressive illness. *Br. J. Psychiat.*, 1964, 110: 786–799.

Creutzfeldt, O.D., Fromm, G.H. and Kapp, H. Influence of transcortical d-c currents on cortical neuronal activity. *Exp. Neurol.*, 1962, 5: 436–452.

Dymond, A.M., Coger, R.W. and Serafetinides, E.A. Intracerebral current levels in man during electrosleep therapy. *Biol. Psychiatry*, 1975, 10: 101–104.

Elbert, T., Lutzenberger, W., Rockstroh, B. and Birbaumer, N. The influence of low-level transcortical DC-currents on response speed in humans. *Int. J. Neurosci.*, 1981, 14: 101–114.

Gartside, I.B. Mechanisms of sustained increases of firing rate of neurones in the rat cerebral cortex after polarization: reverberating circuits or modification of synaptic conductance? *Nature*, 1968a, 220: 382–383.

Gartside, I.B. Mechanisms of sustained increases of firing rate of neurones in the rat cerebral cortex after polarization: Role of protein synthesis. *Nature*, 1968b, 220: 383–384.

Hattori, Y., Moriwaki, A. and Hori, Y. Biphasic effects of polarizing current on adenosine-sensitive generation of cyclic AMP in rat cerebral cortex. *Neurosci. Lett.*, 1990, 116: 320–324.

Hayashi, Y. and Hori, Y. Effect of methamphetamine on rotational behavior induced by anodal polarization of the substantia nigra in rats. *Jpn J. Physiol.*, 1990, 40: 929–933.

Hori, Y. and Yamaguchi, K. Prolonged formation of a cortical dominant focus by anodal polarization. *Med. J. Osaka Univ.*, 1975, 12: 27–38.

Islam, N., Aftabuddin, M., Moriwaki, A., Hattori, Y. and Hori, Y. Increase in the calcium level following anodal polarization in the rat brain. *Brain Res.*, 1995a, 684: 206–208.

Islam, N., Moriwaki, A., Hattori, Y., Hayashi, Y., Lu. Y.F. and Hori, Y. c-Fos expression mediated by N-methyl-D-aspartate receptors following anodal polarization in the rat brain. *Exp. Neurol.*, 1995b, 133: 25–31.

Islam, N., Aftabuddin, M., Moriwaki, A. and Hori, Y. Effects of anodal polarization on protein kinase Cgamma (PKCgamma) in the rat brain. *Indian J. Physiol. Pharmacol.*, 1997, 41: 204–210.

Jaeger, D., Elbert, T., Lutzenberger, W. and Birbaumer, N. The effects of externally applied transcephalic weak direct currents on lateralization in choice reaction tasks. *J. Psychophysiol.*, 1987, 1: 127–133.

Korsakov, I.A. and Matveeva, L.V. Psychophysical characteristics of perception and of brain electrical activity during occipital micropolarization. *Hum Physiol*, 1982, 8: 259–266.

Kupfermann, I. Effects of cortical polarization on visual discriminations. *Exp. Neurol.*, 1965, 12: 179–189.

Kyazimova, K.M. Interaction of two "polarization" dominant foci in the mortor cortex. *Neurosci. Behav. Physiol.*, 1999, 5: 547–553.

Landau, W.M., Bishop, G.H. and Clare, M.H. Analysis of the form and distribution of evoked cortical potentials under the influence of polarizing currents. *J. Neurophysiol.*, 1964, 27: 788–813.

Liebetanz, D., Nitsche, M.A., Tergau, F. and Paulus, W. Pharmacological approach to the mechanisms of transcranial DC-stimulation-induced after effects of human motor cortex excitability. *Brain*, 2002, 125: 2238–2247.

Lifshitz, K. and Harper, P. A trial of transcranial polarization in chronic schizophrenics. *Brit. J. Psychiatry*, 1968, 114: 635–637.

Lippold, O.C.J. and Redfearn, J.W.T. Mental changes resulting from the passage of small direct currents through the human brain. *Brit. J. Psychiatry*, 1964, 110: 768–772.

Lolas, F. Brain polarization: behavioral and therapeutic effects. *Biol. Psychiatry*, 1977, 12: 37–47.

Lu, Y.F., Hattori, Y., Hayashi, Y. and Hori, Y. Dual effects of cortical polarization on peripheral motor activity in the rabbit. *Acta. Med. Okayama*, 1994, 48, 81–86.

Luchkova, T.I. Effect of anodal polarization of deep brain structures on spatial synchronization of cortical potentials during defensive conditioning in rabbits. *Neurosci. Behav. Physiol.*, 1981, 11: 543–549.

Lukhanina, E.P. and Litvinova, A.N. Spontaneous and evoked activity of neurons in deep structures of the brain during their anodal polarization. *Neurosci. Behav. Physiol.*, 1986, 16: 506–512.

McCreery, D.B., Agnew, W.F., Yuen, T.G. and Bullara, L. Charge density and charge per phase as cofactors in neural injury induced by electrical stimulation. *IEEE Trans. Biomed. Eng.*, 1990; 37: 996–1001.

Morrell, F. Effect of anodal polarization on the firing pattern of single cortical cells. *Ann. NY Acad. Sci.*, 1961, 92: 860–876.

Morrell, F. and Naitoh, P. Effect of polarization on a conditioned avoidance response. *Exp. Neurology*, 1962, 6: 507–523.

Murik, S.E. The relation of emotions to polarization processes in sensory systems. *Int. J. Neurosci.*, 1996, 88: 185–197.

Nitsche, M.A. and Paulus, W. Excitability changes induced in the human motor cortex by weak transcranial direct current stimulation. *J. Physiol.*, 2000, 527: 633–639.

Nitsche, M.A. and Paulus, W. Sustained excitability elevations induced by transcranial DC motor cortex stimulation in humans. *Neurology*, 2001, 57: 1899–1901.

Nitsche, M.A., Nitsche, M.S., Klein, C.C., Tergau, F., Rothwell, J. and Paulus, W. Level of action of cathodal DC polarisation induced inhibition of the human motor cortex. *Clin. Neurophys.*, 2003, 114: 600–604.

Nitsche, M.A., Schauenburg, A., Lang, N., Liebetanz, D., Exner, C., Paulus, W. and Tergau, F. Facilitation of implicit motor learning by weak transcranial direct current stimulation of the primary motor cortex in the human. *J. Cog. Neurosci.*, 2003b, 15: 619–626.

Pfurtscheller, G. [Changes in the evoked and spontaneous brain activity of man during extracranial polarization]. *Z. Gesamte Exp. Med.*, 1970, 152: 284–293.

Priori, A., Berardelli, A., Rona, S., Accornero, N. and Manfredi, M. Polarization of the human motor cortex through the scalp. *NeuroReport*, 1998, 9: 2257–2260.

Proctor, F., Pinto-Hamuy, T. and Kupferman, I. Cortical stimulation during learning in rabbits. *Neuropsychologia*, 1964, 2: 305–310.

Purpura, D.P. and McMurtry, J.G. Intracellular activities and evoked potential changes during polarization of motor cortex. *J. Neurophysiol*, 1965, 28: 166–185.

Richter, F., Fechner, R., Haschke, W. and Fanardijan, V.V. Transcortical polarization in rat inhibits spreading depression. *Int. J. Neurosci.*, 1994, 75: 145–151.

Richter, F., Fechner, R. and Haschke, W. Initiation of spreading depression can be blocked by transcortical polarization of rat cerebral cortex. *Int. J. Neurosci.*, 1996, 86: 111–118.

Rioult-Pedotti, M.S., Friedman, D. and Donoghue, J.P. Learning-induced LTP in neocortex. *Science*, 2000, 290: 533–536.

Rosen, S.C. and Stamm, J.S. Transcortical polarization: facilitation of delayed response performance by monkeys. *Exp. Neurol.*, 1972, 35: 282–289.

Rosenkranz, K., Nitsche, M.A., Tergau, F. and Paulus, W. Diminution of training-induced transient motor cortex plasticity by weak transcranial direct current stimulation in the human. *Neurosci. Lett.*, 2000, 296: 61–63.

Rush, S. and Driscoll, D.A. Current distribution in the brain from surface electrodes. *Anaest. Analg. Curr. Res.*, 1968, 47: 717–723.

Rusinova, E.V. Coherent EEG analysis during development of trace processes of the polarization dominant in rabbits. *Neurosci. Behav. Physiol.*, 1988, 18: 50–56.

Rusinova, E.V. Cortico-hippocampal relations of electrical activity in rabbits with a polarization-induced motor dominant focus. *Neurosci. Behav. Physiol.*, 1989, 19: 241–248.

Rusinova, E.V. The structure of cortical-subcortical relationships between electrical processes of the brain during a motor polarization dominant. *Neurosci. Behav. Physiol.*, 1999, 29: 539–545.

Scholfield, C.N. Properties of K-currents in unmyelinated presynaptic axons of brain revealed revealed by extracellular polarisation. *Brain Res.*, 1990, 507: 121–128.

Shelyakin, A.M., Preobrazhenskaya, I.G., Pisar'kova, E.V., Pakhomova, Z.M. and Bogdanov, O.V. Effects of transcranial micropolarization of the frontal cortex on the state of motor and cognitive functions in extrapyramidal pathology. *Neurosci. Behav. Physiol.*, 1998, 28: 468–471.

Stamm, J.S. and Rosen, S.C. Cortical steady potential shifts and anodal polarization during delayed response performance. *Acta. Neurobiol. Exp.*, 1972, 32: 193–209.

Steinhoff, B.J., Tumani, H., Otto, M., Mursch, K., Wiltfang, J., Herrendorf, G., Bittermann, H.J., Felgenhauer, K., Paulus, W. and Markakis, E. Cisternal S100 protein and neuron-specific enolase are elevated and site-specific markers in intractable temporal lobe epilepsy. *Epilepsy Res.*, 1999, 35: 75–82.

Szeligo, F. Electrophysiological and behavioral effects of transcortical polarizing current: comparison with the behaviorally determined characteristics of learning. *Brain Res.*, 1976, 103: 463–475.

Ward, R. and Weiskrantz, L. Impaired discrimination following polarisation of the striate cortex. *Exp. Brain Res.*, 9: 346–356.

Weiss, S.R., Eidsath, A., Li, X.L., Heynen, T. and Post, R.M. Quenching revisited: low level direct current inhibits amygdala-kindled seizures. *Exp. Neurol.*, 1998, 154: 185–192.

Wieser, H.G. Electrophysiological aspects of forced normalization. In: M.R. Trimble and B. Schmitz (Eds.), *Forced Normalization and Alternative Psycoses of Epilepsy*. Wrightson Biomedical Publishing Ltd., 1998.

Yamaguchi, K. and Hori, Y. Long lasting retention of cortical dominant focus in rabbit. *Med. J. Osaka Univ.*, 1975, 26: 39–50.

Yuen, T.G.H, Agnew, W.F., Bullara, L.A., Jacques, S. and McCreery, D.B. Histological evaluation of neural damage from electrical stimulation: Considerations for the selection of parameters for clinical application. *Neurosurgery*, 9, 292–298.

Transcranial Magnetic Stimulation and Transcranial Direct Current Stimulation (Supplements to Clinical Neurophysiology, Vol. 56)
Editors: W. Paulus, F. Tergau, M.A. Nitsche, J.C. Rothwell, U. Ziemann, M. Hallett

Chapter 28

Modulation of motor consolidation by external DC stimulation

Nicolas Lang[a,b]*, Michael A. Nitsche[a], Martin Sommer[a], Frithjof Tergau[a] and Walter Paulus[a]

[a] *Department of Clinical Neurophysiology, University of Göttingen, Robert-Koch-Strasse 40, D-37075 Göttingen (Germany)*

[b] *Sobell Department of Motor Neuroscience and Movement Disorders, Institute of Neurology, University College London, Queen Square, London WC1N 3BG (UK)*

1. Introduction

Cortical excitability can be modulated by constant application of weak electrical currents. Depending on direct current (DC) polarity, neuronal firing rates increase or decrease, presumably due to DC induced changes of the resting membrane potential (Purpura and McMurtry, 1965). If applied sufficiently long, DC can cause excitability changes outlasting the stimulation for several minutes or hours (Bindman et al., 1962). In humans it was shown that motor responses to transcranial magnetic stimulation (TMS) can be modified in a polarity-specific manner when DC is given transcranially over the primary motor cortex (M1) (Nitsche and Paulus, 2000). This relatively new method, referred to as transcranial direct current stimulation (tDCS), has become an interesting tool to selectively modify the excitability of cortical areas for longer periods after stimulation (Nitsche and Paulus, 2001; Nitsche et al., 2003a). It appears that tDCS after-effects are induced by alterations of neuronal membrane excitability and stabilized by NMDA-receptor efficacy changes (Liebetanz et al., 2002). As to the functional effects of tDCS, it was shown that anodal tDCS over the primary motor cortex (M1) facilitates implicit motor learning in a serial reaction time task (SRTT) (Nitsche et al., 2003b). However, different neuronal networks are thought to be involved in implicit, and explicit, motor sequence learning (Honda et al., 1998). Here we address the question of whether tDCS ovcr M1 would also affect memory acquisition and consolidation in an explicit motor sequence task.

2. Methods

Twenty-one healthy, right-handed subjects aged 24–44 years (11 males, mean age 30) participated in the experiments. Their degree of right-handedness was assessed by the 10-item version of the Edinburgh Handedness Inventory (Oldfield, 1971), the subjects gave written informed consent and the study was approved by the local Ethics Committee. All subjects participated in three different sessions separated

* *Correspondence to*: Dr. Nicolas Lang, Department of Clinical Neurphysiology, University of Göttingen, Robert-Koch-Strasse 40, D-37075 Göttingen, Germany.
Tel: +49-551-398457; Fax: +49-551-398126;
E-mail: nlang@gwdg.de

by at least 1 week. Each session consisted of a learning phase and two subsequent recall tests. Recall 1 was tested immediately after learning, whereas recall 2 was carried out 24 h after learning. tDCS conditions (anodal, cathodal or none) and learning sequences were balanced between sessions and subjects.

The subjects sat in a comfortable chair with their right arm lying on a desk and their right hand placed over a computer keyboard. About 60 cm before them was placed a display with a 10-item numerical sequence (black on white, font size 72 pts, i.e. ca. 2.5 cm high) at eye level. Four different sequences of similar complexity were used in the experiments. Learning sequences were "1-3-2-1-2-4-2-1-3-4", "2-3-1-2-4-3-1-2-4-1" and "3-4-2-1-3-1-4-2-1-2", and a test sequence, which was used for familiarisation with the task prior to the first session, was "2-4-1-4-2-1-3-2-1-3" ("1" referring to the index finger, "2" the middle finger, "3" the ring finger and "4" the little finger). The subjects were instructed beforehand that they had to type the sequence during learning sessions as fast and as accurate as possible and that they had to learn the displayed sequence in order to reproduce it later from their memory.

After an auditory start signal (500 ms), which was repeated every 8 s, the subjects had to type the displayed sequence once with their right fingers and then wait for the next signal. The interval between two start signals was defined as one trial. Whenever a typing error occurred during learning, a distinct auditory error signal sounded. In that case subjects were told to continue without correcting their typing. The complete learning phase consisted of 72 trials and lasted approximately 10 min. After every 24 trials, a break of 8 s interrupted the learning phase in order to maintain attention and to prevent development of hand muscle cramps. Immediately after learning, the program was restarted for the first recall test (recall 1). Both recall tests (recall 1 and recall 2) were identical to the learning phase, except that during recall tests (to avoid re-learning) no sequence was displayed to the subjects, no error signals sounded at false typing and only five trials were carried out per recall test.

Motor learning and recall testing were carried out with a self-written computer program run on DOS. The program recorded timing of all key presses and rated presses as incorrect if they were not carried out in the correct sequence or if additional presses were done after completion of the full sequence. All incorrect key presses and all missed key presses were counted as errors. Performance output files transferred data into spreadsheet analysis, where movement length (ML) and error rate (ER) were calculated. ML was defined as the interval between first and last key presses in one trial and ER as the number of errors per trial. Data from each learning phase were grouped into six blocks of 12 trials each (block 1–6), while data from the recall tests were grouped into one block for each test (recall 1, recall 2). The effect of tDCS on ML and ER was evaluated with repeated-measures ANOVAs separately for learning data with tDCS (cathodal, anodal, none) and time (block 1–6) and for recall data with tDCS (cathodal, anodal, none) and time (recall 1, recall 2) as within-subject factors. Paired-samples two-tailed tests were used for post hoc analysis and a p value of < 0.05 was considered significant for all statistical analysis.

For anodal or cathodal tDCS conditions, DC was applied during the entire learning phase (i.e. for about 10 min) by a specially developed, battery-driven DC stimulator (Schneider Electronic, Gleichen, Germany). A constant current flow of 1 mA was controlled by build-in ampere- and voltmeters and applied through 7×5 cm, wet sponge-electrodes. One electrode was placed on the scalp over the left M1 at C3 (according to the international 10-20 system) and the other on the contralateral forehead above the eyebrow. tDCS polarity in the text refers to the electrode placed over C3.

3. Results

With the parameters of stimulation used, none of the subjects reported any adverse effects after tDCS.

During learning phases, ML values consistently decreased regardless of tDCS conditions (Fig. 1). ANOVA on ML during learning revealed a significant effect for time (ANOVA, $df = 5$, $F = 40.683$,

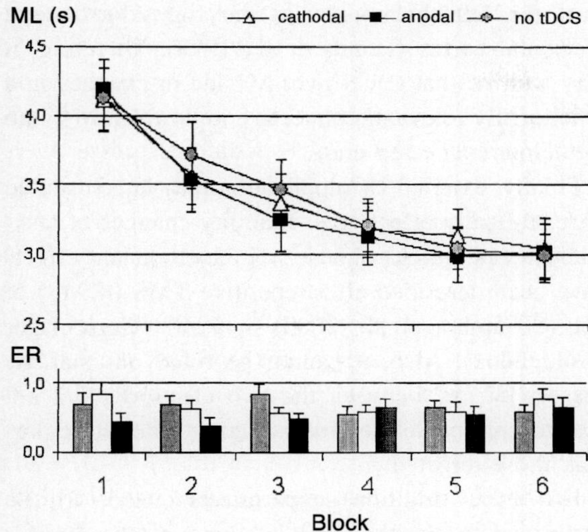

Fig. 1. Motor sequence learning shown by a rapid decline of the movement length (ML) while error rates (ER) remain constant. tDCS has no significant effect on ML and ER during the course of learning. Mean data (± SEM) from 21 subjects.

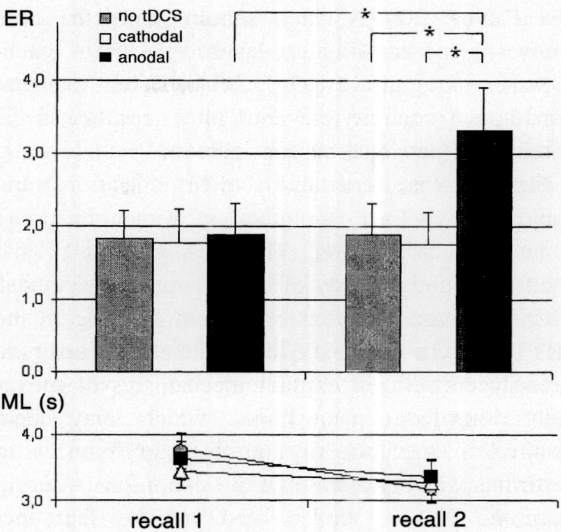

Fig. 2. Comparison of error rates (ER) and movement lengths (ML) produced in a free recall situation immediately after learning (recall 1) and 24 h later (recall 2). In recall 2, subjects produced significantly more errors after anodal tDCS than after cathodal or none, Also, only after anodal tDCS did the error rate significantly increase between recall 1 and recall 2, indicating an impairment of motor consolidation. tDCS had no significant effect on ML during recalls. Mean data (± SEM) from 21 subjects ($*p < 0.05$).

$p < 001$). Mean ML values during both anodal and cathodal tDCS in block 2, and mainly during anodal tDCS in block 3, were slightly lower than in the non-tDCS condition, but ANOVA on ML during learning did not show a significant effect for tDCS or for tDCS*time. In contrast, ER values remained low and fairly stable during learning (Fig. 1). ANOVA on ER during learning did not reveal a significant effect for time and there was no effect for tDCS or for tDCS*time.

However, ANOVA on ER during recall revealed a significant effect for tDCS*time (ANOVA, $df = 2$, $F = 5.455$, $p = 0.008$). Post hoc comparison showed that ER values significantly increased between recall 1 and 2 after anodal tDCS only (t-test, $p = 0.009$) and that ER values within recall 2 were significantly higher after anodal tDCS than after cathodal (t-test, $p = 0.013$) and after no tDCS (t-test, $p = 0.022$) (Fig. 2). ANOVA on ML during recall did not reveal a significant effect for tDCS*time. The Kolmogorov–Smirnov test confirmed normal distribution of all ER and ML values.

4. Discussion

The main finding of the present study is a pronounced recall deficit 24 h after motor sequence learning under anodal tDCS. Performance of finger sequences during learning and in the immediate recall situation did not vary, irrespective of whether tDCS was given or not or whether the current was anodal or cathodal. In contrast, after 24 h recall performance had significantly deteriorated in terms of accuracy if subjects had been exposed to anodal tDCS during learning. This should be interpreted as an impairment of motor consolidation caused by the external DC application. Anodal DC is known to increase neuronal firing rates (Bindman et al., 1964; Purpura and McMurtry, 1965) and, if applied over M1 for 10 min, to produce a motor cortical excitability elevation outlasting the learning phase for approximately 30–60 min (Nitsche and Paulus, 2001), which should cover the time course of consolidation, at least to a certain extent (Brashers-Krug et al., 1996). Still, different explanations how excitability elevation in M1 resulted in the observed effect must be considered.

First, increased excitability in M1 during learning could have helped strengthen movement-encoding connections within M1. This is suggested by the results of another study of our group, where anodal tDCS facilitated implicit movement learning in the SRTT (Nitsche et al., 2003b). Yet the task used here strongly encouraged explicit mechanisms of movement knowledge acquisition, which may have resulted in the lack of significant differences in performance between tDCS conditions during learning. This is underscored by the fact that additional learning-independent reduction of reaction time, known to be caused by anodal tDCS (Elbert et al., 1981; Nitsche et al., 2003b), was also not observed in the task used here. In contrast to learning, a different effect can be assumed for the consolidation period. Here, a lasting and non-specific increase of spontaneous neural background activity may have reduced the signal-to-noise ratio of the task-specific neuronal firing pattern leading to impaired consolidation. However, so far it is not known if M1 actually plays such an important role in consolidating motor memory after explicit learning, as has been proposed for implicit learning (Muellbacher et al., 2002).

Another possible explanation is that functional connectivity between M1 and other task-relevant regions may have been affected by tDCS. It is thought that as a result of consolidation new brain regions are engaged to perform a task and there is evidence that this change in neuronal representation may underlie its increased functional stability (Shadmehr and Holcomb, 1997). Imaging data has demonstrated that right-handed, explicit finger sequence learning, shown as a positive correlation with the correct recall of the sequence, was associated with increased activity in a distributed network of brain areas, including the posterior parietal cortex and premotor cortex (PMC) bilaterally, the supplementary motor area predominantly in the left anterior part, the left thalamus, and the right dorsolateral prefrontal cortex (Honda et al., 1998). Therefore, it may well be that tDCS over M1 led to changes in a functionally relevant, connective input from M 1 into these interconnected areas.

Finally, external DC application may have resulted in functionally effective excitability changes of task-relevant brain areas outside M1. Such distant effects have been described after repetitive TMS (rTMS) of M1 (Schambra et al., 2003) or PMC (Gerschlager et al., 2001). Also, it cannot be ruled out that the passage of DC between the two electrodes did not lead to current distribution affecting other structures than those targeted.

However, addition experiments need to be performed to clarify which of these mechanisms is responsible for the tDCS-induced impairment of motor consolidation.

Conclusions

The novel finding reported here is that external DC stimulation over M1 can affect motor consolidation in normal human subjects, leaving the course of learning mostly unchanged. We propose that the observed effect is due to tDCS-induced prolonged modulation of M1-related neuronal network excitability during the period essential for motor consolidation. It shows that tDCS is evolving into an interesting technique for studying cognition in the human brain.

References

Bindman, L.J., Lippold, O.C.J. and Redfearn, J.W.T. Long-lasting changes in the level of the electrical activity of the cerebral cortex produced by polarizing currents. *Nature*, 1962, 196: 584–585.

Bindman, L.J., Lippold, O.C.J. and Redfearn, J.W.T. The action of brief polarizing currents on the cerebral cortex of the rat (1) during current flow and (2) in the production of long-lasting after-effects. *J. Physiol.* (*Lond.*), 1964, 172: 369–382.

Brashers-Krug, T., Shadmehr, R. and Bizzi, E. Consolidation in human motor memory. *Nature*, 1996, 382: 252–255.

Elbert, T., Lutzenberger, W., Rockstroh, B. and Birbaumer, N. The influence of low-level transcortical DC-currents on response speed in humans. *Int. J. Neurosci.*, 1981, 14: 101–114.

Gerschlager, W., Siebner, H.R. and Rothwell, J.C. Decreased corticospinal excitability after subthreshold 1 Hz rTMS over lateral premotor cortex. *Neurology*, 2001, 57: 449–455.

Honda, M., Deiber, M.P., Ibanez, V., Pascual-Leone, A., Zhuang, P. and Hallett, M. Dynamic cortical involvement in implicit and explicit motor sequence learning. A PET study. *Brain*, 1998, 121: 2159–2173.

Liebetanz, D., Nitsche, M.A., Forgau, F. and Paulus W. Pharmacological approach to the mechanisms of transcranial DC-stimulation-induced after-effects of human motor cortex excitability. *Brain*, 2002, 125, 2238–2247.

Muellbacher, W., Ziemann, U., Wessel, J., Dang, N., Kofler, M., Facchini, S. et al. Early consolidation in human primary motor cortex. *Nature*, 2002, 415: 640–644.

Nitsche, M.A. and Paulus, W. Excitability changes induced in the human motor cortex by weak transcranial direct current stimulation. *J. Physiol.*, 2000, 527: 633–639.

Nitsche, M.A. and Paulus, W. Sustained excitability elevations induced by transcranial DC motor cortex stimulation in humans. *Neurology*, 2001, 57: 1899–1901.

Nitsche, M., Klein, C., Tergau, F., Rothwell, J. and Paulus, W. Level of action of cathodal DC polarisation induced inhibition of the human motor cortex. *Clin. Neurophysiol.*, 2003a, 114: 600–604.

Nitsche, M.A., Schauenburg, A., Lang, N., Liebetanz, D., Exner, C., Paulus, W. et al. Facilitation of implicit motor learning by weak transcranial direct current stimulation of the primary motor cortex in the human. *J. Cogn. Neurosci.*, 2003b, 15(4): 619–626.

Oldfield, R.C. The assessment and analysis of handedness: the Edinburgh inventory. *Neuropsychologia*, 1971, 9: 97–113.

Purpura, D.P. and McMurtry, J.C. Intracellular activities and evoked potential changes during polarization of motor cortex. *J. Neurophysiol.*, 1965; 28: 166–185.

Schambra, H.M., Sawaki, L. and Cohen, L.G. Modulation of excitability of human motor cortex (M1) by 1 Hz transcranial magnetic stimulation of the contralateral M1. *Clin. Neurophysiol.*, 2003, 114: 130–133.

Shadmehr, R. and Holcomb, H.H. Neural correlates of motor memory consolidation. *Science*, 1997, 277: 8215.

Transcranial Magnetic Stimulation and Transcranial Direct Current Stimulation (Supplements to Clinical Neurophysiology, Vol. 56)
Editors: W. Paulus, F. Tergau, M.A. Nitsche, J.C. Rothwell, U. Ziemann, M. Hallett

Chapter 29

Pharmacology of transcranial direct current stimulation: missing effect of riluzole

D. Liebetanz*, M.A. Nitsche and W. Paulus

Department of Clinical Neurophysiology, Georg-August University, Robert-Koch Strasse 40, D-37075 Göttingen (Germany)

1. Introduction

During the middle of the last century, animal studies explored the capability of weak direct current (DC) stimulation for inducing long-lasting alterations in cortical excitability. They related these effects to acute and lasting changes of neuronal activity (Bindman et al., 1962, 1964; Creutzfeldt et al., 1962; Landau et al., 1963; Purpura and McMurtry, 1965; Gartside, 1968). Almost at the same time, Lippold and colleagues applied weak transcranial DC stimulation in humans and described mental changes and therapeutic effects in psychiatric patients (Costain et al., 1964; Lippold and Redfearn, 1964; Redfearn et al., 1964).

Recently, the after-effects of weak transcranial direct current stimulation (tDCS) have been successfully transferred to the human motor cortex (Nitsche and Paulus, 2000, 2001; Nitsche et al., 2003). The direction of excitability changes depends on the polarity of the currents, i.e. anodal tDCS leads to an increase and cathodal tDCS leads to a decrease of cortical excitability (polarity refers to the electrode over the motor cortex). At an intensity of 1 mA (applied via an electrode of 35 cm^2) the duration of the after-effects, which so far may last up to about one hour, are mainly determined by the length of the stimulation (Nitsche and Paulus, 2001; Nitsche et al., 2003).

Because of these exciting features, it is possible that tDCS may serve as a therapeutic tool in disorders associated with hypo- or hyperexcitable cortex, like medication refractory epilepsy, dystonia or Tourette's syndrome. Identifying the mechanisms of tDCS-induced after-effect excitability changes represents an important step towards its rationally founded therapeutic use. However, so far the mechanisms of tDCS are only partially understood. One previous pharmacological study was designed to gain indirect information on the cortical action of tDCS by premedication with two different classes of CNS-active drugs: the voltage-gated sodium channel blocker carbamazepine (CBZ) and the NMDA-receptor blocker dextromethorphan (DMO). The polarity-specific action of CBZ, which selectively suppressed anodal tDCS after-effects, together with the interference of DMO with both cathodal and anodal after-effects, suggests that a combination of glutamatergic and membrane mechanisms is necessary to induce after-effects by tDCS (Liebetanz et al., 2002).

* *Correspondence to*: Dr. David Liebetanz, Department of Clinical Neurophysiology, Georg-August University, Robert-Koch Strasse 40, D-37075 Göttingen, Germany. Tel: +49 551 396650; Fax: +49 551 3988126; E-mail: dliebet@gwdg.de

Since CBZ is active and stabilizes the membrane potential only when the membrane potential is reduced (McLean and Macdonald, 1986), we further hypothesize that polarity-driven alterations of resting membrane potentials represent the crucial mechanism of the tDCS-induced after-effects. According to animal experiments, these changes of resting potentials would consequently lead to an inverse change of spontaneous discharge rates (Bindman et al., 1962; Bindman et al., 1964; Purpura and McMurtry, 1965; Gorman, 1966).

The suppression of the after-effects of both anodal and cathodal tDCS by DMO strongly suggests an involvement of NMDA receptors in both types of tDCS-induced neuroplasticity. The known voltage sensitivity of the NMDA receptor particular supports the proposed mechanism of anodal tDCS after-effects: the capability of NMDA receptors to mediate an increase in synaptic strength is voltage-dependent. Moreover, above the resting membrane potential, the inward current induced by a particular concentration of glutamate increases with depolarization of the resting membrane potential (MacDonald and Wojtowicz, 1982; Artola et al., 1990). A theoretical mechanism for the initiation of long-term effects thus includes a voltage-dependent activation of NMDA receptors by the tDCS-induced alteration of membrane potentials. The correlated changes of firing rates and enhanced synaptic input would then lead to an NMDA receptor-mediated augmentation of synaptic strength (Liebetanz et al., 2002). In the present pharmacological study, in order to determine whether the above-mentioned effects are specific for DMO, we evaluate the interference of the drug riluzole (RLZ) with the after-effect excitability changes of cathodal and anodal tDCS. RLZ, like DMO, is a glutamate antagonist that blocks NMDA receptor transmission (Bryson et al., 1996).

2. Materials and Methods

Eight right-handed healthy volunteers were tested in four sessions. They received a single dose of 150 mg RLZ or placebo tablets 2 h prior to tDCS. 150 mg RLZ have been effective in suppressing intracortical facilitation in a previous study (Liepert et al., 1997). Both conditions were tested for anodal and cathodal tDCS. Direct currents were applied for 5 min at a current intensity of 1 mA via a pair of surface sponge electrodes (35 cm^2) connected to a battery-driven stimulator. One electrode was placed over the representational field of the right abductor digiti minimi muscle (ADM) as determined by transcranial magnetic stimulation (TMS). The other electrode was placed above the contralateral orbit. Cortical excitability changes were recorded by TMS before and directly after tDCS at a frequency of 0.25 Hz for a period of 10 min. A figure-of-8 magnetic coil was placed over the representational field of the right ADM, from which surface EMG was recorded (for details see Nitsche and Paulus, 2000; Liebetanz et al., 2002). MEP amplitudes after tDCS were averaged over 1 min. The normalized data of each session are given as a percentage of the corresponding baseline, where the intensity of the stimulator output was adjusted for a peak-to-peak MEP size of 1 mV. A three-way repeated measurement analysis of variance (ANOVA) was performed with drug intake, polarity and time course after current stimulation as independent variables, the MEP amplitude served as dependent variable. Then post-hoc tests (Fisher's PLSD, level of significance < 0.05) were performed to compare the baseline MEP amplitudes with post-stimulation values.

3. Results

The results of the ANOVA showed a significant main effect of the applied tDCS polarity on the MEP size ($P < 0.05$, Table 1) but not of the drug. In addition, the interaction between time and polarity was significant ($P < 0.05$). When the placebo was administered, anodal tDCS caused a definite elevation of MEP sizes during the first two minutes with an post-stimulation maximum of nearly 140% of baseline level (Fig. 1). After a few minutes, the MEP size returned to baseline level, where it remained stable during the following measurements. In contrast to DMO, which previously has been shown to suppress the anodal after-effect excitability changes (Liebetanz et al. 2002), RLZ left

TABLE 1

RESULTS OF THE THREE-WAY-FACTORIAL REPEATED MEASUREMENT ANOVA

Variables	*d.f.*	*F* values	*P* values
Polarity of current stimulation	1	67.118	< 0.0001*
Time course	9	0.705	0.717
Drug	1	0.935	0.362
Time course × polarity	9	29.270	< 0.0001*
Time course × drug	9	0.675	0.745
Drug × polarity	1	0.01	0.921
Drug × polarity × time course	9	1.05	0.41

The results of the three-way-factorial repeated measurement analysis of variance show that the effects of the current flow depend on the polarity of current flow. Significant interactions of time and polarity indicate that the time course of DC after-effects depends on stimulation polarity. *d.f.* = degrees of freedom. * $P < 0.05$.

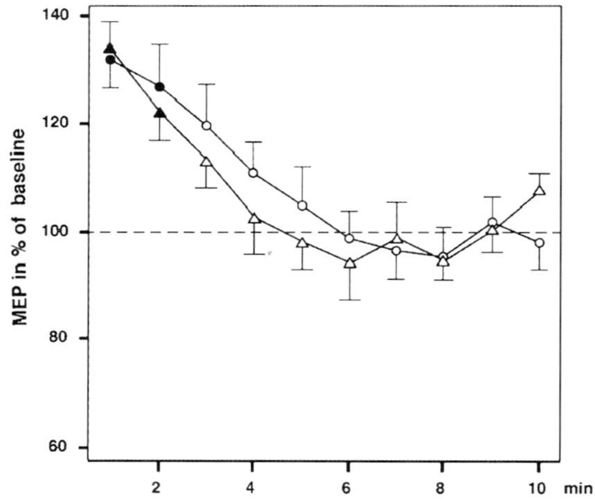

Fig. 1. Comparison of MEP amplitudes after anodal tDCS under pre-medication of riluzole or placebo. Time-course of TMS-assessed persisting changes of motor cortical excitability is shown after 5 min of anodal tDCS with 1 mA. Riluzole (triangles) taken 2 h previous to tDCS did not interfere significantly with excitability changes induced by anodal tDCS as compared to the placebo condition (circles). Significant MEP-size alterations from baseline level are labelled with closed symbols (Fisher's PLSD, $P < 0.05$; bars show standard errors of the MEP amplitudes).

the magnitude as well as the time-course of the post-anodal MEP elevation unchanged when compared to the placebo condition. After 5 min of cathodal tDCS, the MEP size was significantly decreased during the first 3 min in the placebo condition. This MEP reduction vanished steadily within the following minutes, so that baseline level was re-established after five minutes (Fig. 2). Again, the RLZ pre-medication did not alter the amplitudes or the time-course of the of MEP decrease in the placebo condition.

4. Discussion

The aim of this study was to investigate whether the glutamate antagonist RLZ interferes with the capability of the motor cortex to react with excitability changes to tDCS in a manner similar to the previously tested NMDA receptor blocker DMO. DMO, which likewise antagonises glutamate, has been shown to prevent hyperexcitability after anodal as well as hypoexcitability after cathodal tDCS (Liebetanz et al., 2002). Surprisingly, the second tested glutamate antagonist, RLZ, did not produce any effect on the lasting excitability changes induced by five minutes of cathodal or anodal tDCS.

In contrast to DMO, which blocks NMDA receptors non-competitively (Wong et al., 1988; Tortella et al., 1989; Franklin and Murray, 1992), RLZ is assumed to influence different pre- and postsynaptic processes of glutamate transmission (Bryson et al., 1996; Doble, 1997). In addition to a non-competitive blockade of NMDA receptors analogous to DMO, RLZ has been shown to produce a presynaptic inhibition of glutamate release. Although RLZ like DMO suppresses intracortical facilitation, RLZ exerts no

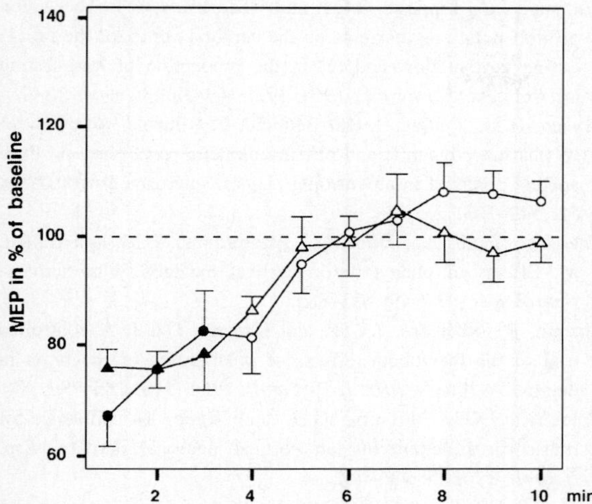

Fig. 2. Comparison of MEP amplitudes after cathodal tDCS under pre-medication of riluzole or placebo. Time-course of TMS-assessed persisting changes of motor cortical excitability is shown after 5 min of cathodal tDCS with 1 mA. Riluzole (triangles) taken 2 h previous to tDCS did not interfere significantly with the excitability diminution induced by cathodal tDCS as compared to the placebo condition (circles). Significant MEP-size alterations from baseline level are labelled with closed symbols (Fisher's PLSD, $P < 0.05$; bars show standard errors of the MEP amplitudes).

significant enhancement of intracortical inhibition, as has been shown for DMO (Liepert et al., 1997; Ziemann et al., 1998; Schwenkreis et al., 2000).

Different non-glutamatergic actions of RLZ and DMO could be responsible for the dissimilar interference of these drugs with the tDCS after-effects. In addition to the blockade of NMDA receptors, DMO causes a partial inhibition of voltage-dependent calcium and sodium channels. However, this effect should be expected only in much higher doses than used in our previous study (Netzer et al., 1993; Liebetanz et al., 2002). If DMO has contributed to the results with a relevant inhibition of calcium and sodium channels, the drug should affect membrane excitability and consequently should alter MEP threshold and MEP size on its own (Ziemann et al., 1996; Chen et al., 1997). However, as a single dose of 150 mg DMO does not affect motor thresholds and MEP recruitment (Ziemann et al., 1998; Liebetanz et al., 2002), it is very unlikely that channel-blocking properties of DMO contributed relevantly to the suppression of tDCS effects. RLZ also inactivates voltage-dependent sodium channels in vitro (Urenjak and Obrenovitch, 1997). Likewise, the lack of an effect of a single dose of RLZ on membrane excitability, as assessed by MEP threshold, argues against the idea that its sodium channel-blocking properties may be significant in vivo (Liepert, 1997). However, RLZ has been shown to reduce motor excitability to some extent after 7 days of administration, which possibly is due to a sodium channel-blocking effect (Schwenkreis et al., 2000). An alternative explanation for the lack of RLZ effect in our study is that, in the given dose, DMO may be a more potent agent than RLZ. This is supported by the fact that 150 mg RLZ did not cause any side effects in the present study, in contrast to DMO (Ziemann et al., 1998; Liebetanz et al., 2002). Furthermore, at least some cortical effects of RLZ, i.e. the normalisation of intracortical inhibition in patients suffering from amyotrophic lateral sclerosis seem to appear first after a delay of 5 days of treatment (Stephan et al., 1998; Sommer et al., 1999). However, smaller doses were given in those studies (100 mg × 1; 2 × 50 mg/day × 5). Further studies are needed to determine whether the partial differences in their modes of action or different pharmacokinetics account for the present disparity in the effects of RLZ and DMO on DC-induced excitability alterations. Nevertheless, assuming that RLZ's anti-glutamatergic effect in vivo may be primarily located at the presynaptic site, one could speculate that the suppressive action of DMO on tDCS effects is particularly a postsynaptic one.

To gain insight into the functionality of tDCS by unravelling receptor and channel effects on the basis of pharmacological interactions with tDCS-induced after-effects has been the major objective of hitherto performed and ongoing pharmacological tDCS studies. Although tDCS mechanisms are still only partially understood, future pharmacological tDCS studies should also aim at identifying possible drug effects that optimize tDCS protocols for clinical application: (1) tDCS after-effects may be prolonged and stabilized by certain drugs, e.g. amphetamines; (2) drug-enhanced tDCS regimes may enhance the safety of tDCS by a possible reduction of the duration and repetition rate of tDCS sessions and (3) intended tDCS after-effects may be optimised and focused by the prevention of undesired effects at the distant electrode. Since the direction of tDCS after-effects not only depends on the current polarity, but also on the anatomical placement and orientation of the affected neurones (Landau et al., 1963; Purpura and McMurtry, 1965), reverse DC effects are inevitably induced at sites where neurones are divergently orientated, e.g. at the opposite wall of a sulcus. For the prevention of these undesired effects, the antiepileptic drug CBZ seems to represent a promising pharmacological candidate, since it exerts a polarity specific effect on the tDCS-induced cortical excitability changes. While CBZ suppresses excitability enhancement after anodal tDCS, it leaves the excitability decrease after cathodal tDCS unchanged (Liebetanz, 2002). Cathodal tDCS, in addition to the intended lasting diminution of motor cortical excitability, theoretically may also induce opposite effects at sites that have a different geometrical orientation with respect to the current flow or are placed at the opposite electrode. By its anodal tDCS-specific effect, pre-medication with CBZ could possibly suppress these undesired "anodal" excitability increases. However, so far CBZ has only been tested in a tDCS study investigating the after-effects over the motor cortex monitored by TMS. Further studies using techniques that allow simultaneous whole brain detection of activity changes like PET or fMRI should be performed to test this hypothesis.

References

Artola, A., Brocher, S. and Singer, W. Different voltage-dependent thresholds for inducing long-term depression and long-term potentiation in slices of rat visual cortex. *Nature*, 1990, 347: 69–72.

Bindman, L.J., Lippold, O.C.J. and Redfearn, J.W.T. Long-lasting changes in the level of the electrical activity of the cerebral cortex activity produced by polarizing currents. *Nature*, 1962, 196: 584–585.

Bindman, L.J., Lippold, O.C.J. and Redfearn, J.W.T. The action of brief polarizing currents on the cerebral cortex of the rat (1) during current flow and (2) in the production of long-lasting after-effects. *J. Physiol.*, 1964, 172: 369–382.

Bryson, H.M., Fulton, B. and Benfield, P. Riluzole. A review of its pharmacodynamic and pharmacokinetic properties and therapeutic potential in amyotrophic lateral sclerosis. *Drugs*, 1996, 52: 549–563.

Chen, R., Samii, A., Canos, M., Wassermann, E.M. and Hallett, M. Effects of phenytoin on cortical excitability in humans. *Neurology*, 1997, 49: 881–883.

Costain, R., Redfearn, J.W.T. and Lippold, O.C.J. A controlled trial of the therapeutic effects of polarization of the brain in depressive illness. *Brit. J. Psychiat.*, 1964, 110: 786–799.

Creutzfeldt, O.D., Fromm, G.H. and Kapp, H. Influence of transcortical dc-currents on cortical neuronal activity. *Exp. Neurol.*, 1962, 5: 436–452.

Doble, A. Effects of riluzole on glutamatergic neurotransmission in the mammalian central nervous system, and other pharmacological effects. *Rev. Contemp. Pharmacother.*, 1997, 8: 213–225.

Franklin, P.H. and Murray, T.F. High affinity [3H]dextrorphan binding in rat brain is localized to a noncompetitive antagonist site of the activated N-methyl-D-aspartate receptor-cation channel. *Mol. Pharmacol.*, 1992, 41: 134–146.

Gartside, I.B. Mechanisms of sustained increases of firing rate of neurons in the rat cerebral cortex after polarization: reverberating circuits or modification of synaptic conductance? *Nature*, 1968, 220: 382–383.

Gorman, A.L. Differential patterns of activation of the pyramidal system elicited by surface anodal and cathodal cortical stimulation. *J. Neurophysiol.*, 1966, 29: 547–564.

Landau, W.M., Bishop, G.H. and Clare, M.H. Analysis of the form and distribution of evoked cortical potentials under the influence of polarizing currents. *J. Neurophysiol.*, 1963, 27: 788–813.

Liebetanz, D., Nitsche, M.A., Tergau, F. and Paulus, W. Pharmacological approach to the mechanisms of transcranial DC-stimulation-induced after-effects of human motor cortex excitability. *Brain*, 2002, 125: 2238–2247.

Liepert, J., Schwenkreis, P., Tegenthoff, M. and Malin, J.P. The glutamate antagonist riluzole suppresses intracortical facilitation. *J. Neural. Transm.*, 1997, 104: 1207–1214.

Lippold, O.C.J. and Redfearn, J.W.T. Mental changes resulting from the passage of small direct currents through the human brain. *Brit. J. Psychiat.*, 1964, 110: 768–772.

Mcdonald, R.L. Carbamazepine. Mechanisms of action. In: R.H. Levy, R.H. Mattson and B.S. Meldrum (Eds.), *Antiepileptic Drugs*. New York: Raven, 1995: 491–498.

McLean, M.J. and Macdonald, R.L. Carbamazepine and 10,11-epoxycarbamazepine produce use- and voltage-dependent limitation of rapidly firing action potentials of mouse central neurons in cell culture. *J. Pharmacol. Exp. Ther.*, 1986, 238: 727–738.

Netzer, R., Pflimlin, P. and Trube, G. Dextromethorphan blocks N-methyl-D-aspartate-induced currents and voltage-operated inward currents in cultured cortical neurons. *Eur. J. Pharmacol.*, 1993, 238: 209–216.

Nitsche, M.A. and Paulus, W. Excitability changes induced in the human motor cortex by weak transcranial direct current stimulation. *J. Physiol.*, 2000, 527: 633–639.

Nitsche, M.A. and Paulus, W. Sustained excitability elevations induced by transcranial DC motor cortex stimulation in humans. *Neurology*, 2001, 57: 1899–1901.

Nitsche, M.A., Nitsche, M.S., Klein, C.C., Tergau, F., Rothwell, J.C. and Paulus, W. Level of action of cathodal DC polarisation induced inhibition of the human motor cortex. *Clin. Neurophysiol.*, 2003, 114: 600–604.

Purpura, D.P. and McMurtry, J.G. Intracelluar activities and evoked potential changes during polarization of motor cortex. *J. Neurophysiol.*, 1965, 28: 166–185.

Redfearn, J.W.T., Lippold, O.C.J. and Costain, R. A preliminary account of the clinical effects of polarizing the brain in certain psychiatric disorders. *Brit. J. Psychiat.*, 1964, 110: 773–785.

Schwenkreis, P., Liepert, J., Witscher, K., Fischer, W., Weiller, C., Malin, J.P. et al. Riluzole suppresses motor cortex facilitation in correlation to its plasma level. A study using transcranial magnetic stimulation. *Exp. Brain Res.*, 2000, 135: 293–299.

Sommer, M., Tergau, F., Wischer, S., Reimers, C.D., Beuche, W. and Paulus, W. Riluzole does not have an acute effect on motor thresholds and the intracortical excitability in amyotrophic lateral sclerosis. *J. Neurol.*, 1999, 246 (Suppl. 3): III22–III26.

Stephan, K., Kunesch, E. and Benecke, R.. Riluzole restores impaired intracortical inhibition in patients with ALS. *J. Neurol.*, 1998, 245: 401.

Tortella, F.C., Pellicano, M. and Bowery, N.G. Dextromethorphan and neuromodulation: old drug coughs up new activities. *Trends Pharmacol. Sci.*, 1989, 10: 501–507.

Urenjak, J. and Obrenovitch, T. Pharmacological modulation of sodium channels by riluzole: an alternative to antiexcitotoxic actions. *Rev. Contemp. Pharmacother.*, 1997, 8: 237–246.

Wong, B.Y., Coulter, D.A., Choi, D.W. and Prince, D.A. Dextrorphan and dextromethorphan, common antitussives, are antiepileptic and antagonize N-methyl-D-aspartate in brain slices. *Neurosci. Lett.*, 1988, 85: 261–266.

Ziemann, U., Lonnecker, S., Steinhoff, B.J. and Paulus, W. Effects of antiepileptic drugs on motor cortex excitability in humans: a transcranial magnetic stimulation study. *Ann. Neurol.*, 1996, 40: 367–378.

Ziemann, U., Chen, R., Cohen, L.G. and Hallett, M. Dextromethorphan decreases the excitability of the human motor cortex. *Neurology*, 1998, 51: 1320–1324.

Section V

Interaction with Perception and Cognition

Transcranial Magnetic Stimulation and Transcranial Direct
Current Stimulation (Supplements to Clinical Neurophysiology, Vol. 56)
Editors: W. Paulus, F. Tergau, M.A. Nitsche, J.C. Rothwell, U. Ziemann, M. Hallett

Chapter 30

Transcranial magnetic and direct current stimulation of the visual cortex

Andrea Antal*, Michael A. Nitsche and Walter Paulus

Department of Clinical Neurophysiology, Georg-August University, D-37075 Göttingen (Germany)

1. Introduction

Of all human senses, vision is probably the most crucial and most dominant among sensory functions in shaping our perceptions of the world. Animal and human studies have delineated many cortical areas that are important for the processing of visual information. One of the most challenging problems in neuroscience is to understand how the visual input is processed in primary and secondary visual areas and how it is transferred to higher cortical areas. Another one is to correlate visual perception with brain function. In previous years, significant achievements have been made in characterizing visual information processing in humans, using several neurophysiological techniques.

The first systematic studies of electrical stimulation of the visual cortex were carried out by intracranial electrical stimulation of the brains of neurological patients during neurosurgery (Penfield and Rasmussen, 1957). Occipital stimulation produced light sensations called phosphenes whose position, color and shape varied according the position of the electrodes. Brindley and Lewin (1968) stimulated the occipital cortex of a blind subject with implanted electrodes and described the properties of elicited phosphenes in detail.

These early invasive approaches were followed by non-invasive stimulation methods: the first stimulation technique through the intact skull, transcranial electrical stimulation (TES), was developed by Merton and Morton in 1980. Compared to the invasive methods, they had to increase voltage and shorten discharge duration. They showed that stimulation of the scalp over the occipital cortex could produce phosphenes. The main problem with this type of stimulation is that the electric current flowing between the electrodes on the scalp causes pain and contraction of the scalp muscles. In contrast, transcranial magnetic stimulation (TMS), which also influences the brain electrically, is a powerful, non-invasive, non-painful tool for activating neurons in the cortex. In the last two decades, TMS has become established as a valuable method for studying the brain function over the motor and sensory cortices. Stimulation occurs when a brief current pulse is passed through a wired coil placed on the scalp, producing an electric field in the brain by electromagnetic induction. The duration of the effects depends on the mode of stimulation. Single-pulse

* *Correspondence to*: Dr. Andrea Antal, Department of Clinical Neurophysiology, Georg-August University, Robert Koch Straße 40, D-37075 Göttingen, Germany. Tel: +49-551-398461; Fax: +49-551-398126
E-mail: Aantal@gwdg.de

TMS can produce a brief excitation or inhibition in the brain for a few milliseconds. Repetitive TMS (rTMS) refers to regularly repeated stimuli to a single scalp site. With rTMS longer lasting effects from hundreds of milliseconds to several seconds and minutes can be elicited, some of which outlast the period of stimulation. Mapping studies within the motor and visual cortex using single-pulse TMS showed a spatial resolution down to 0.5–1.0 cm at the scalp surface (for reviews see: Walsh and Cowey, 1998; Jahanshahi and Rothwell, 2000; Cowey and Walsh, 2001). However, during prolonged rTMS, the effects along cortico-cortical connections may well lead to less focal effects.

In one of the first reports on TMS in humans, Barker et al. (1985) not only described its excitatory effect on the motor cortex but also mentioned that light sensations were evoked by stimulation of the occipital cortex. Since that time several studies have demonstrated that TMS of the visual cortex is able to modify visual perception, imagination, motion processing and cognition (for reviews see: Amassian et al., 1998b; Walsh and Cowey, 1998).

Recently, another non-invasive method has gained significant importance in studying human brain function. Transcranial direct current stimulation (tDCS) applied through the skull was shown to modulate directly the excitability of the motor (Nitsche and Paulus, 2000, 2001; Rosenkranz et al., 2000; Baudewig et al., 2001; Nitsche et al., 2003) and visual (Antal et al., 2001, 2003) cortices in human subjects. Weak cathodal stimulation, which causes membrane hyperpolarization, as shown in animals (Purpura and McMurtry, 1964), has been shown to decrease cerebral excitability while, conversely, anodal stimulation increases excitability, probably by membrane depolarization (Purpura and McMurtry, 1964). According to present data, these effects evolve during tDCS and can remain for up to an hour after the end of stimulation (Nitsche and Paulus, 2000, 2001; Nitsche et al., 2003). Few studies have been made concerning the application of tDCS over the human visual cortex, however, recent data show that a modulation of the visual perception threshold and phosphene thresholds are produced by this technique (Antal et al., 2001, 2003).

Here, we summarize results derived from the use of TMS and tDCS on visual perception and compare characteristics of the two methods.

2. Transcranial magnetic stimulation

In general, the application of TMS to sensory, mainly visual areas of the cortex has developed more slowly than for the motor areas. The main reason for this is the more time-consuming set-up required to quantify visual effects of stimulation. TMS may influence a variety of visual-perceptual aspects. After Barker's pioneer work (1985), Amassian et al. were the first to demonstrate the effect of TMS on visual cortex systematically (1989). Single-pulse TMS was delivered over the occipital cortex of subjects while they were performing a letter-identification task. Performance was impaired when the TMS pulse was applied between 60 and 140 ms after the stimulus onset. They hypothesized that during and after magnetic stimulation of the visual cortex, an inhibitory postsynaptic potential component evoked by the magnetic pulse via polysynaptic circuits causes the suppression of visual perception (Fig. 1). Since then, it has become obvious that this technique can mimic the effect of neurological lesions on visual perception. Impairment of visual perception by TMS has been demonstrated by several investigators using different visual recognition tasks (Beckers and Hömberg, 1991; Masur et al., 1993; Miller et al., 1996). Perceptual impairments induced by TMS were also extended to extrafoveal positions (Epstein and Zangaladze, 1996; Kastner et al., 1998).

2.1. Time course of action and effectiveness

Three separate periods for suppression of vision have been described when single pulse TMS is applied to the occipital cortex (Corthout et al., 1999a, b, 2000a, b). A first period of TMS-induced suppression occurs when the magnetic stimulus precedes the visual stimulus by 50–70 ms. This could be interpreted as a forward-masking mechanism. This time period is,

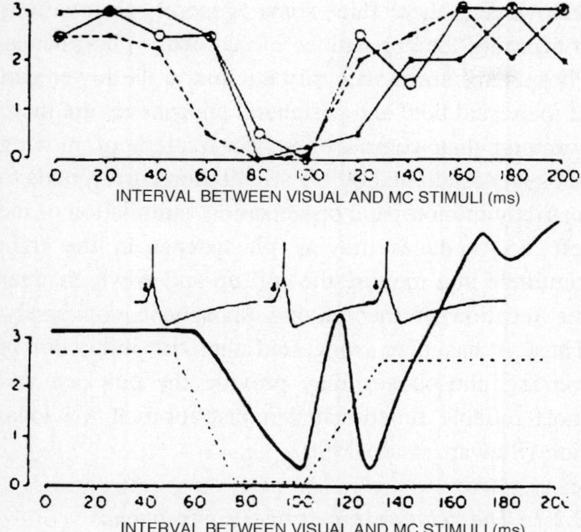

Fig. 1. Top: visual suppression curve in three subjects. The proportion of three briefly flashed dark letters on a light background that were correctly reported, plotted as a function of the delay for the magnetic stimulus. Bottom: hypothetical mechanism of suppression by an inhibitory postsynaptic potential (IPS). The solid line is the visual evoked response, the dashed line is the suppression. (Amassian et al., 1989. Reproduced with permission.)

however, particularly vulnerable for TMS-induced blink artefacts, which have to be considered when the parieto-occipito-temporal junction is stimulated (Beckers and Zeki, 1995). The second period, a magnetic stimulus after 20–30 ms of visual stimulus onset, seems to be related to the first stage of visual processing in V1 and maybe in V2/V3. The third period, 80–120 ms after the visual stimulus onset, could involve some of the feedback projections to V1 from extrastriate areas (Corthout et al., 1999a, b, 2000a, b). However, the latter effects are not stable: the TMS-induced suppression in the second and third periods progressively disappeared during 3 weeks of repeated TMS experiments. This is probably due to practice-induced increase in neuronal activity in the visual cortex (Corthout et al., 2000) that cannot be suppressed by identical TMS pulses. It was also proven that the latest suppression period (80–120 ms) depended more on the coil position on the head than the previous periods: the TMS-induced suppression was effective only when the coil was placed 1–3 cm above the inion, while in the first period, perception was also suppressed when the coil was placed 5–7 cm above the inion.

rTMS blocks different visuo-cognitive processes during stimulation more effectively than single pulse TMS, and the elicited effects of cortical stimulation may outlast the actual stimulation period (Pascual-Leone et al., 1993, 1994; Boroojerdi et al., 2000). However, the cost of using rTMS rather than single-pulse TMS is the diminution in temporal resolution.

Using 1 Hz stimulation frequency, decreased visual cortex excitability was demonstrated, expressed as an increase in phosphene threshold (Boroojerdi et al., 2000). The effect lasted for at least 10 min after the end of stimulation. Similarly, impaired performance was observed in a visual perception and imagery task when 1 Hz rTMS was applied to the visual cortex (Kosslyn et al., 1999). Antal et al. (2002) showed that low frequency (1 Hz) rTMS applied to the occipital cortex could impair contrast perception, and that the effect depended on current waveform and direction: monophasic stimulation with posterior-anterior current direction in the coil, current flow was more effective than biphasic stimulation. Switching current direction resulted in an increased efficacy of biphasic and decreased efficacy of monophasic stimulation, however, both effects were smaller compared to the original stimulation condition.

High frequency rTMS (> 5 Hz) produces increased neuronal excitability which can last for some minutes after the end of stimulation (Pascual-Leone et al., 1993, 1994). With the facilitatory effect of rTMS, it became possible to improve performance in cognitive tasks involving the visual system. Boroojerdi et al. (2001) observed decreased response times in a task involving matching analogous positions of four colored shapes (analogous reasoning task) during stimulation of the left prefrontal cortex.

2.2. *Phosphenes and their topography*

Phosphenes are sensations of light that can be evoked by single pulse or repetitive magnetic stimulation of the occipital cortex. They are commonly described as spots of light or stars that tend to persist for the duration of the stimulation and disappear with its cessation (Fig. 2). Phosphenes can be produced in almost every subject, either with closed or open eyes, if the stimulation intensity is high enough. The stimulation over V1 results in stationary phosphenes while stimulation over V5 produces moving light sensations (Stewart et al., 1999; Pascual-Leone and Walsh, 2001). Phosphenes are relatively variable in position or form, their induction is also somewhat dependent on the orientation and movement of the coil (Meyer et al., 1991; Marg and Rudiak, 1994; Epstein et al., 1996). Generally, the prevalence of phosphenes varies with varying stimulation characteristics (Meyer et al., 1991; Kammer, 1998, 1999; Ray et al., 1998; Pascual-Leone and Walsh, 2001; Stewart et al., 2001).

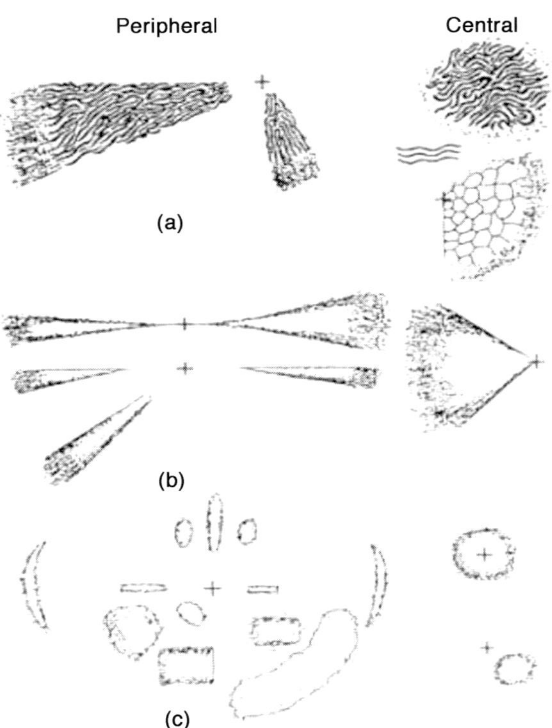

Fig. 2. Artistic impressions of phosphenes reported by different subjects. (a) Structured phosphenes, (b) light flashes, (c) blobs. (Marg and Rudiak, 1994. Reproduced with permission.)

However, there are some general observations concerning the appearance of stationary phosphenes. Phosphenes are most easily elicited in the lower part of the visual field and peripheral phosphenes are more common than central ones. The pattern of moving phosphenes elicited by V5 stimulation corresponds to a strictly retinotopical organization: stimulation of the left V5 produces moving phosphenes in the right hemifield and moving the coil up and down changes the location of the moving phosphene conversely. Thus, it has been suggested that the induction of moving phosphenes may provide the quickest and most reliable functional demonstration of V5 location (Stewart et al., 1999).

2.2.1. The relationship between phosphene threshold and the excitability of the visual cortex

Stationary phosphene thresholds were highly reproducible across test sessions held at least a week apart (Fig. 3), did not correlate with the motor threshold (Kammer et al., 2001; Stewart et al., 2001) and did not change with variations in ambient light (Kammer and Beck, 2002). However, light deprivation – which is known to increase cortical excitability – for up to 180 min causes significant phosphene threshold reduction (Boroojerdi et al., 2000), suggesting that phosphene

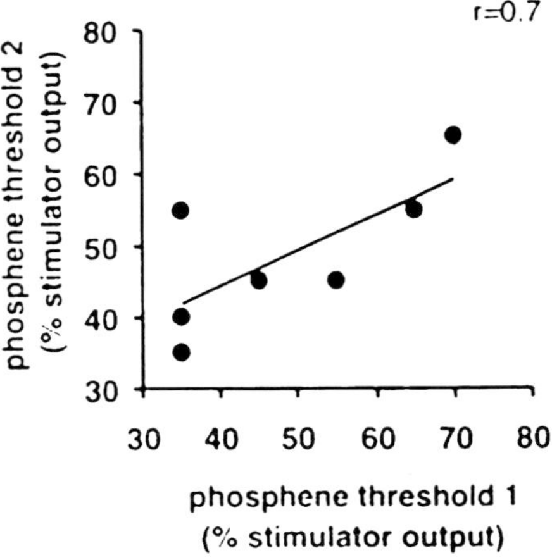

Fig. 3. Stationary phosphene thresholds in a percentage of maximum stimulator output of seven subjects. Phosphene thresholds were stable over 1 week. (Stewart et al., 2001. Reproduced with permission.)

threshold measurements provide information about excitability changes in the human visual cortex. In migraine patients, whose visual cortex is thought to be hyperexcitable between and during migraine attacks, lower phosphene thresholds were found than in healthy subjects (Afra et al., 1998; Aurora et al., 1998).

Based on these results, several studies have applied TMS mapping in partially blind subjects, to study the changes of cortical excitability by analyzing phosphene thresholds (Cowey and Walsh, 2000; Gothe et al., 2002). In a peripherally blind subject, stimulation of V1 resulted in easily elicited and reproducible phosphenes with normal thresholds but the spatial distribution was coarser compared to normal subjects (Cowey and Walsh, 2000). The perception of moving phosphenes when V5 was stimulated was also normal. Thus, in peripheral blindness, most TMS studies do not reveal abnormal function of the visual cortex. However, in a hemianopic subject with central lesion, extensive magnetic stimulation did not evoke phosphenes at all – neither at V1 nor at V5 (Cowey and Walsh, 2000). Gothe et al. (2002) compared phosphene thresholds in subjects with some residual vision (measurable with Snellen test charts), subjects with very poor residual vision (only light or movement perception but not measurable acuity) and without any residual vision. In agreement with previous data, phosphene thresholds were normal in all of the subjects compared to healthy persons, but the number of effective stimulation sites was significantly reduced in subjects who had very poor or no residual vision. These results suggest that long-term visual deafferentation causes a reorganization of the visual system that reduces, but does not eliminate, the ability of blind subjects to perceive cortically elicited phosphenes.

2.2.2. Where do phosphenes or conscious perception of phosphenes emerge?

The individual variability of the exposed surface of the striate cortex (Brindley, 1972) and the fact that phosphenes can be evoked from sites up to 5 cm lateral to the interhemispheric cleft making the answer difficult to ascertain. Meyer et al. (1991) suggested that the probable stimulation site for evoking phosphenes is the supracalcarine part of the occipital lobe. Others (Marg and Rudiak, 1994; Epstein et al., 1996) argue that phosphenes are not evoked in the visual cortex, but rather within the underlying white matter by the activation of the optic radiation, in which adjacent fibers project to occipital cortical neurons. Marg and Rudiak (1994) calculated the depth of stimulation, which in the visual cortex was approximately 4 cm. Kammer et al. (2001) have suggested that unilateral phosphenes are generated in V2 and V3, while the stimulation of V1 yields phosphenes in both visual fields. Possibly in the case of V2/V3 stimulation, these extrastriate areas are first activated and then evoke activity in V1 via backprojection fibers, the latter causing the perception of phosphenes. This may explain the observation that no phosphenes could be evoked in a patient with a lesion of V1 (Cowey and Walsh, 2000). A study conducted by Pascual-Leone and Walsh also underlines the "V1 hypothesis" (2001). Here a dual-pulse paradigm was used to study the role of V1 in the elaboration of the conscious illusory percept of a moving phosphene generated by stimulation of V5. Perception was disrupted by subthreshold stimulation applied to V1 5–40 ms after the suprathreshold stimulus to V5. No effect was observed when stimulation was applied to V1 before the V5 pulse.

Amassian et al. have suggested that frontal lobe outputs modulate conscious perception of phosphenes (Amassian et al., 1998a). When the occipital cortex was stimulated with a low intensity, very few, if any, phosphenes were reported. Similarly, stimulation of the frontal lobe did not elicit phosphenes when applied alone. When stimulation of the frontal lobe was preceded at 0–75 ms by TMS over the occipital cortex, complex chromatic and achromatic phosphenes were reported. The authors hypothesize that frontal lobe outputs facilitate phosphene perception by opening a thalamic gate for occipital outputs, possibly through thalamocortical reverberations.

The effects of TMS depend on the direction of induced current: it was demonstrated that phosphene thresholds were significantly lower if the direction of induced current is oriented from lateral to medial in the occipital cortex, rather than vice versa (Meyer et al., 1991; Amassian et al., 1994; Kammer et al., 2001).

2.2.3. Paired-pulse and repetitive stimulation eliciting phosphenes

Using paired-pulse stimulation with intervals ranging up to 1000 ms, it was found that for the interstimulus interval 2–100 ms, interaction of two pulses significantly reduces the threshold for perception of phosphenes (Ray et al., 1998). This effect is probably due to priming, in which the appearance of the first stimulus facilitates the perception of the second stimulus. Above 100 ms interstimulus interval the second pulse possibly activates neurons and neuronal pathways too late to interact with the effect of the first pulse.

Increasing the frequency of TMS up to 40 Hz is accompanied by a decrease in the phosphene threshold (Ray et al., 1998). Ray et al. applied trains of one-second duration at frequencies of 5, 10, 20 and 40 Hz. The threshold intensity necessary to produce phosphenes decreased as frequency of stimulation increased. When only one 40 Hz train lasting 25–2000 ms was administered, the threshold intensity needed to elicit phosphenes was about the same for stimulus trains from 250 ms to 2000 ms, but increased dramatically for shorter durations (< 250 ms), which shows that a certain threshold exists for eliciting phosphenes.

2.3. Scotomas

Single TMS pulses can induce transient visual field defects called scotomas. Kastner et al. (1998) have described peripheral and central scotomas. They have suggested that the transient scotomas at 1–3° induced by TMS are due to the stimulation of mainly V1 and V2/V3, while visual field defects at 4–9° are due to stimulation of V2/V3 but not V1 (Kastner et al., 1998). They implied that phosphenes do not contribute to scotomas, because at the high intensity (95–100% of stimulator output) which was necessary to induce visual field deficits, subjects did not perceive phosphenes.

Kammer and Nusseck (1998) and Kammer (1999) demonstrated, using lower stimulation intensities, that in most of the cases a transient scotoma produced by TMS was within the area where phosphenes were elicited. The transient scotoma did not mean complete blindness, but rather the elevation of the visual detection threshold. These studies suggest that single pulse TMS given over the occipital pole 60–120 ms after the visual stimulus onset does not completely disrupt visual processing but modulates perception threshold (Miller et al., 1996; Kammer and Nussek, 1998).

As stated earlier, the literature on the relationship between the topography of the phosphenes elicited by TMS and the inhibition of visual function is still contradictory. In the case of a complete overlap, the phosphene locations given by the subject would be in the exact place where sensory processes are interrupted. When scotomas and phosphenes under certain conditions are not elicited simultaneously, this does not necessarily mean that they are differently located: Suppression of perception by magnetic pulses might be due to the decrease of the signal-to-noise ratio, which can come from suppressing the retinal signal and/or increasing the cortical noise. Thus, maybe the total disruption of cortical activity by high intensity stimulation results in scotoma without phosphene generation, but when lower intensities are used, it can be demonstrated that phosphenes and scotomas are localized in the same region.

Kamitani and Shimojo's work (1999) raises the possibility that the effect of TMS-induced scotomas may not only be the disruption of perception, but include further processes: they briefly presented a large grid pattern to subjects and applied a single magnetic pulse to the occipital pole with 80–170 ms delay. The subjects observed a disk-shaped patch in the patterned stimulus in the lower quadrant of the visual field contralateral to the coil. The suppressed region appeared homogenous and gray, while the size of the patch varied across subjects between 1.2–5.6°. When the visual stimulus was a vertical or horizontal grating pattern, the shape of the scotoma was distorted and an ellipse appeared, compressed vertically with a vertical pattern and horizontally with a horizontal pattern. When the stimulus was presented temporally between colored fields and followed by a magnetic pulse, the color perceived inside the scotoma was consistent with that of the background, which was presented after the grid or grating. This shows a filling-in backwards phenomenon, which probably means a compensation for the local information blocked by TMS. These results suggest that TMS-induced suppression does not produce only a local and immediate perceptual interference. The initial reaction to the induced electric field triggers dynamic interactions of neural signals in the visual cortex, resulting in temporal and spatial characteristics of the TMS induced suppression.

2.4. Suppression of color perception

Colored phosphenes have been reported during TMS (Marg and Rudiak, 1994; Kastner et al., 1998) but reports on the effect of TMS on color perception are rare. The reason for this most probably is that it is difficult to selectively disturb color perception by external stimulation because V4, the area assumed to be responsible mainly for color vision, is located far from the skull surface. However, it is possible to separate the time course of achromatic and chromatic perception by TMS. Magnetic stimuli applied over the occipital cortex resulted in later suppression periods when chromatic stimuli (green letters against a red background) were used compared with those with achromatic stimuli (Maccabee et al., 1991). Using threshold detection of chromatic and achromatic Gaussian filtered dots and applying TMS to the primary visual cortex, Paulus et al. (1999) have shown that the magnocellular (achromatic) system has significantly higher susceptibility to TMS than the parvocellular (chromatic) system, probably due to the larger axonal and neuronal size. Using achromatic stimuli, TMS was effective even given 30–45 ms after the onset of the stimuli, but also with a second peak of 90 ms. When chromatic stimuli were shown, the suppression was most effective when the magnetic pulse was applied between 60–120 ms after the stimulus presentation (Fig. 4).

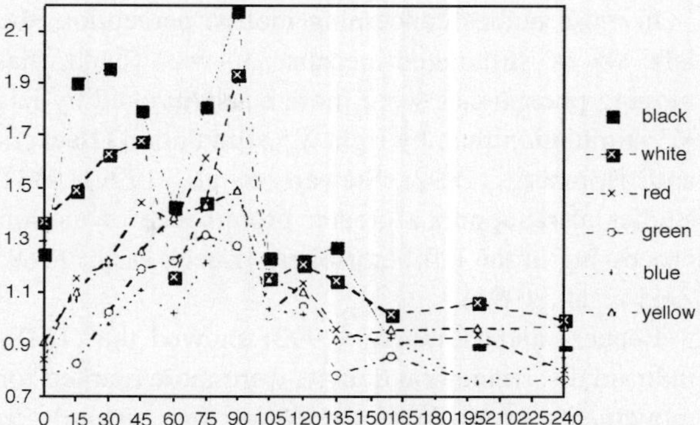

Fig. 4. The differential inhibition of six different colored Gaussian dots by TMS is demonstrated. When the visual stimulus and TMS are applied simultaneously, color perception is facilitated, whereas achromatic perception is inhibited. When TMS is applied 30 ms after presentation of the visual stimulus, a selective inhibition of black and white perception is apparent, whereas color perception is continuously more inhibited with a maximum at 75 and 90 ms interstimulus-interval. Overall, color perception is less susceptible to TMS than achromatic perception. (Paulus et al., 1999. Reproduced with permission.)

2.5. Suppression of motion perception

Several studies have examined the effects of TMS applied to V5 and found that motion perception could be impaired by TMS (Becker and Hömberg, 1992; Hotson et al., 1994; Beckers and Zeki, 1995; Amassian et al., 1998; Walsh et al., 1998; Hotson and Anand, 1999). Stimulation of this area could also shorten motion after-effects (Stewart et al., 1999) and affect learning in a movement perception task (Stewart et al., 1999). In accordance, human brain imaging studies performed with a multiplicity of different moving stimuli suggest that the extrastriatal area responding most convincingly to moving objects is V5 (Watson et al., 1993; Tootell et al., 1995a, b; McKeefry et al., 1997; Braddick et al., 2001), and neurological patients with cortical damage including area V5 suffer from a wide range of deficits in motion perception (Newsome and Pare, 1988; Hess et al., 1989; Shipp et al., 1994).

In most studies concerning motion perception, the left V5 is stimulated because it was found that moving phosphenes were more easily evoked by left V5 stimulation than by right V5 stimulation (Beckers and Hömberg, 1992; Stewart et al., 1999). PET studies also support a greater prominence of motion processing in the left hemisphere (Lueck et al., 1989; Zeki et al., 1991).

Beckers and Hömberg (1992) showed that TMS-induced discrimination deficits were more marked for movements away from the fovea than towards it. These findings are consistent with previous monkey's data showing that V5 includes more neurons tuned for motion away from the fovea than towards it (Albright, 1989).

Hotson et al. (1994) have applied TMS pulses over the left V5 while subjects performed motion-direction discrimination tasks (Fig. 5). TMS elevated the discrimination threshold in both visual hemifields, suggesting that unilateral stimulation could have bilateral physiological effects, probably via trans-callosal connections (Paus et al., 1997). In contrast to this finding, the study by Becker and Hömberg (1992), found TMS over V5 disrupted direction-discrimination only when the stimulus appeared contralateral to the stimulated area.

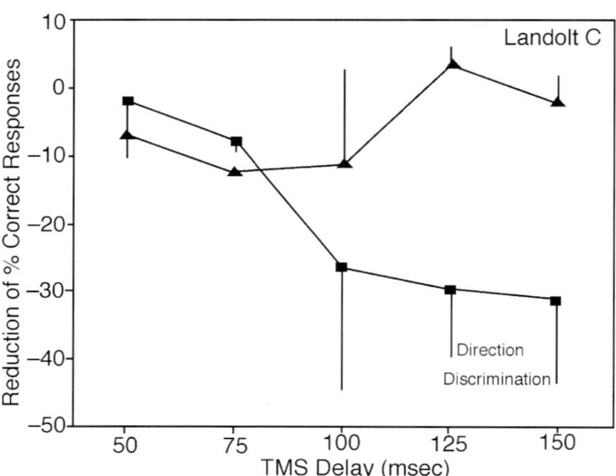

Fig. 5. Plot of the average reduction of the percentage of correct responses produced by TMS over the left V5 in the Landolt C spatial acuity and motion direction task. (Hotson et al., 1994. Reproduced with permission.)

TMS of V1 differentially affects speed and direction judgments, suggesting that sensory information processing constraining speed discrimination is localized differently from the sensory information constraining direction discrimination (Matthews et al., 2001): in a motion perception task, speed discriminability was significantly impaired while direction discriminability remained intact when TMS was applied to this area.

In addition, it was found that TMS could improve performance in non-motion search tasks when motion serves as a distractor (Walsh et al., 1998). In a visual search task in which motion was present but irrelevant and attention to color or form was required, TMS applied over the left V5 improved performance, probably by disruption of motion perception.

Also rTMS was used to modulate V5 function. In a visual motion priming task, rTMS using 10 Hz frequency of 500 ms duration over V5, applied in the intertrial interval of a motion discrimination task, disrupted visual priming of motion while motion perception was not affected when V1 or the posterior-parietal cortex were stimulated (Campana et al., 2002).

Stewart et al. (1999) have shown that rTMS can affect the degree of learning in a visual motion task in a frequency-dependent manner. Subjects had to identify a moving stimulus, which was defined by the conjunction of shape and movement direction. Subjects who were stimulated with 3 Hz frequency over the left V5 learned significantly less during a 4-day session than the control group or the group receiving 10 Hz stimulation (Stewart et al., 1999). These frequency-dependent learning effects were also found during and after stimulation of the motor cortex, suggesting that rTMS effects on learning are generalized across modalities.

3. Transcranial direct current stimulation (tDCS)

As discussed above, single pulse TMS produces a brief (in the range of milliseconds), strong excitation or inhibition in the brain and in that way *stimulates or interrupts* ongoing cortical activity to a spatially and temporally restricted extent. In contrast, transcranial direct current stimulation (tDCS) is usually applied for a much longer duration (at least seconds), *modulates* cortical activity and in this way induces functional changes in the human brain. In this, it shares certain similarities with rTMS. tDCS offers the possibility of inducing acute and persistent neuronal excitability changes without local discomfort, probably by shifting neuronal resting membrane potential (Purpura and McMurtry, 1964). Although this simple method has been used since the 1960s, mainly in animals, human studies were rare up to 1998, when Priori et al. first used TMS to evaluate tDCS-induced changes of human cortex excitability. In rats and cats it was shown that applying an anodal DC stimulus to the surface of both the motor and the visual cortex increased cortical excitability, probably by depolarizing neuronal membranes at subthreshold level and thus increasing the spontaneous firing rate of the cells, while a cathodal current resulted in the reverse effect, most probably due to hyperpolarizing neurons (Creuztfeldt et al., 1962; Bindman et al., 1964; Purpura and McMurtry, 1964; Ward and Weiskrantz, 1969). In cats the stimulation effect on the visual cortex was less pronounced than on the motor cortex, probably due to the different structures of the cortices and different spatial orientations of the neurons (Creuztfeldt et al., 1962). The elicited effects were not restricted to the duration of stimulation itself but could outlast it for several hours if stimulation intensity and duration were high enough (Bindman et al., 1964).

3.1. Functional aspects

Learning processes are accompanied by changes of neuronal activity and excitability, therefore these basic neurophysiological studies have raised the possibility that cortical excitability changes induced by weak direct current stimulation could modify higher order cognitive processes. Indeed, early animal experiments demonstrated that DC stimulation affects behavior in an effective and reversible manner. Cathodal polarization of the striate cortex in the rabbit led to a large decrement in the performance of a conditioned response when light flashes were used as the conditioning stimuli (Morell and Naitoh, (1962). The same effect was found in pattern or brightness discrimination tasks in rats (Kupfermann, 1965). Here, cathodal stimulation most probably compromised perception and impaired performance by decreasing the cortical firing rate. However, Ward and Weiskrantz (1969) found that also anodal polarization applied to the surface of the striate cortex of monkeys resulted in impaired visual discrimination. At first glance, this surprising result can be explained by the specific structure of the task: in visual discrimination tasks, the correct decision must be met by comparing very similar stimuli, thus an overall cortical activity enhancement or increased cortical "noise" caused by anodal DC stimulation would make decision-making more difficult. This interpretation is supported by further studies in animals and humans: in a study using a perceptual discrimination task in humans, anodal polarization of the visual cortex diminished the psychophysical sensitivity of perception and moreover the subjects used a stricter criterion of decision-making (Korsakov and Matveeva, 1982). Choosing a more strict decision criterion would be the possibly preferable strategy if the signal-to-noise ratio decreases. Moreover, as shown in animal experiments, anodal stimulation enhances performance in a delayed reaction time task, which does not include any "noisy" aspects (Rosen and Stamm, 1972). Apparently, an externally induced cortical excitability enhancement supports the activation of task-relevant engrams.

Most early human studies concentrated on possible therapeutic applications of tDCS and described some beneficial effects in psychiatric patients after stimulation (Constain et al., 1964; Lippold and Readfearn, 1964; Readfearn et al., 1964). However, these effects could not be replicated by all later studies, mainly due to different patient subgroups and technical differences (Lifshitz and Harper, 1968; Lolas, 1977). The main problem was to determine the psychophysiological and electrophysiological effects of tDCS objectively, and thus, to define optimal stimulation conditions. Recently it was shown directly that transcranially applied direct current can modulate excitability and activity of the motor cortex in healthy subjects, both during and after stimulation, as measured by TMS and fMRI (Priori et al., 1998; Nitsche and Paulus, 2000, 2001; Rosenkranz et al., 2000; Baudewig et al., 2001; Nitsche et al., 2003). The after-effects can last from minutes to hours, beyond the end of the stimulation, depending on intensity of current and the duration of the stimulation (Nitsche and Paulus, 2000, 2001).

3.2. tDCS studies on visual perception

The number of studies on modification of visual perception by tDCS in humans is low, however, they have particular importance in the context presented here. In a recent study, we measured phosphene thresholds before, 10 and 20 min after the end of tDCS applied to the occipital cortex (Antal et al., 2003). Phosphenes were elicited by both mono- and biphasic short trains of TMS pulses when the coil was placed 3–5 cm over the Oz. tDCS was applied for 10 min. Significantly reduced phosphene thresholds were detected immediately and 10 min after the end of anodal stimulation while cathodal stimulation resulted in an opposite effect.

In another study static and dynamic contrast sensitivities (sCS and dCS) were evaluated before, during, immediately and 10 min after anodal or cathodal tDCS applied to the occipital cortex of healthy subjects (Antal et al., 2001). Significant sCS and dCS loss was found during and immediately after 7 min of cathodal stimulation, which is known to elicit short lasting after-effects in the motor cortex. Ten minutes after the end of the stimulation the sCS and dCS values had reached the baseline levels (Fig. 6). Anodal stimulation had no effect. The stimuli used in this study were black and white sinusoidal gratings with a spatial frequency of 4 cycles/degree which is just at the top of the human CS curve. Thus, the lack of an effect of anodal tDCS in this study is possibly caused by a ceiling effect. These results show that not only motor but also primary visual functions can be transiently altered by tDCS, most probably by modulating neural excitability.

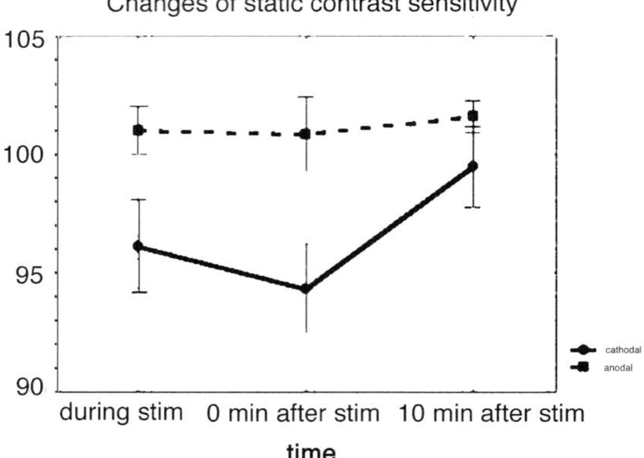

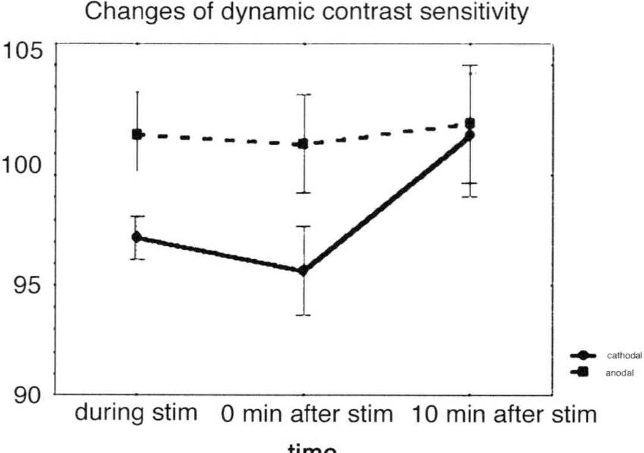

Fig. 6. Effects of transcranial direct current stimulation on static and dynamic contrast sensitivities (CS). Visual stimuli were Gabor patches (vertical Gaussian filtered black and white sinusoidal gratings). The spatial frequency of the pattern was 4 cycles/degree, the temporal frequency in the dynamic condition 4 Hz. For the CS measurement a method of adjustment (MOA) was used. CS are depicted in percentage during, immediately after and 10 min after cathodal and anodal stimulation. (Antal et al., 2001. Reproduced with permission.)

Although the underlying cellular/molecular changes induced by tDCS are at present largely unknown, the elicited effects are most probably localized intra-cortically, as shown for the motor cortex (Nitsche and Paulus, 2001; Nitsche et al., 2003). Also recently it was shown that the evoked after-effects are NMDA receptor-dependent (Liebetanz et al., 2002), and thus, share a certain similarity with other well-known neuroplastic mechanisms (Bennett, 2000). In summary, tDCS offers a non-invasive, non-painful method that can induce rapid plastic changes when it is applied to the occipital cortex, however, further research is necessary to clarify its mode of action and effectiveness in higher order visuo-cognitive processes.

4. Conclusions

One major aim of vision research is to find methods which are suitable to induce functional changes in the human brain in a controlled, safe way in order to explore visual perceptual and visuo-cognitive functions. TMS and tDCS allow a manipulation of cortical network activity in humans and in parallel, a psychophysical evaluation of correlated perceptual changes. They influence the brain's activity electrically and change the organized cortical activity transiently and reversibly in a non-invasive, non-painful way. However, in the mode of action, both techniques are at least partly complementary. In the last decade single pulse TMS has been applied to elicit reversible "virtual lesions" and thus mimic "classical" brain lesions to a certain extent in humans. While single pulse TMS induces externally triggered changes in the neuronal spiking pattern and *interfere* with cortical activity in a spatially and temporally restricted fashion, tDCS most probably modulates the spontaneous firing of neurons by changing resting membrane potential and thus not disrupts but *modifies* ongoing neuronal activity. rTMS stands in between the aforementioned methods, dependent on the strength, frequency and duration of stimulation.

Single pulse TMS possesses a good temporal resolution and produces short-lasting effects, mapping studies within the motor and visual cortex showed a spatial resolution down to 0.5–1.0 cm at the scalp surface (for reviews see: Jahanshahi and Rothwell, 2000; Cowey and Walsh, 2001). The effect of tDCS is probably intracortical (Nitsche and Paulus, 2001; Nitsche et al., 2003) and may be focally restricted (Rush and Driscoll, 1968), however, its temporal resolution is poor.

Thus, single pulse TMS is ideally suited to deliver information about the global involvement of a given cortical area in the performance of a task and its time course. However, specific gradual changes in performance caused by tDCS-induced cortical excitability modulations may deliver additional information about the specific functional role of a given area and help to gain insight into details of cortical information processing.

TMS is an essential tool in studying the effects of abnormal reorganization of the visual cortex (Cohen et al., 1997) or for examining visual learning effects (Walsh et al., 1998). Efforts have been made to combine TMS and tDCS with other techniques, such as fMRI and PET (Paus et al., 1997; Kosslyn et al., 1999; Baudewig et al., 2001). The combination of these techniques seems to be a very promising approach to learn more about localization, time course and functional specifications of a given brain area involved in visual and visuo-cognitive tasks. Moreover, the combination of TMS and electroencephalography (EEG) is able to elicit and to trace neuronal activity and corticocortical connections (Ilmoniemi et al., 1997). TMS and tDCS may elucidate or even modulate plastic changes in the nervous system in order to influence behavior (for a review see: Pascual-Leone et al., 1999; Nitsche et al., this volume). As investigative tools, both methods have the potential to widen our knowledge concerning the underlying neuronal mechanisms of different neurological and neuropsychiatric disorders.

Acknowledgement

Supported by the VW Foundation (I/76 712). We thank Chris Crozier for the English corrections.

References

Afra, J., Mascia, A., Gerard, P., Maertens de Noordhout, A. and Schoenen, J. Interictal cortical excitability in migraine: a study using transcranial magnetic stimulation of motor and visual cortices. *Ann. Neurol.*, 1998, 44: 209–215.

Albright, T.D. Centrifugal directional bias in the middle temporal visual area (MT) of the macaque. *Vis. Neurosci.*, 1989, 2: 177–188.

Amassian, V.E., Cracco, R.Q., Maccabee, P.J., Cracco, J.B., Rudell, A. and Eberle, L. Suppression of visual perception by magnetic coil stimulation of human occipital cortex. *Electroencephalogr. Clin. Neurophysiol.*, 1989, 74: 458–462.

Amassian, V.E., Maccabee, P.J, Cracco, R.Q., Cracco, J.B., Somasundaram, M., Rothwell, J.C., Eberle, L., Henra, K. and Rudell, A.P. The polarity of the induced electric field influences magnetic coil inhibition of human visual cortex: implications for the site of excitation. *Electroencephalogr. Clin. Neurophysiol.*, 1994, 93: 21–26.

Amassian, V.E., Cracco, R.Q., Vergara, M., Maccabee, P.J., Somasundaram, M. and Cracco, J.B. Magnetic transcranial stimulation studies on the roles of frontal and occipital lobes in perception, on estimating perceptual delay, and on temporary relief with parietal stimulation. In: A.V. Apkarian and S.N. Ayrapetian (Eds.), *Pain Mechanisms and Management*. IOS Press, Boston, 1998a: 260–282.

Amassian, V.E., Cracco, R.Q., Maccabee, P.J., Cracco, J.B., Rudell, A.P. and Eberle, L. Transcranial magnetic stimulation in study of the visual pathway. *J. Clin. Neurophysiol.*, 1998b, 15: 288–304.

Antal, A., Nitsche, M.A. and Paulus, W. External modulation of visual perception in humans. *NeuroReport*, 2001, 12: 3553–3555.

Antal, A., Kincses, T., Nitsche, M.A., Bartfai, O., Demmer, I., Sommer, M. and Paulus, W. Pulse configuration dependent effects of repetitive transcranial magnetic stimulation on visual perception. *NeuroReport*, 2002, 13: 2229–2233.

Antal, A., Kincses, Z.T., Nitsche, M.A. and Paulus, W. Manipulation of phosphene thresholds by transcranial direct current stimulation in man. *Exp. Brain Res.*, 2003, 150: 375–378.

Aurora, S.K., Ahmad, B.K., Welch, K.M., Bhardhwaj, P. and Ramadan, N.M. Transcranial magnetic stimulation confirms hyperexcitability of occipital cortex in migraine. *Neurology*, 1998, 50: 1111–1114.

Barker, A.T., Jalinous, R. and Freeston, I.L. Non-invasive magnetic stimulation of the human motor cortex. *Lancet*, 1985, 8: 1106–1107.

Baudewig, J., Nitsche, M.A., Paulus, W. and Frahm, J. Regional Modulation of BOLD MRI responses to human sensorimotor activation by transcranial direct current stimulation. *Magn. Res. Med.*, 2001, 45: 196–201.

Beckers, G. and Hömberg, V. Impairment of visual perception and visual short term memory scanning by transcranial magnetic stimulation of the occipital cortex. *Exp. Brain Res.*, 1991, 87: 421–432.

Beckers, G. and Hömberg, V. Cerebral visual motion blindness: transitory akinetopsia induced by transcranial magnetic stimulation of human visual area V5. *Proc. Roy. Soc. Lond. Ser. B.*, 1992, 249: 173–178.

Beckers, G. and Zeki, S. The consequences of inactivating areas V1 and V5 on visual motion perception. *Brain*, 1995, 118: 49–60.

Bennett, M.R. The concept of long term potentiation of transmission at synapses. *Prog. Neurobiol.*, 2000, 60: 109–137.

Bindman, L.J., Lippold, O.C. and Redfearn, J.W.T. The action of brief polarizing currents on the cerebral cortex of the rat (1) during current flow and (2) in the production of long-lasting after-effects. *J. Physiol.*, 1964, 172: 369–382.

Boroojerdi, B., Prager, A., Muellbacher, W. and Cohen, L.G. Reduction of human visual cortex excitability using 1 Hz transcranial magnetic stimulation. *Neurology*, 2000, 54: 1529–1531.

Boroojerdi, B., Phipps, M., Kopylev, L., Wharton, C.M., Cohen, L.G. and Grafman, J. Enhancing analogic reasoning with rTMS over the left prefrontal cortex. *Neurology*, 2001, 56: 526–528.

Braddick, O.J., O'Brien, J.M.D., Wattam-Bell, J., Atkinson, J., Hartley, T. and Turner, R. Brain areas sensitive to coherent visual motion. *Perception*, 2001, 30: 61–72.

Brindley, G.S. The variability of the human striate cortex. *J. Physiol.* (Lond), 1972, 225: 1P.

Brindley, G.S. and Lewin, W.S. The visual sensations produced by electrical stimulation of the medial occipital cortex. *J. Physiol.*, 1968, 194: 54–5P.

Campana, G., Cowey, A. and Walsh, V. Priming of motion direction and area V5/MT: a test of perceptual memory. *Cereb Cortex.*, 2002, 12: 663–669.

Cohen, L.G., Celnik, P., Pascual-Leone, A., Corwell, B., Falz, L., Dambrosia, J., Honda, M., Sadato, N., Gerloff, C., Catala, M. D. and Hallett, M. Functional relevance of cross-modal plasticity in blind humans. *Nature*, 1997, 389: 180–183.

Constain, R., Redfearn, J.W. and Lippold, O.C. A controlled trial of the therapeutic effect of polarisation of the brain depressive illness. *Br. J. Psych.*, 1964, 110: 786–799.

Corthout, E., Uttl, B., Ziemann, U., Cowey, A. and Hallett, M. Two periods of processing in the (circum) striate visual cortex as revealed by transcranial magnetic stimulation. *Neuropsychol.*, 1999a, 37: 137–145.

Corthout, E., Uttl, B., Walsh, V., Hallett, M. and Cowey, A. Timing of activity of early visual cortex as revealed by transcranial magnetic stimulation. *NeuroReport*, 1999b, 10: 2631–2634.

Corthout, E., Uttl, B., Juan, C.H., Hallett, M. and Cowey, A. Plasticity revealed by transcranial magnetic stimulation of early visual cortex. *NeuroReport*, 2000a, 11: 1–5.

Corthout, E., Uttl, B., Juan, C. H., Hallett, M. and Cowey, A. Suppression of vision by transcranial magnetic stimulation: a third mechanism. *NeuroReport*, 2000b, 11: 2345–2349.

Cowey, A. and Walsh, V. Magnetically induced phosphenes in sighted, blind and blindsighted observers. *NeuroReport*, 2000, 11: 3269–3273.

Cowey, A. and Walsh, V. Tickling the brain: studying visual sensation, perception and cognition by transcranial magnetic stimulation. *Prog. Brain Res.*, 2001, 134: 411–425.

Creutzfeld, O.D., Fromm, G.H. and Kapp, H. Influence of transcortical dc-currents on cortical neuronal activity. *Exp. Neurol.*, 1962, 5: 436–452.

Epstein, C.M. and Zangaladze, A. Magnetic Coil suppression of extrafoveal visual perception using disappearance targets. *J. Clin. Neurophysiol.*, 1996, 13: 242–246.

Epstein, C.M., Verson, R. and Zangaladze, A. Magnetic coil suppression of visual perception at an extracalcarine site. J. *Clin. Neurophysiol.*, 1996, 13: 247–252.

Gothe, J., Brandt, S.A., Irlbacher, K., Roricht, S., Sabel, B.A. and Meyer, B.U. Changes in visual cortex excitability in blind subjects as demonstrated by transcranial magnetic stimulation. *Brain*, 2002, 125(3): 479–490.

Hess, R.H., Baker, C.L. and Zihl, J. The ,motion blind' patient: low-level spatial and temporal filters. *J. Neurosci.*, 1989, 9: 1628–1640.

Hotson, J.R. and Anand, S. The selectivity and timing of motion processing in human temporo-parieto-occipital cortex: a transcranial magnetic stimulation study. *Neuropsychologia*, 1999, 37: 169–179.

Hotson, J., Brain, D., Herzberg, W. and Boman, D. Transcranial magnetic stimulation of extrastriate cortex degrades human motion direction discrimination. *Vis. Res.*, 1994, 34: 2115–2123.

Ilmoniemi, R.J., Virtanen, J., Ruohonen, J., Karhu, J., Aronen, H. J., Naatanen, R. and Katila, T. Neuronal responses to magnetic stimulation reveal cortical reactivity and connectivity. *NeuroReport*, 1997, 8: 3537–3540.

Jahanshahi, M. and Rothwell, J. Transcranial magnetic stimulation studies of cognition: an emerging field. *Exp. Brain Res.*, 2000, 131: 1–9.

Kamitani, Y. and Shimojo, S. Manifestation of scotomas created by transcranial magnetic stimulation of human visual cortex. *Nat. Neurosci.*, 1999, 2: 767–771.

Kammer, T. Phosphenes and transient scotomas induced by magnetic stimulation of the occipital lobe: their topographic relationship. *Neuropsychologia*, 1999, 37: 191–198.

Kammer, T. and Beck, S. Phosphene thresholds evoked by transcranial magnetic stimulation are insensitive to short-lasting variations in ambient light. *Exp. Brain Res.*, 2002, 145: 407–410.

Kammer, T. and Nusseck, H.G. A recognition deficits following occipital lobe TMS explained by raised detection threshold? *Neuropsychologia*, 1998, 36: 1161–1166.

Kammer, T., Beck, S., Erb, M. and Grodd, W. The influence of current direction on phosphene thresholds evoked by transcranial magnetic stimulation. *Clin. Neuropyhsiol.*, 2001, 112: 2015–2021.

Kastner, S., Demmer, I. and Ziemann, U. Transient visual field defects induced by transcranial magnetic stimulation over human occipital pole. *Exp. Brain Res.*, 1998, 118: 19–26.

Korsakov, I.A. and Matveeva, L.V. Psychophysical characteristics of perception and of brain electrical activity during occipital micropolarization. *Fiziologiya Chaloveka.*, 1982, 8: 595–603.

Kosslyn, S.M., Pascual-Leone, A., Felician, O., Camposano, S., Keenan, J.P., Thompson, W.L., Ganis, G., Sukel, K.E. and Alpert, N.M. The role of area 17 in visual imagery: Convergent evidence from PET and rTMS. *Science*, 1999, 284: 167–170.

Kupferman, I. Effects of cortical polarization on visual discrimination. *Exp. Neurol.*, 1965, 12: 179–189.

Liebetanz, D., Nitsche, M.A., Tergau, F. and Paulus, W. Pharmacological approach to the mechanisms of transcranial DC-stimulation-induced after-effects of human motor cortex excitability. *Brain*, 2002, 125: 1–10.

Lifshitz, K. and Harper, P. A trial of transcranial polarization in chronic schizophrenics. *Br. J. Psychiatry*, 1968, 114: 635–637.

Lippold, O.C. and Redfearn, J.W. Mental changes resulting from the passage of small direct currents trough the human brain. *Br. J. Psych.*, 1964, 110: 768–772.

Lolas, F. Brain polarization: behavioral and therapeutic effects. *Biol. Psych.*, 1977, 12: 37–47.

Lueck C.J., Zeki, S., Friston, K.J., Deiber, M.P., Cope, P., Cunningham, V.J., Lammertsma, A.A., Kennard, C. and Frackowiak, R.S. The colour centre in the cerebral cortex of man. *Nature*, 1989, 340; 386–389.

Maccabee, P.J., Amassian, V.E., Cracco, R.Q., Cracco, J.B., Rudell, A.P., Eberle, L.P. and Zemon, V. Magnetic coil stimulation of human visual cortex: studies of perception. *Electroencephalogr. Clin. Neurophysiol.*, 1991 (Suppl.) 43, 111–120.

Marg, E. and Rudiak, D. Phosphenes induced by magnetic stimulation over the occipital brain: description and probable site of stimulation. *Optom. Vis. Sci.*, 1994, 71: 301–311.

Masur, H., Papke, K. and Oberwittler, C. Suppression of visual perception by transcranial magnetic stimulation – experimental finding in healthy subjects and patients with optic neuritis. *Electroencephalogr. Clin. Neurophysiol.*, 1993, 86: 259–267.

Matthews, N., Luber, B., Qian, N. and Lisanby, S.H. Transcranial magnetic stimulation differentially affects speed and direction judgments. *Exp. Brain Res.*, 2001, 140: 397–406.

McKeefry, D.J., Watson, J.D.G., Frackowiak, R.S.J., Fong, K. and Zeki, S. The activity in human areas V1/V2, V3 and V5 during the perception of coherent and incoherent motion. *NeuroImage*, 1997, 5: 1–12.

Merton, P.A. and Morton, H.B. Stimulation of the cerebral cortex in the intact human subject. *Nature*, 1980, 285: 227.

Meyer, B.U., Diehl, R.R., Steinmetz, H., Britton, T.C. and Benecke, R. Magnetic stimuli applied over motor cortex and visual cortex: Influence of coil position and field polarity on motor responses, phosphenes and eye movements. *Electroencephalogr. Clin. Neurophysiol.*, 1991, 43: 121–134.

Miller, M.B., Fendrich, R., Eliassen, J.C., Demirel, S. and Gazzaniga, M.S. Transcranial magnetic stimulation: delays in visual suppression due to luminance changes. *NeuroReport*, 1996, 7: 1740–1744.

Morell, F. and Naitoh, P. Effect of cortical polarization on a conditioned avoidance response. *Exp. Neurol.*, 1962, 6: 507–523.

Nitsche, M.A., and Paulus, W. Excitability changes induced in the human motor cortex by weak transcranial direct current stimulation. *J. Physiol.*, 2000, 527: 633–639.

Nitsche, M.A. and Paulus, W. Sustained excitability elevations induced by transcranial DC motor cortex stimulation in humans. *Neurology*, 2001, 57: 1899–1901.

Nitsche, M.A., Nitsche, M.S., Klein, C.C., Tergau, F., Rothwell, J.C. and Paulus, W. Level of action of cathodal DC polarisation induced inhibition of the human motor cortex. *Clin. Neurophysiol.*, 2003, 114: 600–604.

Nitsche, M.A., Schauenburg, A., Lang, N., Liebetanz, D., Exner, C., Paulus, W. and Tergau, F. Facilitation of implicit motor learning by weak transcranial direct current stimulation of the primary motor cortex in the human. *J. Cogn. Neurosci.*, 2003, 15: 619–626.

Newsome, W.T. and Pare, E.B. A selective impairment of motion perception following lesions of the middle temporal visual area (MT). *J. Neurosci.*, 1988, 8: 2201–2211.

Pascual-Leone, A. and Walsh, V. Fast backprojections from the motion to the primary visual area necessary for visual awareness. *Science*, 2001, 292: 510–512.

Pascual-Leone, A., Houser, C.M., Reese, K., Shotland, L.I., Grafman, J., Sato, S., Valls-Sole, J., Brasil-Neto, J.P., Wassermann, E.M. and Cohen, L.G. Safety of rapid-rate transcranial magnetic stimulation in normal volunteers. *Electroencephalogr. Clin. Neurophysiol.*, 1993, 89: 120–130.

Pascual-Leone, A., Gomez-Tortosa, E., Grafman, J., Always, D., Nichelli, P. and Hallett, M. Induction of visual extinction by rapid-rate transcranial magnetic stimulation of parietal lobe. *Neurology*, 1994, 44: 494–498.

Pascual-Leone, A., Tarazona, F., Keenan, J., Tormos, J.M., Hamilton, R. and Catala, M.D. Transcranial magnetic stimulation and neuroplasticity. *Neuropsychologia*, 1999, 37: 207–217.

Paulus, W., Korinth, S., Wischer, S. and Tergau, F. Differentiation of parvo- and magnocellular pathways by TMS at the occipital cortex. In: W. Paulus, M. Hallett P.M. Rossini and J.C. Rothwell (Eds.), Transcranial magnetic stimulation. *Electroencephalogr. Clin. Neurophysiol.*, 1999 (Suppl.), 51: 351–360.

Paus, T., Jech, R., Thompson, C.J., Comeau, R., Peters, T. and Evans, A.C. Transcranial magnetic stimulation during positron emission tomography: a new method fort studying connectivity of the human cerebral cortex. *J. Neurosci.*, 1997, 17: 3178–3184.

Penfield, W. and Rasmussen, W. *The cerebral cortex of man.* Macmillan, New York, 1998, 1–248.

Priori, A., Berardelli, A., Rona, S., Accornero, N. and Manfredi, M. Polarization of the human motor cortex through the scalp. *NeuroReport*, 1998, 9: 2257–2260.

Purpura, D.P. and McMurtry, J.G. Intracellular activities and evoked potential changes during polarization of the motor cortex. *J. Neurophysiol.*, 1965, 28: 166–185.

Ray, P.G., Meador, K.J., Epstein, C.M., Loring, D.W. and Day, L.J. Magnetic stimulation of visual cortex: factors influencing the perception of phosphenes. *J. Clin. Neurophysiol.*, 1998, 15, 351–357.

Rosen, S.C. and Stamm, J.S. Cortical polarization: facilitation of delayed response performance by monkeys. *Exp. Neurol.*, 1972, 35, 282–289.

Redfearn, J.W., Lippold, O.C. and Constain, R. A preliminary account of the clinical effects of polarizing the brain in certain psychiatric disorders. *Br. J. Psychiatry*, 1964, 110: 773–785.

Rosenkranz, K., Nitsche, M.A., Tergau, F. and Paulus, W. Diminution of training-induced transient motor cortex plasticity by weak transcranial current stimulation in the human. *Neurosci. Lett.*, 2000, 296: 61–63.

Rush, S. and Driscoll, D.A. Current distribution in the brain from surface electrodes. *Anesth. Analg.*, 1968, 47: 717–723.

Shipp, S., de Jong, B.M., Zihl, J., Frackowiak, R.S.J. and Zeki, S. The brain activity related to residual motion vision in a patient with bilateral lesions of V5. *Brain*, 1994, 117: 1023–1038.

Stewart, L., Battelli, L., Walsh, V. and Cowey, A. Motion perception and perceptual learning studied by magnetic stimulation. In: W. Paulus, M. Hallett, P.M. Rossini and J.C. Rothwell (Eds.), Transcranial magnetic stimulation. *Electroenceph. Clin. Neurophys.*, 1999 (Suppl.), 51: 334–350.

Stewart, L.M., Walsh, V. and Rothwell, J.C. Motor and phosphene thresholds: a transcranial magnetic stimulation correlation study. *Neurophsychologia*, 2001, 39: 415–419.

Tootell, R.B.H., Teppas, J.B., Dale, A.M., Look, R.B., Serano, M.I., Malach, R., Brady, T.J. and Rosen, B.R. Visual motion aftereffect in human cortical area MT revealed by functional magnetic resonance imaging. *Nature*, 1995a, 375: 139–141.

Tootell, R.B.H., Teppas, J.B., Kwong, K.K., Malach, R., Born, R.T., Brady, T.J., Rosen, B.R. and Belliveau, J.W. Functional analysis of human MT and related visual cortical areas using magnetic resonance imaging. *J. Neurosci.*, 1995b, 15: 3215–3230.

Walsh, V. and Cowey, A. Magnetic stimulation studies of visual cognition. *Trends Cogn. Neurosci.*, 1998, 2: 103–110.

Walsh, V., Ellison, A., Battelli, L. and Cowey, A. Task-specific impairments and enhancements induced by magnetic stimulation of human visual area V5. *Proc. R. Soc. Lond. B.*, 1998, 265: 537–543.

Ward, R. and Weiskrantz, L. Impaired discrimination following polarization of the striate cortex. *Exp. Brain Res.*, 1969, 9: 346–356.

Watson, J.D.G., Myers, R., Frackowiak, R.S.J., Hajnal, J.V., Woods, R.P., Mazziotta, J.C., Shipp, S. and Zeki, S. Area V5 of the human brain: Evidence from a combined study using positron emission tomography and magnetic resonance imaging. *Cereb Cortex.*, 1993, 3: 79–94.

Zeki, S., Watson, J.D., Lueck, C.J., Friston, K.J., Kennard, C. and Frackowiak, R.S. A direct demonstration of functional specialization in human visual cortex. *J. Neurosci.*, 1991, 11: 641–649.

Transcranial Magnetic Stimulation and Transcranial Direct Current Stimulation (Supplements to Clinical Neurophysiology, Vol. 56)
Editors: W. Paulus, F. Tergau, M.A. Nitsche, J.C. Rothwell, U. Ziemann, M. Hallett

Chapter 31

Neural correlates of phosphene perception

Ingo G. Meister[a], Juergen Weidemann[b], Nina Dambeck[a], Henrik Foltys[a], Roland Sparing[a], Timo Krings[b], Armin Thron[b] and Babak Boroojerdi[a,*]

[a] *Departments of Neurology and* [b]*Neuroradiology, University Hospital Aachen, D-52057 Aachen (Germany)*

1. Introduction

Phosphenes are elementary light perceptions which can be elicited by transcranial magnetic stimulation (TMS) over the occipital cortex (Meyer et al., 1991; Marg and Rudiak, 1994). Phosphene threshold, which is the minimum magnetic stimulation intensity capable of eliciting phosphenes has been used as a measure of the excitability of the visual cortex (Afra et al., 1998; Aurora et al., 1998). In addition, phosphene perception has been utilized to assess short-term plasticity of the visual cortex and its underlying mechanisms (Boroojerdi et al., 2000a, b, 2001).

Single pulse focal TMS does not elicit phosphenes in all normal subjects. The percentage of investigated subjects perceiving phosphenes varies across studies. Our results, along with those of Meyer et al. (1991) indicate that about two-thirds of the subjects tested with TMS report phosphenes. The mechanism underlying the absence of phosphene perception in the remaining third is still unknown.

Furthermore, the neural correlates underlying phosphene perception are not well understood. Studies investigating the cortical site of phosphene perception using different TMS coil positions are yet to determine the exact site in the visual system (Kammer, 1999; Kammer et al., 2001). Although it is widely agreed that phosphenes are evoked within the central visual system, the exact mechanism of phosphene perception could not be characterised, mainly due to methodological limitations.

The present study adopted a new approach to further characterise the neural correlates of phosphene perception. Whereas, previous studies investigated only those subjects who reported phosphene perception, we sought to investigate differences in visual cortex excitability between subjects with, and without, phosphene perception. We addressed this issue by combining the TMS data with functional magnetic resonance imaging (fMRI) measurements of the activated visual network in response to a standard checkerboard stimulus. Previous studies locating the primary motor area of the hand using TMS mapping and fMRI activation found a high coherence between the two methods (Krings et al., 1997, 2001a, b; Boroojerdi et al., 1999), and TMS and fMRI can be seen as complimentary approaches in the evaluation of cortical

* *Correspondence to*: Dr. Babak Boroojerdi, Neurologische Klinik, Universtätsklinikum, Pauwelsstr. 30, D-52074 Aachen, Germany
Tel: +49/241 80 89630; Fax: +49/241 8082444
E-mail: bboroojerdi@ukaachen.de

function. We utilized the comparison of visual fMRI activation between subjects with, and without, phosphene perception to determine the possible cortical areas, where TMS phosphenes are elicited. As an additional method to investigate the properties of the cortical visual system in the two groups, we used Visual Evoked Potentials (VEP) to measure the excitability of the visual system (Bonmassar et al., 1999; Kashikura et al., 2001). Recent studies have demonstrated that the dominant component of the VEP, the N1 component, is generated in the primary visual cortex (Slotnick et al., 1999; Di Russo et al., 2002), whereas the origin of the early P1 component lies within dorsal extrastriate cortex. Thus, the N1-P1 amplitude reflects the excitability of both striate and early extrastriate areas. However, Slotnick et al. investigating retinotopic maps of the primary visual cortex with VEP, showed that N1 is the major component of the VEP amplitude.

2. Methods

2.1. Subjects

We investigated 27 healthy normal volunteers (18 men, nine women, age 19–36 years). All subjects gave written informed consent and the protocol was approved by the local ethics Review Board.

2.2. Transcranial magnetic stimulation

During the determination of phosphene perception, subjects were blindfolded in a dark room. TMS was applied over a grid of nine points centered over Oz, according to the International 10-20 EEG electrode system, each point 2 cm apart. Magnetic stimulation was applied using a Magstim 200 magnetic stimulator (Magstim Co, Whitland, UK), equipped with a figure-of-8 coil (outer diameter of each wing 9.8 cm). Phosphene perception was tested with single pulse TMS with up to 90% of maximum stimulator output over all grid points. The subjects were asked to indicate the perception of phosphenes and the stimulation site where a given TMS intensity evoked the brightest phosphene. This point was determined as the optimal point for eliciting phosphenes. The phosphene threshold was then determined as the minimum intensity over the optimal point capable of eliciting phosphenes in three out of five trials. As a control, subjects who reported phosphenes also received TMS applied additionally over P3 and P4, and sham stimulation was performed over the optimal point (coil tilted away from the head to reproduce the stimulator sound and the cutaneous perception without brain stimulation). Subjects reporting phosphenes in one of the control conditions were excluded from further studies.

2.3. Functional magnetic resonance imaging

Twenty-two subjects participated in the fMRI experiment, 11 of whom reported phosphenes while 11 lacked phosphene perception.

The cerebral activation was studied with functional magnetic resonance imaging employing blood oxygen level-dependent contrast on a 1.5 T Philips Gyroscan scanner (Philips Co., Best, The Netherlands) with a standard headcoil. An epoch design was used with eight experimental epochs (checkerboard) and eight baseline epochs (black screen with a central fixation crosshair). The fMRI sessions comprised four Dummy scans followed by 96 whole-brain scans (four scans for the checkerboard and eight scans for the baseline epochs) using single-shot gradient-refocused echo-planar imaging (EPI) (TR = 3.2 s, TE = 50 ms, flip angle = 90°, 24 slices).

During the experimental condition, a checkerboard alternating with a frequency of 8 Hz was presented via MRI compatible high-resolution 3-D glasses. The frequency of 8 Hz for the fMRI experiment was chosen to optimize the fMRI BOLD signal. In a previous study (Hoge et al., 1999) comparing different frequencies for a checkerboard, 8 Hz turned out to elicit a larger BOLD signal than 1 Hz. A checkerboard of 10 horizontal and eight vertical fields was chosen comprising a 30° field of view; it was presented at a resolution of 1024 × 768 pixels. The subjects were asked to look carefully at the presented checkerboard.

2.4. *Visual evoked potentials*

Visual evoked potentials were measured in 16 subjects (eight reporting phosphenes, eight without phosphene perception). The VEP were evoked by an alternating checkerboard pattern (frequency 1.3 Hz); the cortical response was measured using an electrode placed 4 cm above inion in the midline and referenced to an electrode over Fz (according to the International 10–20-EEG electrode system) using a Nicolet Electrodiagnostic System (Nicolet Co, USA). Each VEP was averaged across 120 single runs for both eyes separately. For further analysis the VEP amplitude (N1-P1 amplitude) was determined.

2.5. *Statistical analysis*

2.5.1. *fMRI data*

The fMRI data were analysed using Statistical Parametric Mapping software (SPM99, www.fil.ion.ac.uk/spm, London, UK). The dummy scans were discarded. The remaining scans were realigned and spatially normalised to a stereotactic space using an EPI-template (Montreal Neurological Institute (MNI), www.bic.mni.mcgill.ca/brainweb). The voxel size was 1.5 × 1.5 × 1.5 mm. The normalised data were smoothed using a Gaussian kernel of 3 × 3 × 3 mm in order to improve the signal-to-noise ratio. For the following parameter estimation an appropriate design matrix was specified using a box-car function as reference waveform. According to the general linear model, the voxel-by-voxel parameter estimation for the smoothed data was carried out. In order to test hypotheses about regionally specific effects, the resulting estimated beta-maps were compared by means of linear contrasts of each active and control condition. From this analysis resulted a map of *t*-statistic values (SPM(t)-map). To correct for the inference drawn by multi-subject fMRI data, a random effect model was applied (Friston et al., 1999), comparing the raw data of the subjects with a one-sample-*t*-test ($p = 0.001$). The resulting activations were corrected within boxes of 30 × 30 × 30 mm around activated voxels found to be activated in previous studies (Bonmassar et al., 1999; Kashikura et al., 2001).

The data of the two groups of subjects were analysed separately. To investigate those regions which were activated in subjects perceiving phosphenes but not in subjects lacking phosphenes, a masked activation map was created out of the SPM(t)-maps of the contrasts "checkerboard vs. baseline" of the two group activation maps resulting in a SPM(t) map "phosphene perception [masked by] no phosphene perception".

2.5.2. *TMS and VEP data*

To investigate whether there is a correlation between phosphene threshold and cluster size in fMRI activity, the linear regression coefficient between these values was calculated.

Comparing VEP amplitudes over the right and left visual cortex using a *t*-test, there were no significant side differences in neither group ($P = 0.2$). Therefore, the VEP amplitudes of the right and the left eye were averaged for each subject and pooled. The VEP amplitudes of the two subject groups were then compared using Student's *t*-test.

3. Results

3.1. *TMS and VEP data*

Fifteen of the subjects (56%) tested reported phosphene perception, 11 (41%) lacked any phosphene perception, while one subject was excluded because she did not report phosphenes consistently. In the phosphene perceiving subgroup, the average phosphene threshold was 58.1% (3.36% (SEM) of the maximum stimulator output. Only one subject reported Oz as optimal stimulation site, whereas in the other subjects the lateral stimulation sites were optimal (seven subjects right side vs. three subjects left side). The optimum point was located above Oz in three and below Oz in five subjects. None of the subjects showed optimal stimulus sites at points of the grid in the midline rostral and caudal to Oz. All subjects perceived phosphenes contralaterally, most describing them as small spots of light, while in some cases there were larger phosphenes commonly described as stripes in the contralateral hemifield.

The average VEP amplitude was 5.03 ± 0.78 µV (SEM) for phosphene perceiving subjects and 9.09 ± 1.25 µV for the non-perceiving group. VEP amplitudes were significantly higher in the group lacking phosphene perception than in the group perceiving phosphenes ($t(7) = 3.17$, $p = 0.016$) (Fig. 1). The latencies of the N1 and P1 component did not differ significantly between the two groups (no phosphene group N1: 68.82 ± 1.69 ms (SEM), P1: 104.51 ± 1.93 ms; phosphene group N1: 70.33 ± 2.52 ms, P1: 101.74 ± 2.3 ms; $p > 0.1$).

3.2. MRI data

Analysis of the fMRI data revealed bilateral activations comprising the whole striate and extrastriate visual network in response to the checkerboard pattern for both subject groups (Fig. 2). Analysis of the cluster size and the peak activations in the group data showed that the network activated in the phosphene perceiving group was larger than in the non-perceiving group (total size of the clusters activated in the visual network was 1870 voxels in the phosphene group and 1026 voxels in the no phosphene group). In contrast, the peak fMRI activation, which was located in the striate cortex in both groups, was slightly higher in the group lacking phosphene perception compared to the perceiving subjects (t-value phosphene group: $t = 12.83$; no phosphene group: $t = 14.53$, $p > 0.1$).

The analysis using a masked activation map to determine the regions which were activated solely in the phosphene group but not in the no phosphene group revealed that bilateral extrastriate areas comprising Brodmann Area 18 and 19 (V2, V3) were activated in association with phosphene perception (Fig. 3).

There was no significant correlation between phosphene threshold and size of the whole activated cluster in fMRI ($r = 0.169$).Because it is not possible in SPM to determine the size of subclusters belonging to a certain Brodmann Area within a greater cluster,

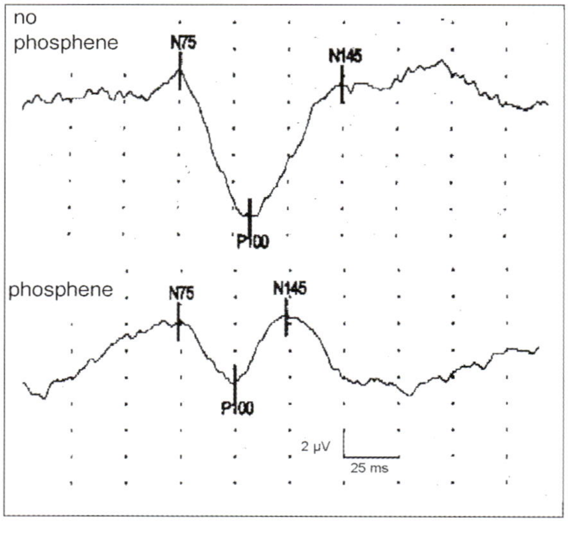

Fig. 1. Visual evoked potentials. Left: examples of right-eye VEP of a subject lacking phosphene perception (above) and a subject reporting phosphenes. Right: the average VEP amplitudes of the two groups. Error bars indicate standard errors.

No phosphene perception

Phosphene perception

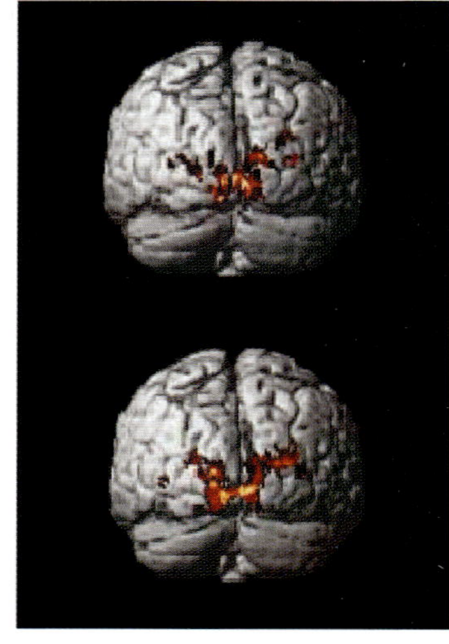

Fig. 2. fMRI group activations of subjects without (above) and with phosphene perception (bottom). Whereas subjects reporting phosphenes activated a larger visual network in response to checkerboard stimuli, the peak amplitude was slightly (not significantly) higher in subjects lacking phosphene perception.

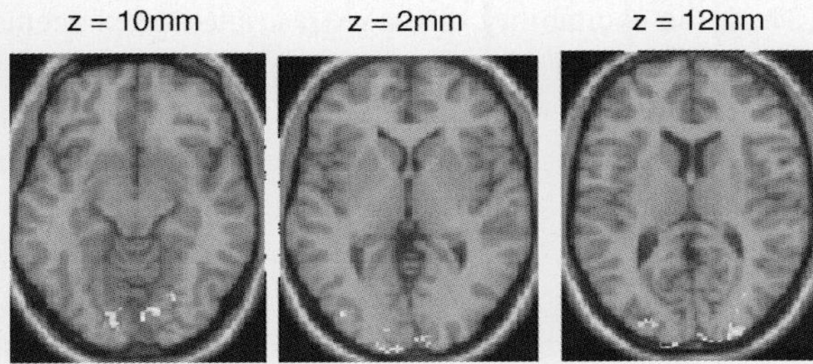

Fig. 3. Three slices showing fMRI activations, which were only present in subjects perceiving phosphenes but not in subjects lacking phosphene perception. This activation comprises part of the extrastriate cortex.

we performed a correlation analysis between the size of the whole activated fMRI cluster including V1 and phosphene threshold.

4. Discussion

The present study revealed remarkable differences in visual network activation in response to a standard checkerboard pattern between subjects perceiving phosphenes and those lacking phosphene perception. The activated bilateral visual network in response to the standard visual stimulus was larger in subjects who perceived phosphenes, comprising a greater part of the exstrastriate cortex. Both the peak activation measured with fMRI and VEP amplitudes, however, were higher in subjects who did not report phosphene perception. This suggests that the excitability of the primary visual cortex (and possibly early extrastriate areas) is higher in subjects who do not perceive phosphenes, whereas the excitability of higher extrastriate areas is higher in subjects who do report them. In our study, N1-P1 VEP amplitude was measured. It has been shown before, that generators in V1 and early extastriate areas contribute to this amplitude (Di Russo et al., 2002). Therefore, a conclusive distinction between V1 and early extrastriate excitability is not possible using N1-P1 VEP amplitude.

Although a wide range of paradigms have been employed for phosphene induction, and it is generally accepted that phosphenes are generated in the central visual system and provide a measure of visual cortex excitability, there is no consistent theory concerning the anatomical site where TMS induced phosphenes are elicited. Meyer et al. (1991) performed a topographical analysis of phosphenes under different TMS coil positions, asking subjects to rate the brightness of the induced phosphenes. Comparing the position of the coil with the phosphene location within the visual field reported by the subjects, they concluded that the rostral part of the calacarine sulcus may be the region where TMS induced phosphenes are likely to be generated.

Marg and Rudiak (1994) used a different approach to the problem: in their study, two TMS coils of different diameters were used to evoke phosphenes. TMS intensity was adjusted to induce phosphenes of the same brightness with both coils. Comparison of the electrical field revealed a depth of stimulation of 4 cm, suggesting the optic radiation as locus of phosphene perception. This was supported by the finding that phosphenes were reported to the same extent in the periphery and the foveal part of the visual field.

Three recent studies (Cowey and Walsh, 2000; Fernandez et al., 2002; Gothe et al., 2002) have employed transcranial magnetic stimulation in blind subjects. In the first study, TMS was applied to sighted subjects, one retinally blind subject and one subject lacking V1 in one hemisphere due to trauma at young age. Whereas the retinally blind subject reported phosphenes, the latter subject did not report phosphene perception when stimulated over the damaged hemisphere. Cowey and Walsh claimed that an intact V1 is essential for phosphene perception. However, it remains unclear if an intact V1 is also sufficient for phosphene perception. The second and third studies have shown that phosphene perception may be present in peripherally blind subjects. In the study of Fernandez et al., 13 blind participants were studied, seven of whom were able to perceive phosphenes. Gothe et al. (2002) compared phosphene perception in subjects with or without residual vision and fully sighted individuals and found that phosphenes could be elicited in all sighted subjects and those with residual vision but only in 20% of blind subjects. The two latter studies included only subjects with blindness due to pregeniculate lesions preserving the integrity of the occipital cortex without visual input.

The fact that phosphenes can be elicited in subjects suffering from blindness due to pregeniculate lesions show that phosphene perception is independent of intact visual perception, however, the phosphene threshold is usually higher than in healthy controls.

In accordance with the studies by Cowey and Walsh (2000), Kammer et al. (2000) noted that phosphenes can be induced from multiple target sites over the striate and extrastriate (V2/V3) cortex without qualitative differences, and concluded that either the target structure for TMS is the optic radiation or that the extrastriate cortex evokes activity in V1 which results in phosphene perception.

Taken together, there are several hypotheses but no clear evidence concerning the cortical site of phosphene perception. In the present study a standard alternating checkerboard stimulus elicited a stronger BOLD response in V2/V3 in the phosphene group compared to the no phosphene group which favours an involvement of the exstrastriate cortex in phosphene perception. If, as suggested by Cowey and Walsh (2000), V1 is also critical for phosphene perception, then phosphenes could be a product of signals originating in V1 (or the optic radiation) which are then transmitted to secondary visual areas.

Our finding that subjects lacking phosphene perception tend to have a higher excitability in V1 would be in accordance with the notion that only a certain level of excitability in V2/V3, where the incoming information from V1 is processed, can lead to perception of phosphenes. This is supported by the finding of Fernandez et al. (2002) that phosphenes differ remarkably in size, from a "pinpoint" to almost the whole visual field, and that phosphene size is not correlated with phosphene intensity: if there were a distinct cortical site within V1 generating phosphenes, one would expect a greater uniformity of phosphene perception.

In conclusion, subjects reporting phosphenes activate a larger extrastriate cortex network when exposed to a standard checkerboard stimulus compared to subjects lacking phosphene perception. Thus, the excitability of the extrastriate cortex seems to be related to phosphene perception, whereas the level of striate cortex excitability does not play a critical role for phosphene perception. This has implications on studies using phosphene threshold to measure the excitability of the visual cortex: studies which found short-term plasticity within the visual system due to light deprivation (Boroojerdi et al., 2000a) or changes of phosphene threshold in migraine patients (Aurora et al., 1998) measure changes likely to occur also in the extrastriate cortex. However, properties of phosphene perception need to be further characterised. An interesting approach would be to investigate phosphenes using separate TMS stimuli to V1 and V2/V3 at different time intervals.

Acknowledgements

This study was supported partly by the IZKF "BIOMAT" "Interdisciplinary Center for Clinical Research (BMBF project No. 01 KS 9503/9)", START-programs of the University of Aachen, and by Deutsche Forschungsgemeinscahft (KFO 112/1). The authors are grateful to Dr. Stuart Fellows for skillful editing of the manuscript.

References

Afra, J., Mascia, A., Gerard, P., Maertens de Noordhout, A. and Schoenen, J. Interictal cortical excitability in migraine: a study using transcranial magnetic stimulation of motor and visual cortices. *Ann. Neurol.*, 1998, 44: 209–215.

Aurora, S.K., Ahmad, B.K., Welch, K.M., Bhardhwaj, P. and Ramadan, N.M. Transcranial magnetic stimulation confirms hyperexcitability of occipital cortex in migraine. *Neurology*, 1998, 50: 1111–1114.

Bonmassar, G., Anami, K., Ives, J. and Belliveau, J.W. Visual evoked potential (VEP) measured by simultaneous 64-channel EEG and 3T fMRI. *NeuroReport*, 1999, 10: 1893–1897.

Boroojerdi, B., Foltys, H., Krings, T., Spetzger, U., Thron, A. and Topper, R. Localization of the motor hand area using transcranial magnetic stimulation and functional magnetic resonance imaging. *Clin. Neurophysiol.*, 1999, 110: 699–704.

Boroojerdi, B., Bushara, K.O., Corwell, B., Immisch, I., Battaglia, F., Muellbacher, W. and Cohen, L.G. Enhanced excitability of the human visual cortex induced by short-term light deprivation. *Cereb. Cortex*, 2000a, 10: 529–534.

Boroojerdi, B., Prager, A., Muellbacher, W. and Cohen, L.G. Reduction of human visual cortex excitability using 1-Hz transcranial magnetic stimulation. *Neurology*, 2000b, 54: 1529–1531.

Boroojerdi, B., Battaglia, F., Muellbacher, W. and Cohen, L.G. Mechanisms underlying rapid experience-dependent plasticity in the human visual cortex. *Proc. Natl. Acad. Sci. USA*, 2001, 98: 14698–14701.

Cowey, A. and Walsh, V. Magnetically induced phosphenes in sighted, blind and blindsighted observers. *NeuroReport*, 2000, 11: 3269–3273.

Di Russo, F., Martinez, A., Sereno, M.I., Pitzalis, S. and Hillyard, S.A. Cortical sources of the early components of the visual evoked potential. *Hum. Brain Mapp.*, 2001, 15: 95–111.

Fernandez, E., Alfaro, A., Tormos, J.M., Climent, R., Martinez, M., Vilanova, H., Walsh, V. and Pascual-Leone, A. Mapping of the human visual cortex using image-guided transcranial magnetic stimulation. *Brain Res. Protoc.*, 2002, 10: 115–124.

Friston, K.J., Holmes, A.P., Price, C.J., Buchel, C. and Worsley, K.J. Multisubject fMRI studies and conjunction analyses. *Neuroimage*, 1999, 10: 385–396.

Gothe, J., Brandt, S.A., Irlbacher, K., Röricht, S., Sabel, B.A. and Meyer, B.U. Changes in visual cortex excitability in blind subjects as demonstrated by transcranial magnetic stimulation. *Brain*, 2002, 125: 479–490.

Hoge, R.D., Atkinson, J., Gill, B., Crelier, G.R., Marrett, S. and Pike, G.B. Stimulus-dependent BOLD and perfusion dynamics in human V1. *Neuroimage*, 1999, 9: 573–585.

Kammer T. Phosphenes and transient scotomas induced by magnetic stimulation of the occipital lobe: their topographic relationship. *Neuropsychologia*, 1999, 37: 191–198.

Kammer, T., Erb, M., Beck, S. and Grodd, W. Multimodal mapping of the visual cortex: comparison of functional fMRI and stereotactic TMS. *Eur. J. Neurosci.*, 2000, 12 (Suppl. 11): 192.

Kammer, T., Beck, S., Erb, M. and Grodd, W. The influence of current direction on phosphene thresholds evoked by transcranial magnetic stimulation. *Clin. Neurophysiol.*, 2001, 112: 2015–2021.

Kashikura, K., Kershaw, J., Yamamoto, S., Zhang, X., Matsuura, T. and Kanno, I. Temporal characteristics of event-related BOLD response and visual-evoked potentials from checker-board stimulation of human V1: a comparison between different control features. *Magn. Reson. Med.*, 2001, 45: 212–216.

Krings, T., Buchbinder, B.R., Butler, W.E., Chiappa, K.H., Jiang, H.J., Cosgrove, G.R. and Rosen, B.R. Functional magnetic resonance imaging and transcranial magnetic stimulation: complementary approaches in the evaluation of cortical motor function. *Neurology*, 1997, 48: 1406–1416.

Krings, T., Schreckenberger, M., Rohde, V., Foltys, H., Spetzger, U., Sabri, O., Reinges, M.H., Kemeny, S., Meyer, P.T., Moller-Hartmann, W., Korinth, M., Gilsbach, J.M., Buell, U. and Thron, A. Metabolic and electrophysiological validation of functional MRI. *J. Neurol. Neurosurg. Psychiatry*, 2001a, 71: 762–771.

Krings, T., Foltys, H., Reinges, M.H., Kemeny, S., Rohde, V., Spetzger, U., Gilsbach, J.M. and Thron, A. Navigated transcranial magnetic stimulation for presurgical planning – correlation with functional MRI. *Minim. Invasive Neurosurg.*, 2001b, 44: 234–239.

Marg, E. and Rudiak, D. Phosphenes induced by magnetic stimulation over the occipital brain: description and probable site of stimulation. *Optom. Vis. Sci.*, 1994, 71: 301–311.

Meyer, B.U., Diehl, R., Steinmetz, H., Britton, T.C. and Benecke, R. Magnetic stimuli applied over motor and visual cortex: influence of coil position and field polarity on motor responses, phosphenes, and eye movements. *Electroencephalogr. Clin. Neurophysiol.*, 1991 (Suppl.), 43: 121–134.

Slotnick, S.D., Klein, S.A., Carney, T., Sutter, E. and Dastmalchi, S. Using multi-stimulus VEP source localization to obtain a retinotopic map of human primary visual cortex. *Clin. Neurophysiol.*, 1999, 110: 1793–1800.

Transcranial Magnetic Stimulation and Transcranial Direct Current Stimulation (Supplements to Clinical Neurophysiology, Vol. 56)
Editors: W. Paulus, F. Tergau, M.A. Nitsche, J.C. Rothwell, U. Ziemann, M. Hallett

Chapter 32

The causal role of the prefrontal cortex in episodic memory as demonstrated with rTMS

C. Miniussi[a,*], S.F. Cappa[b], M. Sandrini[a], P.M. Rossini[c] and S. Rossi[d]

[a] *IRCCS S. Giovanni di Dio – FBF, Via Pilastroni 4, 25125 Brescia (Italy)*
[b] *Centro di Neuroscienze Cognitive, Università Vita-Salute S. Raffaele, Milan (Italy)*
[c] *Neurologia, Università Campus Biomedico, Rome (Italy)*
[d] *Dipartimento di Neuroscienze, Sezione Neurologia, Università di Siena, Siena (Italy)*

1. Imaging episodic memory

Episodic memory refers to the ability to memorize and recollect specific events in our lives. This memory system accumulates daily experiences to form the conscious story of our existence and its functioning requires the encoding and subsequent retrieval of information from long-term memory (for a review see Tulving 2002). As such, it plays an important role in many cognitive processes. In the last few years, many researchers have moved toward the investigation of its neural basis by means of neuroimaging techniques. Brain imaging studies in humans, performing an episodic memory task have shown a consistent engagement of lateral prefrontal areas during the encoding and retrieval of information. These data, point out that prefrontal cortex is not only active while subjects perform working memory tasks, as shown previously (Goldman-Rakic, 1996; Ungerleider et al., 1998; Fuster, 2001), but also in long-term episodic learning (see Fletcher and Henson, 2001). However, the causal relationship between prefrontal cortex activations and episodic memory processes still needs to be established.

Quite unexpectedly, on the basis of findings in lesional patients, early investigations with positron emission tomography have also indicated a hemispheric functional asymmetry pattern during episodic memory tasks with verbal material. Namely the left prefrontal cortex appeared to be mostly involved in encoding processes, while a right prefrontal predominance was observed during retrieval. These findings led Tulving et al. (1994) to propose a general model of brain function subserving episodic memory, the hemispheric encoding retrieval asymmetry (HERA). According to the HERA model, the left prefrontal cortex plays a crucial role in encoding, whereas the right prefrontal cortex is involved in the retrieval of information from episodic memory. The HERA model, initially corroborated only for verbal tasks, was later proposed also for non-verbal material by Nyberg et al. (1996).

In the last few years, a number of imaging studies have indicated that the hemispheric asymmetry pattern during episodic memory is not an absolute feature, but rather is influenced by several task-related and individual factors, such as the verbal or non-verbal nature of the stimulus, its novelty for the subjects, the difficulty of the task, the outcome of

* *Correspondence to*: Dr. C. Miniussi, IRCCS "San Giovanni di Dio – FBF", Via Pilastroni 4, 25125 Brescia, Italy.
Tel: +39 0303501597; Fax:. +39 0303533513;
E-mail: c.miniussi@oh-fbf.it

the memory process and the age of subjects (Wagner et al., 1998; Cabeza, 2002; Johnson et al., 2003).

A recent review by Cabeza and Nyberg (2000) conclude that in encoding conditions of verbal materials, prefrontal activation was often left lateralized. In contrast, for nonverbal stimuli a bilateral or right-lateralized activation is generally observed. Regarding the retrieval conditions, it has been shown that prefrontal activation is sometimes bilateral, although most of the studies point to a right-sided lateralization (Kelley et al., 1998; Wagner et al., 1998; McDermott et al., 1999; Golby et al., 2001). Kelley et al. (1998) investigated the involvement of dorsal frontal regions during the encoding of words, nameable line-drawn objects, and unfamiliar faces. Encoding of words produced left-lateralized dorsal frontal activation, whereas encoding of unfamiliar faces produced homologous right-lateralized activation. Encoding of nameable objects yielded bilateral dorsal frontal activation. Golby et al. (2001) found that, while verbal encoding resulted in left-lateralized activation of prefrontal cortex, abstract pattern encoding activated the right prefrontal cortex whereas scenes (indoor and outdoor) and unfamiliar faces resulted in approximately symmetrical activation in both regions. Wagner et al. (1998) found asymmetrical activation in the prefrontal cortex when directly comparing words and patterns during both encoding and retrieval. McDermott et al. (1999) found that words produced predominantly left-sided activation and faces produced predominantly right-sided activation during both encoding and retrieval. Thus, both the material and type of memory process may affect the lateralization of frontal activation during memory tasks (Fletcher and Henson, 2001).

The functional significance of right-lateralization during retrieval has been the subject of much debate. It has for example been interpreted as reflecting the adoption of a "retrieval mode" (Nyberg et al., 1995), the expenditure of "retrieval effort", the right (and left) prefrontal cortex being more active when retrieval is difficult (Schacter et al., 1996), and the engagement of "postretrieval" processing (Rugg et al., 1996). According to postretrieval hypothesis, right prefrontal activation reflects demands placed upon cognitive operations responsible for acting on the products of memory retrieval. These operations are thought to include the integration of retrieved information into a coherent episodic representation, and the monitoring of retrieved information for its relevance to task-related behavioral goals.

On the whole, differences in task demand, stimulus type, cognitive strategy and overall difficulty of these experiments places limits on what we can conclude from this analysis. Moreover, the activation of these brain circuits recruited during different tasks does not show that there are functional consequences of these activations in terms of playing a crucial role in a given task (i.e. lack of causality).

This widely acknowledged limitation of neuroimaging studies in establishing a critical role beyond greater precision in mapping a process (Price and Friston, 1999) suggests that the HERA model should also endorse using other sources of information. Repetitive TMS can be directly used to test the prediction of the HERA model, that is neural activity of prefrontal cortex during an episodic memory task is asymmetric. So the first aim of the present study was to better clarify the role of the DLPFC(s) during encoding and retrieval memory process using TMS technique. The second aim was to evaluate possible changes in the hemispheric pattern of lateralization related to the verbal or non-verbal nature of the material and to its novelty.

Despite the increasing interest for TMS, a technique that is seen as one of the most useful research tools to "interact directly" with brain activity (Helmuth, 2001; Chicurel, 2002), its application to the investigation of episodic long-term memory is still limited. The first mention of an induction of a free recall deficit induced by rTMS dates back to 1994, when Grafman et al. (1994) investigated whether they could selectively interfere with an immediate recall task of verbal information, depending on the site and timing of TMS. Recall was consistently significantly diminished only after left mid-temporal and bilateral dorsofrontal rTMS. However, limitations of this study were the lack of a sham-controlled condition and the several scalp sites stimulated during the memory task, a factor that makes it hard to disentangle whether the decremental effect on the memory performance was actually due to the stimulation of a specific region or to the summation of the effects of several rTMS trains sequentially applied to several scalp positions along the whole task.

We performed two recognition memory studies with pictures and word pairs; the implementation of the same experimental design for both types of memoranda allows to better disentangle the role of the attributes of the presented material on the functional lateralization of PFC involvements, by measuring individual behavioral performances, during episodic memory tasks.

2. Visual episodic memory studied with rTMS

The first study showed that using an interference approach, it was possible to obtain an asymmetric performance pattern, during encoding and retrieval, consistent with the HERA model. Moreover, in the same experiment we were able to induce interference (i.e. worsen the performance) only in subjects who were unfamiliar with the material used. This effect suggests that the prefrontal cortex takes part actively in encoding and retrieval process only with novel material. In the second study, additional evidences are presented using verbal material underlying the asymmetrical role of prefrontal cortex in episodic memory of novel information.

A total of eighteen subjects aged 22–41 years free from family history of epilepsy or other neurological disorders participated in this study (these data are partially reported in Rossi et al., 2001). They were right-handed, with a mean Edinburgh Handedness Inventory score of 91.1%. For this, and all the other experiments, informed consent was obtained, and the local ethics committee approved the protocols. Thirteen of the subjects were naïve to experiments with rTMS and were blinded to the aims of the study, except that it was designed "to investigate memory". The other five subjects were extremely familiar with TMS recordings as well as with the pictures of the task, due to picture scanning operation, preparation and assistance during the experimental task. However, their degree of familiarity with memoranda was not specifically scored.

The subjects sat in front of a computer monitor in a dimly illuminated room. During the encoding phase the subjects were asked to classify a set of pictures as indoor or outdoor (six encoding blocks, each one containing eight indoor and eight outdoor images). One hour later, six paired retrieval blocks were again presented, each one containing 16 pictures, eight of which being novel indoor pictures (distractors) and eight indoor pictures presented in the previous phase (tests). In this second part they were ask to press a button to differentiate between "test" and "distractor" pictures. The six encoding/retrieval blocks were labeled according to the type (active or sham) and the side (left/right) of the rTMS applied on dorsolateral prefrontal areas (see Table 1). The course of the experiment can be found in Fig. 1. Trains of rTMS (20 Hz, 500 ms) were delivered at 10% below individual resting motor threshold, immediately after each picture presentation over the left or right DLPFC.[1]

[1] Relatively to the cerebral site of stimulation a common problem of most TMS studies regards the location of the stimulating coil with respect to the anatomy of the targeted cortex, in the single subject. In this regard recently developed neuronavigated TMS systems seem to be promising tool (Herwig et al. 2001; Fernandez et al., 2002) but not always the subjects' MRIs are available. In this study left and right DLPFCs were stimulated by placing the anterior end of the junction of the two coil wings on F3 or F4 (10-20 international EEG system). F3 and F4 locations on the subject's scalp were automatically identified using SofTaxic Navigator system, on the basis of digitised skull landmarks (nasion, inion and two pre-auricular points) and about 40 scalp points (Fastrak Polhemus digitiser). Although individual radiological head images (i.e. magnetic resonance images – MRIs) were not available, Talairach coordinates of cortical sites underlying F3 and F4 locations were automatically estimated by the SofTaxic Navigator Stereotaxic Navigator System (E.M.S. Italy. www.emsmedical.net), on the basis of an MRI-constructed stereotaxic template (accuracy of ± 1 cm, Talairach space) (Talairach and Tournoux, 1988). This method represents a good compromise among the localization accuracy, the high economical demands of neuronavigation devices, and the availability of the single subject MRI.

TABLE 1

EXPERIMENTAL BLOCKS

Label	Description
Baseline	Absence of stimulation in encoding and in retrieval
Sham	rTMS* applied on left DLPFC in encoding and right DLPFC in retrieval
R-Enc	Right rTMS in encoding, applied on the DLPFC; no stimulation in retrieval
L-Enc	Left rTMS in encoding, applied on the DLPFC; no stimulation in retrieval
R-Ret	No stimulation in encoding; right rTMS, applied on the DLPFC, in retrieval
L-Ret	No stimulation in encoding; left rTMS, applied on the DLPFC, in retrieval

* The coil was handled perpendicular to the scalp surface, by using the same intensity of stimulation (10% below the individual resting motor threshold) of the other conditions.

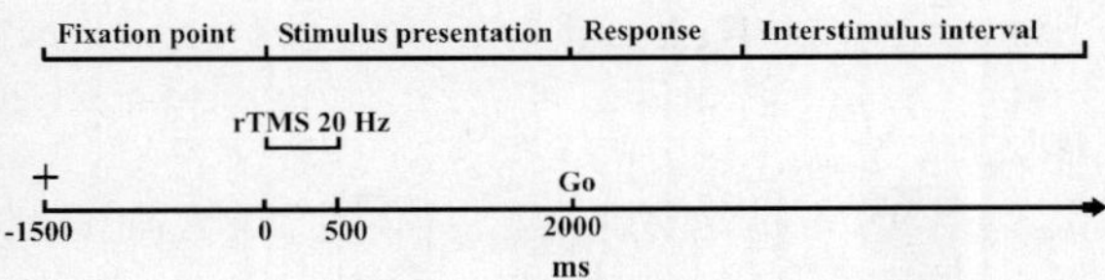

Fig. 1. Time course of the experimental conditions with respect to visual and rTMS stimulation. Subjects fixated a small cross at centre of the screen, which preceded images for 1500 ms, and monitored for the appearance of target stimuli. In the encoding phase subjects had to classify stimuli in relation to a category by a choice response. One hour later, in the retrieval phase, they had to recognize stimuli previously presented (tests) among new stimuli (distractors). The stimuli were present on the monitor for 2000 ms. Trains of rTMS (500 ms, 20 Hz, 10% subthreshold) were delivered simultaneously with the visual stimulus presentation to the left or right DLPFC, when required by the experimental design.

Behavioral findings of this study in the group of 13 naïve subjects directly demonstrated that the prefrontal cortex was actively participating both to encoding and episodic retrieval, and basically reproduced what could be predicted on the basis the neuroimaging-derived HERA model. Indeed, the highest number of recognition errors was induced in the R-Ret block (42%), when the right DLPFC was stimulated during retrieval (Fig. 2a). This suggested that the disrupting effect of rTMS was direct, since it took place immediately after the stimulation period and lasted at least 1.5 s, that is the time in which the picture was displayed on the monitor without concurring rTMS. Such right-sided prevalence of the PFC during episodic retrieval is in line with most of neuroimaging findings (Fletcher and Henson, 2001). A less expected finding, given the material presented, was a left functional prevalence during the encoding phase. Indeed, the probability to correctly remember the encoded information was significantly lower (versus sham and baseline blocks) when the left DLPFC had been stimulated during the encoding. Given the material used (essentially a visuospatial stimulus) a right side functional prevalence could be expected (see, for example, Kirkhoff et al., 2000), although individual strategies of stimulus verbalization could not be excluded. Nevertheless, this finding might reflect a less efficient encoding (more “shallow” processing) and/or to a faster decay of the information due to the concomitant interference of the rTMS.

Notably, in the sub-group of subjects who were familiar with pictures, the effects of the rTMS on the performance were almost lacking (Fig. 2b). An analyses of variance with training as between-subjects factor and condition as within-subjects factor, showed a significant training by condition interaction [$F = 4.59$; $p < 0.00$], arising from a different effect of the rTMS in naïve and trained subjects: in fact, there was no behavioural interference of rTMS on trained subjects for any site of stimulation [$F = 2.08$; $p = 0.11$], whereas clear modulation was detected in subjects naïve to the stimuli. As expected, the factor of training was also significant as main effect, because errors were significantly lower in trained than naïve subjects [$F = 23.57$; $p < 0.00$].

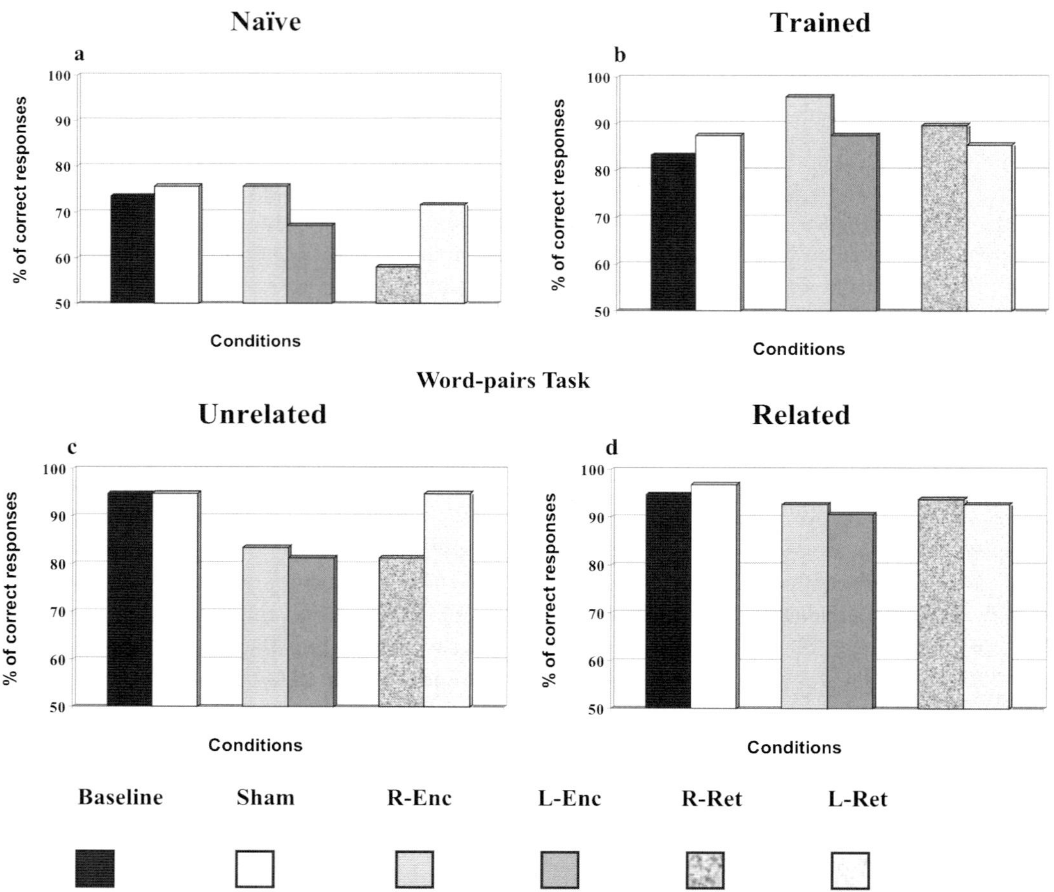

Fig. 2. Results of picture and word recognition experiments. The graphs show percentages of correct detection of target stimuli in the retrieval phase for the six conditions divided by type of material. In the following experiments (a) recognition of picture in the naive group (b) recognition of picture in the trained group (c) recognition of unrelated word-pairs (d) recognition of related word-pairs.

The maximal error rate during encoding was present in the Baseline block (16.7%) without rTMS stimulation, in other words rTMS did not interfered with subjects performance suggesting that the functional specialization of the left and right DLPFC in encoding and retrieval, respectively, likely occurs mainly when new material has to be used. This supports the idea that the prefrontal cortex decrease its competence to subserve encoding and retrieval of information, once they are previously stored. Moreover, these data are compatible with reports of progressively reduced frontal activation with task repetition (Petersen et al., 1996), and may be related to the requirement of more elaborate information processing during encoding of novel information, as well as to the different retrieval demands of the non-practiced task (Rugg and Wilding, 2000).

3. Verbal episodic memory studied with rTMS

In the second study (Sandrini et al., 2003), we tested the functional DLPFC asymmetries in a verbal episodic memory task, in order to confirm with the rTMS approach the HERA model in the verbal domain and to verify the observation that only novel material engages the prefrontal cortex during encoding and retrieval. Twelve healthy young Italian-speaking subjects, aged between 20 and 34 years (Handedness 85.2%), were tested using the same experimental design as in previous experiment (Fig. 1 and Table 1). In the current setting, pairs of Italian nouns with high imagery content replaced complex pictures. For each block of the six encoding phase blocks, 16 word pairs (eight semantically related and eight unrelated) were randomly presented on the monitor, with two inter-trial intervals (7000 or 8000 ms). During the encoding phase the subjects were asked to classify word pairs as highly associated (e.g. bread-butter, garlic-onion), or non-associated (cow-table), according to norms collected for this experiment. One hour later, they were presented with the first word of each pair, and a choice between the second and a novel word (distractor). Events of the retrieval and encoding phases occurred with the same timing (see Fig. 1). Subjects were instructed to press the left or right key according to the position of the word which had been seen previously. The correct responses during the encoding and retrieval phases were evenly distributed across left and right button presses (eight each), thus avoiding rules effects.

Both left and right DLPFC rTMS interfered with the encoding phase, only to semantically unrelated word pairs (Fig. 2c), therefore, suggesting a specific role of DLPFC(s) only when novel information had to be memorized. Such bilateral reliance on DLPFCs for encoding process was somewhat unexpected, since most of previous neuroimaging literature pointed to a left-lateralization, at least for verbal materials (see Fletcher and Henson, 2001). We therefore speculated that the current task might have required participants to perform a deep manipulation, in agreement with the predictions of the "dual-coding theory". According to it, processing of abstract nouns would rely almost exclusively on left-sided verbal code representations, whereas concrete nouns additionally would access a second image-based processing system in the right hemisphere (Paivio, 1986). The involvement of the right DLPFC during encoding (that is, increased errors induced by right rTMS) of word pairs of high imagery content could parallel this strategy. Therefore, bilateral DLPFC involvement might result from the combined engagement of verbal as well as non-verbal strategies in the context of episodic encoding. Comparison with our previous study indicates that only the retrieval effect is largely material-independent; during encoding, both hemispheres are engaged, with a relative contribution modulated by the nature of the material. The prefrontal contribution to episodic memory is crucial only in the case of "novel" information, such as unusual word combinations.

4. Conclusions

By means of rTMS we were able to interfere transiently with ongoing tasks subserved by cortical networks involved in specific cognitive processes; this offers advantages for the investigation of the neurophysiological mechanisms underlying cognitive task performance. Perfusion-based neuroimaging techniques, such as functional magnetic resonance, are very useful to provide a spatially precise correlation of neural activity with a dependent variable, such as attention to a selected visual stimulus or behavioral performance in a given task. However, after this initial correlation TMS can be use as a direct test of the causal role of a given cerebral area in a task. In other words, we can verify if regions that are "functionally active" are also "functionally relevant", and in this instance, rather than asking whether activity is correlated with some dependent variable, TMS assess whether or not it is necessary for a specified task (Stewart et al., 2001).

The present findings of prefrontal cortical involvement during encoding and retrieval are consistent with data from animal studies (Goldman-Rakic, 1987, 1996) as well as neuropsychological investigations of brain-damaged patients (Warrington and Weiskrantz, 1982; Milner et al., 1985; Schacter, 1987), pointing to an involvement of the prefrontal cortex in episodic memory. In addition, they consistently show that functional hemispheric asymmetries can be observed for encoding and retrieval processes. In line with this observation, prefrontal activations during episodic memory tasks have been demonstrated in numerous neuroimaging studies (for a review, see Cabeza and Nyberg, 2000). The number of TMS studies addressing episodic long-term memory in humans is still limited; however all of them converge in indicating that the PFC plays an important role in long-term episodic memory. These results, therefore, extend the concept that the prefrontal regions are mainly devoted to short-term and working memory processes. An important qualification is that the functional role of PFC appears to be limited to the memory processing of novel information.

Previous investigations on the effects of rTMS on memory are limited and focused mainly on verbal tasks: the recall of a 12-word list was impaired after rTMS of the left mid-temporal or dorsofrontal regions (Grafman et al., 1994). A more recent study by Epstein et al. (2002) used an associative memory task involving pairs of Kanji pictographs and unfamiliar abstract patterns. The authors found a significant impairment during recall only with TMS over right DLPFC. On the basis of theses results, the authors (Epstein et al., 2002) conclude that the right DLPFC is important in encoding mechanisms of non-verbal material. Some methodological factors, like the type of TMS protocol used, could account for partial discrepancies of these results with other findings on episodic memory in encoding (Rossi et al., 2001; Sandrini et al., 2003). An alternative hypothesis is that the functional relevance of the right DLPFC might be in relation to working memory processes required for the maintenance of paired associations until the recall phase.

The regions affected by rTMS in our study are probably the same as those engaged in working memory tasks (Callicott et al., 1999; Wagner, 1999; Fletcher et al., 2001). In the two-stage model of working memory, ventrolateral prefrontal regions are specialized for the maintenance and comparison of representations held in working memory, while dorsolateral areas are posited to subserve more complex or effortful monitoring and manipulation (Petrides, 1995). The operations of working memory and encoding/retrieval may in fact be closely linked, in the sense that prefrontal activation during learning and remembering might represent the contribution of working memory operations to episodic memory. A recent study by Ranganath et al. (2003) supports the view that the same regions are engaged by working memory and episodic memory, similar results were reported also by Nyberg et al. (2003). Notably, rTMS of the same prefrontal regions is able to impair behaviorally both working memory (Mottaghy et al., 2000, 2002) and episodic memory (Rossi et al., 2001). rTMS might transiently disable the processing contribution of DLPFC and adjacent structures to the circuitry of working memory, inducing a dramatic decrement of its role in the active manipulation of information (Fletcher and Henson, 2001).

To summarize, the important role of the right prefrontal areas in the retrieval of verbal and nonverbal material is confirmed by TMS. The causal role of prefrontal cortex in encoding is also supported by rTMS studies. Other variables, such as the type of process tested and individual strategies of memorization and retrieval may account for the inconsistent lateralisation of these encoding effects (Johnson et al., 2003). Therefore, lateralization differences among tasks may be due to the reliance on a mixture of verbal as well as nonverbal strategies in the context of episodic encoding (dual-coding). This interpretation is in line with findings that unfamiliar faces activated the right prefrontal cortex, whereas nameable famous faces activated bilateral prefrontal cortical areas (Kelley et al., 1998). Other variables, which should be taken into account, are those related to the experimental design, to the timing and parameters of TMS, and to the accuracy of coil positioning with respect to the underlying cortical anatomy.

Acknowledgements

This research was supported by a grant provided by the Italian Ministry of Health. We thank for experimental help Drs P. Pasqualetti, K. Sosta, F. Carducci and C. Babiloni.

References

Cabeza, R. Hemispheric asymmetry reduction in older adults: the HAROLD model. *Psychol. Aging*, 2002, 17: 85–100.

Cabeza, R. and Nyberg, L. Imaging Cognition II: An empirical review of 275 PET and fMRI studies. *J. Cogn. Neurosci.*, 2000, 12: 1–47.

Callicott, J.H., Mattay, V.S., Bertolino, A., Finn, K., Coppola, R., Frank, J.A., Goldberg, T.E. and Weinberger, D.R. Physiological characteristics of capacity constraints in working memory as revealed by functional MRI. *Cereb. Cortex*, 1999, 9(1): 20–26.

Chicurel, M. Magnetic mind games. *Nature*, 2002, 417: 114–116.

Epstein, C.M., Sekino, M., Yamaguchi, K., Kamiya, S. and Ueno, S. Asymmetries of prefrontal cortex in human episodic memory: effects of transcranial magnetic stimulation on learning abstract patterns. *Neurosi. Lett.*, 2002, 320: 5–8.

Fernandez, E., Alfaro, A., Termos, J.M., Climent, R., Martinez, M., Vilanova; H., Walsh, V. and Pascual-Leone, A. Mapping of the human visual cortex using image-guided transcranial magnetic stimulation. *Brain Res. Protoc.*, 2002, 10(2): 115–24.

Fletcher, P.C. and Henson, R.N.A. Frontal lobes and human memory. Insights from functional neuroimaging. *Brain*, 2001, 124: 849–881.

Funster, J.M. The prefrontal cortex-an update: time is the essence. *Neuron*, 2001, 30(2): 319–333.

Golby, A.J., Poldrack, R.A., Brewer, J., Spencer, D., Desmond, J.E., Aron, A.P. and Gabrieli, J.D.E. Material-specific lateralization in the medial temporal lobe and prefrontal cortex during memory encoding. *Brain*, 2001, 124: 1841–1854.

Goldman-Rakic, P.S. Circuitry of primate prefrontal cortex and regulation of behaviour by representational memory. In: V.B. Mountcastle and F. Plum (Eds.), *Handbook of Physiology*, Sect 1, Vol, 5, American Physiological Society, Bethesda (MD), 1987: 373–417.

Goldman-Rakic, P.S. The prefrontal landscape: Implications of functional architecture for understanding human mentation and central executive. *Philos. Trans. R. Soc Lond. B Biol. Sci.*, 1996, 351: 1445–1453.

Grafman, J., Pascual-Leone, A., Always, D., Nichelli, P., Gomez-Tortosa, E. and Hallett, M. Induction of a recall deficit by rapid-rate transcranial magnetic stimulation. *NeuroReport*, 1994, 9: 1157–1160.

Helmuth, L. Neuroscience. Boosting brain activity from the outside in. *Science*, 2001, 292(5520): 1284–1286.

Herwig, U., Schönfeldt-Laucona, C., Wunderlich, A.P., Von Tiesenhausen, C., Thielscher, A., Walter, H. and Spitzer, M. The navigation of transcranial magnetic stimulation. *Psychiatr. Res.*, 2001, 108: 123–131.

Johnson, M.K., Raye, C.L., Mitchell, K.J., Greene, E.J. and Anderson A.W. fMRI evidence for an organization of prefrontal cortex by both type of process and type of information. *Cereb. Cortex*, 2003, 13(3): 265–273.

Kelley, W.M., Miezin, F.M., McDermott, K.B., Buckner, R.L., Raichle, M.E., Cohen, N.J., Ollinger, J.M., Akbudak, E., Conturo, T.E., Snyder, A.Z. and Petersen, S.E. Hemispheric specialization in human dorsal frontal cortex and medial-temporal lobe for verbal and nonverbal memory encoding. *Neuron*, 1998, 20: 927–936.

Kirchhoff, B.A., Wagner, A.D., Maril, A. and Stern, C.E. Prefrontal-temporal circuitry for episodic encoding and subsequent memory. *J. Neurosci.*, 2000, 20: 6173–6180.

McDermott, K.B., Buckner, R.L., Petersen, S.E., Kelley, W.M. and Sanders, A.L. Set- and code-specific activation in frontal cortex: an fMRI study of encoding and retrieval of faces and words. *J. Cogn. Neurosci.*, 1999, 11: 631–640.

Milner, B., Petrides, M. and Smith, M.L. Frontal lobes and the temporal organization of memory. *Hum. Neurobiol.*, 1985, 4(3): 137–142.

Mottaghy, F.M., Krause, B.J., Kemma, L.J., Topper, R., Tellmann, L., Beu, M., Pascual-Leone, A. and Muller-Gartner, H. Modulation of the neural circuitry subserving working memory in healthy human subjects by repetitive transcranial magnetic stimulation. *Neurosci. Lett.*, 2000, 280: 167–170.

Mottaghy, F.M., Gangitano, M., Krause, B.J. and Pascual-Leone, A. Segregation of areas related to visual working memory in prefrontal cortex revealed by rTMS. *Cereb. Cortex.*, 2002, 12: 369–375.

Nyberg, L., Tulving, E., Habib, R., Nilson, L.G., Kapur, S., Cabeza, R. and McIntosh, A.R. Functional brain maps of retrieval mode and recovery of episodic information. *NeuroReport*, 1995, 7: 249–252.

Nyberg, L., Cabeza, R. and Tulving, E. PET studies of encoding and retrieval: The HERA model. *Psychonom. Bull. Rev.*, 1996, 3: 135–148.

Nyberg, L., Marklund, P., Persson, J., Cabeza, R., Forkstam, C., Petersson, K.M. and Ingvar, M. Common prefrontal activations during working memory, episodic memory, and semantic memory. *Neuropsychologia.*, 2003, 41(3): 371–377.

Paivio, A. *Mental representations: A dual coding theory.* University Press, Oxford.

Petersen, S.E., Van Mier, H., Fiez, J.A. and Raichle, M.E. The effects of practice on the functional anatomy of task performance. *Proc. Natl. Acad. Sci. USA*, 1998, 95: 853–860.

Petrides, M. Frontal lobes and working memory: evidence from investigation of the effects of cortical excisions in nonhumans primates. In: F. Boller and J. Grafmann (Eds.), *Handbook of Neuropsychology*. Elsevier, Amsterdam, 1994.

Petrides, M. Impairments on non-spatial self-ordered and externally ordered working memory tasks after lesions of the mid-dorsal part of the lateral frontal cortex in the monkey. *J. Neurosci.*, 1995, 15: 359–375.

Price, C.J. and Friston, K.J. Scanning patients with tasks they can perform. *Hum. Brain Mapp.*, 1999, 8: 102–108.

Ranganath, C., Johnson, M.K. and D'Esposito, M. Prefrontal activity associated with working memory and episodic long-term memory. *Neuropsychologia*, 2003, 41(3): 378–379.

Rossi, S., Cappa, S.F., Babiloni, C., Pasqualetti, P., Miniussi, C., Carducci, F., Babiloni, F. and Rossini, P.M. Prefrontal cortex in long-term memory: an "interference" approach using magnetic stimulation. *Nat. Neurosci.*, 2001, 9: 948–952.

Rugg, M.D. and Wilding, E.L. Retrieval processing and episodic memory. *Trends in Cogn. Sci.*, 2000, 4: 108–115.

Rugg, M.D., Fletcher, P.C., Frith, C.D., Frackowiak, R.S. and Dolan, R.J. Differential activation of the prefrontal cortex in successful and unsuccessful memory retrieval. *Brain*, 1996, 119: 2073–2083.

Sandrini, M., Cappa, S.F., Rossi, S., Rossini, P.M. and Miniussi C. The role of prefrontal cortex in verbal episodic memory: rTMS evidence. *J. Cogn. Neurosci.*, 2003, 15(6): in press.

Schacter, D.L. Implicit expressions of memory in organic amnesia: learning of new facts and associations. *Hum. Neurobiol.*, 1987, 6(2): 107–118.

Schacter, D.L., Alpert, N.M., Savage, C.R., Rauch, S.L. and Albert, M.S. Conscious recollection and the human hippocampal formation: evidence from positron emission tomography. *Proc. Natl. Acad. Sci. USA*, 1996, 93: 321–325.

Stewart, L., Ellison, A., Walsh, V. and Cowey, A. The role of transcranial magnetic stimulation (TMS) in studies of vision, attention and cognition. *Acta Psychol.*, 2001, 107(1–3): 275–291.

Tailarach, J. and Tournoux, P. *Coplanar stereotaxic atlas of the human brain.* Stuggart, NY: Thieme, 1998.

Tulving, E. Episodic memory: from mind to brain. *Annu. Rev. Psychol.*, 2002, 53: 1–25.

Tulving, E., Kapur, S., Craik, F.I.M., Moscovitch, M. and Houle, S. Hemispheric encoding/retrieval asymmetry in episodic memory: positron emission tomography findings. *Proc. Natl. Acad. Sci.* USA, 1994, 91: 2016–2020.

Ungerleider, L.G., Courtney, S.M. and Haxbym J.V. A neural system for human visual working memory. *Proc. Natl. Acad. Sci. USA*, 1998, 95(3): 883–890.

Wagner, A.D. Working memory contributions to human learning and remembering. *Neuron.*, 1999, 22(1): 19–22.

Wagner, A.D., Poldrack, R.A., Eldridge, L.L., Desmond, J.E., Glover, G.H. and Gabrieli, J.D. Material-specific lateralization of prefrontal activation during episodic encoding and retrieval. *NeuroReport*, 1998, 9: 3711–3717.

Warrington, E.K. and Weiskrantz, L. Amnesia: a disconnection syndrome? *Neuropsychologia*, 1982, 20(3): 233–248.

Transcranial Magnetic Stimulation and Transcranial Direct Current Stimulation (Supplements to Clinical Neurophysiology, Vol. 56)
Editors: W. Paulus, F. Tergau, M.A. Nitsche, J.C. Rothwell, U. Ziemann, M. Hallett

Chapter 33

The parietal cortex in visual search: a visuomotor hypothesis

Amanda Ellison[a], Matthew Rushworth[b] and Vincent Walsh[c,*]

[a] *Cognitive Neuroscience Research Unit, Wolfson Research Institute, University of Durham Queen's Campus, University Boulevard, Stockton-on-Tees TS17 6BH (UK)*
[b] *Department of Experimental Psychology, University of Oxford, South Parks Road, Oxford OX1 3UD (UK)*
[c] *Institute of Cognitive Neuroscience, University College London, Alexandra House, 17 Queen Square, London WC1N 3AR (UK)*

1. Introduction

There seems to be little doubt that the right posterior parietal cortex (rPPC) has a special role in visual search tasks, a role most commonly attributed to feature binding (in the sense described as "property binding" by Treisman, 1996; Robertson, 1999). In support of this, patients with damage to rPPC have difficulty identifying targets defined by a conjunction of two different features such as form and colour (Arguin et al., 1994; Friedman-Hill et al., 1995; Wocjiulik and Kanwisher, 1998). These findings have been corroborated by neuroimaging (Corbetta et al., 1998; Donner et al., 2000, 2002) and magnetic stimulation studies of visual search (Ashbridge et al., 1997; Walsh et al., 1998).

The apparent need to bind two features is, perhaps, the most salient visual component of a conjunction search task. However, search tasks can be difficult in the absence of the need for binding, for example when the target and distractors are very similar (Duncan and Humphreys, 1989; Wolfe, 1994). We were therefore concerned to examine whether rPPC is important in *any* difficult visual search task irrespective of the need for feature binding. A second concern of the work reported in this chapter was to question the prevailing view that rPPC makes its contribution only in relation to the visual aspects of search. Our motivation for raising this question lies in the anatomy and physiology of the PPC; anatomically, it is poised between the visual and motor cortices; physiologically, PPC neurons do not posses the receptive field properties that would be consistent with a higher visuo-visual role. We thus propose the hypothesis that the contribution of rPPC to search lies in visuo-motor transformations, for example in forming spatially encoded stimulus response associations. This possibility is neglected because the emphasis in search experiments is usually on the visual aspects of the task and also because the reports of illusory conjunctions in patients are compelling (Friedman-Hill et al., 1995). Illusory conjunctions are false positive reports and therefore do not yield information about search on target absent trials. Using transcranial magnetic stimulation (TMS) to disrupt search performance, we have shown elsewhere (Ashbridge et al., 1997; Walsh et al., 1998, 1999)

* *Correspondence to*: Dr. Vincent Walsh, Institute of Cognitive Neuroscience, University College London, Alexandra House, 17 Queen Square, London WC1N 3AR, UK.
Tel: 0044 207 679 1162;
E-mail: v.walsh@ucl.ac.uk

that rPPC is required for normal performance on target absent trials in search (i.e. in the absence of target binding).

To discriminate between the visuo-visual and visuo-motor accounts of the role of PPC in search, we used repetitive TMS (rTMS) to selectively disrupt visual search performance in four experiments. We first manipulated the difficulty of feature tasks that did not require binding and conjunction tasks that did; we then manipulated the spatial requirements of target detection, the set size to be searched, and finally the visuomotor requirements of the task. The results concur with the view that, in some sense, visuospatial elements of search depend on PPC. However, our results also show that binding does not always require PPC and that the *motor* requirements in search tasks are a key determinant of the extent of PPC involvement these tasks.

2. Materials and methods

In all four experiments stimuli were presented on a computer monitor subtending 33.7° of visual angle and divided into a virtual array of 8×6 boxes in each of which a stimulus could be presented. Stimuli were drawn to be constrained in these boxes and the location of stimulus was jittered by ± 3 pixels in the x and y axes to prevent alignment of stimuli. On each trial, subjects were presented with a fixation spot (500 ms) followed by the search array for 1000 ms. Subjects made a button press response to indicate whether they thought the target was present or absent in the array. They were instructed to respond as quickly and as accurately as possible. The dependent variable was reaction time on correct trials. We have reported TMS effects on visual search in several earlier papers and therefore, for simplicity, we analyse only target present trials (which emphasise the visual aspects of search) in Experiments 1–3 and only report absent data in Experiment 4, because that experiment emphasises motor responses and a comparison between present and absent trials is therefore critically informative. Biphasic repetitive pulse TMS (rTMS) (Magstim 200 Super Rapid, Whitland, Dyffed, Wales, UK) was delivered at 10 Hz for 500 ms, beginning at the onset of the visual stimulus, at 60% of stimulator output and using a 70 mm figure-of-8 coil oriented with the handle pointing backwards and parallel to the floor. Subjects received 100 trials in each condition of each experiment. Stimulus conditions were blocked both for stimulus type and delivery of TMS. The sequence of events in a TMS trial is shown in Fig. 1 (a) and have been detailed elsewhere (Ashbridge et al., 1997; Walsh et al., 1998, 1999; Rushworth et al., 2001). Figure 1 (b) shows the localisation of the TMS stimulation site with anatomical MRI scans. All subjects gave informed consent in line with permissions granted by the Oxford Research Ethics Committee (OxREC C99.178).

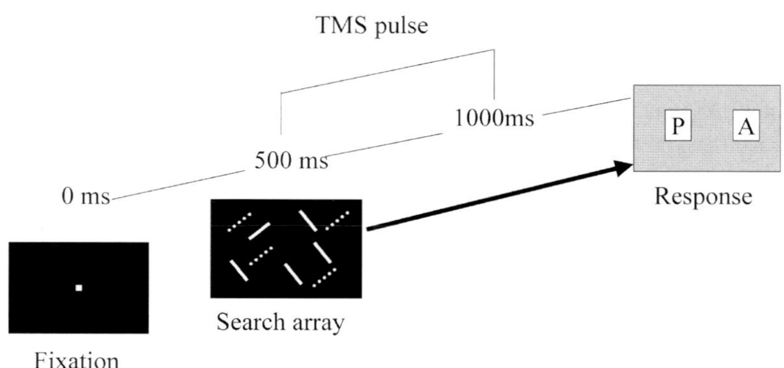

Fig. 1a. A schematic of the visual search task. Visual stimuli were presented following a fixation spot and TMS was applied for 500 ms beginning with the onset of the visual stimulus.

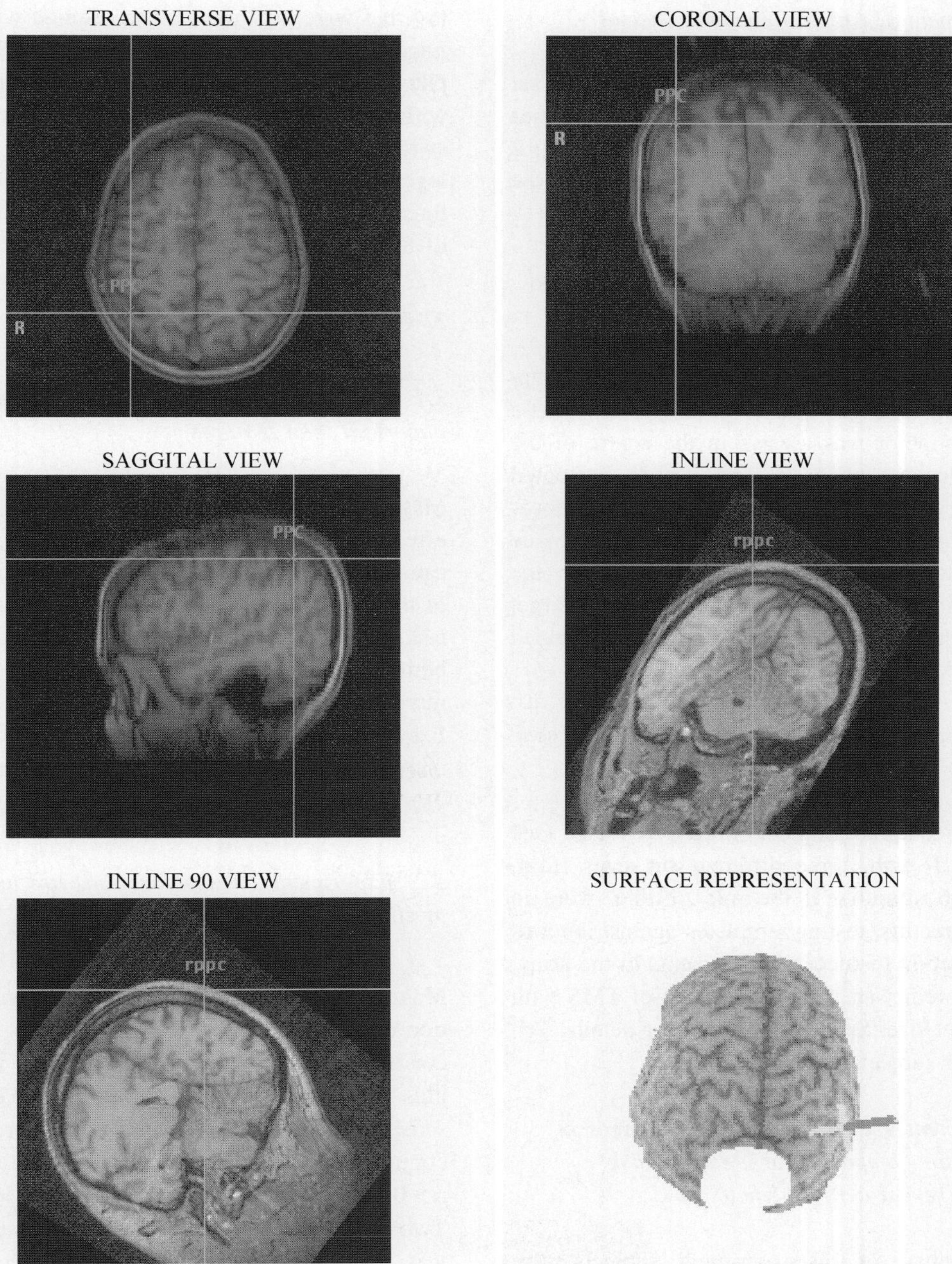

Fig. 1b. Using Brainsight™, the right PPC was localised in each subject by co-registering subjects' structural MRI scans and coil position on the scalp and the trajectory of a TMS pulse into the cortex from a figure-of-8 TMS coil was calculated from the scalp position. The area functionally localised by impairment with TMS in a conjunction search task is seen in the sections above, with the trajectory of the pulse most clearly seen in the Inline and Inline 90 views.

2.1. Experiment 1. Are conjunctions special?

Four search tasks were used, each with a single set size of eight stimuli: easy and hard feature searches and easy and hard conjunction searches. See Fig. 2 and legend for details. Eight subjects took part in the experiments, all right handed (aged 17–39).

2.2. Experiment 2. Is spatial uncertainty a special factor?

Four tasks were used: two feature and two conjunction detection tasks. In one of each type the single target or distractor was always in the centre of the array and in one of each type it was presented randomly in any one of the 48 possible screen locations. See Fig. 3 and legend for details. Subjects made "target/non-target" key press decisions and in the stream of single stimuli the probability of a target being the stimulus was 0.25. Five right handed subjects took part in this experiment.

2.3. Experiment 3. Does the number of non-targets affect the role of PPC?

A colour orientation conjunction task was used (see Experiment 1) with three different set sizes (four, eight and 16 stimuli). If the role of PPC were in filtering distractors, testing templates against input or guiding selection to successive elements in the array, one would predict an increasing effect of TMS with increasing set size. See Fig. 4 legend for details. Ten right handed subjects took part.

2.4. Experiment 4. Are responses to changes in only the motor component of a search task sufficient to reveal a PPC deficit?

In the first phase of this experiment, subjects were presented with a single visual search task and received rTMS over right PPC. In the second phase, they trained on the visual search task for 2500 trials, after which they were highly efficient. Following training they were retested with TMS. In the third and final phase subjects saw the same visual search task but were now required to respond with different fingers than in the original test phase or the training phase. In this third phase, subjects received 50 trials, without TMS, to assess the behavioural cost of finger switching, followed by 100 TMS trials. See Fig. 5 legend for details. All training was carried out with three set sizes and TMS testing with a single set size of 8 stimuli. Six right handed subjects took part.

3. Results

3.1. Experiment 1 – Conjunctions are more important than features

Magnetic stimulation over the rPPC did not have any effect on either of the feature tasks (Fig. 2) but did cause a significant increase in reaction times in both of the conjunction tasks. There was a main effect of task ($F = 85.12$, $df = 5$, $p < 0.0001$) and post hoc, bonferroni corrected t tests showed the reaction time increases on the conjunction tasks to be significant. Easy conjunction: $t = 5.376$, $df = 7$, $p < 0.001$, RT increase = 48.9 ms. Hard conjunction: $t = 3.224$, $df = 7$, $p < 0.02$, RT increase = 78.23 ms.

3.2. Experiment 2 – Conjunctions are insufficient to elicit a rPPC TMS deficit

Magnetic stimulation over rPPC only disrupted detection of target presence or absence in one of the four conditions in Experiment 2. When the single stimulus was presented, predictably, in the centre of the screen rTMS had no effect on either feature or conjunction detection (Feature task $t = 1.103$, $df = 4$, $p > 0.1$; conjunction task $t = 1.099$, $df = 4$, $p > 0.1$. Two-tailed, bonferroni corrected). When the stimulus was presented at a random, unspecified location, however, rTMS over rPPC elevated reaction times to detect the conjunction target from 561 ms (SD 77 ms, SEM 34 ms) without TMS to 620 ms (SD 118 ms, SEM 52 ms) with TMS ($t = 3.234$, $df = 4$, $p < 0.05$) but had no effect on the feature task ($t = 0.223$, $df = 4$, $p > 0.1$) (Fig. 3).

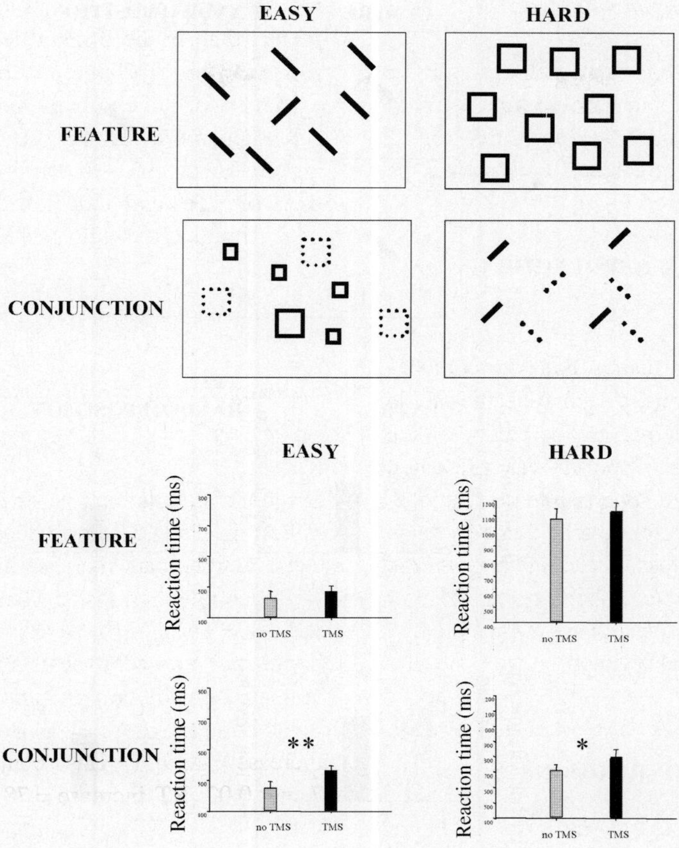

Fig. 2 PPC is involved in conjunction but not in feature search. This is true for both serial and parallel search. PPC is not involved even when serial search is required for feature items. * = $p < 0.05$, ** = $p < 0.01$

3.3. Experiment 3 – Increasing set size does not increase the induced deficit

Magnetic stimulation over rPPC disrupted conjunction search performance on all three set sizes, but the deficit did not increase with increasing numbers of distractors. With four stimuli, mean RT increased from 669 ms (no TMS. SD 134 ms, SEM 42 ms) to 759 ms (SD 143 ms, SEM 45 ms), $t = 2.439$, $df = 9$, $p < 0.02$. With eight stimuli, mean RT increased from 762 ms (no TMS, SD 126 ms, SEM 40 ms) to 862 ms (SD 128 ms, SEM 40 ms) $t = 2.937$, $df = 9$, $p < 0.009$). With 16 stimuli in the array, RT increased from 895 ms (no TMS, SD 171 ms, SEM 54 ms) to 1030 ms (SD 173 ms, SEM 54 ms) $t = 2.519$, $df = 9$, $p < 0.02$. As Fig. 4 shows there was no significant change in the magnitude of the TMS effect with increasing set size.

3.4. Experiment 4 – Changing motor factors elicits a PPC deficit

When TMS was applied over rPPC during a conjunction search task (with a single set size of eight stimuli) reaction times were elevated relative to the no TMS condition ($t = 3.451$, $df = 5$, $p < 0.02$). Following training on the task with three set sizes (4, 8 and 16 stimuli) subjects were much more efficient

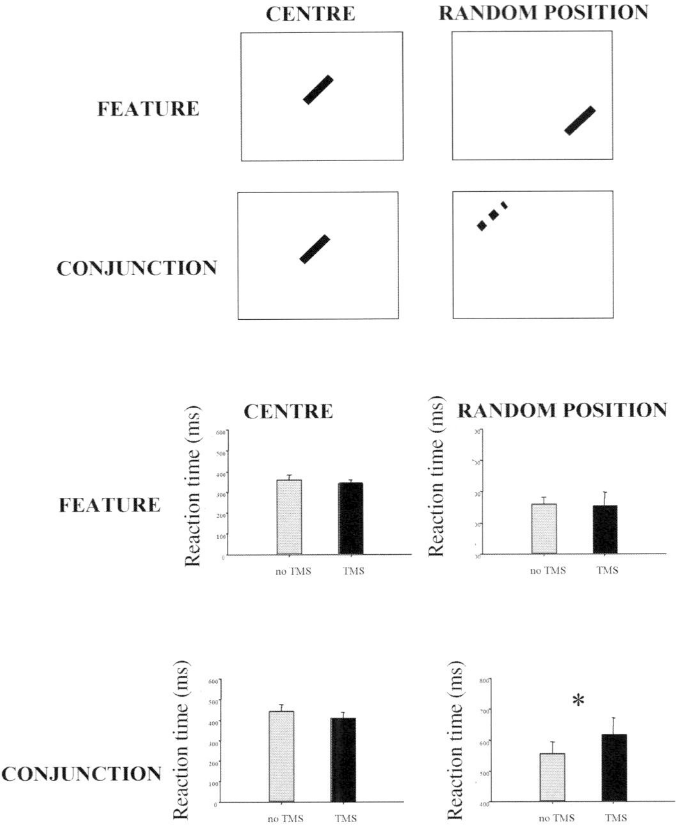

Fig. 3. PPC is not involved when no spatial search is required, i.e. the target is presented centrally. However, if the single target is randomly presented in around the display area, PPC is involved only in the conjunction condition. * = $p < 0.05$.

(pre-training slope = 45.34 ms per item, post-training slope = 6.53 ms per item). When TMS was applied over rPPC following this training improvement, there was no longer an effect on reaction times ($t = 0.358$, $df = 5$, $p > 0.07$). When subjects were required to reverse the finger of response on the now highly efficient search task, there was a cost in baseline performance of over 10 ms per item slope = 17.49 ms per item) and a return of the TMS effect ($t = 5.701$, $df = 5$, $p < 0.002$).

4. Discussion

From the results of Experiment 1 we can conclude that the right posterior parietal cortex is important in visual conjunction tasks even when the tasks are easy, but it is not needed when the search target is defined by a single feature regardless of whether it is detected with ease (Fig. 2, top right panels) or difficulty (Fig. 2, bottom right panels). This may seem to support the standard view that rPPC contributes to feature binding. However, from Experiment 2 we can assert that if the conjunction to be detected is presented in a central location and in the absence of distractors, rPPC is not required for fast and accurate performance. Experiment 3 further strengthens the case that rPPC may not be critical for visual aspects of conjunction search tasks. With increasing set size, baseline reaction times increased from 669 ms (four stimuli) to 762 ms (eight stimuli) to 895 ms (16

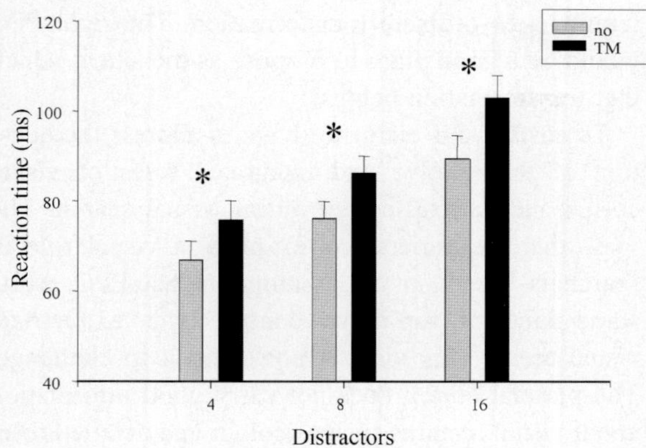

Fig. 4. PPC is involved to the same degree over all set sizes. The slope of the cost of TMS is less than 4 ms per item, suggesting that the RT costs of between 90 and 135 ms are not related to increments in visual analysis, which would predict greater costs per item.

stimuli) (Fig. 4). Despite the increase in baseline reaction time of 19 ms for each additional item in the array, rTMS over PPC yielded a relatively constant cost in RTs. The slope of the RT increase × set size is less than 3 ms per item. We interpret this as evidence that rPPC does not contribute to a process that involves selection or comparison of visual attributes. Rather a constant cost implies a function that is independent of visual factors. We have argued this previously (Ashbridge et al., 1997; Walsh et al., 1998) when single pulse TMS has disrupted performance at specific times that correlate with response time rather than the visual elements of the task. Finally, in Experiment 4, we established that the effects of rTMS on visual search can be manipulated as a function of changes only in the motor requirements of the task.

The search tasks we have used in these experiments have been standard tasks similar to those used in many other studies, but whereas search is usually discussed as an example of a visual task (hence the concentration on the visual requirements), we would now argue that it is best considered in its motor context as the beginnings of selection for action. One usually searches for an object for two reasons – to fixate it or to move towards/away from it. Maioli et al. (2001) have argued cogently that there is no need to postulate attentional mechanisms separate from eye movements in visual search tasks. Indeed, James (1890/1964), though often cited for knowing what attention is, also argued that attention and action are inseparable; attending he argued "is the *fiat*; . . . and immediate motor consequences should ensue". We would agree with James in this context and extend the argument of Maioli et al. (see also Allport, 1987) to other motor behaviours such as reaching. The importance of pointing and grasping in a 3-D search environment has been shown by Bekkering et al. (2002) and also by Humphreys and Riddoch (2001). In a previous study (Walsh et al., 1998) we showed that rPPC rTMS effects on visual search could be "trained away" in a task specific manner, to return with the presentation of a novel visual search array. In that experiment, however, by presenting subjects with a new visual search array we also presented them with a new visuomotor association to perform. We could not know, therefore, whether the return of the TMS effect with a new task was due to visual or visuomotor factors. The results of Experiment 4 clearly demonstrate the visuomotor nature of the effect. In the light of the work of Bekkering (2002) and Humphreys and Riddoch (2001), we would interpret the results of Experiment 4 as showing that when an affordance is easily defined or automated by repetition, the parietal cortex is not needed in the translation from vision to action.

Our findings help to bring together a number of recent, seemingly unconnected reports of visual search, binding and action intention. As noted above, the behavioural and neuropsychological studies have highlighted convincingly the role of action affordance in search. Some recent single unit recording studies also suggest a visuomotor association role for parietal cortex (Zhang and Barash, 2000; Assad and Toth, 2002). Wocjiulik and Kanwisher (1998), in noting that bilateral parietal patient RM could implicitly bind features, suggest that the parietal lobe is only necessary for explicit binding "available to other functional domains (e.g. action, language), such that the system as a whole can use it for goal directed action" (1998, p. 179). Elsewhere, we have

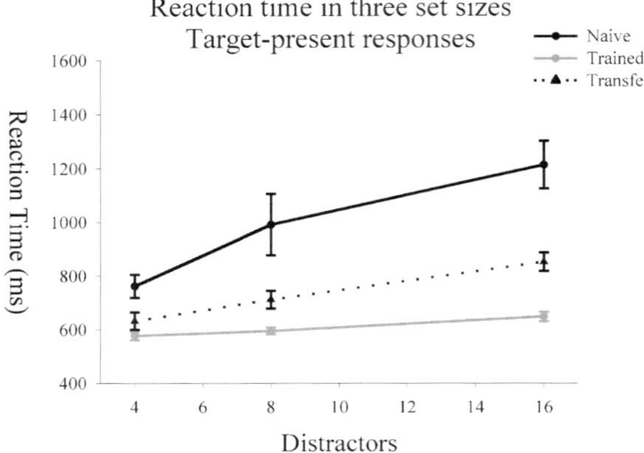

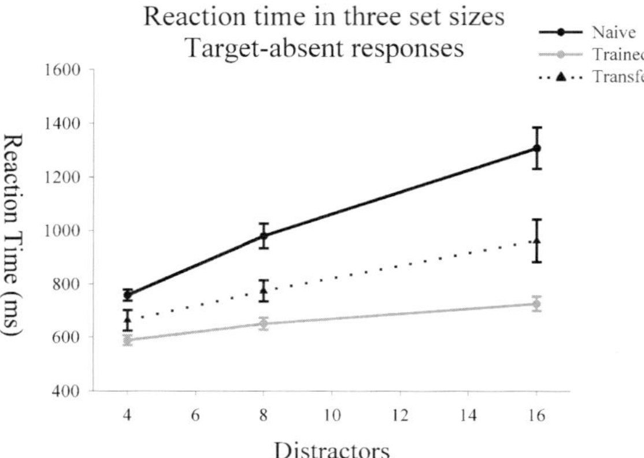

Fig. 5a. Behaviourally, following training on a conjunction visual search task requiring serial search, the search function becomes flat. However, when the visuomotor response association is changed the search slope returns.

demonstrated complementary lateralisation of visual and motor orienting (Rushworth et al., 2001). This group of findings strongly suggests that the role of parietal cortex in visual search is post-visual, and specifically is to transform visual inputs into a metric useful for an action system. While there is a consensus that left anterior and right posterior parietal mechanisms may be responsible for orienting respectively to an act and a location, there has not been a proposal to explain how the visual and motor orienting systems communicate. At some stage this communication will require a co-ordinate transformation. The right PPC would be a good place to propose as the site at which that transformation begins.

To sustain this claim we have to address the question of the relative and integrated roles of visual cortex and parietal cortex during visual search. The view that the parietal cortex plays a visual role in search is based on the assumption that PPC exerts some kind of top-down control over extrastriate visual areas. This view is not difficult to challenge. The parietal cortex does not carry good information about visual features such as colour and detailed form so it is difficult to see how a top down, feature based mechanisms may work. The stronger assumption is that PPC directs spatial selection. This too is difficult to sustain. PPC neurons have large receptive fields and it is not clear why (or how) these would convey spatial information to direct selection by the smaller and malleable receptive field sizes of extrastriate neurons (Moran and Desimone, 1985; Desimone and Duncan, 1995). We therefore propose, contrary to the common assumption that the PPC exerts some top down influence on the extrastriate cortex, that PPC merely acts on information coming from extrastriate cortex to generate a response-weighted transformation into the appropriate body co-ordinate system required to act (the act can be eye, head, limb or hand movements). In a conjunction visual search task, e.g. colour and orientation, the neurons in extrastriate cortex which give the best responses to colour and orientation will independently respond to the elements in the task. These neurons' outputs to the parietal cortex will carry target-weighted information i.e. the correct colour response is weighted greater than the incorrect colour and the correct orientation greater than the distractor orientation. The task of the parietal cortex is to read these incoming signals and to detect the target weighted inputs from the two feature inputs. When there is only one feature to distinguish the target, as in feature search, (however similar to the distractors) there is only one channel of input for the PPC to read. Thus, even when a task is *visually* very difficult, as in our hard feature in Experiment 1, the output from visual cortex will be less noisy than when there

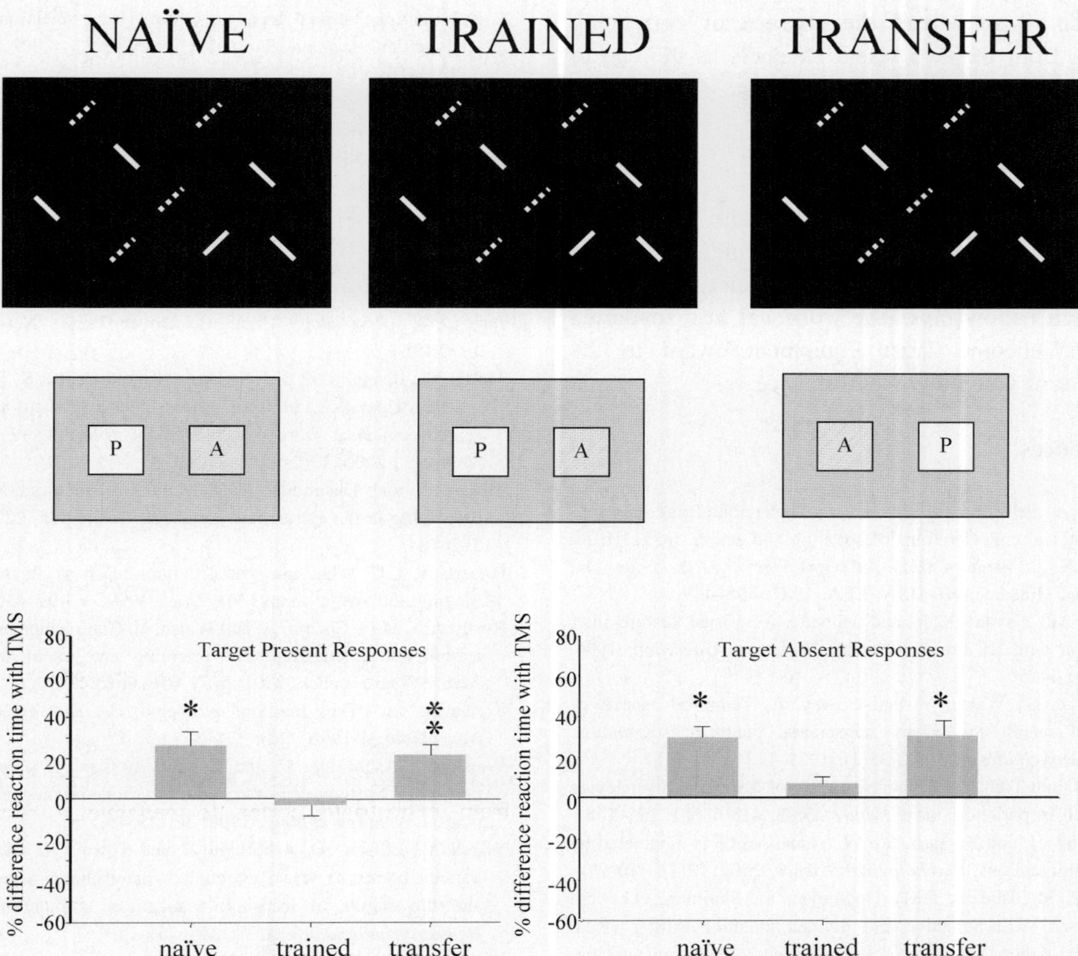

Fig. 5b. Following extensive training on a conjunction visual search task, TMS over PPC no longer causes an impairment. However, if the motor response requirements are changed, i.e. the finger response is switched, an impairment with TMS is again apparent.

are two channels to be read. One incoming stimulus channel requires a single co-ordinate transformation from visual to motor space whereas two incoming channels, even if each is less noisy than a single feature channel, require two accurate transformations. In this sense, one may say the PPC acts on two response-weighted signals, but this is not property binding. To this extent we agree that the PPC is critical to deciding which regions of space carry the best target signals for each of the two features. Thus we can dissociate visual difficulty from the visuomotor transformations that are required of parietal cortex. If the PPC were concerned with visual components of the tasks, deficits would correlate simply with task difficulty, but this is not the case. It is also important to note that the effects of TMS over PPC are the same for target absent trials as for target present trials (see our previous demonstrations – Ashbridge et al., 1998; Walsh et al., 1998). This too is difficult to reconcile with a visuo-visual account of the role of PPC. In our visuomotor account, however, if PPC operated a temporal cut off for a decision, it may read the absence of correlating signals from the two visual channels as the cue to make a negative motor response.

Acknowledgements

Amanda Ellison was supported by the Dr Hadwen Research Trust. Matthew Rushworth and Vincent Walsh are supported by Royal Society University Research Fellowships. The work was also supported by a Wellcome Trust Equipment award to the Institute of Cognitive Neuroscience.

References

Allport, A. Selection for action: some behavioural and neurophsyiological considerations of attention and action. In: H. Heuer and A. F. Sanders (Eds.), *Perspectives on Perception and Action.* Hillsdale, NJ, USA: LEA, 1987: 395–419.

Arguin, M., Cavanagh, P. and Joanette, Y. Visual feature integration with an attention deficit. *Brain and Cognition*, 1994, 24(1): 44–56.

Ashbridge, E., Walsh, V. and Cowey, A. Temporal aspects of visual search studied by transcranial magnetic stimulation. *Neuropsychologia.*, 1997, 35(8): 1121–1131.

Assad, J. and Toth, L.J. Dynamic coding of behaviourally relevant stimuli in parietal cortex. *Nature*, 2002, 415(6868): 165–168.

Bekkering, H. and Neggers, S.F.W. Visual search is modulated by action intentions. *Psychological Science*, 2002, 13(4): 370–374.

Corbetta, M., Miezin, F.M., Dobmeyer, S., Shulman, G.L. and Petersen, S.E. Selective and divided attention during visual discriminations of shape, color and speed: functional anatomy by positron emission tomography. *J. Neurosci.*, 1991, 11: 1202–1226.

Desimone, R. and Duncan, J. Neural mechanisms of selective visual attention. *Ann. Rev. Neurosci.*, 1995, 18: 193–222.

Donner, T., Kettermann, A., Diesch, E., Ostendorf, F., Villringer, A. and Brandt, S.A. Involvement of the human frontal eye field and multiple parietal areas in covert visual selection during conjunction search. *Europ. J. Neurosci.*, 2002, 12(9): 3407–3414.

Duncan, J. and Humphreys, G.W. Visual search and stimulus similarity. *Psychological Rev.*, 1989, 96(3): 433–458.

Friedman Hill, S.R., Robertson, L.C. and Treisman, A. Parietal contributions to visual feature binding: evidence from a patient with bilateral lesions. *Science*, 1995, 269(5225): 853–855.

Humphreys, G. and Riddoch, J. Detection by action: neuropsychological evidence for action-defined templates in search. *Nat. Neurosci.*, 2001, 4(1): 84–88.

James, W. *Psychology,* Vol. II. Dover Press, New York, 1890/1964.

Maioli, C., Benaglio, I., Siri, S., Sosta, K. and Cappa, S. The integration of parallel and serial processing mechanisms in visual search: evidence from eye movement recording. *Europ. J. Neurosci.*, 2000, 13(2): 364–372.

Moran, J. and Desimone, R. Selective attention gates visual processing in the extrastriate cortex. *Science*, 1985, 229(4715): 782–784.

Robertson, L.C. What can spatial deficits teach us about feature binding and spatial maps? *Vis. Cog.*, 1999, 6: 409–430.

Rushworth, M.F., Ellison, A. and Walsh, V. Complementary localization and lateralization of orienting and motor attention. *Nature Neuroscience*, 2001, 4(6): 656–661.

Treisman, A. The binding problem. *Current Opinion in Neurobiology*, 1996, 6(2): 171–178.

Walsh, V., Ashbridge, E. and Cowey, A. Cortical plasticity in perceptual learning demonstrated by transcranial magnetic stimulation. *Neuropsychologi*, 1998, 36: 45–49.

Walsh, V., Ellison, A., Ashbridge, E. and Cowey, A. The role of parietal cortex in visual attention – hemispheric asymmetries and the effects of learning: a magnetic stimulation study. *Neuropsychologia*, 1999, 37: 245–251.

Wocjiulik, E. and Kanwisher, N. Implicit but not explicit feature binding in a Balint's patient. *Vis. Cog.*, 1998, 5: 157–181.

Wolfe, J. Guided search 2.0: a revised model of visual search. *Psychonomic Bulletin and Review*, 1994, 1: 202–238.

Zhang, M. and Barash, S. Neuronal switching of sensorimotor transformations for antisaccades. *Nature*, 2000, 408(6815): 971–975.

Transcranial Magnetic Stimulation and Transcranial Direct Current Stimulation (Supplements to Clinical Neurophysiology, Vol. 56)
Editors: W. Paulus, F. Tergau, M.A. Nitsche, J.C. Rothwell, U. Ziemann, M. Hallett

Chapter 34

Effects of repetitive transcranial magnetic stimulation (rTMS) on slow cortical potentials (SCP)

Ahmed A. Karim[a,b,*], Thomas Kammer[c], Martin Lotze[a], Thilo Hinterberger[a], Ben Godde[a], Leonardo Cohen[d] and Niels Birbaumer[a,e]

[a] *Institute of Medical Psychology and Behavioral Neurobiology, University of Tübingen, D-72072 Tübingen (Germany)*
[b] *International Max Planck Research School of Neural and Behavioral Sciences, Tübingen (Germany)*
[c] *Department of Neurology, University of Tübingen, Tübingen (Germany)*
[d] *Human Cortical Physiology Section, NINDS, National Institutes of Health, Bethesda, MD 20892 (USA)*
[e] *Center for Cognitive Neuroscience, University of Trento, Trento (Italy)*

1. Introduction

Negative slow cortical potential shifts are thought to reflect depolarization of the apical dendrites of layer I cortical pyramidal cells, and hence to indicate cortical excitability (Rockstroh et al., 1993). Studies testing reaction time (Rockstroh et al., 1982) and mental arithmetic (Lutzenberger et al., 1982) have shown performance enhancement following biofeedback trained increases in negativity. Studies in epileptic patients have shown that a learned decrease in cortical negativity reduces seizure rate and severity when employed during early aura (Rockstroh et al., 1993; Kotchoubey et al., 2001). Birbaumer et al. (1999) have proposed that a brain-computer interface (Thought Translation Device; see Hinterberger, 1999), controlled by self-regulation of slow cortical potentials (SCP) can contribute to communication of completely paralyzed patients. Following operant learning principles, a shaping procedure enables the patients to select letters in a Language Support Program by producing SCP amplitude changes (Birbaumer et al., 1999). However, one of the main barriers to the efficacy of neurofeedback training is that some subjects (about 30%) have not been able to gain sufficient control over their SCP even after extended training. Accordingly, we are searching for a possibility to support self-regulation of SCP and hence to facilitate the learning process. A promising approach seems to lie in the application of repetitive transcranial magnetic stimulation (rTMS). Repetitive TMS uses trains of magnetic pulses to induce an electrical field in the neural tissue below the coil (Walsh and Rushworth, 1999; Hallett, 2000). Thereby, one important parameter is the frequency of repeatedly

* *Correspondence to*: Dr. Ahmed A. Karim, Institute of Medical Psychology and Behavioral Neurobiology, University of Tübingen, Gartenstrasse 29, D-72072 Tübingen, Germany.
Tel: +49-7071-2974220; Fax: +49-7071-95956;
E-mail: ahmed.karim@uni-tuebingen.de.

delivered TMS pulses. Several studies report an inhibitory effect of low-frequency (1 Hz or less) rTMS (Chen et al., 1997a; Boroojerdi et al., 2000) while high-frequency (5 Hz and more) rTMS has been shown to lead to an increase of cortical excitability (Pascual-Leone et al., 1994; Mottaghy et al., 1999). Another important factor is the temporal relationship between task performance and magnetic stimulation. Application of fast rTMS (at a frequency of 5 Hz or higher) during task performance (or the presentation of the task relevant stimulus) usually has detrimental effects on cognitive processes (Grafman et al., 1994; Wassermann et al., 1999). If, however, fast rTMS is delivered in a period preceding a task (Hamilton and Pascual-Leone, 1998) or in short periods during processing of a task (Boroojerdi et al., 2001), enhanced performance can be observed. In the current study we investigated if rTMS contributes to voluntarily induced modulation of SCP. Since negative SCP shifts were shown to reflect an increase, and positive SCP shifts a decrease in the excitability of the underlying cortical networks (Birbaumer et al., 1992), we hypothesized that high-frequency rTMS would enhance negative SCP shifts, whereas low-frequency rTMS would enhance positive SCP.

2. Methods

2.1. Subjects

Ten right-handed healthy volunteers (9 men, aged between 20 and 33 years) gave their informed consent according to the standards of the local ethics committee and were trained for four sessions (within 2 weeks) to self-regulate their SCP amplitude using the Thought Translation Device (Hinterberger, 1999; Kübler et al., 1999).

2.2. EEG recording

The electroencephalogram (EEG) was recorded from the following positions against both mastoids: Cz, FC3, CP3, FC4, CP4. The vertical electrooculogram (vEOG) and respiration (respiratory sensor) were recorded additionally and the EEG was corrected on-line for vEOG artifacts. Low-conductivity small Ag-AgCl electrodes prevented possible TMS induced heating artifacts (Ilmoniemi et al., 1997). An eight-channel EEG amplifier (EEG 8, Contact Precision Instrument) was used with a time constant of 16 s and a low pass filter of 40 Hz. Data were sampled at 256 Hz.

2.3. Experimental procedure

Participants sat in a comfortable chair viewing the neurofeedback monitor. Training included 11 blocks on each of the four sessions, each block comprised 34 feedback trials. A Medtronic-Dantec Magnetic Stimulator (Skovlunde, Denmark) was used to generate repetitive biphasic magnetic pulses with a focal figure-of-eight magnetic coil (MC-B70). At the beginning of each session the individual resting motor threshold (MT) was registered from the right abductor pollicis brevis muscle (APB). MT was defined as the minimal intensity of stimulation capable of inducing MEPs greater than 50 μV peak-to-peak amplitude in at least five out of 10 consecutive trials.

Figure 1 shows the chosen rTMS parameters for the activation (a) and the inhibition (b) condition.

In the activation condition subjects received 15 Hz rTMS for 2 s preceding each feedback trial. After a 500 ms pause (in order to let the EEG amplifier recover from the TMS artifact) a baseline (BL) was recorded. A feedback phase followed lasting 3.5 s, in which visual feedback of SCP was provided as a cursor movement on a PC screen. The cursor moved up and down proportionally to the current SCP amplitude compared to the previously recorded baseline (the algorithm is described in Kübler et al., 2001). In each trial participants had to move the cursor towards the top (by producing a negative shift of their SCP) or towards the bottom of the feedback screen (by producing a positive SCP shift). The required direction was randomised over trials and was indicated by highlighting a corresponding rectangle at the top or bottom of the screen. If the subject was successful, a reinforcement stimulus (a smiling face) appeared for 500 ms on the feedback screen.

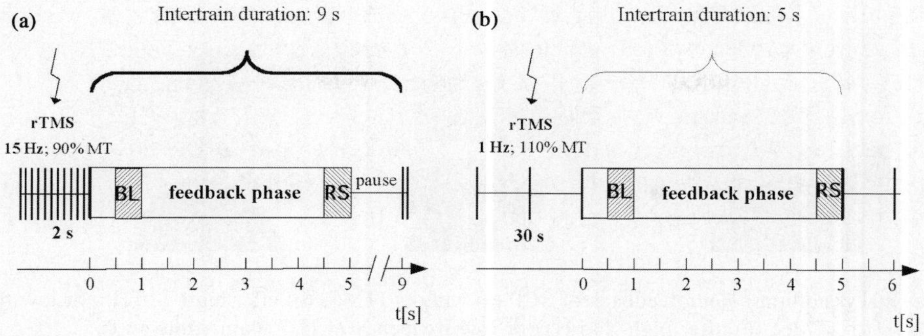

Fig. 1. Scheme of the experimental paradigm with the excitatory (a) and inhibitory (b) condition. (a) In the excitatory condition subjects received 15 Hz repetitive transcranial magnetic stimulation (rTMS) with a duration of 2 s and an intensity of 90% of the resting motor threshold (MT) preceding each feedback trial. (b) In the inhibitory condition subjects received 1 Hz rTMS with a duration of 30 s and an intensity of 110% of the resting motor threshold (MT). Note that in both conditions a fixed number of 30 pulses were applied before each feedback trial. After rTMS application a pause of 500 ms was added in order to let the EEG amplifier recover from the TMS induced artifact. The following 500 ms served as actual baseline (BL) for the SCP-feedback calculation. During the feedback phase, in which visual feedback of SCP was provided as a cursor movement on a PC screen, subjects had to move the cursor towards the top (by producing a negative SCP shift) or towards the bottom of the screen (by producing a positive SCP shift). If the subject was successful, a reinforcement stimulus (RS; a smiling face) appeared for 500 ms on the screen.

In order to increase the safety of the subjects during high-frequency stimulation, a pause of 4 s was added, so that the next rTMS train never started earlier than 9 s after the previous stimulation. Furthermore, the stimulation intensity was set at 90% of the MT (cf. Chen et al., 1997b; Jalinous, 2001). In the inhibition condition (Fig. 1(b)) subjects received 1 Hz rTMS for 30 s preceding each feedback trial. In both the activation and inhibition condition subjects received a fixed number of 30 pulses before each feedback trial. In order to maximise the inhibitory effect of the 1 Hz stimulation, rTMS was delivered at an intensity of 110% of the MT (cf. Fritzgerald et al., 2002). RTMS was delivered centro-frontally over the supplementary motor area (SMA) for two reasons. First, fMRI data show that self-regulated negative SCP shifts are associated with activation of the SMA (Birbaumer et al., 2001); and second, SCP amplitudes are highest over the centro-frontal region of the cortex (Birbaumer et al., 1990). The TMS coil was positioned tangentially to the skull on FCz, according to the international 10-20 system of electrode placement, with the handle parallel to the sagittal axis, and with the center of the figure-eight over the site to be stimulated. The junction region of the double squared coil straddled the midline. This coil orientation is assumed to be most effective for stimulating the SMA (Deecke et al., 1990; Cunnington et al., 1996; Verwey et al., 2002). FCz is the scalp position in between Cz and Fz, 10% of the distance between the inion and the nasion (i.e. about 4 cm) anterior of Cz. During sham stimulation the magnetic coil was also positioned on the SMA, but in a 90° angle to the scalp in order to prevent the magnetic field reaching the brain tissue (Loo et al., 2000; Verwey et al., 2002).

The experimental design contained the following conditions: (1) feedback without rTMS; (2) feedback immediately after high-frequency rTMS (15 Hz for 2 s with an intensity of 90% of the resting motor threshold); (3) feedback after low-frequency rTMS (1 Hz for 30 s with an intensity of 110% of the resting motor threshold); (4) feedback after high-frequency sham stimulation (15 Hz for 2 s) and (5) feedback after low-frequency sham stimulation (1 Hz for 30 s). The order of these conditions was counterbalanced across the training sessions.

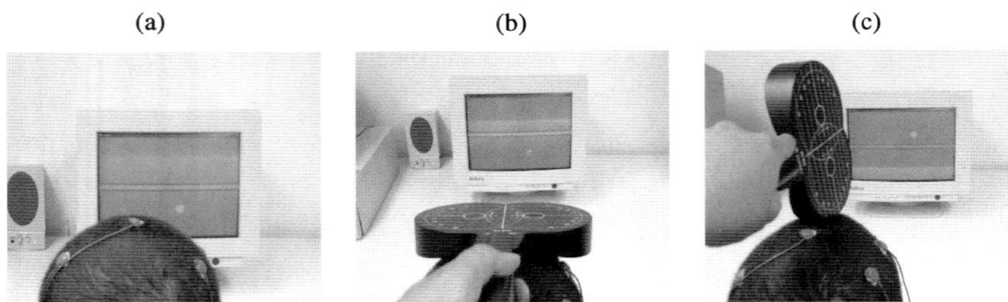

Fig. 2. Experimental conditions. Neurofeedback of SCP (a) without rTMS, (b) after high- (15 Hz) or low-frequency (1 Hz) rTMS, (c) after high- (15 Hz) or low-frequency (1 Hz) sham stimulation.

3. Results

To investigate differential effects of high- and low-frequency rTMS on SCP shifts, trials were separated according to the task requirement (positive vs. negative shifts). A multifactorial repeated measures ANOVA with correct response as dependent variable, the applied frequency (1 Hz vs. 15 Hz) and the experimental condition (real TMS, sham TMS, without TMS) as fixed factors and the task as repeated measures revealed a significant task effect [$F_{(1,235)} = 78.70$; $p < 0.001$]. Post hoc *t*-test showed that subjects were in general better able to produce negative SCP shifts than positive ones ($p < 0.001$; cf. Fig. 3). Both frequency [$F_{(1,235)} = 3.16$; $p = 0.90$] and experimental condition main effects [$F_{(2,235)} = 1.17$; $p = 0.31$] were (independent of the task requirement) not significant, however the interaction between frequency, experimental condition and task was in accordance with our hypotheses significant [$F_{(2,235)} = 15.62$; $p < 0.001$], indicating a differential effect of the stimulation conditions on required positive and negative SCP shifts, respectively.

Duncan post hoc tests revealed a significant increase of positive SCP shifts ($p < 0.01$) and a significant decrease of negative SCP shifts ($p < 0.05$) after 1 Hz rTMS compared to *all* other conditions. 15 Hz rTMS, in turn, caused numerically the highest amount of negative SCP shifts and the lowest amount of positive SCP shifts, however this effect was not consistently significant compared to the other stimulation conditions. 15 Hz rTMS led to a significant increase of negative SCP shifts compared to 1 Hz rTMs ($p < 0.001$), sham 1 Hz rTMS ($p < 0.01$) and to sham 15 Hz rTMS ($p < 0.05$), however there was no significant difference to the condition without stimulation ($p = 0.20$). After 15 Hz rTMS positive SCP shifts were significantly fewer than negative ones ($p < 0.001$). Positive SCP shifts after 15 Hz rTMS were also significantly reduced compared to sham 1 Hz ($p < 0.05$), but there was no significant difference compared to the other two control conditions (sham 1 Hz and without stimulation). Among the control conditions sham 1 Hz rTMS didn't lead to a significant increase of positive SCP shifts compared to the condition without stimulation ($p = 0.05$) and sham 15 Hz rTMS didn't lead to a significant increase of negative SCP shifts compared to the condition without stimulation ($p = 0.16$). Figures 3 and 4 summarize the main results: low-frequency (1 Hz) rTMS enhanced positive SCP but reduced negative SCP in comparison to *all* other conditions, whereas high-frequency (15 Hz) rTMS enhanced negative SCP and reduced positive SCP only partially compared to the other conditions. A modulating effect of high- and low-frequency rTMS on SCP shifts could be found, whereby the inhibitory effect of low-frequency stimulation seems to be more consistent than the excitatory effect of high-frequency stimulation.

4. Discussion

We have reported here, for the first time, the modulating effect of high- and low-frequency rTMS

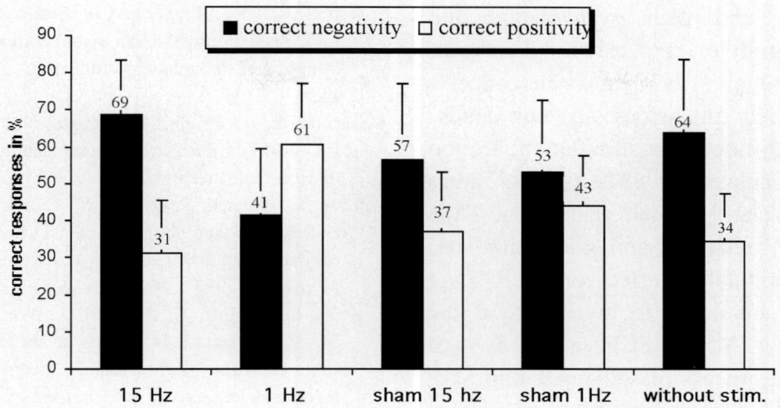

Fig. 3. Percentage of correct responses according to the stimulation condition. Error bars indicate the standard deviation.

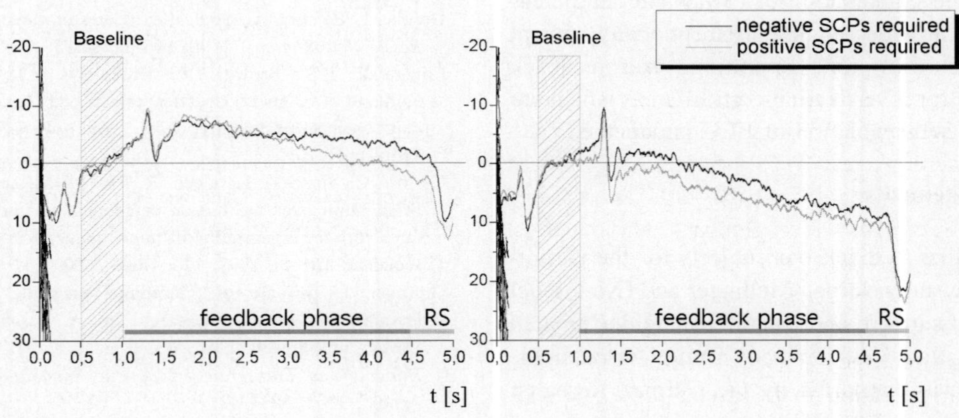

Fig. 4 Averaged SCP curves for 5 s (a) after 15 Hz rTMS and (b) after 1 Hz rTMS. A differential modulating effect can be observed: 15 Hz rTMS enhanced negative SCP shifts but reduced positive SCP shifts, whereas 1 Hz rTMS enhanced positive SCP shifts and reduced negative SCP shifts. The end of the feedback phase elicited a positive evoked potential with a latency of 300 ms. RS = reinforcement stimulus (a smiling face).

on SCP shifts as used in our brain-computer interface. The observed effects are in line with findings of several researchers, who describe facilitating effects of high-frequency and inhibiting effects of low-frequency rTMS (e.g. Mottaghy et al., 1999; Boroojerdi et al., 2000). The finding that the assumed inhibitory effect of low-frequency stimulation leads to more consistent results than the facilitating effect of high-frequency stimulation has already been reported by different research groups (cf. Grafman, 2002; Lappin and Ebmeier, 2002). Besides the question of the temporal relationship between the onset of the task and magnetic stimulation, a further escrow issue may lie in the fact that every attempt to enhance the effectiveness of high-frequency rTMS (by applying higher intensities or longer stimulation trains) can potentially be at the expense of the subjects safeness. Interestingly, Mottaghy et al. (1999) assume that there might be a cut-off point, where the facilitating effect of rTMS with higher intensities disappears and might even change into disruption of cognitive processes. However, according to Gerloff et al. (1997) it may be conceivable that the applied intensities in our study, especially during high-frequency stimulation, are too low in order to stimulate the SMA. Thus, future studies will have to clarify which changes of TMS parameters (intensity, frequency and stimulation site) will optimise the modulating effect on SCP. In a follow-up study we are going to investigate if the modulating effect of rTMS on SCP can be used to facilitate the learning process of self-regulating SCP shifts. It would mean a new hope for non-learners among patients with locked-in syndrome to support self-regulation of SCP and hence to re-establish communication through a Brain-Computer Interface. The presented combination of rTMS and neurofeedback may provide a new, exceptionally potent non-invasive tool for supporting neurofeedback training and for investigating cortical areas which are involved in self-regulation of EEG parameters.

Acknowledgements

We would like to thank our subjects for the participation in the study, Jürgen Mellinger and Eva Friedel for technical support, and Kuno Kirschfeld, Christian Gerloff and Ralf Veit for many fruitful discussions. This study was supported by the German Research Society (DFG) and the Volkswagen Foundation.

References

Birbaumer, N., Elbert, T., Canavan, A.G.M. and Rockstroh, B. Slow potentials of the cerebral cortex and behavior. *Physiological Rev.*, 1990, 70: 1–41.

Birbaumer, N., Roberts, L.E., Lutzenberger, W., Rockstroh, B. and Elbert, T. Area-specific self-regulation of slow cortical potentials on the sagittal midline and its effects on behavior. *Electroencephalogr. Clin. Neurophysiol.*, 1992, 84: 351–361.

Birbaumer, N., Flor, H., Ghanayim, N., Hinterberger, T., Iverson, I., Taub, E., Kotchoubey, B., Kübler, A. and Perelmouter, J. A Spelling Device for the Paralyzed. *Nature*, 1999, 398: 297–298.

Birbaumer, N., Strehl, U., Veit, R., Neumann, N. and Brener, J. Self-regulation of slow cortical potentials (SCP) and functional magnetic resonance imaging (fMRI). *Psychophysiology*, 2001, 38: 26.

Boroojerdi, B., Prager, A., Muellbacher, W. and Cohen, L.G. Reduction of human visual cortex excitability using 1-Hz transcranial magnetic stimulation. *Neurology*, 2000, 54: 1529–1531.

Boroojerdi, B., Phipps, M., Kopylev, L., Wharton, C.M., Cohen, L.G. and Grafman, J. Enhancing analogic reasoning with rTMS over the left prefrontal cortex. *Neurology*, 2001, 56: 526–528.

Chen, R., Classen, J., Gerloff, C., Celnik, P., Wassermann, E.M., Hallett, M. and Cohen, L.G. Depression of motor cortex excitability by low-frequency transcranial magnetic stimulation. *Neurology*, 1997a, 48: 1398–1403.

Chen, R., Gerloff, C., Classen, J., Wassermann, E.M., Hallett, M. and Cohen, L.G. Safety of different inter-train intervals for repetitive transcranial magnetic stimulation and recommendations for safe ranges of stimulation parameters. *Electroencephalogr. Clin. Neurophysiol.*, 1997b, 105: 415–421.

Cunnington, R., Iansek, R., Thickbroom, G.W., Laing, B.A., Mastaglia, F.L. and Bradshaw, J.L. Effects of magnetic stimulation over the supplementary motor area on movement in Parkinson's disease. *Brain*, 1996, 119: 815–822.

Deecke, L. Electrophysiological correlates of movement initiation. *Revue Neurologique*, 1990, 146: 609–612.

Fritzgerald, P.B., Brown, T.L., Daskalakis, Z.J., Chen, R. and Kulkarni, J. Intensity-dependent effects of 1 Hz rTMS on human corticospinal excitability. *Clin. Neurophysiol.*, 2002, 113: 1136–1141.

Gerloff, C., Corwell, B., Chen, R., Hallett, M. and Cohen, L.G. Stimulation over the human supplementary motor area interferes with the organisation of future elements in complex motor sequences. *Brain*, 1997, 120: 1587–1602.

Grafman, J. The use of transcranial magnetic stimulation in learning and memory research. In: A. Pascual-Leone, N.J. Davey, J. Rothwell, E.M. Wassermann and B.K. Puri (Eds.), *Handbook of Transcranial Magnetic Stimulation*. New York: Arnold, 2002: 303–312.

Grafman, J., Pascual-Leone, A., Always, D., Nichelli, P., Gomez-Tortosa, E. and Hallett, M. Induction of a recall deficit by rapid-rate transcranial magnetic stimulation. *NeuroReport*, 1994, 5: 1157–1160.

Hallett, M. Transcranial magnetic stimulation and the human brain. *Nature*, 2000, 406: 147–150.

Hamilton, R. and Pascual-Leone, A. Cortical plasticity associated with Braille reading. *Trends Cogn. Sci.*, 1998, 2: 168–174.

Hinterberger, T. Optimierungsmethoden für die Kommunikation durch Selbstkontrolle langsamer kortikaler Potentiale. Tübingen: Schwäbische Verlagsgesellschaft, 1999.

Ilmoniemi, R.J., Virtanen, J., Ruohonen, J., Karhu, J., Aronen, H.J., Näätänen, R. and Katila, T. Neural responses to magnetic stimulation reveal cortical reactivity and connectivity. *NeuroReport*, 1997, 8: 3537–3540.

Jalinous, R. A guide to magnetic stimulation. Available: http://www.magstim.com/Documents.html, 2001.

Kotchoubey, B., Strehl, U., Uhlmann, C., Holzapfel, S., König, M., Fröscher, W., Blankenhorn, V. and Birbaumer, N.

Modification of slow cortical potentials in patients with refractory epilepsy: A controlled outcome study. *Epilepsia*, 2001, 42: 406–416.

Kübler, A., Kotchoubey, B., Hinterberger, T., Ghanayim, N., Perelmouter, J., Schauer, M., Fritsch, C., Taub, E. and Birbaumer, N. The Thought Translation Device: A neurophysiological approach to communication in total motor paralysis. *Exp. Brain Res.*, 1999, 124: 223–232.

Kübler, A., Neumann, N., Kaiser, J., Kotchoubey, B., Hinterberger, T. and Birbaumer, N. Brain-computer communication: Self-regulation of slow cortical potentials for verbal communication. *Arch. Phys. Med. Rehab.*, 2001, 82: 1533–1539.

Lappin, J. and Ebmeir, K.P. Transcranial magnetic stimulation in psychiatric disorders: does TMS affect cortical function by long-term potentation? In: A. Pascual-Leone, N.J. Davey, J. Rothwell, E.M. Wassermann, B.K. Puri (Eds.), *Handbook for Transcranial Magnetic Stimulation*. New York: Arnold, 2002: 361–375.

Lutzenberger, W., Elbert, T., Rockstroh, B. and Birbaumer, N. Biofeedback produced slow brain potentials and task performance. *Biol. Psychol.*, 1982, 14: 99–111.

Mottaghy, F.M., Hungs, M., Brugmann, M., Sparing, R., Boroojerdi, B., Foltys, H., Huber, W. and Topper, R. Facilitation of picture naming after repetitive transcranial magnetic stimulation. *Neurology*, 1999, 53: 1806–1812.

Pascual-Leone, A., Valls-Sole, J., Wassermann, E.M. and Hallett, M. Responses to rapid-rate transcranial magnetic stimulation of the human motor cortex. *Brain*, 1994, 117: 847–858.

Rockstroh, B., Elbert, T., Lutzenberger, W. and Birbaumer, N. The effects of slow cortical potentials on response speed. *Psychophysiology*, 1982, 19: 211–217.

Rockstroh, B., Elbert, T., Birbaumer, N., Wolf, P., Düchting-Röth, A., Reker, M., Daum, I., Lutzenberger, W. and Dichgans, J. Cortical self-regulation in patients with epilepsies. *Epilepsy Res.*, 1993, 14: 63–72.

Verwey, W.B., Lammens, R. and Van Honk, J. On the role of the SMA in the discrete sequence production task: a TMS study. *Neuropsychologia*, 2002, 40: 1268–1276.

Walsh, V. and Rushworth, M. A primer of magnetic stimulation as a tool for neuropsychology. *Neuropsychologia*, 1999, 37: 125–135.

Wassermann, E.M., Blaxton, T.A., Hoffman, E.A., Berry, C.D., Oletsky, H., Pascual-Leone, A. and Theodore, W.H. Repetitive transcranial magnetic stimulation of the dominant hemisphere can disrupt visual naming in temporal lobe epilepsy patients. *Neuropsychologia*, 1999, 37: 537–544.

Section VI

Neurological and Psychiatric Diseases

Transcranial Magnetic Stimulation and Transcranial Direct Current Stimulation (Supplements to Clinical Neurophysiology, Vol. 56)
Editors: W. Paulus, F. Tergau, M.A. Nitsche, J.C. Rothwell, U. Ziemann, M. Hallett

Chapter 35

Transcranial magnetic stimulation in brainstem lesions and lesions of the cranial nerves

Peter P. Urban

Department of Neurology, University of Mainz, Langenbeckstr. 1, D-55101 Mainz (Germany)

1. Introduction

Transcranial magnetic stimulation (TMS) represents a non-invasive, safe, and painless method of motor cortex activation for the functional assessment of the rapid conducting corticobulbar and corticospinal projections. TMS delivered to different levels of the motor system can provide information on the excitability of the motor cortex, the functional integrity of intracortical neuronal structures, the conduction along corticospinal, corticonuclear, and callosal fibres, as well as on the function of nerve roots and the peripheral motor pathway to the muscles. Brain stem lesions may lead to corticonuclear and/or corticospinal tract involvement. It is therefore useful to examine both tracts, which can be identified following the accurate selection of the respective recording and stimulation site.

The focus of this chapter is not only on TMS applications in brainstem pathology, but also on the description of TMS techniques for the evaluation of motor cranial nerve function, which is an essential measure in the diagnostic workup of brainstem lesions. Applications of TMS to the cranial nerve innervated muscles have been the objective of numerous investigations, ranging from basic neuroanatomic studies to determine the central course of corticonuclear projections to clinical applications carried out to determine the location of lesions, investigate the pathophysiology of ischemic dysarthria, detect clinically silent lesions in multiple sclerosis, obtain prognostic information regarding persistent motor deficits following cerebral ischemia, and to identify corticonuclear tract involvement in motor neuron diseases. TMS is also of clinical relevance in the evaluation of those peripheral cranial nerve lesions which most frequently affect the facial nerve.

* Correspondence to: Dr. Peter P. Urban, Department of Neurology, University of Mainz, Langenbeckstr. 1, D-55101 Mainz, Germany.
Tel.: +49-6131-175162, Fax: +49-6131-173271;
E-mail: urban@neurologie.klinik.uni-mainz.de

2. Methods

Brainstem lesions may affect the corticospinal and/or corticobulbar projections. A description of the stimulation and recording technique from the limbs is given in the IFCN recommendations (Rossini et al., 1994; Rothwell et al., 1999), as well as by a number of recently published reviews (Rossini and Rossi, 1998; Weber and Eisen, 2002; Kobayashi and Pascual-Leone, 2003). In contrast to their application in limb muscles, fractionated examinations of the projections to the cranial nerve muscles are less commonly performed, and frequently require special recording and stimulation techniques, which are described in greater detail in this review. Recordings from the facial muscles and the tongue are particularly useful in the assessment of corticonuclear function due to the relatively large size of the cortical representation area of these structures.

3. Masticatory muscles (N. V)

Motor evoked potentials (MEP) of the masticatory muscles by TMS have been described for healthy subjects and patients with hemiplegia, trigeminal neuralgia, amyotrophic lateral sclerosis (ALS), and multiple sclerosis (e.g. Cruccu et al., 1989; Türk et al., 1994; Trompetto, 1998). However, reliable recordings of TMS evoked MEPs of the masseter muscle are more difficult to achieve than those of the facial, tongue or intrinsic hand muscles due to methodological problems associated with the recording and stimulation technique.

3.1. Recording technique

Recordings from the masseter muscle are performed most frequently, although recordings from other masticatory muscles as, e.g. the anterior digastric muscle (Gooden et al., 1999), and the medial pterygoid muscle (Türk et al., 1994) have been reported. A relevant methodological problem is the presence of volume conducted potentials from the overlying facial muscles which are also activated in the course of cortical stimulation. To avoid recording of volume conducted facial muscle activity, both an enoral recording technique (Türk et al., 1994) and a very short distance between active and reference electrodes have been recommended (Guggisberg et al., 2001). Furthermore, selective preactivation of the masticatory muscles is required to focus on the target muscle and to reduce the relative influence of the relaxed neighboring muscles.

3.2. Stimulation technique

3.2.1. Stimulation of the motor cortex

Due to the relatively small cortical representation area for masticatory muscles, the correct placement of the magnetic coil is essential (Guggisberg et al., 2001). The masticatory muscles also have a higher motor threshold compared to facial muscles and the tongue. This may be accounted for by the presence of fewer cortical connections to the pyramidal cells (Guggisberg et al., 2001). The location of the optimal stimulation site using a circular coil, has been described as 2–4 cm paramedially to the vertex (Türk et al., 1994). For the figure-of-eight coil, a coil orientation of 120° relative to a fronto-dorsal line in an area 4–10 cm lateral to the vertex and 0–4 cm frontal to the bi-auricular line has been shown to have the lowest motor threshold, the highest amplitudes, and shortest MEP latencies from the masseter muscle (Guggisberg et al., 2001).

3.2.2. Peripheral nerve stimulation

The proximal part of the trigeminal motor nerve can be activated with an ipsilateral coil position 6 cm lateral to the vertex. The responses occur at a mean latency of about 2 ms (Cruccu et al., 1989; Guggisberg et al., 2001). Comparing the responses of direct electrical trigeminal nerve stimulation during microvascular decompression operations with TMS evoked responses preoperatively, it has been shown that TMS activates the trigeminal nerve distal to the root entry zone within the cerebrospinal fluid near the porus trigeminale. However, the activation site was not constant and migrated distally at increasing stimulus intensities (Schmid et al., 1995). Electrical stimulation of the distal trigeminal nerve at the zygomatic arch evokes peripheral compound muscle action potentials (CMAP) with a latency of about 1.5 ms. However, due to the small distance between stimulation and recording site, the presence of a substantial stimulus artefact often interferes with the determination of the CMAP onset.

4. Facial muscles (N. VII)

Recordings from the facial muscles allow reliable conduction measurements across the central and peripheral motor pathways. Clinical applications include supranuclear and infranuclear facial palsies of different etiologies, and the detection of a clinically silent involvement of the supranuclear tract in multiple sclerosis and ALS.

4.1. Recording technique

There are no firm recommendations regarding the recording site, and CMAPs have been recorded from the nasalis, mentalis, orbicularis oculi, frontalis, triangularis, levator labii, and buccinator muscles. A systematic comparison of these recording sites as to the elicitation of a CMAP, stimulus artefact, interferences with the R1-component of the blink reflex, cross-talk from the contralateral face, interside differences of the amplitudes and intraindividual reproducibility showed clear advantages for the buccinator and triangularis muscles under facial nerve stimulation, and for the buccinator and levator labii muscles under motor cortex stimulation (Urban et al., 2002a). These findings are consistent with results of recently published neuroanatomic studies demonstrating that only the lateral facial nucleus, which contains neurons for the orofacial muscles, receives contralateral projections from the contralateral primary motor cortex, while the upper face muscles receive projections from the supplementary motor cortex and rostral parts of the gyrus cinguli (Morecraft et al., 2001). Thus, the orofacial muscles are especially suitable for the evaluation of the central facial motor pathway.

We prefer the use of an enoral technique for recordings from the buccinator muscle, because it is characterized by a high CMAP amplitude caused by the large muscle volume, no volume conduction from the contralateral side as a result of the lateral position, no relevant stimulus artefact associated with the enoral recording technique, no R1-component of the blink reflex resulting from the caudal position, and a distinct negative deflection of the CMAP due to the clearly defined nerve entry zone (motor point). For this purpose, pairs of Ag/AgCl-surface disc electrodes are embedded at a distance of 18 mm in a specially designed fork-shaped metacrylate device adapted to the oral vestibulum (Urban et al., 1997a). The electrodes are in contact with the insides of the cheeks and a slight contraction of the buccinator muscles during motor cortex stimulation is achieved by pursing the lips.

4.2. Stimulation technique

4.2.1. Stimulation of the motor cortex

The center of a circular coil is positioned tangentially 2–4 cm (buccinator muscle) lateral of Cz for motor cortex stimulation. Using a figure-of-eight coil, the most effective site for stimulation has been described as 8–10 cm lateral to the vertex, with a coil orientation allowing the current induced into the brain to flow in a posterior to anterior direction (Meyer et al., 1994). Stimulation intensity is increased stepwise during slight preactivation until stable latencies (total motor conduction time: TMCT) are achieved. Recording of volume-conducted activity from the adjacent masticatory muscles is negligible due to their higher motor threshold, as may be observed in the presence of absent activity in complete peripheral facial palsy.

4.2.2. Peripheral nerve stimulation

The proximal peripheral facial nerve is stimulated magnetically at the extra-axial intracranial segment. A comparison of the responses to direct electrical facial nerve stimulation during microvascular decompression operations with preoperatively recorded TMS findings showed that TMS activates the facial nerve at the end of the labyrinthine segment (canalicular stimulation) on leaving the low-resistance cerebrospinal fluid and entering the high resistance petrous bone (Schmid et al., 1991). To achieve excitation of the proximal facial nerve, the circular coil is placed in a parieto-occipital position ipsilaterally to the facial nerve. For stimulation of the left (right) peripheral nerve, side "B" ("A") of the circular coil is viewed from the outside. The peripheral motor conduction time (PMCT) is about 5 ms and serves to calculate the central motor conduction time (CMCT) (TMCT – PMCT = CMCT). Only a relatively low stimulation intensity (about 30–50%

of the maximal stimulator output) should be applied for magnetic stimulation to avoid stimulation of the distal nerve at the stylomastoid foramen. Inadvertent facial nerve stimulation at the stylomastoid foramen can be identified by comparing the PMCT with the distal motor latency (DML), which is equal to the conduction time on electrical stimulation of the distal facial nerve at the stylomastoid foramen. The normal value for the difference between PMCT and DML (i.e. the transosseal conduction time) is about 1–1.5 ms (Rösler et al., 1989; Urban et al., 1997a), although it is lower in the presence of inadvertent distal nerve stimulation. In the latter case, the stimulation intensity should be reduced and the coil position ought to be moved to a more parietal site.

4.2.3. Interpretation

Because stimulation of the motor cortex yields varying ipsilateral responses in healthy subjects, only the contralateral responses should be considered (Urban et al., 1997a). A supranuclear lesion of the corticofacial pathways is assumed, when: (1) no responses are obtained on motor cortex stimulation (no reproducible response at four consecutive trials with a gain of 200 (V/div); (2) the amplitude correlation between motor cortex response and M-wave amplitude with electrical stimulation is (10% (MEP/M-wave-ratio); and (3) a delayed CMCT or interside difference of the CMCT (> 2.5 SD from the normal mean) is present. An infranuclear facial nerve lesion may be assumed when the interside amplitude difference of the M-wave is (50% compared to the normal side) 10 days after the acute lesion.

5. Sternocleidomastoid muscle and trapezius muscle (N. XI)

A clinical application of motor evoked potentials (MEP) of the sternocleidomastoid (SCM) and trapezius muscles evoked by TMS has recently been described for the differentiation of amyotrophic lateral sclerosis and cervical spondylotic myelopathy (Truffert et al., 2000).

5.1. Recording technique

Recordings from both the sternocleidomastoid and trapezius muscles have been reported in the literature. However, using surface electrode recordings, additional volume conducted activity from the overlying platysma (SCM) (Thompson et al., 1997), and the underlying neck muscle activity (trapezius muscle) (Berardelli et al., 1991) has to be considered during motor cortex stimulation.

5.2. Stimulation technique

5.2.1. Stimulation of the motor cortex

The results of a number of studies using magnetic and electric transcranial stimulation (Gandevia and Applegate, 1988; Berardelli et al., 1991; Odergren and Rimpiläinen, 1996; Thompson et al., 1997; Strenge and Jahns, 1998), and clinical observations during hemispheric suppression of one hemisphere by amytal during the Wada test (DeToledo and Dow, 1998) have shown that stimulation of the motor cortex evokes both bilateral, but predominantly contralateral responses in the SCM and trapezius muscle. The center of a circular coil is positioned tangentially 3–4 cm lateral of Cz and 1–2 cm anterior to the interaural line for motor cortex stimulation. Mapping studies using a figure-of-eight coil for motor cortex stimulation and dual monopolar shielded needles for muscle activity recordings demonstrated that the SCM is represented at the cerebral convexity medial to the upper limb representation, leading to short latency (mean 2.2 ms) responses in the contralateral SCM and longer latency (mean 9.3 ms) responses in the ipislateral SCM (Thompson et al., 1997).

5.2.2. Peripheral nerve stimulation

The accessory nerve may be magnetically stimulated by placing the centre of the coil below the mastoid (Priori et al., 1991). No comparative intraoperative and preoperative studies on the most suitable stimulation site have been publisheded thus far. The distal accessory nerve is generally stimulated electrically at the midpoint of the posterior border of the

SCM, and the CMAP is recorded from the trapezius muscle (e.g. Petrera and Trojaborg, 1984).

6. Tongue muscles (N. XII)

Recordings from the tongue enable reliable conduction measurements across the central and peripheral motor pathways. Clinical applications include the identification of supranuclear lesions of the corticolingual pathway of different etiologies in dysarthria, and the detection of clinically silent corticonuclear tract involvement in multiple sclerosis and ALS.

6.1. Recording technique

Non-invasive recordings from the genioglossus muscle can be performed reliably with an enoral surface electrode technique. For this purpose, pairs of Ag/AgCl-surface disc electrodes are embedded at a distance of 18 mm in a specially designed spoon-shaped metacrylate device, which is adapted to the oral vestibulum (Urban et al., 1994, 1996, 1997c; Muellbacher et al., 1994). The electrodes are in contact with the surface of the tongue, and slight contraction of the genioglossus during motor cortex stimulation is achieved by pressing the device gently against the hard palate.

6.2. Stimulation technique

6.2.1. Stimulation of the motor cortex

The centre of a circular coil is positioned tangentially 4–6 cm lateral of Cz for motor cortex stimulation. The optimal reported stimulation site using a focal 8-shaped coil (outside diameter of one half-coil: 8.5 cm) is 8–10 cm lateral to the midline, and 2–4 cm anterior to the interaural line (Meyer et al., 1997). Stimulation strength is increased stepwise during slight preactivation until stable latencies (total motor conduction time: TMCT) are achieved.

6.2.2. Peripheral nerve stimulation

Magnetic stimulation is assumed to activate the hypoglossal nerve at the intracranial segment or around the hypoglossal canal, although a comparison with intraoperative stimulation findings has not yet been performed in man. However, in the cat it has been shown that the site of magnetic excitation of the hypoglossal nerve is at the exit of the hypoglossal canal (Kobayashi et al., 1999). In clinical practice, the proximal hypoglossal nerve can be excited with the circular coil in a suboccipital position ipsilaterally to the hypoglossal nerve. For stimulation of the left (right) peripheral nerve, side "B" ("A") of the circular coil is viewed from the outside. However, magnetic suboccipital stimulation fails to evoke responses in about 25% of subjects (Urban et al., 1997c), which is most probably due to the anatomical position of the hypoglossal nerve deep at the base of the skull. High voltage electrical stimulation using surface electrodes over the occipital skull may serve to overcome this problem as suggested by the results of a recently published study showing that supramaximal stimulation of the proximal hypoglossal nerve using this technique was possible in all 10 subjects (Kobayashi et al., 1999). The distal hypoglossal nerve can easily be stimulated supramaximally medial and posterior to the angle of the jaw with a conventional surface electrical stimulator (Redmond and Di Benedetto, 1988).

6.2.3. Interpretation

In healthy subjects, stimulation of one hemisphere evokes bilateral responses at both halves of the tongue (Muellbacher et al., 1994; Urban et al., 1994; Meyer et al., 1997). Muellbacher et al. (1998) reported significantly higher amplitudes and shorter latencies for the contralateral projections, while others did not find significant differences for these parameters between the ipsilateral and contralateral projections (Meyer et al., 1997; Urban et al., 1997c). Since supramaximal electrical hypoglossal nerve stimulation also elicits a slight muscle response (25–30% of the ipsilateral response) at the contralateral half of the tongue due to volume conduction (Meyer et al., 1997; Chen et al., 1999), the presence of some cross-talk has to be considered on cortical stimulation.

A supranuclear lesion of the corticolingual pathways may be assumed, when: (1) no responses are obtained on motor cortex stimulation (no reproducible response for four consecutive trials with a gain of 200 (V/div); (2) the amplitude relation between motor cortex response and M-wave amplitude with electrical stimulation is 10%; and (3) a delayed CMCT or interside difference of the CMCT (> 2.5 SD from the normal mean) is observed.

7. Neuroanatomic studies

7.1. The course of corticofacial projections in the human brainstem

The course of corticofacial projections in the human brainstem was reconstructed in 53 patients with unifocal brainstem infarctions (Urban et al., 2001b). At the midbrain and the pontomesencephalic level, infarctions with a lesion of the corticofacial projections were located at the centre of the cerebral peduncle, while the lesions at the upper and middle pontine levels extended across the centre of the pontine base (Fig. 1). The lesion sites at the lower third of the pons were found at a more ventromedial location close to the midline. The distribution of the lesions within the pons indicates that the corticofacial fibres are split into a number of small dispersed fascicles, or show significant variability as to their location within the base of the pons. Since the clinical

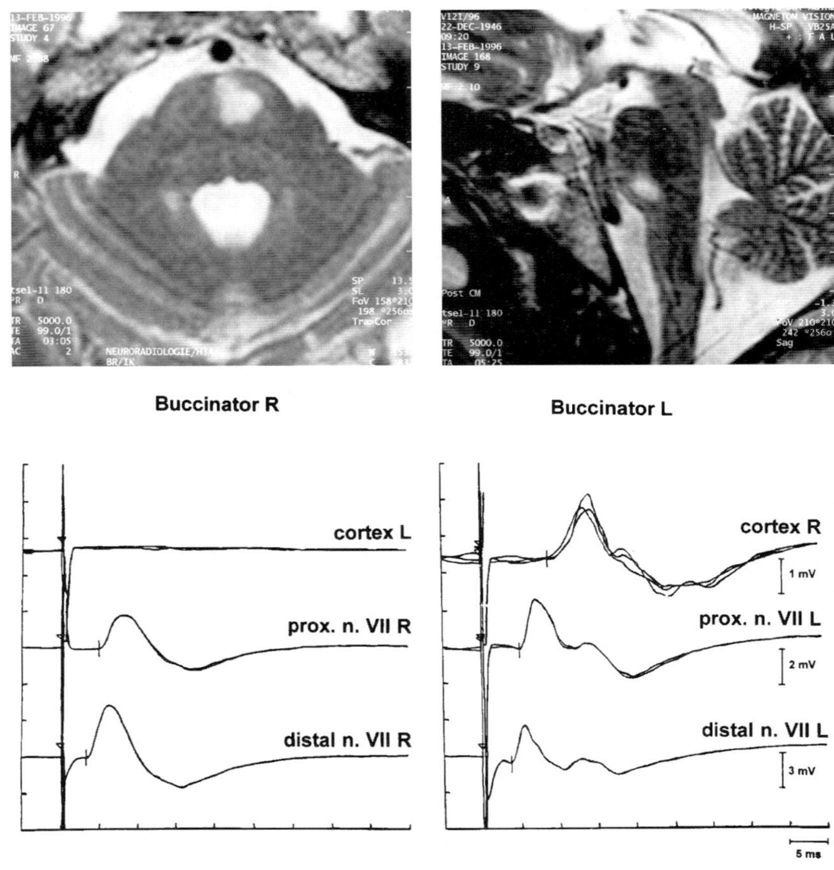

Fig. 1. MRI of a patient with contralateral central facial paresis due to a lesion of the left base of the pons. TMS of the motor cortex and stimulation of the proximal and distal facial nerve with recordings from the buccinator muscles (day 11 after onset of symptoms). Stimulation of the left facial motor cortex (ipsilateral to the pontine lesion) evoked no response in the contralateral buccinator muscle (from Urban et al., 2001b).

picture of patients with a lesion at the lower third of the pons was characterized by contralateral central facial palsy, it may be assumed that the corticofacial fibres cross the midline below this level. In three patients with contralateral facial palsy, the lesions were located in the middle and upper pons in a paralemniscal position at the dorsal edge of the pontine base (Fig. 2). This location correlates with histological descriptions of an 'aberrant bundle', which branches off the main pyramidal tract at the midbrain and upper pontine level and reaches the facial nucleus in a paralemniscal position (Hoche, 1898; Barnes, 1901; Yamashita and Yamamoto, 2001).

Central facial paresis was also observed in five patients with upper medullary infarctions. Two of these patients showed left ventral medullary infarction (Fig. 3) and contralateral central facial paresis, while the remaining three patients with lateral medullary infarctions had central facial paresis ipsilateral to the lesion with a supranuclear lesion pattern on TMS (Fig. 4). The distribution of these medullary lesions suggests that in some individuals

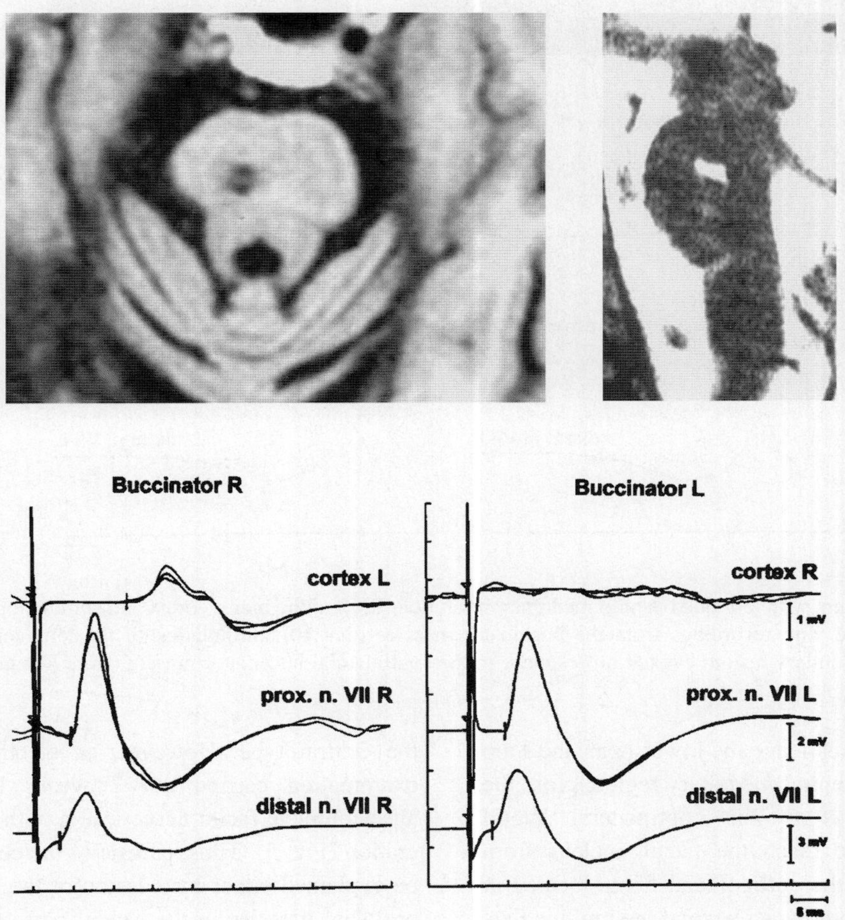

Fig. 2. MRI of a patient with isolated contralateral central facial paresis due to a lesion of the right dorsal base of the pons near the medial lemniscus. TMS of the motor cortex and stimulation of the proximal and distal facial nerve with recordings from the buccinator muscles (day 12). Stimulation of the right facial motor cortex (ipsilateral to the pontine lesion) evoked no response in the contralateral buccinator muscle (from Urban et al., 2001b).

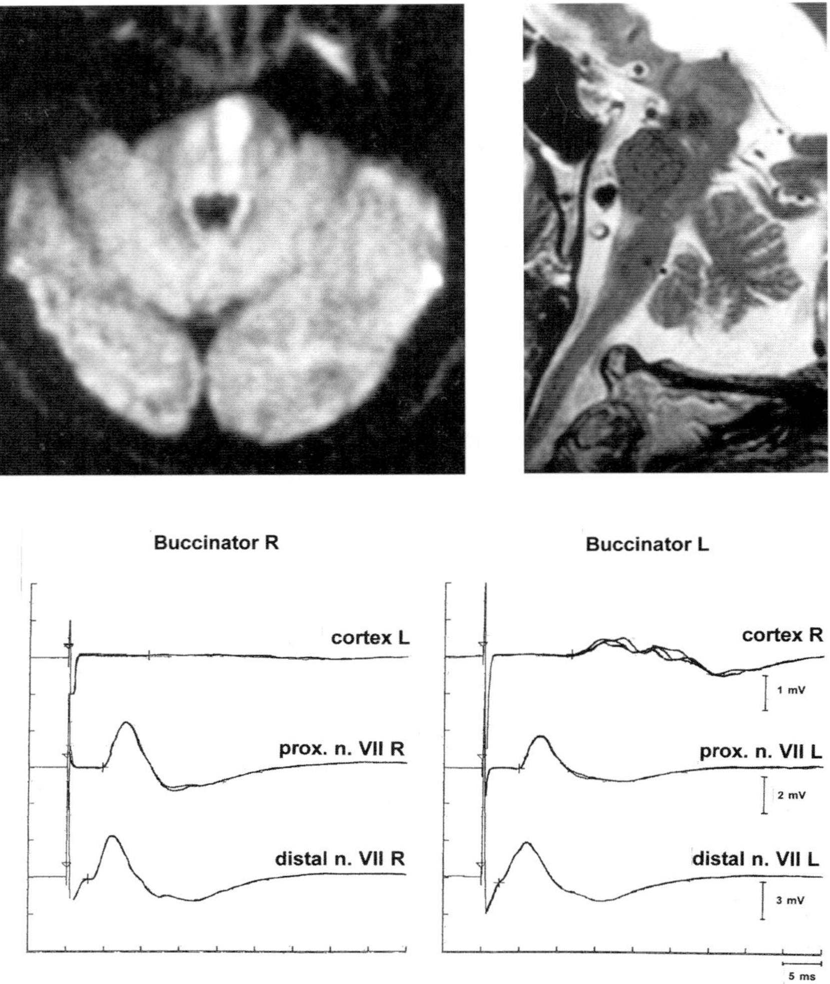

Fig. 3. MRI of a patient with left-sided ventral medullary infarction. TMS of the motor cortex and stimulation of the proximal and distal facial nerve with recordings from the buccinator muscles (day 10). Stimulation of the left facial motor cortex (ipsilateral to the medullary lesion) evoked no response in the contralateral buccinator muscle (from Urban et al., 2001b).

the corticofacial fibres leave the lower pons and loop into the ipsilateral ventral medullary region, cross the midline and ascend to the contralateral lateral medullary region to reach the facial nucleus from below. A lesion of the corticofacial fibres located in the lateral medulla oblongata beyond the midline thus explains the occurrence of central facial palsy ipsilateral to the lesion side.

Two additional patients with dorsolateral medullary infarction also presented with facial paresis of the central type. However, an electrophysiological examination carried out 2 weeks later, revealed an incomplete facial nerve lesion with axonal degeneration (Fig. 5). Thus, paresis of the central type may be explained either by a lesion of the neurons of the orofacial muscles in the caudal part of the musculotopically organized facial nucleus, or by a selective lesion of infranuclear facial nerve fibres occurring along the course of these nerves within the brainstem (Urban et al., 1999a).

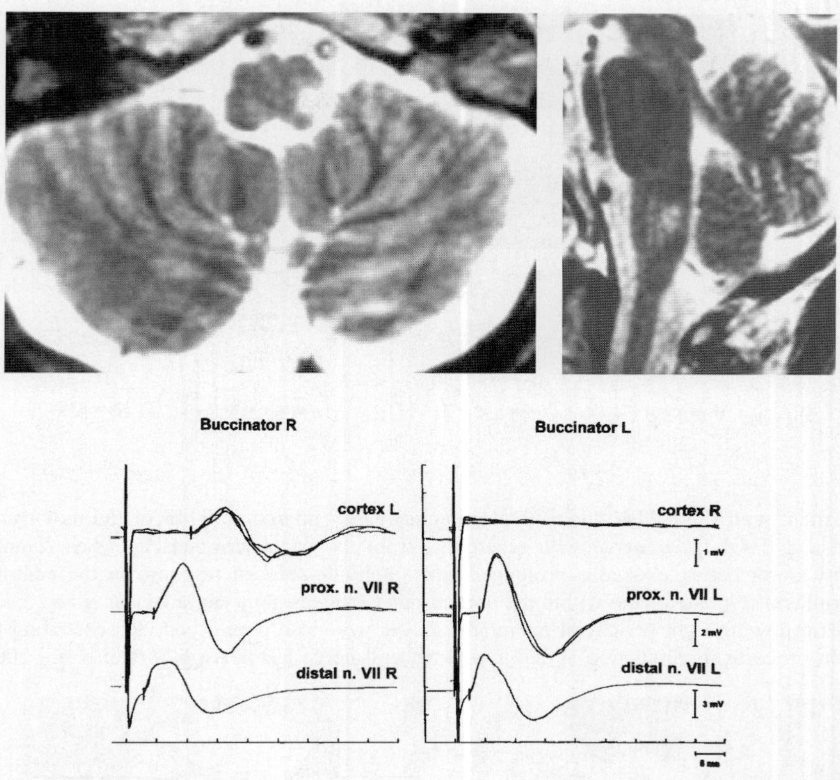

Fig. 4. MRI of a patient with left-sided lateral medullary infarction. TMS of the facial motor cortex and stimulation of the proximal and distal facial nerve from the buccinator muscle (day 10). Stimulation of the right motor cortex evoked no response in the left buccinator muscle (from Urban et al., 2001b).

7.2. The course of corticolingual projections in the human brainstem

The course of corticolingual projections in the human brainstem was reconstructed in 30 patients with unifocal infarctions (Urban et al., 1996, 2001b, 2002b). Similar to the corticofacial projections, infarctions with a lesion of the corticolingual projections were located at the midbrain level at the centre of the cerebral peduncle, while the lesions at the upper and middle pontine levels extended across the centre of the pontine base (Fig. 6). The lesion sites at the lower third of the pons were located in a more ventromedial position close to the midline. In view of the fact that patients with a lesion at the lower third of the pons also showed a lesion of the corticolingual projections, the lesion may be assumed to cross the midline below this level. No patient in this group was found to have a lesion localized along the course of the 'aberrant bundle'.

In three patients with dorsolateral medullary infarction, only the corticolingual fibres to the ipsilateral tongue were affected. This finding suggests that the corticolingual projections were affected after leaving the main pyramidal tract and crossing the midline on their way to the ipsilateral hypoglossal nucleus.

8. Dysarthria

The corticolingual projections are frequently impaired in ischaemic dysarthria (Urban et al., 1997b, 1999b, 2001a). In a prospective study including 106

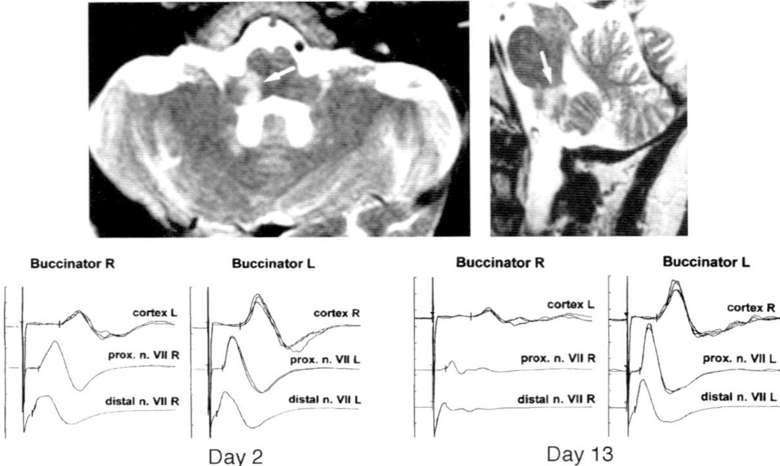

Fig. 5. MRI of a patient with right-sided dorsolateral pontomedullary infarction. TMS of the motor cortex and stimulation of the proximal and distal facial nerve with recordings from the buccinator muscles (days 2 and 13). On day 2, stimulation of the left motor cortex evoked a prolonged and amplitude-reduced response in the contralateral buccinator muscle, while the peripheral responses were within the normal range, suggesting a supranuclear lesion. On day 13, however, the CMAP amplitudes following right peripheral nerve stimulation were also diminished, demonstrating that the amplitude reduction on cortical stimulation is due to a peripheral nerve lesion (from Urban et al., 2001b).

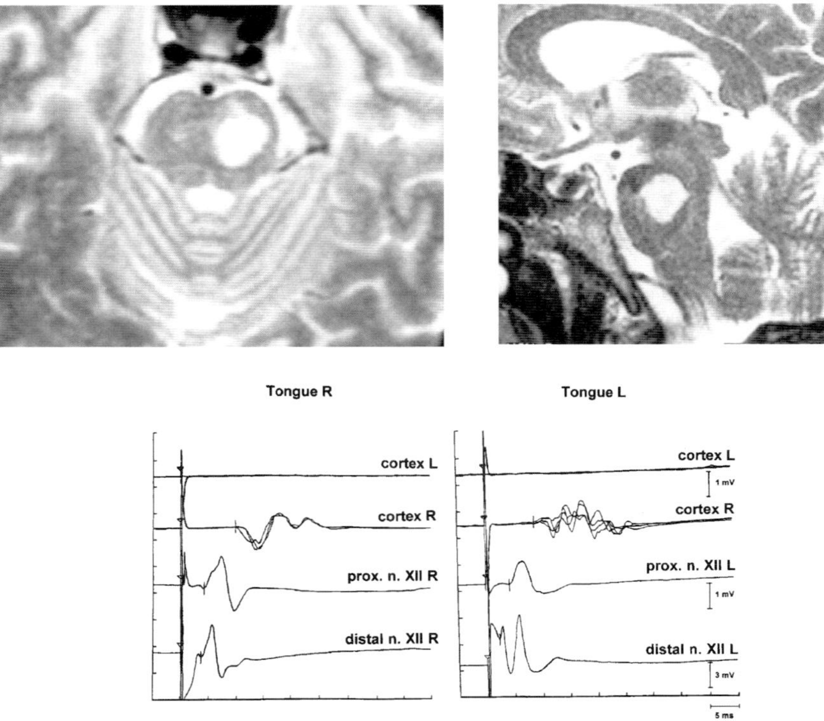

Fig. 6. MRI of a patient with left-sided infarction of the pontine base with central facial palsy and dysarthria. TMS of the left motor cortex (ipsilateral to the pontine lesion) evoked no response in both halves of the tongue.

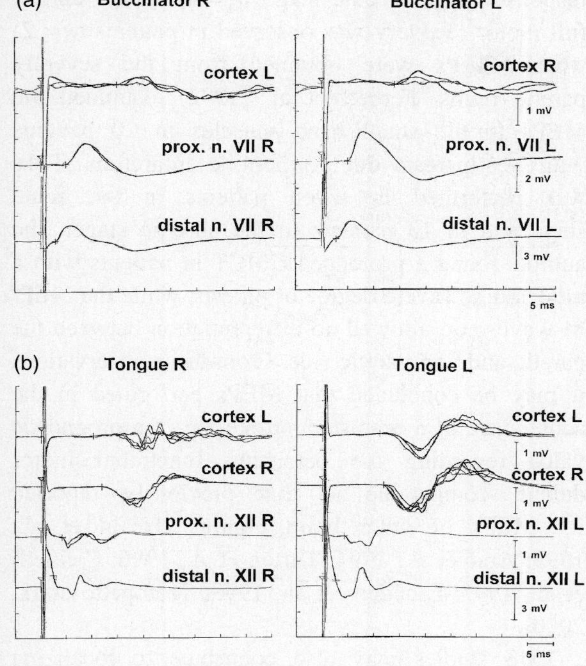

Fig. 7. (a) Multiple sclerosis: Severe bilateral delay of the buccinator response latencies following stimulation of both motor cortices. Normal latencies following stimulation of both the proximal and distal part of the peripheral facial nerve. (b) Multiple sclerosis: Severe bilateral delay of the tongue muscle response latencies following stimulation of both motor cortices. Normal latencies following stimulation of both the proximal and distal part of the peripheral hypoglossal nerve.

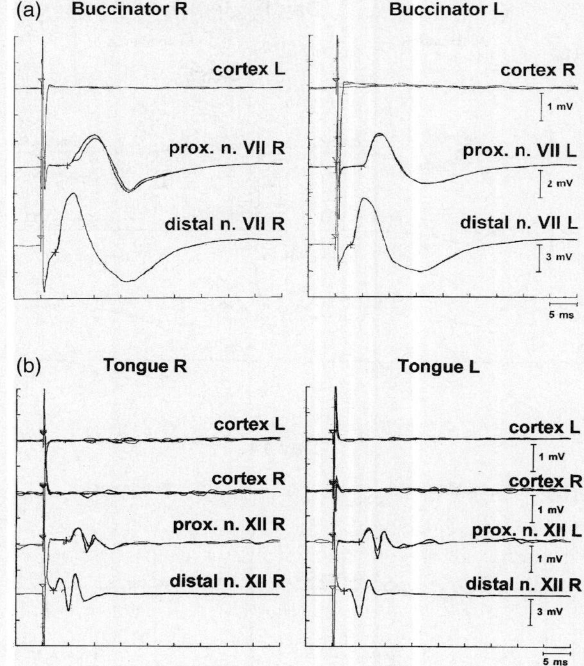

Fig. 8. (a) ALS: Bilaterally absent buccinator muscle responses on cortical stimulation while the CMAPs on peripheral facial nerve stimulation are unaffected. (b) ALS: Bilaterally absent tongue muscle responses on cortical stimulation while the CMAPs on peripheral hypoglossal nerve stimulation are unaffected.

patients with sudden dysarthria due to a single occurrence of ischemia, we showed that the corticolingual projections at extracerebellar locations were affected in 91% of patients, while other potentially speech-relevant projections were spared. However, comparable to ALS (Urban et al., 1998a) and corticobasal degeneration (Thümler et al., 2003), dysarthria of other etiologies may also be associated with abnormal MEPs to the tongue. Thus, in dysarthria without evidence of signs at other locations, TMS of the tongue may contribute to the detection of lesions and the identification of the underlying pathophysiology of dysarthria.

9. Cerebral Ischemia

The typical MEP pattern after cerebral ischemia is characterized by a reduced amplitude-quotient (MEP/M-wave-ratio) or an absent response during motor cortex stimulation, a raised motor threshold, and a slightly prolonged CCT (Weber and Eisen, 2002). TMS findings in brainstem ischemia have rarely been reported. MEPs to the upper limbs only were examined in the largest reported series of 30 patients in an intensive care unit, including patients with brainstem infarction ($n = 15$), space occupying cerebellar infarction ($n = 5$), brainstem or cerebellar hemorrhage ($n = 6$), brainstem concussion ($n = 2$), encephalitis ($n = 1$), and basilar aneurysm ($n = 1$)

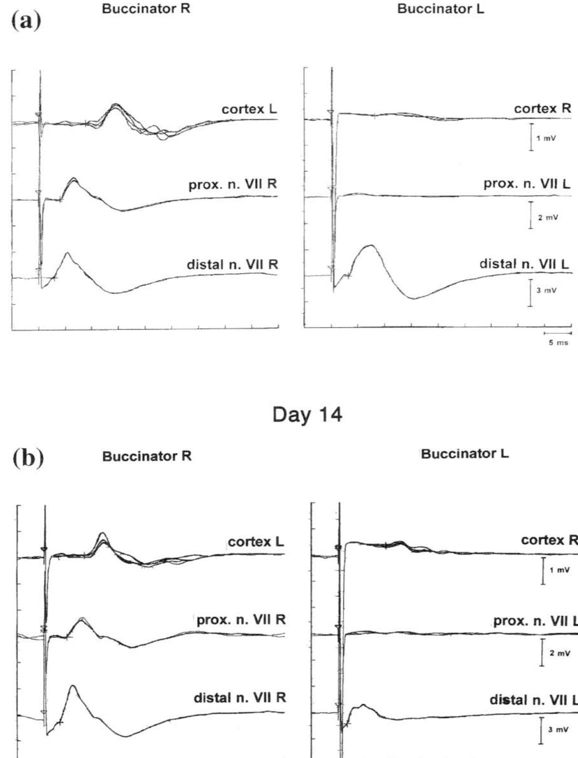

Fig. 9. (a) Bell's palsy of the left side: On day 1, absent CMAP on magnetic stimulation of the proximal facial nerve and amplitude reduction in the buccinator muscle response on stimulation of the right facial motor cortex. (b) Bell's palsy of the left side: On day 14, absent CMAP on magnetic stimulation of the proximal facial nerve and increasing amplitude of the buccinator muscle response on stimulation of the right facial motor cortex. Electrical stimulation of the left distal facial nerve shows amplitude reduction in the CMAP to 30% compared to the unaffected side.

(Schwarz et al., 2000). It has further been shown that an absent response during motor cortex stimulation in the acute stage correlated significantly with a persisting motor deficit 3 months later. Bassetti et al. (1994) reported TMS findings to the upper and lower limbs of six patients with a locked-in syndrome due to bilateral brainstem infarctions. The motor deficit did not improve in the patients with absent responses in the acute stage ($n = 4$), while almost full motor recovery was observed in patients ($n = 2$) where MEPs were obtained from the severely paretic limbs. Ferbert et al. (1992) examined the MEPs to the small hand muscles in 20 patients with hemiparesis due to pontine infarction. TMS was performed in seven patients in the acute stage and in 13 patients in the chronic stage. The authors found a prolonged CMCT in patients with a moderate to severe degree of paresis, while the MEP/M-wave-ratio allowed no differentiation between the paretic and non-paretic side. From these observations it may be concluded that MEPs performed in the acute stage of a brainstem stroke are of a prognostic value regarding the persisting functional motor deficit, comparable to that previously reported for MEPs of other brain regions (Heald et al., 1993; Arac et al., 1994; Turton et al., 1996; Cicinelli et al., 1997; Escudero et al., 1998; Trompetto et al., 2000).

TMS studies may also contribute to localizing lesions within the nervous system. Although TMS enables the identification of the lesion location in the axial plane, it allows only limited conclusions concerning the level at which the lesion is located in the rostro-caudal direction. This is due to the fact that the MEPs fail to show whether the lesion is located within the brainstem or in the supratentorial region. However, if recordings are performed not only from the limbs, but also from cranial nerve innervated muscles (e.g. facial muscles, tongue), the lesion pattern allows some conclusions as to the lesion level, e.g. that the lesion should be located rostral from the uppermost pathological altered segment.

10. Multiple sclerosis

Characteristic TMS findings in patients with multiple sclerosis are prolongation of CMCT, reduced MEP/M-wave ratio, increased variability of onset latency of the MEP (latency jitter), and dispersed morphology of the MEPs on motor cortex stimulation (Weber and Eisen, 2002). Involvement of the corticobulbar projections have also been investigated

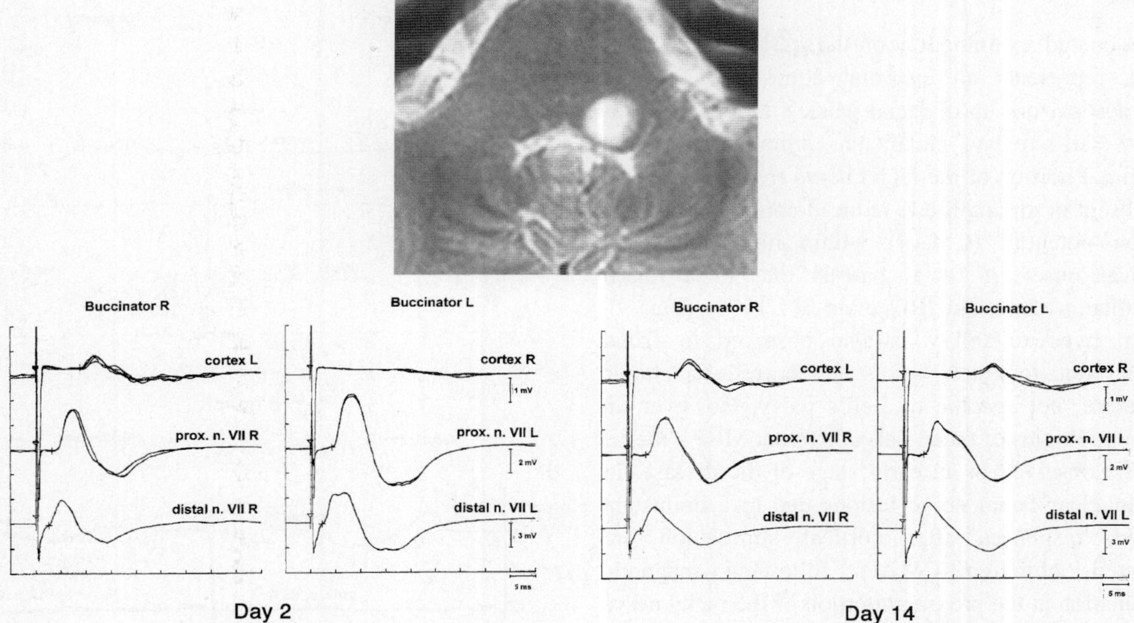

Fig. 10. Multiple sclerosis: MRI showing demyelination in the left dorsolateral pons with peripheral facial palsy on the left side. TMS on day 2 shows no response on cortical stimulation of the right motor cortex and normal peripheral nerve CMAPs, enabling the exclusion of Bell's palsy. Corresponding to the clinical recovery, TMS on day 14 shows a normal motor response following right motor cortex stimulation and no axonal degeneration on peripheral nerve stimulation.

in multiple sclerosis, and demonstrated clinically silent lesions (Fig. 7a, b). However, in 30 patients with known multiple sclerosis, MEPs of the cranial nerve muscles were associated with a lower probability (40%) to disclose clinically silent lesions compared to the upper (67%) and lower (80%) limbs, corresponding to the shorter length of the central projections which may be affected by a demyelinating lesion (Riepe and Ludolph, 1993; Urban et al., 1994).

11. Amyotrophic lateral sclerosis (ALS)

TMS studies to the limbs frequently show a modest prolongation of CMCT, marked MEP/M-wave ratio attenuation and, in some cases, absence of MEPs. It has recently been shown by TMS that corticobulbar tract function to the orofacial muscles (Urban et al., 1998), tongue (Urban et al., 1998a), masseter (Trompetto et al., 1998; Desiato et al., 2002) and trapezius muscle (Truffert et al., 2000) is frequently impaired in the course of ALS (Fig. 8). Because the corticobulbar and corticospinal tracts may be independently involved in ALS (Bonduelle, 1975), the examination of both tracts in the diagnostic work-up is of special value to reveal upper motor neuron involvement (Urban et al., 2001c), and to differentiate ALS from cervical spondylotic myelopathy (Truffert et al., 2000). In a series of 51 consecutive patients with different clinical patterns of ALS, a lesion of the corticolingual projections was observed in 53%, of the corticofacial projections in 47%, and of the corticospinal projections to the upper and lower limbs in 25% and 43% of patients, respectively (Urban et al., 2001c).

12. Facial nerve palsy

Fractionated examination of the corticofacial pathways represents an essential contribution to the diagnostic work-up of facial palsies. Even in incomplete Bell's palsy, canalicular stimulation of the proximal portion of the facial nerve frequently shows an absent or an amplitude reduced compound muscle action potential (CMAP) within hours after the clinical onset of facial paresis due to a raised stimulation threshold (Rösler et al., 1995) (Fig. 9). Local hypoexcitability is also observed in facial palsies due to zoster oticus and borreliosis and is therefore, not specific to Bell's palsy. However, in other etiologies of facial palsy different MEP patterns can be observed in an early stage of the disease. In infranuclear facial nerve lesions due to a brainstem lesion, responses after cortical stimulation are affected, although CMAPs following magnetic stimulation at the proximal portion of the facial nerve are preserved (Urban et al., 1998b) (Fig. 10). In borreliosis or malignant meningeosis, the contralateral facial nerve may also show a subclinical amplitude reduction in the CMAP with magnetic stimulation (Rösler et al., 1995) (Fig. 11). In Guillain–Barré syndrome and hereditary motor and sensory neuropathy type I (Charcot–Marie–Tooth type I) and type III (Déjerine–Sottas), prolonged latencies are observed after cortical stimulation and proximal stimulation of the facial nerve (Rösler et al., 1995, Glocker et al., 1999). Thus, the pattern of MEP abnormalities enables conclusions as to both the lesion site and the etiology. Since the local hypoexcitability on canalicular stimulation may persist for months, even after complete clinical recovery from facial palsy, canalicular stimulation has no prognostic value (Glocker et al., 1994), in contrast to supramaximal electrical stimulation 2 weeks after the onset of facial palsy (Esslen 1977).

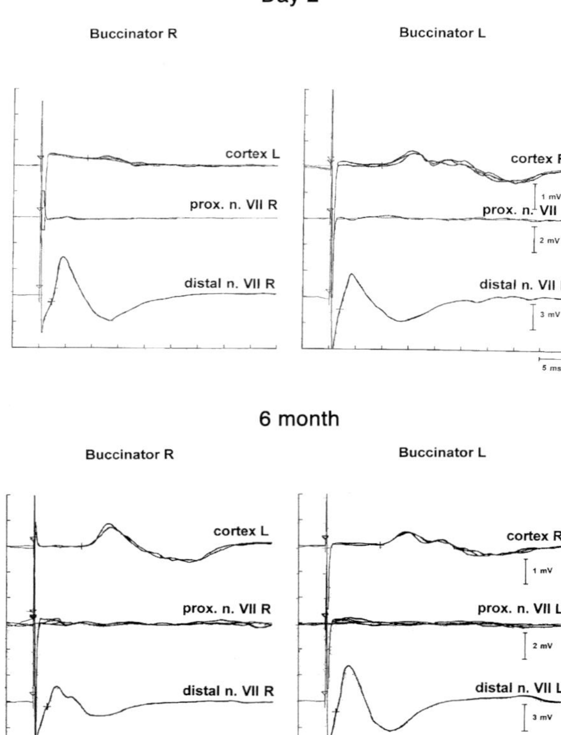

Fig. 11. (a) Borreliosis with facial palsy on the right side. On day 2, bilaterally absent CMAPs on magnetic stimulation of the proximal facial nerve and amplitude reduction of the buccinator muscle response on stimulation of the left facial motor cortex. (b) Borreliosis with facial palsy on the right side. After six months, TMS continues to show bilaterally absent CMAPs on magnetic stimulation of the proximal facial nerve, while the amplitude of the buccinator muscle response on stimulation of the left facial motor cortex is within the normal range. Electrical stimulation of the right distal facial nerve shows amplitude reduction in CMAP to 50% compared to the unaffected side.

13. Hypoglossal nerve palsy

Peripheral hypoglossal nerve palsies occur less frequently compared to facial palsies. In contrast to facial palsies, TMS is less suitable for the electrophysiological assessment of hypoglossal nerve palsies, because magnetic stimulation activates both hypoglossal nerves across the cerebrospinal fluid, and even in the presence of complete unilateral palsy a small volume conducted muscle response from the intact half of the tongue is recorded. However, distal stimulation of the affected hypoglossal nerve leads to an amplitude reduction in the ipsilateral half, reflecting the extent of the axonal degeneration (Chen et al., 1999).

References

Arac, N., Sagduyu, A., Binai, S. and Ertekin, C. Prognostic value of transcranial magnetic stimulation in acute stroke. *Stroke*, 1994, 25: 2183–2186.

Barnes, S. Degenerations in hemiplegia: with special reference to a ventrolateral pyramidal tract, the accessory fillet and Pick's bundle. *Brain*, 1901, 24: 463–501.

Bassetti, C., Mathis, J. and Hess, C.W. Multimodal electrophysiological studies including motor evoked potentials in patients with locked-in syndrome: report of six patients. *J. Neurol. Neurosurg. Psychiatry*, 1994, 57: 1403–1406.

Berardelli, A., Priori, A., Inghilleri, M., Cruccu, G., Mercuri, B. and Manfredi, M. Corticobulbar and corticospinal projections to neck muscle and motoneurons in man. *Exp. Brain Res.*, 1991, 87: 402–406.

Bonduelle, M. Amyotrophic lateral sclerosis. In: P.J. Vinken and G.W. Bruyn (Eds) *Handbook of clinical neurology.* Vol. 22. North Holland Publishing, Amsterdam 1975: 281–338.

Chen, C.H., Wu, T. and Chu, N.S. Bilateral cortical representation of the intrinsic lingual muscles. *Neurology* 1999, 52: 411–413.

Cicinelli, P., Traversa., R. and Rossini, P.M. Post-stroke reorganization of brain motor output to the hand: a 2–4 month follow-up with focal magnetic transcranial stimulation. *Electroenceph. Clin. Neurophysiol.*, 1997, 105: 438–450.

Cruccu, G., Berardelli, A., Inghilleri, M. and Manfredi, M. Functional organization of the trigeminal motor system in man. *Brain*, 1989, 112: 1333–1350.

Desiato, M.T., Bernardi, G., Hagi, A., Boffa, L. and Caramia, M.D. Transcranial magnetic stimulation of motor pathways directed to muscles supplied by cranial nerves in amyotrophic lateral sclerosis. *Clin. Neurophysiol.*, 2002, 113: 132–140.

DeToledo, J.C. and Dow, R. Sternomastoid function during hemispheric suppression by amytal: insights into the inputs to the spinal accessory nerve nucleus. *Mov Disord*, 1998, 13: 809–812.

Escudero, J.V., Sancho, J., Bautista, D., Escudero, M. and Lopez-Trigo, J. Prognostic value of motor evoked potential obtained by transcranial magnetic brain stimulation in motor function recovery in patients with acute ischemic stroke. *Stroke*, 1998, 29: 1854–1859.

Esslen, E. (Ed.). The acute facial palsies. Springer, Berlin 1977.

Ferbert, A., Vielhaber. S., Meincke, U. and Buchner, H. Transcranial magnetic stimulation in pontine infarction: correlation to degree of paresis. *J. Neurol. Neurosurg. Psychiatry*, 1992, 55: 294–299.

Gandevia, S.C. and Applegate, C. Activation of neck muscles from the human motor cortex. *Brain*, 1988, 111: 801–813.

Glocker, F.X., Magistris, M.R., Rösler, K.M. and Hess, C.W. Magnetic transcranial and electrical stylomastoidal stimulation of the facial motor pathways in Bell's palsy: time course and relevance of electrophysiological parameters. *Electroenceph. Clin. Neurophysiol.*, 1994, 93: 113–120.

Glocker, F.X., Rösler, K.M., Linden, D., Heinen, F., Hess, C.W. and Lücking, C.H. Facial nerve dysfunction in hereditary motor and sensory neuropathy type I and III. *Muscle Nerve*, 1999, 22: 1201–1208.

Gooden, B.R., Ridding, M.C., Miles, T.S., Nordstrom, M.A. and Thompson, P.D. Bilateral cortical control of the human anterior digastric muscles. *Exp Brain Res*, 1999, 129: 582–591.

Guggisberg, A.G., Dubach, P., Hess, C.W., Wüthrich, C. and Mathis, J. Motor evoked potentials from the masseter muscle induced by transcranial magnetic stimulation of the pyramidal tract: the importance of coil orientation. *Clin. Neurophysiol.*, 2001, 112: 2312–2319.

Heald, A., Bates, D., Cartlidge, N.E., French, J.M. and Miller, S. Longitudinal study of central motor conduction time following stroke. 1. Natural history of central motor conduction. *Brain*, 1993, 116: 1355–1370.

Hoche, A. Beiträge zur Anatomie der Pyramidenbahn und der oberen Schleife, nebst Bemerkungen über die abnormen Bündel in Pons und Medulla oblongata. *Arch. Psychiat. Nervkrankh.*, 1898, 30: 103–139.

Kobayashi, M. and Pascual-Leone, A. Transcranial magnetic stimulation in neurology. *Lancet Neurology*, 2003, 2: 145–156.

Kobayashi, M., Ohira, T., Ochiai, M., Mihara, B. and Kaease, T. Transcranial magnetic stimulation of the central and peripheral motor pathways to the lingual muscles in cat. *Clin. Neurophysiol.*, 1999, 110: 445–448.

Meyer, B.U., Werhahn, K., Rothwell, J.C., Roericht, S. and Fauth, C. Functional organisation of corticonuclear pathways to motoneurones of lower facial muscles in man. *Exp. Brain Res.*, 1994, 101: 465–472.

Meyer, B.U., Liebsch, R. and Röricht, S. Tongue motor responses following transcranial magnetic stimulation of the motor cortex and proximal hypoglossal nerve in man. *Electroenceph. Clin. Neurophysiol.*, 1997, 105: 15–23.

Morecraft, R.J., Louie, J.L., Herrick, J.L. and Stilwell-Morecraft, K.S. Cortical innervation of the facial nucleus in the non-human primate: a new interpretation of the effects of stroke and related subtotal brain trauma on the muscles of facial expression. *Brain*, 2001, 124: 176–208.

Muellbacher, W., Mathis. J. and Hess CW. Electrophysiological assessment of central and peripheral motor routes to the lingual muscles. *J. Neurol. Neurosurg. Psychiatry*, 1994, 57: 309–315.

Muellbacher, W., Artner, C. and Mamoli, B. Motor evoked potentials in unilateral lingual paralysis after monohemispheric ischemia. *J. Neurol. Neurosurg. Psychiatry*, 1998, 65: 755–761.

Odergren, T. and Rimpiläinen, I. Activation and suppression of the sternocleidomastoid muscle induced by transcranial magnetic stimulation. *Electroenceph. Clin. Neurophysiol.*, 1996, 101: 175–180.

Petrera, J.E. and Trojaborg, W. Conduction studies along the accessory nerve and follow-up of patients with trapezius palsy. *J. Neurol. Neurosurg. Psychiatry*, 1984, 47: 630–636.

Priori, A., Berardelli. A., Inghilleri. M., Crucco, G., Zaccagnini, M. and Manfredi, M. Electrical and magnetic stimulation of the accessory nerve at the base of the skull. *Muscle Nerve*, 1991, 14: 477–478.

Redmond, M.D. and Di Benedetto, M. Hypoglossal nerve conduction in normal subjects. *Muscle Nerve*, 1988, 11: 447–452.

Riepe, M. and Ludolph. A.C. Untersuchungen kortikobulbärer Bahnen und peripherer Hirnnerven bei Normalpersonen und Patienten mit multipler Sklerose: Ergebnisse nach nichtinvasiver elektromagnetischer Reizung. *Z EEG-EMG*, 1993, 24: 269–273.

Rösler, K.M., Hess. C.W. and Schmid, U.D. Investigation of facial motor pathways by electrical and magnetic stimulation: sites and mechanisms of excitation. *J. Neurol. Neurosurg. Psychiatry*, 1989, 52: 1149–1156.

Rösler, K.M., Magistris, M.R., Glocker, F.X., Kohler, A., Deuschl, G. and Hess, C.W. Electrophysiological characteristics of lesions in facial palsies of different etiologies. A study using electrical and magnetic stimulation techniques. *Electroenceph. Clin. Neurophysiol.*, 1995, 97: 355–368.

Rossini, P.M. and Rossi. S. Clinical applications of motor evoked potentials. *Electroenceph. Clin. Neurophysiol.*, 1998, 106: 180–194.

Rossini, P.M., Barker, A.T., Berardelli, A., Caramia, M.D., Caruso, G., Cracco, R.Q., Dimitrijevic, M.R., Hallett, M., Katayama. Y., Lücking, C.H., Maertens de Noordhout, A.L., Marsden, C.D., Murray, N.M.F., Rothwell, J.C., Swash, M. and Tomberg, C. Non-invasive electrical and magnetic stimulation of the brain, spinal cord and roots: basic principles and procedures for routine clinical application. Report of an IFCN committee. *Electroenceph. Clin. Neurophysiol.*, 1994, 91: 79–92.

Rothwell, J.C., Hallett, M., Berardelli, A., Eisen, A., Rossini, P. and Paulus, W. Magnetic stimulation: motor evoked potentials. *Electroenceph. Clin. Neurophysiol.*, 1999 (Suppl.) 52: 97–103.

Schmid, U.D., Møller, A.R. and Schmid, J. Transcranial magnetic stimulation excites the labyrinthine segment of the facial nerve: an intraoperative electrophysiological study in man. *Neurosci. Lett.*, 1991, 124: 273–276.

Schmid, U.D., Møller, A.R. and Schmid, J. Transcranial magnetic stimulation of the trigeminal nerve: intraoperative study on stimulation characteristics in man. *Muscle Nerve*, 1995, 18: 487–494.

Schwarz, S., Hacke, W. and Schwab, S. Magnetic evoked potentials in neurocritical care patients with acute brainstem lesions. *J. Neurol. Sci.*, 2000, 172: 30–37.

Strenge, H. and Jahn. R. Activation and suppression of the trapezius muscle induced by transcranial magnetic stimulation. *Electromyogr. Clin. Neurophysiol.*, 1998, 38: 141–145.

Thompson, M.L., Thickbroom, G.W. and Mastaglia, F.L. Corticomotor representation of the sternocleidomastoid muscle. *Brain*, 1997, 120: 245–255.

Thuemler, B.H., Urban, P.P., Davids, E., Schreckenberger, M., Benz, P., Stoeter, P., Bartenstein, P. and Hopf, H.C. Dysarthria and pathological laughter/crying as presenting symptoms of corticobasal-ganglionic degeneration. *J. Neurol.* (in press).

Trompetto, C., Caponnetto, C., Buccolieri, A., Marchese, R. and Abbruzzese, G. Responses of masseter muscles to transcranial magnetic stimulation in patients with amyotrophic lateral sclerosis. *Electroenceph. Clin. Neurophysiol.* 1998, 109: 309–314.

Trompetto, C., Assini, A., Buccolieri, A., Marchese, R. and Abbruzzese, G. Motor recovery following stroke: a transcranial magnetic stimulation study. *Clin. Neurophysiol.*, 2000, 111: 1860–1867.

Truffert, A., Rösler, K.M. and Magistris, M.R. Amyotrophic lateral sclerosis vs. cervical spondylotic myelopathy: a study using transcranial magnetic stimulation with recordings from the trapezius and limb muscles. *Clin. Neurophysiol.*, 2000, 111: 1031–1038.

Türk, U., Rösler, K.M., Mathis, J., Muellbacher, W. and Hess, C.W. Assessment of motor pathways to masticatory muscles: an examination technique using electrical and magnetic stimulation. *Muscle Nerve*, 1994, 17: 1271–1277.

Turton, A., Wroe, S., Trepte, N., Fraser, C. and Lemon, R.N. Contralateral and ipsilateral EMG responses to transcranial magnetic stimulation during recovery of arm and hand function after stroke. *Electroenceph. Clin. Neurophysiol.*, 1996, 101: 316–328.

Urban, P.P. Vergleichende Untersuchung elektrisch und magnetisch evozierter Potentiale aus unterschiedlichen Fazialis-innervierten Muskeln. *Klin. Neurophysiol.*, 2002a, 33: A27.

Urban, P.P. and Hopf, H.C. Verlauf kortiko-fazialer und kortiko-lingualer Projektionen im Hirnstamm des Menschen. In: J. Bohl (Ed.), *Neuropathology*. Shaker, Aachen 2002b: 1–18

Urban, P.P., Heimgärtner, I. and Hopf, H.C. Transkranielle Stimulation der Zungenmuskulatur bei Gesunden und Patienten mit Encephalomyelitis disseminata. *Z EEG EMG*, 1994, 25: 254–258.

Urban, P.P., Hopf, H.C., Connemann, B., Hundemer, H.P. and Koehler, J. The course of cortico-hypoglossal projections in the human brain-stem. Functional testing using transcranial magnetic stimulation. *Brain*, 1996, 119: 1031–1038.

Urban, P.P., Beer. S. and Hopf, H.C. Cortico-bulbar fibers to orofacial muscles: recordings with enoral surface electrodes. *Electroencephalogr. Clin. Neurophysiol.*, 1997a, 105: 8–14.

Urban, P.P., Hopf, H.C., Fleischer, S., Zorowka, P.G. and Müller-Forell, W. Impaired cortico-bulbar tract function in dysarthria due to hemispheric stroke. *Brain*, 1997b, 120: 1077–1084.

Urban, P.P., Connemann, B., Hundemer, H.P., Koehler, J. and Hopf, H.C. Technical considerations of electromyographic tongue muscle recordings using transcranial magnetic stimulation (letter). *Brain*, 1997c, 120: 1911–1914.

Urban, P.P., Vogt, T. and Hopf, H.C. Corticobulbar tract involvement in amyotrophic lateral sclerosis. A transcranial magnetic stimulation study. *Brain*, 1998a, 121: 1099–1108.

Urban, P.P., Wicht, S., Marx, J., Mitrovic, S., Fitzek, C. and Hopf, H.C. Isolated voluntary facial paresis due to pontine ischemia. *Neurology*, 1998b, 50: 1859–1862.

Urban, P.P., Wicht, S., Fitzek, S., Marx, J., Thömke, F., Fitzek, C. and Hopf, H.C. Ipsilateral facial weakness in upper medullary infarction-supranuclear or infranuclear origin? *J. Neurol.*, 1999a, 246: 798–801.

Urban, P.P., Wicht, S., Hopf, H.C., Fleischer, S. and Nickel, O. Isolated dysarthria due to extracerebellar lacunar stroke: a central monoparesis of the tongue. *J. Neurol. Neurosurg. Psychiatry*, 1999b, 66: 495–501.

Urban, P.P., Wicht, S., Vukurevic, G., Fitzek, C., Stoeter, P., Massinger, C. et al. Dysarthria in ischemic stroke - Localization and etiology. *Neurology*, 2001a, 56: 1021–1027.

Urban, P.P., Wicht, S., Vucorevic, G. et al. The course of corticofacial projections in the human brainstem. *Brain*, 2001b, 124: 1866–1876.

Urban, P.P., Wicht, S. and Hopf, H.C. Sensitivity of transcranial magnetic stimulation of cortico-bulbar vs. cortico-spinal tract involvement in amyotrophic lateral sclerosis (ALS). *J. Neurol.*, 2001c, 248: 850–855.

Weber, M. and, Eisen, A.A. Magnetic stimulation of the central and peripheral nervous system. *Muscle Nerve*, 2002, 25: 160–175.

Yamashita, M. and Yamamoto, T. Aberrant pyramidal tract in the medial lemniscus of the human brainstem: normal distribution and pathologiacl changes. *Eur. Neurol.*, 2001, 45: 75–82.

Transcranial Magnetic Stimulation and Transcranial Direct
Current Stimulation (Supplements to Clinical Neurophysiology, Vol. 56)
Editors: W. Paulus, F. Tergau, M.A. Nitsche, J.C. Rothwell, U. Ziemann, M. Hallett

Chapter 36

Modulation of sensorimotor performances and cognition abilities induced by RPMS: clinical and experimental investigations

Albrecht Struppler,* Bernhard Angerer and Peter Havel

Sensorimotor Integration Research Group, Klinikum Rechts der Isar der TUM, Psychiatrische Klinik, Ismaningerstr. 22, 81675 Munich (Germany)

1. Introduction

Recent studies on healthy subjects demonstrated that somatosensory input due to peripheral nerve stimulation or muscle stretch results in functional changes in corticomotor excitability. Ridding et al. (2000) showed that a prolonged period of peripheral nerve stimulation can induce a lasting increase in corticomotoneuronal excitability concerning the stimulated body parts. The importance of the conjoint activity of somatosensory afferents and intrinsic motor cortical circuits was shown by using low frequency median nerve stimulation paired with transcranial magnetic stimulation. If the effects of these stimuli are synchronous at the level of the motor cortex, this results in a long-lasting increase in the motor evoked potential (MEP) (Stefan et al., 2000). Kaelin-Lang et al. (2002) concluded that electrical ulnar nerve stimulation elicits a focal increase in corticomotoneuronal excitability which outlasts the stimulation period and probably occurs at cortical sites. Active training of fast wrist flexion-extension movements was more effective than passive movements of the same kinematics elicited by a torque motor to activate the contralateral motor cortex as measured by functional magnetic resonance imaging (fMRI) and MEP intensity curves, and to improve motor performance (Lotze et al., 2003).

Earlier studies under normal and pathological conditions showed that the proprioceptive inflow induced by repetitive peripheral magnetic stimulation (RPMS) elicits conditioning effects on various levels of the sensorimotor and cognitive systems (Struppler et al., 1996, 2003a, b). In central paresis morphological and functional investigations revealed that even in adults the sensorimotor cortex retains the capability to adapt to altered afferent input (Merzenich et al., 1983; Sanes et al., 1990; Brasil-Neto et al., 1992; Sadato et al., 1995; Ziemann et al., 1998a, b). The cortical representations of the limbs are neither static nor fixed in structure, but are subject to a permanent, dynamic balance in an extended, redundant and overlapping network of neuronal circuits (Liepert and Weiller, 1999; Cramer and Basting, 2000). Also the mature brain is capable of considerable and partly structural modifications (Dettmers et al., 1996; Weiller and Rijntjes, 1999; Stefan et al., 2000). The adaptation to changes in input or output can occur quickly, first only as a

* Correspondence to: Dr. A. Struppler, Sensorimotor Integration Research Group, Klinikum Rehts der Isar der TUM, Psychiatrische Klinik (7/0), Ismaningerstr. 22, D-81675 Munich, Germany.
Tel: +49 89 4140 6183; Fax: +49 89 4140 4888;
E-mail: struppler@lrz.tum.de (Albrecht Struppler)

functional modulation (Classen et al., 1998), later as a lasting reorganization (Nicolelis et al., 1998). The cellular basis of reorganization is neuronal synaptic plasticity: a change of synaptic effectiveness is caused by classic synaptic transduction and neuromodulation (Binder et al., 1993). These mechanisms can result in activation of already existing, but inactive neuronal pathways (unmasking of pre-existing connections) (Jakobs and Donoghue, 1991). In addition, neuronal sprouting which produces new synapses has to be discussed (Dettmers et al., 1996).

The overall target of our research is to improve the rehabilitation of learned goal-directed hand and finger movements like reaching and grasping following localized brain lesions of vascular or traumatic origin. It is a well-known fact that highly controlled fine skilled motor tasks, especially manipulation and exploration, seldom recover sufficiently. Basically the rehabilitation of these motor tasks has to achieve a reduction of spasticity and a facilitation of voluntary movement activity.

The concept that we employed here is based on the generation of proprioceptive input to the central nervous system (CNS). This input should be virtually the same as the physiological input generated by active movements, in order to activate modulatory and plasticity processes in the CNS.

For the induction of such aproprioceptive input, RPMS proved to be the best stimulation method at present, since even small muscle groups can be activated without any unpleasant sensation. The magnetic field impulses depolarize thick myelinated nerve fibres. RPMS applied to the area of the muscle supplying terminal nerve branches elicits a proprioceptive input to the CNS in two different ways:

- Adequate (indirect) activation of mechanoreceptors (fiber groups Ia, Ib, II) during the rhythmic contraction and relaxation as well as vibration of the muscles.
- Inadequate (direct) activation of sensorimotor nerve fibres with an orthodromic and antidromic conduction.

This afferent input leads to sensations like movement, and vibration, and is conveyed simultaneously to higher CNS levels. However, it should be considered that fibres of the groups III and IV, like nociceptor as well as mechanoreceptor afferents from the skin, may not be activated by RPMS.

In contrast to transcutaneous electrical stimulation, the biologically effective electrical field is considerably lower. This avoids activation of cutaneous receptors, like nociceptors. The spatial field distributions are also different in terms of spreading. The magnetic field depends upon the ion environment and penetrates to deeper regions of the muscle, whereas the current caused by the electrical field will take the way of lowest resistance, thus being largely limited to the surface.

In this chapter, we present an overview of clinical and experimental investigations on normal and pathological conditions. These investigations were designed to gain more insight into the modulatory mechanisms underlying the effects of RPMS on sensorimotor performances and cognitive abilities.

In the following investigations the conditioning RPMS is always applied in an identical manner: RPMS is transcutaneously performed to the area of muscle supplying terminal nerve branches by a conventional stimulation coil (magstim double coil). For every conditioning RPMS single magnetic field impulses at an average amplitude of 1.2 T[1] are applied. After every impulse a break of 3 s is required in order to delay heating of the coil. The field impulses are generated by a self-built stimulator (Schmid, 1992). RPMS frequency (20 Hz) was adopted according to the physiological activation frequency (in the range of 15 Hz to 25 Hz). With this method repetitive contractions and relaxations are induced to the target muscles simultaneously with the sensation of movement, vibration and proprioceptive inflow to the CNS which causes the effects described in the following sections.

2. Spasticity

It is a well-known fact that spasticity independent of the level of origin is one of the major factors for the

[1] $1.2\ T = 12{,}000 \times g$.

patients quality of life and rehabilitation efforts after lesions of the CNS. In order to develop an innovative rehabilitation method by using RPMS, first of all the influence of RPMS on spasticity was investigated in a clinical and experimental study.

Clinical outcome: RPMS caused a reduction of spasticity in 47 out of 52 patients as can be seen in Fig. 1. The depicted results were based on the modified Ashworth-Scale (Bohannon and Smith, 1987). There was no correlation between the reduction of spasticity and the level of lesion, the time interval between the lesion and the first stimulation as well as the age of the patients (Struppler et al., 2003b).

In a clinical experimental investigation of voluntary index finger movements in a group of eight patients who were able to move the index finger of the paretic hand, RPMS resulted in the following effects: index finger extensions could be performed faster, with a larger displacement and at a greater velocity with a rather diminished amount of muscle activity in the flexor and extensor muscles. These effects increased within 2–4 h following RPMS and were still to be observed after 72 h. These findings demonstrate a decrease of spasticity and an increase of voluntary goal-directed movements. However, it cannot be distinguished if these effects are only due to reduced spasticity or due to facilitation of voluntary motor activity at the level of the sensorimotor cortex (Struppler et al., 2003b).

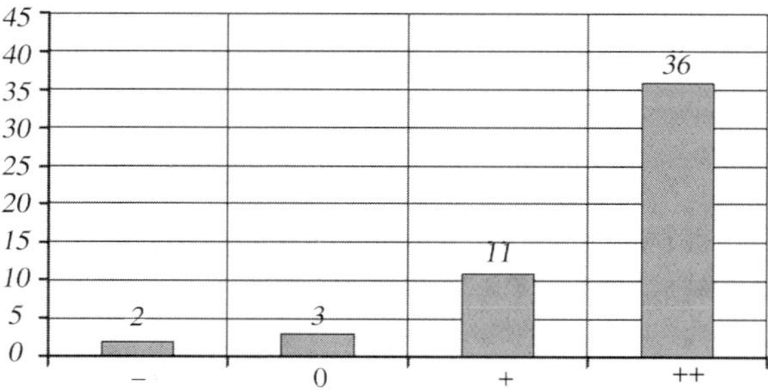

Fig. 1. Effect of RPMS on spasticity: number of patients classified according to outcome on the modified Ashworth-Scale: "–" worsening; "0" no change; "+" improvement of up to minus one Ashworth point; "++" improvement of minus 1.5 and more Ashworth points.

This uncertainty led to a PET study in order to clarify, if RPMS has an influence on cortical level. The study on eight patients showed that areas of the fronto-parietal circuits are activated after RPMS performed to the upper extremity (Spiegel et al., 2000). These findings strongly suggest that not only transient spinal mechanisms are responsible for the improvement of voluntary motor tasks but also cortical neuroplasticity. Therefore, it is assumed that RPMS primarily facilitates the well-known parieto-frontal neuronal circuits involved in goal-directed controlled movements (for review see Binkofski et al., 1999; Seitz et al., 2000).

3. Gripping task and grasping trajectory

Clinical observations showed that disturbed goal-directed motor performances, like reaching and grasping, can be improved also by an increase in the regularity of the movement trajectory as a result of RPMS. This finding was associated an improvement of gripping tasks.

A pilot study on gripping tasks was performed to establish, if voluntarily intended motor tasks can be improved independently of the concomitant spasticity.

For the data registration of the displacement, the electromyogram (EMG) and the gripping force a special registration set-up was developed. This set-up contains a video-device[2] and a data acquisition device[3] which are coordinated by an especially developed software based on a real-time operating system.[4] The principle arrangement of this registration set-up is depicted in Fig. 2. The set-up is capable of up to 20 pictures per second and 5 k samples of EMG and gripping force per second.

The main advantage of this set-up is the time correlation between the EMG, the gripping force and the video. This means, that each EMG sample is combined with a picture of the video sequence.

An additional advantage is the clinical evaluation of the effects of the RPMS since the video sequence

[2] Logitech QuickCam 3000 pro.
[3] National Instruments NI 6023 E.
[4] RTAI Linux 24.1.7 Linux-Kernel 2.4.16.

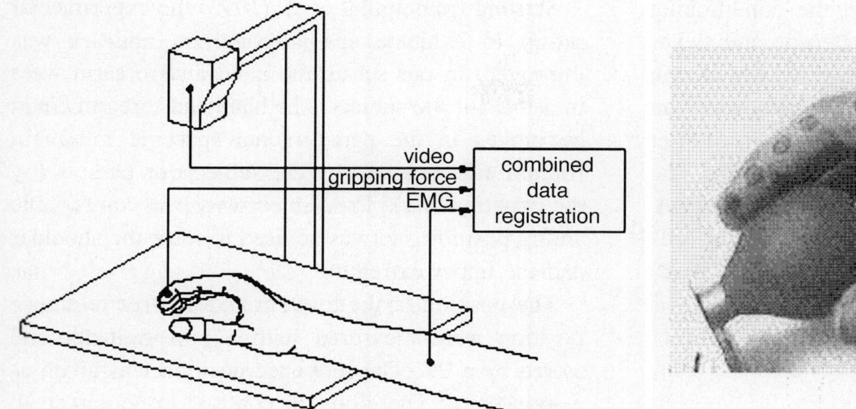

Fig. 2. Schematic arrangement and sample picture of the coordinated video, gripping force and EMG data registration. The rubber ball is filled with water and connected to a pressure sensor for gripping force measurement.

can be repeated in original speed and in slow motion. The patients index finger is marked with (blue) points as can be seen on the right side of Fig. 2. Therefore, it is possible to extract the index finger displacement based on the idea of a blue-box.

A detailed evaluation of the algorithms for this information extraction has been developed by Weber (2002).

Since, so far, only a pilot study was conducted, only the video stream was evaluated clinically. The complete study including all measurements (displacement, EMG and gripping force) is currently in preparation. The ten patients were asked to grip (and hold for a few seconds) the rubber ball depicted in Fig. 2. This task is clinically evaluated by five independent judging physiotherapists before and after RPMS performed to the finger and hand extensor or flexor muscles respectively. Hence each conditioning RPMS is described by 50 points (10 patients × 5 evaluators) distributed to the evaluation-classes "worsening", "no effect" and "improvement". The results of this evaluation can be seen in Fig. 3. If these results are summarized, it may be assumed that the voluntary gripping task can be obviously improved even if the RPMS is applied to the flexor or the extensor muscles as well as independent of the cause of the underlying spasticity.

In addition, the regularity of a reaching task was judged by the same method. Therefore, nine patients were asked to reach a given target (rubber ball). This

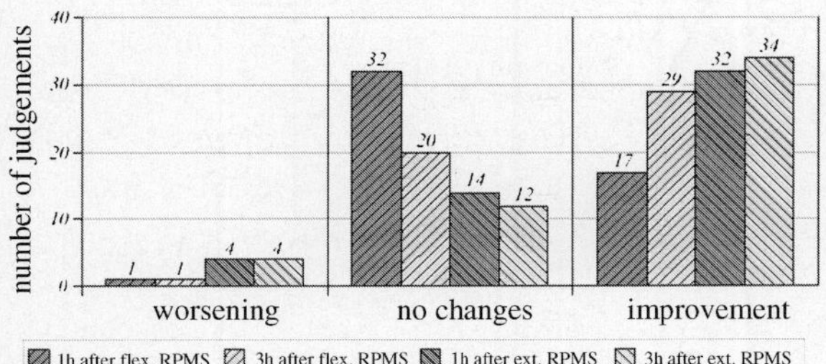

Fig. 3. Results of the clinical evaluation of the gripping task – evaluated is the degree of coordination of the compound movement (i.e. first and second finger).

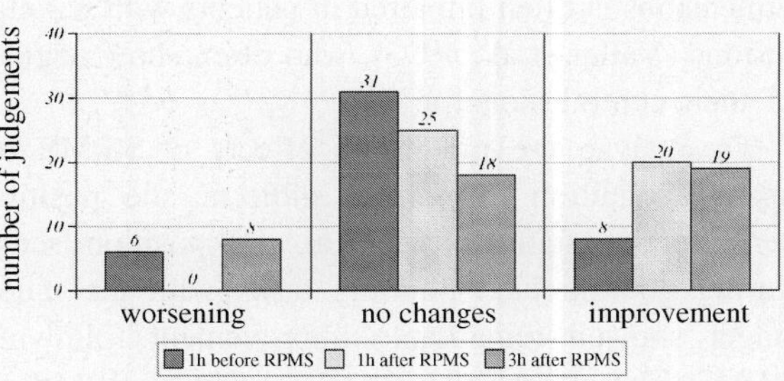

Fig. 4. Results of the clinical evaluation of the reaching task – evaluated is the accuracy of the reaching trajectory.

was carried out before, and after, the conditioning RPMS of the finger and hand extensor and flexor muscles. The results of this evaluation are depicted in Fig. 4. According to our clinical dexterity-score an improvement of the reaching task was observed after RPMS was applied. Of note, the number of "no changes" decreased dramatically after RPMS in comparison to the evaluation before RPMS (see Fig. 4).

4. Cognition

4.1. Perception cognition

Besides the improvement of motor performances, an improvement of cognitive functions was observed clinically in many patients. To investigate the influence of RPMS on a pure cognition ability, the effect of RPMS on local tactile extinction in patients after right sided brain lesions was analyzed. For quantification of the perception of different tactile stimuli, using the model of local tactile extinction was investigated. This is defined as the inability to attend to a stimulus on the affected side when simultaneously a stimulus is applied to the unaffected side. We found that RPMS clearly reduced the number of recognition errors (Heldmann et al., 2000).

4.2. Spatial cognition (position sense/body scheme)

The results of our PET study (Spiegel et al., 2000) together with the findings of Wolpert et al. (1998), Vallar et al. (1999), Cabeza and Nyberg (2000), led to an investigation of special cognitive abilities. Postural control of arm position in the three spatial dimensions is often impaired in patients with parietal lesions (Vallar et al., 1993), who often show neglect of their contralesional arm.

To analyze the modifying effects of RPMS on spatial cognition in normal subjects, the position sense under static as well as the position sense during goal-directed pointing tasks with the index finger showed remarkable improvement following RPMS. The effects of a single session of RPMS on 12 healthy subjects (ages from 21–44, all dominant right-handed) were studied.

Starting from Vallar et al. (1993) the experimental set-up to evaluate spatial cognition abilities was improved. In our set-up the hand and forearm were invisible for the subject. The hand and forearm could be moved in the peri-personal space at minimum friction either active (by the subject) or passive (by the experimenter). The subject was in a comfortable sitting position and was advised to relax the shoulder and the upper extremity.

The position of the forearm and the free reference position were measured with a potentiometer and stored by a PC. The reference position was given as a light-point. Therefore, in contrast to Vallar et al. (1993) – the direction of the reference was invisible for the subject. The mechanical arrangement is depicted in Fig. 5.

In the first task the subject was asked to localize the right index finger (positioned very slowly by the experimenter) by placing the reference point above the index finger tip.

In the second task the subject was asked to place actively the invisible index finger tip under the reference point given by the experimenter.

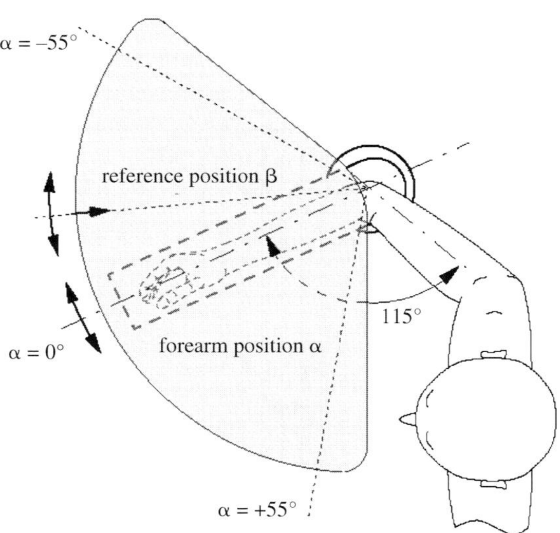

Fig. 5. Mechanical arrangement and definition of the reference for the position α of the hand; the figure shows the subject in a comfortable sitting position with the forearm hidden by a rounded table.

These two tasks were recorded at four different angular positions on a total of 20 trials in each condition (hence five trials in each spatial position). After a first baseline test of position sense the subject received a single session of RPMS on the dorsal palm of the right hand. The second test of position sense was conducted 45 min post stimulation, and a late post-test was performed 120 min after the end of RPMS.

Three weeks after the first experiment all 12 subjects were retested in the same experiment. However, in this experiment RPMS was applied to the left hand, while position sense was tested again on the right hand as in the first experimental session. Statistical evaluation showed a significant reduction of the angular deviation in position sense from the baseline (pre) to the early post-test 45 min after RPMS to the right hand ($p > 0.007$; see Fig. 6). The late post-test did not differ significantly from the baseline ($p > 0.05$). No significant effect was obtained in the position sense of the right arm when RPMS was applied to the left arm ($p > 0.05$; see Fig. 6).[5]

In summary, the results of this pilot study clearly show that RPMS applied to the arm significantly improves the arm position sense in the stimulated arm whereas it has no effect on arm position in the non stimulated arm. The time course of this improvement ranges up to 45 min after cessation of stimulation and thus produces a clear after-effect. However, this effect is no longer evident two hours after stimulation. This indicates that sensory inflow via RPMS improves temporarily postural control for the stimulated arm by lowering the threshold by some 30%. This improvement is not due to mere test repetition or learning of the task as no such effects were obtained when the non-stimulated arm was tested (left-sided RPMS, see Fig. 6). In conclusion, the data indicates that somatosensory inflow updates postural arm control in healthy subjects. Following these promising results, it is currently being tested as to whether RPMS can also be used for rehabilitative purposes in patients with neglect from parietal lesions who often show impaired postural control, extinction and body neglect (Kerkhoff, 2003).

5. Joint stabilization – postural component of motor performance

The effect of RPMS on the postural component of goal-directed motor performances of 13 healthy subjects was investigated. This study was also undertaken to clarify if RPMS modifies skeletal muscle intrinsic factors like visco elasticity or if it operates purely on the central, i.e. cortical level.

[5] With respect to Maike Kiehl for the data recordings.

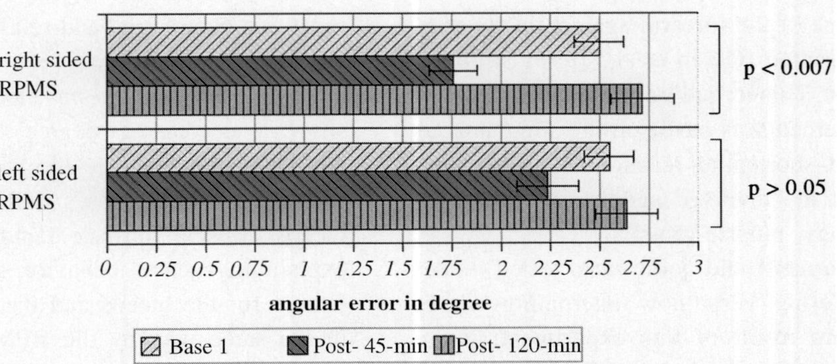

Fig. 6. Effect of RPMS performed to the right arm (right sided RPMS) on position sense (2D; 12 healthy subjects). Note the significant reduction of the angular error in the stimulated arm (RPMS, $p < 0.006$) whereas no effect occurs when RPMS is performed to the opposite arm (left-sided RPMS).

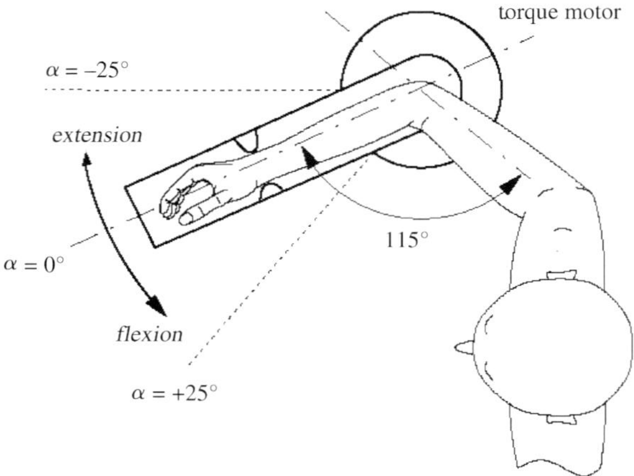

Fig. 7. Mechanical arrangement and definition of the reference for the position of the TM; the figure shows the subject in a comfortable sitting position; the forearm is fixed at the lever of the torque motor.

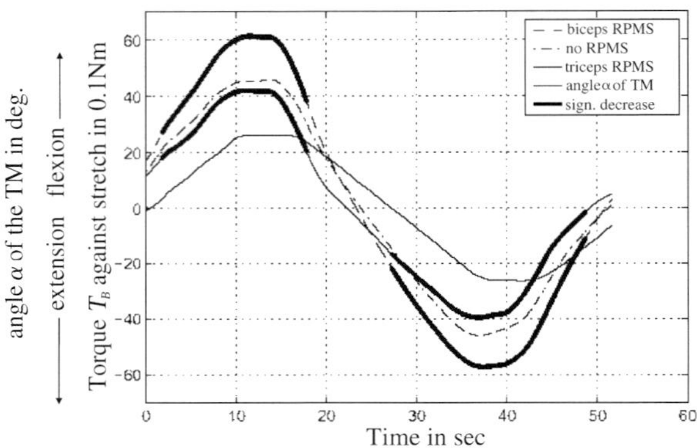

Fig. 8. Significant descrease ($p < 0.05$) of the stabilization of the elbow joint after RPMS performed to the triceps in comparison to the stabilization of the elbow joint after RPMS performed to the biceps; the dash-dotted line corresponds to the reference group with no RMPS intervention.

The schematic mechanical arrangement depicted in Fig. 7 shows the subject in a comfortable sitting position. The subject was advised to relax the shoulder and the upper extremity.

To evaluate the resistance against very slow alternating movements a torque motor (TM) was used. This TM is controlled by a closed-loop position control to impose slow alternating movements to the subject's forearm. The reference of the TM is equivalent to a relaxed position of the forearm, which is approximately 115° at the elbow joint.

For evaluation purposes, the angle of the TM as well as the torque of the forearm against the lever of the TM are measured (Given et al., 1995; Struppler and Jakob, 1995). This torque (resistance against slow alternating movements) is based on the simultaneous lengthening and shortening reactions (stiffness and muscle tone) of the involved agonistic and antagonistic, respectively, muscle groups.

The torque around the joint was tested under relaxed state during very slow alternating movements. The main result of this experiment was a correspondence between the stabilization of the elbow joint (resistance against very slow movements) and the conditioning RPMS. RPMS performed on the biceps (flexor muscles) induced a higher resistance whereas RPMS applied to the triceps (extensor muscles) caused a decrease of the resistance around the elbow joint as depicted in Fig. 8. This is a reciprocal coherence between location of the conditioning RPMS on one side and the stabilization of the elbow joint on the other side (Struppler et al., 2003a).

6. Discussion

Skeletal Muscle intrinsic factors like viscosity and elasticity could be directly modified via induced repetitive contraction and relaxation of the *extrafusal skeletal muscle fibres*.

The investigations on elbow joint stabilization show a decreasing degree of stabilization when RPMS is performed to the triceps while the degree of stabilization increases if RPMS is applied to the biceps. Muscle intrinsic factors are not capable of explaining such a behavior since muscle intrinsic factors for the biceps and the triceps are influenced in the same way by the RPMS. Therefore, muscle intrinsic factors can be excluded from the stabilization of the elbow joint, while the effects depending on neuronal activity (skeletal muscle tone) must be taken into account.

The repetitive induced movements might modify the thixotropic behavior of the **mechanoreceptor** bearing *intrafusal muscle fibers* due to after-effects of repetitive stretch and/or contractions (Hagbarth et al., 1995; Jahnke et al., 1989). However, since the conditioning effect is long lasting and independent of intermediate movements it seems that neuromodulaton on the CNS (intraneuronal) level must be involved.

Direct effects of the induced movements on the extrafusal skeletal muscle fibres seems to be excluded by the data. Therefore, the effects on neuronal commands should be considered. The RPMS induced proprioceptive inflow has modifying effects on spinal, supraspinal and cortical level as described in the introduction.

Spasticity can always be suppressed by RPMS independent of its level of origin (Ashworth scale). In a clinical experimental investigation with spastic paresis of finger and hand extensor muscles, a dramatic decrease of spasticity and an increase of voluntary movements was demonstrated (Struppler et al., 2003b). The improvement of spasticity is eventually elicited at the spinal level independent of where and which reflex controlling systems are lesioned. This also explains the decrease of spasticity in lower extremity in paraplegia following spinal cord lesion (Krause and Straube, 2003).

Concerning the experiments on voluntary finger extension in spastic paresis (Struppler et al., 1996) the well-known reciprocal effect of the Ia-afferents on spinal (premotoneural) level have to be taken into account. In RPMS, the autogenetic inhibition by the inhibitory Ib neuronal system has to be considered (Jankowska and Lundberg, 1981). These mechanisms are thought to be responsible for the decrease of spasticity in distal hand muscles due to passive finger and hand extensions in physiotherapy (Hummelsheim and Mauritz, 1993). Antidromically induced activation of α-motoneurons may cause a recurrent inhibition (Renshaw inhibition). However, it is not yet known if this mechanism plays a role for hand and finger movements in humans. Inhibitory systems of the brainstem can be activated if the proprioceptive input (e.g. via spinocerebellar systems) is fairly intact. It is assumed that the reduction of spasticity may additionally occur through an activation of descending inhibitory pathways except in paraplegia. A neuromodulator, which may be responsible for the reduction of spasticity on spinal level, can probably belong to the GABA-ergic system (Ziemann et al., 2001).

Concerning the improvement of **voluntary** (i.e. **goal-directed) movements** – besides the decrease of spasticity – an improvement at the level of cortical sensorimotor integration has to be considered. The underlying motor program activates the desired components of the synergic muscle groups in order to perform a selective and regular goal-directed movement.

The presented clinical pilot studies concerning gripping and reaching tasks may partially be explained by the inhibition of coactivation. However, for a more accurate explanation, the underlying muscle activity has to be recorded in a detailed study including a control group.

Postural component. According to our paradigm, the role of the static component of muscle-spindles (group Ia- and II-afferents) for static (slow kinetic) conditions have to be considered. Prochazka showed that group II-afferents follow muscle length changes even more clearly than Ia-afferents, especially during imposed movements (Prochazka and Gorassini, 1998; Prochazka et al., 2002).

Concerning the functional relevance of the elbow joint stabilization, it has to be considered that forearm flexor and extensor muscles are facilitated or inhibited concomitantly depending on the location of the conditioning RPMS. This means that RPMS modulates the stabilization of the elbow joint most likely on the cortical level, corresponding adequately to the planed motor tasks:

- Preceding motor tasks like manipulation, pointing, grasping (postural component in forearm and shoulder) a stabilization of the elbow joint is necessary.
- Preceding goal-directed movements (kinetic component) the stabilization of the joint has to be decreased in order to facilitate the movements.

Increased stabilization may also ameliorate the spatial cognition of the limb due to increased proprioceptive afferent inflow especially from the group II afferents which are responsible for the tonic component.

For the **perceptual-cognitive component** it has to be considered that the movements induced by RPMS are found to be very similar to self-induced movements, than electrically or passively induced movements. The neuromodulatory effect of the RPMS is highly dependent on the function of the activated afferent neuronal systems, like lemniscal and extra-lemniscal systems. This leads to the question, if the improvement of sensorimotor performances by RPMS is primarily due to an improvement of cognitive functions like planning, preparing and initiation of a motor program?

A PET-study (Spiegel et al., 2000) shows an activation of parietal areas following RPMS. These areas are strongly involved in cognitive functions. This activation indicates an facilitatory effect of RPMS also on cognitive functions. This correlates with the improvement of spatial cognition caused by RPMS, which is clear evidence that modulatory effects elicited by RPMS take place at the level of an associative cortex i.e. the superior parietal areas.

7. Summary and conclusion

The investigations presented in this chapter lead to the conclusion that proprioceptive afferent inflow to the CNS induced by RPMS elicits various modulatory effects in sensorimotor and cognitive systems. Since the build-up of the conditioning effects is delayed and the effects itself are long-lasting, it has to be assumed that these effects are caused via neuromodulators. Therefore, the presented approach is promising to improve sensorimotor and congnitive disturbances after lesions in the CNS, e.g. after a stroke, by facilitation of reorganization.

Acknowledgements

This work was supported by the "Deutsche Forschungsgemeinschaft (DFG)" Str 11/33-1 and Ko 2111/2-1 in cooperation with the Institute for Electrical Drive Systems, Prof. Dr.-Ing. Dr.-Ing. h. c. D. Schröder. We would like to thank Barbara Gebhard and Renate Gobitz-Pfeifer for their technical assistance.

References

Binder, M., Heckman, C. and Powers, R. How different afferent inputs control motoneuron discharge and the output of the motoneuron pool. *Current Opinion of Neurobiology*, 1993, 3(6): 1028–1034.

Binkofski, F., Buccin, G., Posse, S., Seitz, R., Rizzolatti, G. and Freund, H. A fronto-parietal circuit for object manipulation in man: evidence from an fMRI-study. *Europ. J. Neurosci.*, 1999, 11(9): 3276–3286.

Bohannon, R. and Smith, M. Interrater reliability of a modified ashworth scale of muscle spasticity. *Physical Therapy*, 1987, 67(2): 206–207.

Brasil-Neto, J., Cohen, L., Pascual-Leone, A., Jabir, F., Wall, R. and Hallett, M. Rapid reversible modulation of human motor outputs after transient deaf-ferentation of the forearm: a study with transcranial magnetic stimulation. *Neurology*, 1992, 42(7): 1302–1306.

Cabeza, R. and Nyberg, L. Imaging cognition II: An empirical review of 275 PET and fMRI studies. *J. Cognitive Neurosci.*, 2000, 12(1): 1–47.

Classen, J., Liepert, J., Wise, S., Hallett, M. and Cohen, L. Rapid plasticity of human cortical movement representation induced by practice. *J. Neurophysiol.*, 1998, 79(2): 1117–1123.

Cramer, S. and Basting, E. (2000). Mapping clinically relevant plasticity after stroke. *Neuropharmacology*, 39(5): 842–851.

Dettmers, C., Stephan, K., Rijntjes, M. and Fink, G. Reorganisation des motorischen kortikalen Systems nach zentraler oder peripherer Schädigung. *Neurologie and Rehabilitation*, 1996, 3: 137–148.

Given, J., Dewald, J. and Rymer, W. Joint dependent passive stiffness in paretic and contralateral limbs of spastic patients with hemiparetic stroke. *J. Neurol., Neurosurg., Psychiat.*, 1995, 59(3): 271–279.

Hagbarth, K., Nordin, M. and Bongiovanni, L. After-effects on stiffness and stretch reflexes of human finger flexor muscles attributed to muscle thixotropy. *J. Physiol.*, 1995, 482(1): 215–223.

Heldmann, B., Kerkhoff, G., Struppler, A., Havel, P. and Jahn, T. Repetitive peripheral magnetic stimulation alleviates tactile extinction. *NeuroReport*, 2000, 11(14): 3193–3198.

Hummelsheim, H. and Mauritz, K. Spasticity: *Mechanisms and Management*. Springer-Verlag, Heidelberg, Ch. Neurophysiological mechanisms of spasticity modification by physiotherapy, 1993: 426–438.

Jahnke, M., Proske, U. and Struppler, A. Measurements of muscle stiffness, the electromyogram and activity in single muscle spindles of human flexor muscles following conditioning by passive stretch or contraction. *Brain Res.*, 1989, 493: 103–112.

Jakobs, K. and Donoghue, J. Reshaping the cortical motor map by unmasking latent intracortical connections. *Science*, 1991, 251: 944–947.

Jankowska, E. and Lundberg, A. Interneurons in the spinal cord. *Trends in Neuroscience*, 1981, 4: 230–233.

Kaelin-Lang, A., Luft, A., Sawaki, L., Burstein, A., Sohn, Y. and Cohen, L. Modulation of human corticomotor excitability by somatosensory input. *J. Physiol.*, 2002, 540(2): 623–633.

Kerkhoff, G. *Neural Control of Space Coding and Action Production*. Vol. 142 of Progress in Brain Research. Elsevier Science BV, Amsterdam, Ch. 16: Modulation and rehabilitation of spatial neglect by sensory stimulation, 2003: 257–271.

Krause, P. and Straube, T. E. A. Lumbar repetitive magnetic stimulation reduces spastic tone increase of the lower limbs. submitted to "Spinal Cord" Department of Neurology, University of Munich, Klinikum Grosshadern, Munich, Germany 2003.

Liepert, J. and Weiller, C. Mapping plastic brain changes after acute lesions. *Current Opinion in Neurology*, 1999, 12(6): 709–713.

Lotze, M., Braun, C., Birbaumer, N., Anders, S. and Cohen, L. Motor learning elicited by voluntary drive. *Brain*, 2003, 126(4): 866–872.

Merzenich, M., Kaas, J., Wall, J., Nelson, R., Sur, M. and Felleman, D. Topographic reorganization of somatosensory cortical areas 3b and 1 in adult monkeys following restricted deafferentation. *Neuroscience*, 1983, 8(1): 33–55.

Nicolelis, M., Katz, D. and Krupa, D. Potential circuit mechanisms underlying concurrent thalamic and cortical plasticity. *Reviews in the Neurosciences*, 1998, 9(3): 213–224.

Prochazka, A. and Gorassini, M. Models of ensemble firing of muscle spindle afferents recorded during normal locomotion in cats. *J. Physiol.*, 1998, 507(1): 277–291.

Prochazka, A., Gritsenko, V. and Yakovenko, S. *Sensorimotor Control of Movement and Posture*. Vol. 508 of Advances in Experimental Medicine and Biology. Kluwer Academic/Plenum Publishers, London, New York, Ch. 41: Sensory Control of Locomotion: Reflexes vs. higher-level control, 2002: 357–367.

Ridding, M., Brouwer, B., Miles, T., Pitcher, J. and Thompson, P. Changes in muscle responses to stimulation of the motor cortex induced by peripheral nerve stimulation in human subjects. *Exp. Brain Res.*, 2000, 131(1): 135–143.

Sadato, N., Zeffiro, T., Campbell, G., Konishi, J., Shibasaki, H. and Hallett, M. Regional cerebral blood flow changes in motor cortical areas after transient anesthesia of the forearm. *Ann. Neurol.*, 1995, 37(1): 74–81.

Sanes, J., Suner, S. and Donoghue, J. Dynamic organization of primary motor cortex output to target muscles in adult rats. I. Long-term patterns of reorganization following motor or mixed peripheral nerve lesions. *Exp. Brain Res.*, 1990, 79(3): 479–491.

Schmid, M. Entwicklung und Bau einer Speisequelle mit verstärkter Leistung zur Nervenstimulation mittels zeitlich veränderlicher Magnetfelder. Diplomarbeit, Lst. für elektrische Maschinen und Geräte, Technische Universität München, Munich, May 1992.

Seitz, R., Stephan, K. and Binkofski, F. Control of action as mediated by the human frontal lobe. *Exp. Brain Res.*, 2000, 133(1): 71–80.

Spiegel, S., Bartenstein, P., Struppler, A., Havel, P., Drzezga, A. and Schwaiger, M. Zentrale Bewegungsverarbeitung bei spastisch-paretischen Patienten nach repetitiver peripherer Magnetstimulation (RPMS): Eine PET – Studie mit H_2O – 15. Nuklearmedizin 2000, 39: 37–55.

Stefan, K., Ans L.G., Cohen, E.K., Benecke, R. and Classen, J. Induction of plasticity in the human motor cortex by paired associative stimulation. *Brain* 2000, 123(3): 572–584.

Struppler, A. and Jakob, C. *Instrumental Methods and Scoring in Extrapyramidal disorders*. Springer-Verlag, Berlin, Heidelberg, Ch. 2. Measurement of Muscle Tone – Demarcation between Spasticity and Rigidity, 1995: 56–70.

Struppler, A., Jakob, C., Müller-Barna, P., Schmid, M., Lorenzen, H.-W., Prosiegel, M. and Paulig, M. Eine neue Methode zur Fr¨ uhrehabilitation zentralbedingter Lähmungen von Arm und Hand mittels Magnetstimulation. Zeitschrift für *EEG und EMG*, 1996, 27: 151–157.

Struppler, A., Angerer, B., Gündisch, C. and Havel, P. Modulatory effect of repetitive peripheral magnetic stimulation (rpms) on the skeletal muscle tone (stabilization of the elbow joint) on healthy subjects. Prepared for *Exp. Brain Res.*, 2003a.

Struppler, A., Havel, P. and Müller-Barna, P. Facilitation of skilled finger movements by repetitive peripheral magnetic stimulation (RPMS) – a new approach in central paresis. *NeuroRehabilitation*, 2003b, 18(1).

Vallar, G., Antonucci, G., Guariglia, C. and Pizzamiglio, L. Deficits of position sense, unilateral neglect and optokinetic stimulation. *Neuropsychologia*, 1993, 31(11): 1191–1200.

Vallar, G., Lobel, E., Galati, G., Berthoz, A., Pizzamiglio, L. and Bihan, D. A fronto-parietal system for computing the egocentric spatial frame of reference in humans. *Exp. Brain Res.*, 1999, 124(3): 281–286.

Weber, A. 2D CCD-Kamera-Messsystem zur Erfassung von Bewegungsabläufen der menschlichen Hand, Bachelor-Thesis, Lst. für Messsystem-und Sensortechnik, Technische Universität München, March 2002.

Weiller, C. and Rijntjes, M. Learning, plasticity, and recovery in the central nervous system. *Exp. Brain Res.*, 1999, 128(1/2): 134–138.

Wolpert, D., Goodbody, S. and Husain, M. Maintaining internal representations: the role of the human superior parietal lobe. *Nat. Neurosci.*, 1998, 1(6): 529–533.

Ziemann, U., Corwell, B. and Cohen, L. Modulation of plasticity in human motor cortex after forearm ischemic nerve block. The *J. Neurosci.*, 1998a, 18(3): 1115–1123.

Ziemann, U., Hallett, M. and Cohen, L. Mechanisms of deafferentation-induced plasticity in human motor cortex. *J. Neurosci.*, 1998b, 18(17): 7000–7007.

Ziemann, U., Müllbacher, W., Hallett, M. and Cohen, L. Modulation of practice-dependent plasticity in human motor cortex. *Brain*, 2001, 124(6), 1171–1181.

Transcranial Magnetic Stimulation and Transcranial Direct Current Stimulation (Supplements to Clinical Neurophysiology, Vol. 56)
Editors: W. Paulus, F. Tergau, M.A. Nitsche, J.C. Rothwell, U. Ziemann, M. Hallett

Chapter 37

TMS in stroke

Joachim Liepert

Department of Neurology, University of Hamburg, D-20246 Hamburg (Germany)

1. Introduction

After a stroke, hemiparesis is the most important and most frequent reason for dependency. A large number of patients (40–67%) remain impaired due to motor deficits (Dijkerman et al., 1996; Broeks et al., 1999). However, substantial recovery may occur even months after the cerebral infarction (e.g. Traversa et al., 2000). The ability to regain motor function depends rather on the site than the size of the lesion (Homberg et al., 1991; Binkofski et al., 1996, 2001). The mechanisms underlying these improvements of motor function are poorly understood. Presumably, they include a recovery of neurons in the penumbra, the activation of previously silent synapses and pathways and the involvement of motor areas in the ipsilesional and contralesional hemisphere (Nelles et al., 2001; Johansen-Berg et al., 2002; Rossini and Liepert, 2003). Further insight into the pathophysiological processes may be useful to develop more specific treatment strategies. Up to now therapy of motor impairments includes a variety of physiotherapeutic approaches (reviews: Van der Lee et al., 2001; Steultjens et al., 2003) and there is some evidence that restitution of motor function can be enhanced by application of noradrenergic and serotonergic drugs (Crisostomo et al., 1988; Walker-Batson et al., 1995; Dam et al., 1996; Grade et al., 1998; Pariente et al., 2001; Scheidtmann et al., 2001). However, guidelines for an individual therapy based on anatomical, pathophysiological or clinical aspects are still lacking.

Transcranial magnetic stimulation in stroke is useful for several reasons:

(1) TMS in the early stage after stroke provides important prognostic informations.
(2) TMS helps to quantify the severity of central motor pathway lesions.
(3) TMS techniques to evaluate intracortical inhibition and intracortical facilitation, stimulus response curves, motor output area mappings, transcallosal inhibition and silent periods increase our understanding of stroke pathophysiology.
(4) TMS serves to describe motor excitability changes associated with spontaneous or therapy-induced improvement of motor functions.

In this chapter, I will discuss different indications for TMS after stroke, and the information that can be obtained by the use of various TMS techniques.

* *Correspondence to:* Prof. Dr. J. Liepert, Department of Neurology, University Hospital Eppendorf, Martini Str. 52, D-20246 Hamburg, Germany.
Tel. #49 40 428033772; Fax: #49 40 428035623;
E-mail: liepert@uke.uni-hamburg.de

2. TMS as an early predictor of recovery

In numerous studies TMS has been used as a predictor of outcome after stroke. However, results are not consistent. For example, Timmerhuis et al. (1996) found that only MEPs measured in the acute stage had predictive value. In contrast, Arac et al. (1994) reported that irrespective of presence or absence of MEPs in the acute stage patients had the same motor function 3 to 6 months later. Catano et al. (1996) suggested that motor threshold determination 30 days after stroke had the best correlation with outcome. However, Di Lazzaro et al. (1999) found motor thresholds within the first 8 h after stroke to be a reasonable predictor of outcome. In agreement with this study, Nardone and Tezzon (2002) also detected high motor thresholds within 24 h after stroke as the most sensitive parameter for a poor outcome. In most studies TMS was performed within the first days (e.g. Heald et al., 1993; Péréon et al., 1995; Escudero et al., 1998; Pennisi et al., 1999; Vang et al., 1999) or even hours (Di Lazzaro et al., 1999) after stroke. Results obtained by TMS were compared to overall functional outcome, measured by Barthel Index or Rankin scale, or to motor recovery. Outcome evaluation was usually performed two to 12 months after stroke. Some studies repeated TMS to compare electrophysiological follow-up with clinical progress (Heald et al., 1993; Péréon et al., 1995; Catano et al., 1996; Rapisarda et al., 1996; Timmerhuis et al., 1996; D'Olhaberriague et al., 1997; Hendricks et al., 1997; Cruz Martinez et al., 1999; Pennisi et al., 1999). In most studies, patients were subdivided into groups according to the TMS results. Patients with existing MEPs were usually compared with those without MEPs. Other investigators defined patient groups according to their clinical symptoms (D'Olhaberriague et al., 1997). In some papers patients were not grouped but statistical analysis was performed to discriminate the most important variables for predicting outcome results (e.g. Feys et al., 2000). Patient populations were quite different: In some studies the number of severely affected patients with poor recovery was particularly high, and in most studies cortical and subcortical infarctions as well as ischemic and hemorrhagic lesions were mixed. The above mentioned different methods probably contribute substantially to the different results that are encountered (Rossini, 2000). However, a majority of studies supports the following statements:

(1) Patients in whom MEPs can be elicited in the paretic limb early after stroke have a significantly better clinical outcome than patients without MEPs at early stage.
(2) Presence or absence of a MEP is a more important variable than a differentiation between normal and delayed central motor conduction times (CMCT) (Heald et al., 1993; Catano et al., 1995; Rapisarda et al., 1996).
(3) TMS should not only be performed while the target muscle is relaxed but also during facilitation (contraction of the target muscle or, if impossible, innervation of the homologous contralateral muscle). Patients without MEPs at rest, but with MEPs during facilitation, have a substantially better prognosis than patients who have no MEPs during facilitation (Heald et al., 1993; Catano et al., 1995).
(4) The inability to obtain MEPs early after stroke is associated with a poor recovery (Rapisarda et al., 1996; Escudero et al., 1998; Vang et al., 1999).
(5) Motor thresholds are often elevated after stroke (particularly in subcortical strokes). They tend to decrease in the subsequent months. The best predictive value was found when determining motor threshold 30 days after stroke (Catano et al., 1996) but even threshold evaluation within the first 8–24 h after stroke may predict outcome (Di Lazzaro et al., 1999, Nardone and Tezzon, 2002).

Several studies have compared the prognostic value of motor evoked potentials with somatosensory evoked potentials (SSEPs) in stroke (Macdonell et al., 1989; Abbruzzese et al., 1991; Péréon et al., 1995; Timmerhuis et al., 1996; Hendricks et al., 1997; Feys et al., 2000). In most studies the authors found MEPs to be more sensitive in the prediction of outcome

(Macdonell et al., 1989; Abbruzzese et al., 1991; Péréon et al., 1995; Timmerhuis et al., 1996; Hendricks et al., 1997). Feys et al. (2000) concluded from their data that in the acute phase a combination of a motor score and SSEP results had the best prognostic value, whereas 2 months after stroke the combination of motor score and MEPs was best for predicting the long-term outcome.

In studies that exclusively included patients with brainstem lesions TMS abnormalities were closely related to the degree of paresis (Ferbert et al., 1992b), and absent MEPs were highly correlated with presence of persisting motor deficit 3 months later (Schwarz et al., 2000).

3. Central motor conduction time (CMCT)

In numerous studies CMCTs were calculated. Heald et al. (1993a) studied 118 stroke victims and subdived them into three groups: a normal response group, a delayed response group and no-response group. The delayed response group was small (6% of all patients) and, after 12 months, had the same clinical outcome as the patients in the normal response group. A similar distribution of patients into the three groups was reported by Berardelli et al. (1987, 1991). Several authors found persisting CMCT prolongations despite clinical improvements (Cicinelli et al., 1997b; Traversa et al., 1997; Traversa et al., 2000; Byrnes et al., 2001; Pennisi et al., 2002). Thus, CMCT abnormalities indicate a lesion or dysfunction of central motor pathways but only have a weak correlation with motor deficits. Thickbroom et al. (2002) described a correlation of MEP amplitudes and motor thresholds with hand strength but not with dexterity. Stroke patients with minor deficits such as impairments of dexterity may even have normal CMCTs (Homberg et al., 1991).

4. Silent periods (SP)

The silent period or postexcitatory inhibition is a measure of motor cortical inhibition. To produce a SP, a suprathreshold TMS pulse is applied during voluntary contraction of the target muscle. The transient interruption of EMG activity is attributed to activation of spinal and cortical inhibitory circuits (Fuhr et al., 1991; Cantello et al., 1992; Inghilleri et al., 1993; Roick et al., 1993; Triggs et al., 1993). SP duration shows a high interindividual variability. However, intraindividual interhemispheric differences are small (Haug et al., 1992; Cicinelli et al., 1997a; Fritz et al., 1997) which makes SP measurements particularly useful for evaluation of unilateral abnormalities. Early after stroke the SP is prolonged on the paretic side (Haug et al., 1992; Kukowski and Haug, 1992; Braune and Fritz, 1995; Liepert et al., 1995; Faig and Busse, 1996; Classen et al., 1997; Ahonen et al., 1998; Nardone and Tezzon, 2002), see Fig. 1. In most studies, SP abnormalities occurred more often than prolongations of central motor latencies, indicating that SP is a more sensitive parameter. Von Giesen et al. (1994) pointed out that small lesions within the primary sensorimotor cortex were associated with a reduction of SP duration whereas

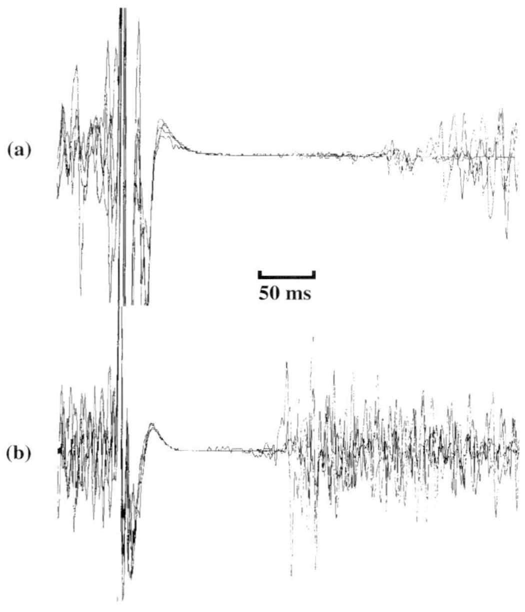

Fig. 1. Silent period in a single stroke patient obtained by TMS during activation of the target muscle with 20% of maximal voluntary contraction. Stimulus intensity: 120% of individual motor threshold. (a) affected side; (b) unaffected side.

patients with subcortical infarcts or lesions in premotor, parietal and temporal areas showed SP prolongations on the affected side. Classen et al. (1997) reported a close association between SP duration and motor performance. Patients with motor disturbances that resembled motor neglect had particularly prolonged SPs.

Spasticity was associated with a shortening of SP duration (Liepert et al., 1995; Catano et al., 1997a; Cruz Martinez et al., 1998), thus reflecting a decreased activity of inhibitory circuits. A SP shortening during a high level of voluntary contaction (as compared to SP duration during low force contractions) predicted the eventual occurrence of spasticity (Catano et al., 1997b).

In conclusion, SP evaluation can be a valuable additional tool to detect subtle sequelae of a stroke. For diagnostic purposes, this method is particularly useful in stroke patients with normal MEPs and normal central motor latencies.

5. TMS as an indicator of ipsilateral motor pathways

A still debated issue is the contribution of ipsilateral uncrossed fibers to recovery. In most functional imaging studies using PET or fMRI activations in the ipsilateral non-lesioned hemisphere were observed during passive or active movements of the paretic hand (Chollet et al., 1991; Weiller et al., 1992; Pantano et al., 1996; Dettmers et al., 1997; Cao et al., 1998; Seitz et al., 1998; Nelles et al., 1999a, b; Marshall et al., 2000). Some of these studies did not control mirror movements performed with the unaffected hand. Thus, it remained unclear if the brain activations were indeed exclusively related to movements with the paretic hand. Moreover, the results did not allow deciding if ipsilateral activations are clinically relevant for motor function or if they are mere epiphenomena. A recent publication by Johansen-Berg et al. (2002) has elegantly demonstrated that TMS over the dorsal premotor cortex of the unaffected hemisphere slowed reaction time finger movements in patients, but had no effect in normal subjects. This finding suggests that premotor areas in the contralesional hemisphere of stroke patients are functionally relevant.

In normal subjects, high-intensity TMS can produce ipsilateral MEPs (iMEPS) during strong muscle contraction (Wassermann et al., 1994; Ziemann et al., 1999; Alagona et al., 2001). As iMEP amplitudes could be modulated by neck rotations it was suggested that these iMEPs are mediated through corticoreticulospinal or corticopropriospinal pathways (Ziemann et al., 1999). Palmer et al. (1992) were unable to stimulate ipsilateral pathways in stroke patients and concluded that ipsilateral corticospinal connections do not contribute to motor recovery. In other studies with stroke patients, iMEPs could either be elicited by TMS over the non-lesioned hemisphere (Caramia et al., 1996, 2000; Turton et al., 1996; Hendricks et al., 1997; Netz et al., 1997; Trompetto et al., 2000) or over the affected hemisphere (Fries et al., 1991; Trompetto et al., 2000; Alagona et al., 2001). In these patients iMEPs were usually obtained by stimulating anteriorly and medially to the primary motor cortex. This probably indicates that corticospinal pathways originating from premotor areas were activated.

Those patients who had iMEPs when stimulating the non-affected hemisphere still had a variable outcome: some authors (Caramia et al., 1996, 2000; Trompetto et al., 2000) found a correlation between iMEPs and motor recovery while other investigators described an association between the occurrence of iMEPS and a poor outcome (Turton et al., 1996; Hendricks et al., 1997; Netz et al., 1997). It remains unclear if clinical, pathophysiological or methodological differences are responsible for these different observations. In any case iMEPs described by Caramia et al. (1996) and Trompetto et al. (2000) seem to differ from those reported by Turton et al. (1996) in some electrophysiological features: iMEPS in Caramia's and Trompetto's patient group had rather low excitability thresholds and rather large amplitudes, while in Turton's patients only small iMEPs could be elicited with high stimulation intensities.

Therefore, it seems possible that two different patient groups exist: one probably small group with a larger portion of ipsilateral, uncrossed corticospinal fibers, which contribute to a quick recovery. However, the majority of patients probably has less ipsilateral corticospinal connections. They may become accessible but may not support restitution of function substantially.

Alagona et al. (2001) found an association between iMEPs produced by stimulation of the affected hemisphere and bimanual dexterity 6 months after stroke. They suggested that the existence of these iMEPs indicates a hyperexcitability of premotor areas in the affected hemisphere. Such a hypothesis corresponds to the results by Johansen-Berg et al. (2002).

6. Mapping of motor output areas

Mapping studies are usually performed using a focal figure-of-eight coil. The motor output area size is determined by shifting the coil systematically in steps of 1 cm over the skull. The output area is represented by the number of positions whose stimulation produces a MEP in the target muscle. Another parameter frequently used is the center of gravity of the output map (Wassermann et al., 1992) or the position of the map in relation to the vertex. It was shown repeatedly that, in normal subjects, map size and location are rather symmetrical when studying both hemispheres (e.g. Cicinelli et al., 1997a; Classen et al., 1998). Presumably, expansions or shrinkage of an output map only indicate a change of corticospinal excitability (Thickbroom et al., 1998). In contrast, shifts of the center of gravity or an asymmetry of the map suggest "true" reorganization.

Several studies have investigated map changes after stroke. Cicinelli et al. (1997b) and Traversa et al. (1997) reported that the motor output map in the affected hemisphere is reduced early after stroke and enlarges within the subsequent weeks. These changes were associated with clinical improvement. The authors also described some abnormally located excitable spots in the affected hemisphere, suggesting some kind of reorganization. Similarily, Byrnes et al. (1999, 2001) demonstrated map size asymmetries in a heterogeneous group of stroke patients. They also interpreted their data as an indicator of functional reorganization. Since the patients had regained almost normal motor functions, the authors postulated that cortical reorganization had contributed to the motor recovery. Rossini et al. (1998) published a case report of a stroke patient with an impressive improvement of motor function who had a much larger motor output map in the affected hemisphere which was expanded into a lateral direction. This report also suggested a perilesional reorganization.

We used the TMS mapping technique to investigate intervention-induced changes of motor cortex excitability (Liepert et al., 1998, 2000a, b, 2001). Chronic stroke patients participated in 2 weeks of constraint-induced movement therapy (CIMT) (Taub et al., 1993). Mapping was performed 2 weeks and 1 day prior to therapy and 1 day, 4 weeks and 6 months after the treatment period (Fig. 2).

Prior to CIMT, the patients had higher motor thresholds and smaller motor output maps in the lesioned hemisphere. After therapy, motor output maps in the affected hemisphere had increased by approximately 40% while those in the non-affected hemisphere were non-significantly decreased. Both changes presumably reflect use-dependent mechanisms: the increased

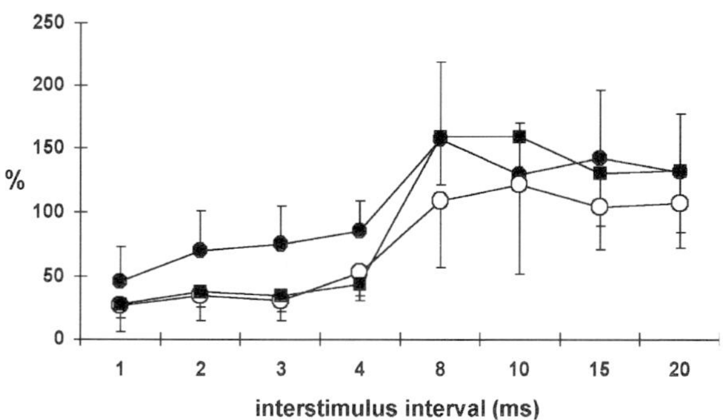

Fig. 2. Intracortical inhibition and intracortical facilitation in stroke patients and healthy subjects expressed as a percentage of the mean MEP amplitude after single TMS. Filled circles, MEP amplitudes after stimulation of the affected hemisphere; open circles, MEP amplitudes after TMS in the unaffected hemisphere in patients; filled squares, MEP amplitudes after TMS in the control group. (From: Liepert, J., Storch, P., Fritsch, A. and Weiller, C. Motor cortex disinhibition in acute stroke. *Clin. Neurophysiol.*, 2000, 111: 671–676.)

amount of use of the paretic hand during the training period and the decreased use of the immobilized non-affected hand. These electrophysiological changes were paralleled by a large improvement of motor function (Fig. 3). Motor thresholds remained identical after CIMT. As motor thresholds are determined in the *center* of the cortical representation area it was concluded that enlargements of the motor output map were due to increases of excitability at the *borders* of the representation area. One of the mechanisms involved in these map changes could be a GABA dependent modulation of horizontal intracortical inhibitory circuits which strongly influence the size of a representation area (Jacobs and Donoghue, 1991).

After CIMT, the amplitude-weighted centers of the motor output maps (center of gravity, CoG) had shifted significantly stronger in the affected than in the non-affected hemisphere. These shifts were mainly observed in the medio-lateral axis. We suggested that CoG shifts indicated an intervention-induced recruitment of additional brain areas that were adjacent to the areas excitable prior to therapy. Similar results have also been reported in monkey studies (Nudo et al., 1996). In the subsequent 6 months after CIMT the motor output map sizes equalized (the area size in the affected hemisphere decreased somewhat, and the map in the non-affected hemisphere increased somewhat) while motor performance remained unchanged. The electrophysiological changes were interpreted as an indicator of increased effective connectivity between neuronal populations, which allows reducing the excitability level while maintaining the same level of performance (Liepert et al., 2000a).

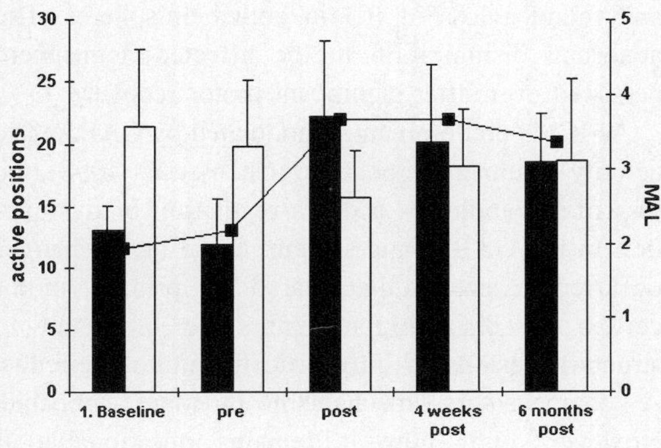

Fig. 3. Number of active TMS positions in the infarcted (black bars) and non-infarcted (grey bars) hemispheres 2 weeks and 1 day pre-treatment and 1 day, 4 weeks and 6 months post-treatment. Black squares indicate the corresponding motor activity log (MAL) data for the paretic limb. (From: Liepert, J., Bauder, H., Miltner, W.H.R., Taub, E. and Weiller, C. Treatment-induced cortical reorganization after stroke in humans. *Stroke*, 2000, 31: 1210–1216.)

In a TMS mapping study in patients 4 to 8 weeks after stroke we found that a single dexterity training (duration: 1.5 h) enhanced corticospinal excitability, as the motor output map of a paretic hand muscle increased. However, since there was no CoG shift, cortical reorganization could not be demonstrated (Liepert et al., 2000b). In another study we compared 1 week of conventional physiotherapy with 1 week of conventional physiotherapy plus forced-use therapy (Wolf et al., 1989). Corticospinal excitability increased significantly stronger during the forced-use treatment period, and CoG shifts indicated a reorganization in the affected hemisphere after 2 weeks of therapy (Liepert et al., 2001). Thus, similar to the study in chronic patients participating in CIMT, this study indicated that increases of motor cortex excitability are closely related to the amount of use of the target muscle.

7. Intracortical inhibition and intracortical facilitation

The paired pulse paradigm first described by Kujirai et al. (1993) allows to test intracortical excitability. Depending on the interstimulus interval between the subthreshold conditioning TMS pulse and the suprathreshold test pulse either inhibitory or excitatory neuronal circuits can be explored. This method has been applied to stroke patients at different stages of their illness and allows to suggest some mechanisms of brain plasticity.

7.1. CI and ICF in the unaffected hemisphere

In patients with hemiplegia due to a large infarction in the territory of the middle cerebral artery the contralateral, non-lesioned hemisphere was studied with single and paired pulse TMS, and recordings were taken from the unaffected first dorsal interosseous muscle. A decrease of ICI was found 2 weeks after stroke (Liepert et al., 2000c). These results were confirmed by Shimizu et al. (2002) and Manganotti et al. (2002). Shimizu et al. (2002) compared a group of patients with cortical stroke with a patient group with subcortical lesions. A loss of ICI in the unaffected hemisphere was only found in cortical infarctions. This finding corresponds to results obtained in animal studies (Buchkremer-Ratzmann et al., 1996, 1997; Reinecke et al., 1999). In rats, the disinhibition was associated with downregulation of GABA (A) receptors and enhancement of glutamatergic activity (Que et al., 1999a, b). As changes of ICI are supposed to be modulated by GABAergic activity (Ziemann et al., 1996; Chen et al., 1998) the decreased ICI in the non-lesioned hemisphere of patients with large territorial infarctions may indicate a downregulation of GABA activity in this hemisphere. Two main mechanisms could be responsible: a damage of transcallosal fibers which could lead to a loss of physiological intercortical inhibition (Ferbert et al., 1992a; Boroojerdi et al., 1996) or an enhanced use of the unaffected arm in all daily activities as ICI is modified in a task- and use-dependent manner (Liepert et al., 1998a). The idea of a disinhibition in the non-lesioned hemisphere is also supported by other groups who found enlarged MEP amplitudes when stimulating the unaffected hemisphere after stroke (Cicinelli et al., 1997b, Trompetto et al., 2000). Butefisch et al. (2003) explored changes of ICI in the unaffected hemisphere of stroke patients and reported that patients and normal controls had similar intracortical excitability when using low intensities for the conditioning stimulus. In contrast, higher intensities of the conditioning pulse were associated with a loss of intracortical inhibition in the patients. This increase of intracortical excitability was only seen in patients with good recovery but not in those with poor recovery. This result is in some contrast to two other studies: Manganotti et al. (2002) described normal intracortical excitability in the unaffected hemisphere of stroke patients with significant motor recovery, and Shimizu et al. (2002) found intracortical disinhibition of the unaffected hemisphere in patients with poor motor recovery.

7.2. ICI and ICF in the affected hemisphere

In a study by Liepert et al. (2000d) ICI and ICF were studied in stroke patients who either had a small motor deficit at onset of symptoms or who underwent a rapid (spontaneous) motor recovery. Thus, the patients were almost recovered at the time of electrophysiological evaluation. In this group, a loss of intracortical inhibition was observed in the affected hemisphere. In contrast, ICI in the unaffected hemisphere was not different from an age-matched control group (Fig. 3). This result corresponds to animal studies which described a loss of GABAergic inhibition in the surround of a cortical lesion (Schiene et al., 1996). Manganotti et al. (2002) reported a similar finding. They investigated stroke patients with a moderate to severe hemiparesis in the acute stage and found a loss of ICI in both hemispheres. The abnormal disinhibition in the affected hemisphere persisted even after significant motor recovery.

As ICI is predominantly modulated by GABAergic activity (Ziemann et al. 1996; Chen et al., 1998), the loss of ICI indicates a down-regulation or dysfunction in the GABAergic system. Since these changes occurred in strokes that spared the primary motor cortex the disinhibition cannot be attributed to structural lesions of intracortical inhibitory circuits. A compensatory mechanism is more probable. However, until now it remains questionable if intracortical disinhibition contributes to motor recovery or is an epiphenomenon.

Recently we observed an intracortical disinhibition *and* an enhancement of ICF in a patient with a somatosensory cortex lesion, suggesting that, under normal conditions, the somatosensory cortex exerts some inhibitory influence on primary motor cortex (Liepert et al., 2003).

8. Stimulus–response curves (SRC)

The technique was first described by Ridding and Rothwell (1997). Pharmacological studies have indicated that SRC are modulated by various neurotransmitters. The GABA A agonist lorazepam depressed SRCs, amphetamine as an indirect agonist of the dopaminergic-adrenergic system enhanced SRCs (Boroojerdi et al., 2001). The serotonine reuptake inhibitor sertraline enhanced SRCs (Ilic et al., 2002). Ketamine also enhanced SRCs, presumably through activation of non-NMDA glutamatergic transmission (Di Lazzaro et al., 2003).

Patients with ischemic subcortical lacunar lesions SRC are significantly depressed on the affected side. This phenomenon becomes more evident with higher stimulus intensities (Fig. 4, Liepert et al., in preparation). Two different hypotheses could explain these findings. (1) The lesion has predominantly affected corticospinal neurons with higher motor thresholds. In that case these neurons are no longer excitable by TMS and could not contribute to an increase in the SRC. (2) Motor neurons that usually have higher motor thresholds have become excitable with stimulus intensities close to the motor threshold. In that case the majority of excitable corticospinal neurons would already be recruited with slightly suprathreshold stimulus intensities. This would rather indicate a compensatory mechanism and would correspond to the finding of intracortical disinhibition in this patient group.

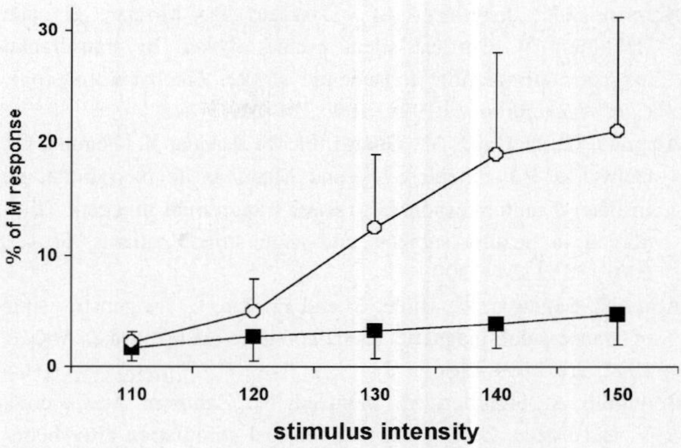

Fig. 4. Stimulus–response curves obtained from transcranial magnetic stimulation of the affected (black squares) and the unaffected (open circles) hemisphere in patients with subcortical lacunar lesions ($n = 5$). Y axis: amplitudes of motor evoked potentials are expressed as percentage of the corresponding M response. X axis: stimulus intensities in relation to the individual motor threshold.

9. TMS as an indicator of interhemispheric interactions

Using a technique first described by Ferbert et al. (1992a) a conditioning TMS pulse applied to one motor cortex induces an inhibition of a second TMS pulse applied to the other motor cortex. The phenomenon occurs with interstimulus intervals of 5–6 ms or more. This interhemispheric inhibition (II) is believed to be mediated through the corpus callosum. Boroojerdi et al. (1996) employed this method to demonstrate that stroke patients with cortical lesions had a loss or a reduction of II. In contrast, subcortical lesions sparing callosal fibers were associated with normal II. These results have recently been reproduced by Shimizu et al. (2002). Presumably, the loss of II is one of the reasons for the loss of ICI in the unaffected hemisphere (Liepert et al., 2000; Shimizu et al., 2002).

In conclusion, the above mentioned techniques have demonstrated perilesional excitability changes, but also effects in the non-lesioned hemisphere. They further support the hypothesis that a single monohemispheric lesion may affect a widespread bihemispherically organized network. TMS methods have also shown that the adult brain is capable of reorganization, and appropriately timed TMS pulses can help to clarify the functional relevance of brain areas activated in PET or fMRI studies. Hopefully, these tools will allow to optimize the treatment of stroke patients in the future.

References

Abbruzzese, G., Morena, M., Dall'Agata, D., Abbruzzese, M. and Favale, E. Motor evoked potentials (MEPs) in lacunar syndromes. *Electroencephalogr. Clin. Neurophysiol.*, 1991, 81: 202–208.

Ahonen, J.P., Jehkonen, M., Dastidar, P., Molnár, G. and Häkkinen, V. Cortical silent period evoked by transcranial magnetic stimulation in ischemic stroke. *Electroencephalogr. Clin. Neurophysiol.*, 1998, 109: 224–229.

Alagona, G., Delvaux, V., Gérard, P., De Pasqua, V., Pennisi, G., Delwaide, P.J., Nicoletti, F. and Maertens de Noordhout, A. Ipsilateral motor responses to focal transcranial magnetic stimulation in healthy subjects and acute-stroke patients. *Stroke*, 2001, 32: 1304–1309.

Arac, N., Sagduyu, A., Binai, S. and Ertekin, C. Prognostic value of transcranial magnetic stimulation in acute stroke. *Stroke*, 1994, 25: 2183–2186.

Berardelli, A., Inghilleri, M., Manfredi, M., Zamponi, A., Cecconi, V. and Dolce, G. Cortical and cervical stimulation after hemispheric infarction. *J. Neurol. Neurosurg. Psychiatry*, 1987, 50: 861–86.5

Berardelli, A., Inghilleri. M., Cruccu, G., Mercuri, B. and Manfredi, M. Electrical and magnetic transcranial stimulation in patients with corticospinal damage due to stroke or motor neurone disease. *Electroencephalogr. Clin. Neurophysiol.*, 1991, 81: 389–396.

Binkofski, F., Seitz, R.J., Arnold, S., Classen, J., Benecke, R. and Freund, H.J. Thalamic metabolism and corticospinal tract integrity determine motor recovery in stroke. *Ann. Neurol.*, 1996, 39: 460–470.

Binkofski, F., Seitz, R.J., Hacklander, T., Pawelec, D., Mau, J. and Freund, H.J. Recovery of motor functions following hemiparetic stroke: a clinical and magnetic resonance-morphometric study. *Cerebrovasc. Dis.*, 2001, 11: 273–281.

Boroojerdi, B., Diefenbach, K. and Ferbert, A.Transcallosal inhibition in cortical and subcortical cerebral vascular lesions. *J. Neurol. Sci.*, 1996, 144: 160–170.

Boroojerdi, B., Battaglia, F., Muellbacher, W. and Cohen, L.G. Mechanisms influencing stimulus-response porperties of the human corticospinal system. *Clin. Neurophysiol.*, 2001, 112: 931–937.

Braune, H.J. and Fritz, C. Transcranial magnetic stimulation-evoked inhibition of voluntary muscle activity (silent period) is impaired in patients with ischemic hemispheric lesion. *Stroke*, 1995, 26: 550–553.

Broeks, J.G., Lankhorst, G.J., Rumping, K. and Prevo, A.J. The long-term outcome of arm function after stroke: results of a follow-up study. *Disabil. Rehabil.*, 1999, 21: 357–364.

Buchkremer-Ratzmann, I., August, M., Hagemann, G. and Witte, O.W. Electrophysiological transcortical diaschisis after acute photothrombosis in rat brain. *Stroke*, 1996, 27: 1005–1111.

Buchkremer-Ratzmann, I. and Witte, O.W. Extended brain disinhibition following small photothrombotic lesions in rat frontal cortex. *NeuroReport*, 1997, 8: 519–522.

Bütefisch, C.M., Netz, J., Wessling, M., Seitz, R.J. and Hömberg, V. Remote changes in cortical excitability after stroke. *Brain*, 2003, 126: 470–481.

Byrnes, M.L., Thickbroom, G.W., Phillips, B.A., Wilson, S.A. and Mastaglia, F.L. Physiological studies of the corticomotor projection to the hand after subcortical stroke. *Clin. Neurophysiol.*, 1999, 110: 487–498.

Byrnes, M.L., Thickbroom, G.W., Phillips, B.A. and Mastaglia, F.L. Long-term changes in motor cortical organisation after recovery from subcortical stroke. *Brain Res.*, 2001, 889: 278–287.

Cantello, R., Gianelli, M., Civardi, C. and Mutani, R. Magnetic brain stimulation: The silent period after the motor evoked potential. *Neurology*, 1992, 42: 1951–1959.

Cao, Y., D'Olhaberriague, L., Vikingstad, E.M., et al. Pilot study of functional MRI to assess cerebral activation of motor function after poststroke hemiparesis. *Stroke*, 1998, 29: 112–122.

Caramia, M.D., Iani, C. and Bernardi, G. Cerebral plasticity after stroke as revealed by ipsilateral responses to magnetic stimulation. *NeuroReport*, 1996, 7: 1756–1760.

Caramia, M.D., Palmieri, M.G., Giacomini, P., Iani, C., Dally, L. and Silvestrini, M. Ipsilateral activation of the unaffected motor cortex in patients with hemiparetic stroke. *Clin. Neurophysiol.*, 2000, 111: 1990–1996.

Catano, A., Houa, M., Caroyer, J.M., Ducarne, H. and Noel, P. Magnetic transcranial stimulation in non-haemorrhagic sylvian strokes: interest of facilitation for early functional prognosis. *Electroencephalogr. Clin. Neurophysiol.*, 1995, 97: 349–354.

Catano, A., Houa, M., Caroyer, J.M., Ducarne, H. and Noel, P. Magnetic transcranial stimulation in acute stroke: early excitation threshold and functional prognosis. *Electroencephalogr. Clin. Neurophysiol.*, 1996, 101: 233–239.

Catano, A., Houa, M. and Noel, P. Magnetic transcranial stimulation: dissociation of excitatory and inhibitory mechanisms in acute strokes. *Electroencephalogr. Clin. Neurophysiol.*, 1997a, 105: 29–36.

Catano, A., Houa, M. and Noel, P. Magnetic transcranial stimulation: Clinical interest of the silent period in acute and chronic stages of stroke. *Electroencephalogr. Clin. Neurophysiol.*, 1997b, 105: 290–296.

Chen, R., Corwell, B., Yaseen, Z., Hallett, M. and Cohen, L.G. Mechanisms of cortical reorganization in lower-limb amputees. *J. Neurosci.*, 1998, 18: 3443–3450.

Chollet, F., DiPiero, V., Wise, R.J., Brooks, D.J., Dolan, R.J. and Frackowiak, R.S. The functional anatomy of motor recovery after stroke in humans: a study with positron emission tomography. *Ann. Neurol.*, 1991, 29: 63–71.

Cicinelli, P., Traversa, R., Bassi, A., Scivoletto, G. and Rossini, P.M. Interhemispheric differences of hand muscle representation in human motor cortex. *Muscle Nerve*, 1997a, 20: 535–542.

Cicinelli P, Traversa R. and Rossini PM. Post-stroke reorganization of brain motor output to the hand: a 2–4 month follow-up with focal magnetic transcranial stimulation. *Electroencephalogr. Clin. Neurophysiol.*, 1997b, 105: 438–450.

Classen, J., Schnitzler, A., Binkowski, F., Werhahn. K.J., Kim, Y., Kessler, K.R. and Benecke, R. The motor syndrome associated with exaggerated inhibition within the primary motor cortex of patients with hemiparetic stroke. *Brain*, 1997, 120: 605–619.

Classen, J., Knorr, U., Werhahn, K., Schlaug, G., Kunesch, E., Cohen, L.G., Seitz, R.J. and Benecke, R. Multimodal output mapping of human central motor representation on different spatial scales. *J. Physiol.*, 1998, 512: 163–179.

Crisostomo, E.A., Duncan, P.W., Probst, M., Dawson, D.V. and Davis, J.N. Evidence that amphetamine with physical therapy promotes recovery of motor function in stroke patients. *Ann. Neurol.*, 1988, 23: 94–97.

Cruz Martinez, A., Munoz, J. and Palacios, F. The muscle inhibitory period by transcranial magnetic stimulation. Study in stroke patients. *Electromyogr. Clin. Neurophysiol.*, 1998, 38: 189–192.

Cruz Martinez, A., Tejada, J. and Dietz Tejedor, E. Motor hand recovery after stroke. Prognostic yield of early transcranial magnetic stimulation. *Electromyogr. Clin. Neurophysiol.*, 1999, 39: 405–410.

Dam, M., Tonin, P., De Boni, A., Pizzolato, G., Casson, S., Ermani, M., Freo, U., Piron, L. and Battistin, L. Effects of fluoxetine and maprotiline on functional recovery in poststroke hemiplegic patients undergoing rehabilitation therapy. *Stroke*, 1996, 27: 1211–1214.

Dettmers, C., Stephan, K.M., Lemon, R.N. and Frackowiak, R.S.J. Reorganization of the executive motor system after stroke. *Cerebrovasc. Dis.*, 1997, 7: 187–200.

Dijkerman, H.C., Wood, V.A. and Hewer, R.L. Long-term outcome after discharge from a stroke rehabilitation unit. *J. R. Coll. Physicians Lond.*, 1996, 30: 538–546.

Di Lazzaro, V., Oliviero, A., Profice, P., Saturno, E., Pilato, F. and Tonali, P. Motor cortex excitability changes within 8 hours after ischaemic stroke may predict the functional outcome. *Eur. J. Emerg. Med.*, 1999, 6: 119–121.

Di Lazzaro, V., Oliviero, A., Profice, P., Pennisi, M.A., Pilato, F., Zito, G., Dileone, M., Nicoletti, R., Pasqualetti, P. and Tonali, P.A. Ketamine increases human motor cortex excitability to transcranial magnetic stimulation. *J. Physiol.*, 2003, 547: 485–496.

D'Olhaberriague, L., Espadaler Gamissans, J.M., Marrugat, J., Valls, A., Oliveras Ley, C. and Seoane, J.L. Transcranial magnetic stimulation as a prognostic tool in stroke. *J. Neurol. Sci.*, 1997, 147: 73–80.

Dominkus, M., Grisold, W. and Jelinek, V. Transcranial electrical motor evoked potentials as a prognostic indicator for motor recovery in stroke patients. *J. Neurol. Neurosurg. Psychiatry*, 1990, 53: 745–748.

Escudero, J.V., Sancho, J., Bautista, D., Escudero, M. and Lopez-Trigo, J. Prognostic value of motor evoked potential obtained by transcranial magnetic brain stimulation in motor function recovery in patients with acute ischemic stroke. *Stroke*, 1998, 29: 1854–1859.

Faig, J. and Busse, O. Silent period evoked by transcranial magnetic stimulation in unilateral thalamic infarcts. *J. Neurol. Sci.*, 1996, 142: 85–92.

Ferbert, A., Priori, A., Rothwell, J.C., Day, B.L., Colebatch, J.G. and Marsden, C.D. Interhemispheric inhibition of the human motor cortex. *J. Physiol.*, 1992a, 453: 525–546.

Ferbert, A., Vielhaber, S., Meincke, U. and Buchner, H. Transcranial magnetic stimulation in pontine infarction: correlation to degree of paresis. *J. Neurol. Neurosurg. Psychiatry*, 1992b, 55: 294–299.

Feys, H., Van Hees, J., Bruyninckx, F., Mercelis, R. and De Weerdt, W. Value of somatosensory and motor evoked potentials in predicting arm recovery after a stroke. *J. Neurol. Neurosurg. Psychiatry*, 2000, 68: 323–331.

Fritz, C., Braune, H.J., Pylatiuk, C. and Pohl, M. Silent period following transcranial magnetic stimulation: a study of intra- and inter-examiner reliability. *Electroencephalogr. Clin. Neurophysiol.*, 1997, 105: 235–240.

Fuhr, P., Agostino, R. and Hallett, M. Spinal motor neuron excitability during the silent period after cortical stimulation. *Electroencephalogr. Clin. Neurophysiol.*, 1991, 81: 257–262.

Grade, C., Redford, B., Chrostowski, J., Toussaint, L. and Blackwell, B. Methylphenidate in early poststroke recovery: a double-blind, placebo-controlled study. *Arch. Phys. Med. Rehabil.*, 1998, 79: 1047–1050.

Haug, B.A., Schönle, P.W., Knobloch, C. and Köhne, M. Silent period measurement revives as a valuable diagnostic tool with transcranial magnetic stimulation. *Electroencephalogr. Clin. Neurophysiol.*, 1992, 85: 158–160.

Heald, A., Bates, D., Cartlidge, N.E., French, J.M. and Miller, S. Longitudinal study of central motor conduction time following stroke. 1. Natural history of central motor conduction. *Brain*, 1993a, 116: 1355–1370.

Heald, A., Bates, D., Cartlidge, N.E., French, J.M. and Miller, S. Longitudinal study of central motor conduction time following stroke. 2. Central motor conduction measured within 72 h after stroke as a predictor of functional outcome at 12 months. *Brain*, 1993b, 116: 1371–1385.

Hendricks, H.T., Hageman, G. and Van Limbeek, J. Prediction of recovery from upper extremity paralysis after stroke by measuring evoked potentials. *Scand. J. Rehabil. Med.*, 1997, 29: 155–159.

Homberg, V., Stephan, K.M. and Netz, J. Transcranial stimulation of motor cortex in upper motor neurone syndrome: ist relation to the motor deficit. *Electroencephalogr. Clin. Neurophysiol.*, 1991, 81: 377–388.

Ilic, T.V., Korchounov, A. and Ziemann, U. Complex modulation of human motor cortex excitability by the specific serotonin re-uptake inhibitor sertraline. *Neurosci. Lett.*, 2002, 319: 116–120.

Inghilleri, M., Berardelli, A., Cruccu, G. and Manfredi, M. Silent period evoked by transcranial stimulation of the human cortex and cervicomedullary junction. *J. Physiol.*, 1993, 466: 521–534.

Jacobs, K.M. and Donoghue, J.P. Reshaping the cortical motor map by unmasking latent intracortical connections. *Science*, 1991, 251: 944–947.

Johansen-Berg, H., Rushworth, M.F., Bogdanovic, M.D., Kischka, U., Wimalaratna, S. and Matthews, P.M. The role of ipsilateral premotor cortex in hand movement after stroke. *Proc. Natl. Acad. Sci. USA*, 2002, 99: 14518–14523.

Kujirai, T., Caramia, M.D., Rothwell, J.C., Day, B.L., Thompson, P.D., Ferbert, A., Wroe, S., Asselman, P. and Marsden, C.D. Corticocortical inhibition in human motor cortex. *J. Physiol.*, 1993, 471: 501–519.

Kukowski, B. and Haug, B. Quantitative evaluation of the silent period, evoked by transcranial magnetic stimulation during sustained muscle contraction, in normal man and in patients with stroke. *Electromyogr. Clin. Neurophysiol.*, 1992, 32: 373–378.

Liepert, J., Tegenthoff, M. and Malin, J.-P. Changes of postexcitatory inhibition after transcranial magnetic stimulation in the course of hemiparesis. *Neurol., Psych. Brain Res.*, 1995, 4: 1–6.

Liepert, J., Classen, J., Cohen, L.G. and Hallett, M. Task-dependent changes of intracortical inhibition. *Exp. Brain Res.*, 1998a, 118: 421–426.

Liepert, J., Miltner, W.H.R., Bauder, H., Sommer, M., Dettmers, C., Taub, E. and Weiller, C. Motor cortex plasticity during constraint-induced movement therapy in stroke patients. *Neurosci. Lett.*, 1998b, 250: 5–8.

Liepert, J., Bauder, H., Miltner, W.H.R., Taub, E. and Weiller, C. Treatment-induced cortical reorganization after stroke in humans. *Stroke*, 2000a, 31: 1210–1216.

Liepert, J., Gräf, S., Uhde, I., Leidner, O. and Weiller, C. Training-induced changes of motor cortex representations in stroke patients. *Acta. Neurol. Scand.*, 2000b, 101: 321–326.

Liepert, J., Hamzei, F. and Weiller, C. Motor cortex disinhibition of the unaffected hemisphere after acute stroke. *Muscle Nerve*, 2000c, 23: 1761–1763.

Liepert, J., Storch, P., Fritsch, A. and Weiller, C. Motor cortex disinhibition in acute stroke. *Clin. Neurophysiol.*, 2000d, 111: 671–676.

Liepert, J., Uhde, I., Gräf, S., Leidner, O. and Weiller, C. Motor cortex plasticity during forced use therapy in stroke patients. *J. Neurol.*, 2001, 248: 315–321.

Liepert, J., Gorsler, A.C., van Eimeren, T., Munchau, A. and Weiller, C. Motor excitability in a patient with a somatosensory cortex lesion. *Clin. Neurophysiol.*, 2003, in press.

Macdonell, R.A., Donnan, G.A. and Bladin, P.F. A comparison of somatosensory evoked and motor evoked potentials in stroke. *Ann. Neurol.*, 1989, 25: 68–73.

Manganotti, P., Patuzzo, S., Cortese, F., Palermo, A., Smania, N. and Fiaschi, A. Motor disinhibition in affected and unaffected hemisphere in the early period of recovery after stroke. *Clin. Neurophysiol.*, 2002, 113: 936–943.

Marshall, R.S., Perera, G.M., Lazar, R.M., et al. Evolution of cortical activation during recovery from corticospinal tract infarction. *Stroke*, 2000, 31:656–661.

Nardone, R. and Tezzon, F. Inhibitory and excitatory circuits of cerebral cortex after ischaemic stroke: prognostic value of the transcranial magnetic stimulation. *Electromyogr. Clin. Neurophysiol.*, 2002, 42: 131–136.

Nelles, G., Spiekermann, G., Jueptner, M., Leonhardt, G., Müller, S., Gerhard, H. and Diener, H.C. Reorganization of sensory and motor systems in hemiplegic stroke patients. A positron emission tomography study. *Stroke*, 1999a, 30: 1510–1516.

Nelles, G., Spiekermann, G., Jueptner, M., Leonhardt, G., Müller, S., Gerhard, H. and Diener, H.C. Evolution of functional reorganization in hemiplegic stroke: a serial positron emission tomographic activation study. *Ann. Neurol.*, 1999b, 46: 901–909.

Nelles, G., Jentzen, W., Jueptner, M., Muller, S. and Diener, H.C. Arm training induced brain plasticity in stroke studied with serial positron emission tomography. *Neuroimage*, 2001, 13: 1146–1154.

Netz, J., Lammers, T. and Hömberg, V. Reorganization of motor output in the non-affected hemisphere after stroke. *Brain*, 1997, 120: 1579–1586.

Nudo, R.J., Wise, B.M., SiFuentes, F. and Milliken, G.W. Neural substrates for the effects of rehabilitative training on motor recovery after ischemic infarct. *Science*, 1996, 272: 1791–1794.

Palmer, E., Ashby, P. and Hajek, V.E. Ipsilateral fast corticospinal pathways do not account for recovery in stroke. *Ann. Neurol.*, 1992, 32: 519–525.

Pantano, P., Formisano, R., Ricci, M. et al., Motor recovery after stroke. Morphological and functional brain alterations. *Brain*, 1996, 119: 1849–1857.

Pariente, J., Loubinoux, I., Carel, C., Albucher, J.F., Leger, A., Manelfe, C., Rascol, O. and Chollet, F. Fluoxetine modulates motor performance and cerebral activation of patients recovering from stroke. *Ann. Neurol.*, 2001, 50: 718–729.

Pennisi, G., Rapisarda, G., Bella, R., Calabrese, V., Maertens de Noordhout, A. and Delwaide, P.J. Absence of response to early transcranial magnetic stimulation in ischemic stroke patients: prognostic value for hand motor recovery. *Stroke*, 1999, 30: 2666–2670.

Pennisi, G., Alagona, G., Rapisardi, G., Nicoletti, F., Costanzo, E., Ferri, R., Malaguarnera, M. and Bella, R. Transcranial magnetic stimulation after pure motor stroke. *Clin. Neurophysiol.*, 2002, 113: 1536–1542.

Péréon, Y., Aubertin, P. and Guihenuc, P. Prognostic significance of electrophysiological investigations in stroke patients: somatosensory and motor evoked potentials and sympathetic skin response. *Neurophysiol. Clin.*, 1995, 25: 146–157.

Que, M., Schiene, K., Witte, O.W. and Zilles, K. Widespread up-regulation of N-methyl-D-aspartate receptors after focal photothrombotic lesion in rat brain. *Neurosci. Lett.*, 1999a, 273: 77–80.

Que, M., Witte, O.W., Neumann-Haefelin, T., Schiene, K., Schroeter, M. and Zilles, K. Changes in GABA (A) and GABA (B) receptor binding following cortical photothrombosis: a quantitative receptor autoradiographic study. *Neuroscience*, 1999b, 93: 1233–1240.

Rapisarda, G., Bastings, E., Maertens de Noordhout, A., Pennisi, G. and Delwaide. P.J. Can motor recovery in stroke patients be predicted by early transcranial magnetic stimulation? *Stroke*, 1996, 27: 2191–2196.

Reinecke, S., Lutzenburg, M., Hagemann, G., Bruehl, C., Neumann-Haefelin, T. and Witte, O.W. Electrophysiological transcortical diaschisis after middle cerebral artery occlusion (MCAO) in rats. *Neurosci. Lett.*, 1999, 261: 85–88.

Ridding, M.C. and Rothwell, J.C. Stimulus/response curves as a method of measuring motor cortical excitability in man. *Electroencephalogr. Clin. Neurophysiol.*, 1997, 105: 340–344.

Roick, H., von Giesen, H.J. and Benecke, R. On the origin of the postexcitatory inhibition seen after transcranial magnetic brain stimulation in awake human subjects. *Exp. Brain Res.*, 1993, 94: 489–498.

Rossini, P.M. Is transcranial magnetic stimulation of the motor cortex a prognostic tool for motor recovery after stroke? *Stroke*, 2000, 31: 1463–1464.

Rossini, P.M. and Liepert, J. Lesion of cortex and post-stroke plastic reorganization. In S. Boniface and U. Ziemann, (Eds.), *Plasticity in the Human Brain: Scientific and Clinical Studies with TMS.* Cambridge University Press, 2003, in press.

Rossini, P.M., Calatagirone, C., Castriota-Scandenberg, A., Cicinelli, P., Del Gratta, C., Demartin, M., Pizzella, V., Traversa, R. and Romani, G.L. Hand motor cortical areas reorganization in stroke: a study with fMRI, MEG and TCS maps. *NeuroReport*, 1998, 9: 2141–2146.

Scheidtmann, K., Fries, W., Muller, F. and Koenig, E. Effect of levodopa in combination with physiotherapy on functional motor recovery after stroke: a prspective, randomized, double-blind study. *Lancet*, 2001, 358: 787–790.

Schiene, K., Bruehl, C., Zilles, K., Qu, M., Hagemann, G., Kraemer, M. and Witte, O.W. Neuronal hyperexcitability and reduction of GABAA-receptor expression in the surround of cerebral photothrombosis. *J. Cereb. Blood Flow Metab.*, 1996, 16: 906–914.

Schwarz, S., Hacke, W. and Schwab, S. Magnetic evoked potentials in neurocritical care patients with acute brainstem lesions. *J. Neurol. Sci.*, 2000, 172: 30–37.

Seitz, R.J., Hoflich, P., Binkofski, F., et al. Role of the premotor cortex in recovery from middle cerebral artery infarction. *Arch. Neurol.*, 1998, 55: 1081–1088.

Shimizu, T., Hosaki, A., Hino, T., Sato, M., Komori, T., Hirai, S. and Rossini, P.M. Motor cortical disinhibition in the unaffected hemisphere after unilateral cortical stroke. *Brain*, 2002, 125: 1896–1907.

Steultjens, E.M., Dekker, J., Bouter, L.M., van de Nes, J.C., Cup, E.H. and Van den Ende, C.H. Occupational therapy for stroke patients: a systematic review. *Stroke*, 2003, 34: 676–687.

Taub, E., Miller, N.E., Novack, T.A., Cook, E.W., Fleming, W.C., Nepomuceno, C.S., Conell, J.S. and Crago, J.E.. Technique to improve chronic motor deficit after stroke. *Arch. Phys. Med. Rehabil.*, 1993, 74: 347–354.

Thickbroom, G.W., Sammut, R. and Mastaglia, F.L. Magnetic stimulation mapping of motor cortex: factors contributing to map area. Electroencephalogr *Clin. Neurophysiol.*, 1998, 109: 79–84.

Thickbroom, G.W., Byrnes, M.L., Archer, S.A. and Mastaglia, F.L. Motor outcome after subcortical stroke: MEPs correlate with hand strength but not dexterity. *Clin. Neurophysiol.*, 2002, 113: 2025–2029.

Timmerhuis, T.P., Hageman, G., Oosterloo, S.J. and Rozeboom, A.R. The prognostic value of cortical magnetic stimulation in acute middle cerebral artery infarction compared to other parameters. *Clin. Neurol. Neurosurg.*, 1996, 98: 231–236.

Traversa, R., Cicinelli, P., Bassi, A., Rossini, P.M. and Bernardi, G. Mapping of motor cortical reorganization after stroke. *Stroke*, 1997, 28: 110–117.

Traversa, R., Cicinelli, P., Oliveri, M., Palmieri, M.G., Filippi, M.M., Pasqualetti, P. and Rossini, P.M. Neurophysiological follow-up of motor cortical output in stroke patients. *Clin. Neurophysiol.*, 2000, 111: 1695–1703.

Triggs, W.J., Cros, D., Macdonell, R.A.L., Chiappa, K.H., Fang, J. and Day, B.J. Cortical and spinal motor excitability during the transcranial magnetic stimulation silent period in humans. *Brain Res.*, 1993, 628: 39–48.

Trompetto, C., Assini, A., Buccolieri, A., Marchese, R. and Abbruzzese, G. Motor recovery following stroke: a transcranial magnetic stimulation study. *Clin. Neurophysiol.*, 2000, 111: 1860–1867.

Turton, A., Wroe, S., Trepte, N., Fraser, C. and Lemon, R.N. Contralateral and ipsilateral EMG responses to transcranial magnetic stimulation during recovery of arm and hand function after stroke. *Electroencephalogr. Clin. Neurophysiol.*, 1996, 101: 316–328.

Van der Lee, J.H., Snels, I.A., Beckerman, H., Lankhorst, G.J., Wagenaar, R.C. and Bouter, L.M. Exercise therapy for arm function in stroke patients: a systematic review of randomized controlled trials *Clin. Rehabil.*, 2001, 15: 20–31.

Vang, C., Dunbabin, D. and Kilpatrick, D. Correlation between functional and electrophysiological recovery in acute ischemic stroke. *Stroke*, 1999, 30: 2126–2130.

Von Giesen, H.-J., Roick, H. and Benecke, R. Inhibitory actions of motor cortex following unilateral brain lesions as studied by magnetic brain stimulation. *Exp. Brain Res.*, 1994, 99: 84–96.

Walker-Batson, D.W., Smith, P., Curtis, S., Unwin, H. and Greenlee, R. Amphetamine paired with physical therapy accelerates motor recovery after stroke. *Stroke*, 1995, 26, 2254–2259.

Wassermann, E.M., McShane, L.M., Hallett, M. and Cohen, L.G. Noninvasive mapping of muscle representations in human motor cortex. *Electroencephalogr. Clin. Neurophysiol.*, 1992, 85: 1–8.

Wassermann, E.M., Pascual-Leone, A. and Hallett, M. Cortical motor representation of the ipsilateral hand and arm. *Exp. Brain. Res.*, 1994, 100: 121–132.

Weiller, C., Chollet, F., Friston, K.J., Wise, R.J.S. and Frackowiak, R.S.J. Functional reorganization of the brain in recovery from striatocapsular infarction in man. *Ann. Neurol.*, 1992, 31: 463–472.

Wolf, S.L., Lecraw, D.E., Barton, L.A. and Jann, B. Forced use of hemiplegic upper extremities to reverse the effect of learned nonuse among chronic stroke and head-injured patients. *Exper. Neurol.*, 1989, 104: 125–132.

Ziemann, U., Lönnecker, S., Steinhoff, B.J. and Paulus, W. The effect of lorazepam on the motor cortical excitability in man. *Exp. Brain Res.*, 1996, 109: 127–135.

Ziemann, U., Ishii, K., Borgheresi, A., Yaseen, Z., Battaglia, F., Hallett, M., Cincotta, M. and Wassermann, E.M. Dissociation of the pathways mediating ipsilateral and contralateral motor-evoked potentials in human hand and arm muscles. *J. Physiol.*, 1999, 518: 895–906.

Transcranial Magnetic Stimulation and Transcranial Direct Current Stimulation (Supplements to Clinical Neurophysiology, Vol. 56)
Editors: W. Paulus, F. Tergau, M.A. Nitsche, J.C. Rothwell, U. Ziemann, M. Hallett

Chapter 38

Cortical silent period is shortened in restless legs syndrome independently from circadian rhythm

K. Stiasny-Kolster[a,*], H. Haeske[a], F. Tergau[b], H.-H. Müller[c], H.-J. Braune[a] and W.H. Oertel[a]

[a] *Department of Neurology, Center of Nervous Diseases, Philipps-University of Marburg, D-35033 Marburg (Germany)*
[b] *Department of Clinical Neurophysiology, University of Göttingen, Göttingen (Germany)*
[c] *Institute for Medical Biometry and Epidemiology, Medical Center for Methodology and Health Research, Philipps-University of Marburg, D-35033 Marburg (Germany)*

1. Introduction

Restless legs syndrome (RLS) is a sensorimotor disorder with unpleasant sensations in the legs associated with an irresistible urge to move. As characteristic features of RLS, symptoms occur at rest, are mostly pronounced in the evening and therefore, may lead to severe sleep disturbances. Almost all patients with RLS have periodic limb movements (PLM) in sleep which additionally contribute to sleep fragmentation as they are frequently associated with arousals or awakenings. PLM also occur during wakefulness and may keep the patient from falling asleep. Very little is known about the origin and pathophysiolology of RLS. The resemblance of PLM to the Babinski sign (Smith, 1985) suggests a failure of higher cortical centers and/or in descending pathways resulting in impaired inhibition to the spinal cord. Hyperactive brainstem and spinal cord reflexes (blink reflex, H-reflex) in patients with pure periodic limb movement disorder (PLMD) (Atlas Task Force of the American Sleep Disorders Association, 1997) also suggest impairment of the corticospinal tract (Wechsler et al., 1986; Martinelli et al., 1987). However, blink reflex or H-reflex abnormalities were not detected in patients with RLS (Bucher et al., 1996). TMS, having both excitatory and inhibitory effects, has proven to be a useful tool to investigate the functional integrity of the corticospinal tract. TMS induces motor evoked potentials (MEPs) predominantly in contralateral muscles which are thought to be transmitted by the fast-conducting pyramidal tract fibers. Also, inhibitory effects can be elicited by TMS in a voluntarily contracted muscle. One of those phenomena is called cortical Silent Period (SP) which directly follows the MEP in the electromyogram. The SP is thought to be due to inhibitory mechanisms mainly at the level of the motor cortex (Hallett, 1995).

* *Correspondence to*: Dr. Karin Stiasny-Kolster, MD, Department of Neurology, Center of Nervous Diseases, Philipps-University of Marburg, Rudolf-Bultmann-Strasse 8, D-35033 Marburg, Germany.
Tel: 0049-6421-28-65217; Fax: 0049-6421-28-65307;
E-mail: stiasny@mailer.uni-marburg.de

Assuming RLS to be caused by an impairment of inhibitory circuits we hypothesized that the SP is shortened in patients with RLS. Since symptomatology of RLS shows a circadian rhythm with aggravation in the evening and night (Trenkwalder et al., 1999) we sought to elucidate the question whether this relevant inhibitory TMS parameter correlates with the diurnal changes of RLS symptoms or whether it is a general phenomenon independent of the physiological pattern of circadian periodicity. Because of the preponderance of RLS symptoms in the legs rather than in the arms we investigated the upper and lower limbs suspecting abnormalities to be present or more pronounced in the legs. To investigate the influence of levodopa, which is known to significantly improve RLS symptoms, we performed TMS before and after the intake of levodopa.

2. Methods

2.1. Patients and subjects

Fifteen patients (10 women and 5 men, mean age 55.4 ± 9.3, range 38–72 years) with idiopathic RLS (Walters, 1995) for 16.8 ± 11.4 years (range 3–40 years) were included. Neurological examination revealed no evidence of other neurological disease. All patients had polysomnography prior to the study to confirm diagnosis and to further determine the severity of RLS. At study entry, the physician rated the patients as extremely ill ($n = 3$), severely ill ($n = 7$), markedly ill ($n = 4$) and moderately ill ($n = 1$) according to the Clinical Global Impression Scale. In all patients, only the legs but not arms were affected. All patients were already on RLS specific medication on presentation to our clinic. Twelve patients had previously been treated with levodopa, one with pergolide, one with levodopa plus pergolide and one patient with zolpidem. In all patients, RLS medication was stopped prior to TMS studies (at least 2 days for levodopa and 1 week for dopamine agonists). The control group consisted of 15 age and sex matched healthy subjects (10 women and five men, mean age 55.4 ± 9.6, range 38–71 years). Patients and controls were not allowed to take any other centrally active drugs apart from RLS medication in the 4 weeks prior to testing. Chronic renal failure, spinal cord lesions, rheumatoid arthritis, polyneuropathy, other diseases of the central nervous system or complaints of other sleep disorders and shift or night work were considered as general exclusion criteria. Experiments were performed in accordance to the Declaration of Helsinki and approved by the local ethics committee. Written informed consent was given by all participants.

2.2. Technique

TMS studies were performed about 8 am in the morning and 8 pm in the evening. The participants reclined on a comfortable bed in a quiet room. Surface electromyographic (EMG) recordings were made from the left abductor digiti minimi (ADM) and tibialis anterior (TA) muscles in a belly-to-tendon montage. The amplified and bandpass filtered (1 Hz to 10 kHz) raw EMG signals were displayed on a screen of a conventional four-channel EMG system (Nihon Kohden Neuropack 4) with a sensitivity of 0.5 mV per division and were recorded on paper. The duration of the analysis time was 100 to 300 ms. Focal TMS was delivered to the right motor cortex through a flat round coil (14 cm outer diameter) using a Novametrix Magstim 200 stimulator. The maximum magnetic field strength was 1.5 T pulsed for 100 μs. Clockwise currents were used as they are preferential for the right hemisphere. The coil was placed tangential to the skull, with its center over the vertex and with the lateral bent of the coil above the hand area crossing the central sulcus over the hand area (for the ADM) or was placed over CPZ with the anterior bent of the coil over the leg area crossing the interhemispheric line for activation of the TA. The optimal position was finally determined by moving the coil in small steps around the presumed area of the right motor cortex and was defined as the site where stimuli of slightly suprathreshold intensity consistently yielded the largest motor evoked potentials (MEPs) in the target muscle. Measurements were reproduced five times for each parameter.

2.3. Active motor threshold, silent period threshold, central motor conduction time

Active motor threshold (AMT) was determined in the isometrically moderately activated ADM and TA muscle (approximately 10% of maximum voluntary contraction) and was defined as the minimum stimulus intensity that produced MEPs of at least 200 μV. Silent period threshold (SPT) was defined as the lowest stimulus intensity that produced a SP in the moderately active muscle. The threshold intensities were approached by increasing stimulus intensity in steps of 5% beginning at 30% of the maximal output of the stimulator. For calculation of the central motor conduction time (CMCT) we recorded the shortest F-wave latency and the corresponding M-latency evoked by supramaximal electrical stimulation of the ulnar nerve at the wrist and peroneal nerve in the popliteal fossa respectively. CMCT was obtained as follows: MEP latency − $[1/2 \times (M + F - 1)]$. Motor potentials were evoked at stimulus intensities 50% above the excitatory threshold.

2.4. Duration of the silent period

The silent period was determined in the isometrically moderately active ADM and TA muscle (approximately 10% of the maximum voluntary contraction, monitored by an auditory feedback of the EMG signal) at stimulus intensities 50% above the silent period threshold. The silent period was defined from the time of the MEP onset to the reoccurrence of continuous voluntary EMG activity (Inghilleri et al., 1993).

2.5. Levodopa administration

In RLS patients ($n = 14$) all measurements were performed again on another day after patients received 200/50 mg levodopa/benserazide 1.5 h prior to the evening measurements.

2.6. Data analysis

Quantitative values were calculated as number of values, mean ± standard deviation, minimum and maximum. In Fig. 1 median and quartiles were plotted for the box instead of mean ± standard deviation for a more adequate presentation of probably non-normally distributed data. Differences between cases and 1:1 matched controls were tested by using Wilcoxon–Mann–Whitney statistics. Intra-individual comparisons were performed by using the Wilcoxon signed rank test. The significance level was set at $\alpha = 5\%$. Interpretation of the results has to be exploratory.

3. Results

3.1. Silent period threshold, active motor threshold, central motor conduction time

Silent period thresholds tended to be higher in RLS patients compared to controls in the evening and the morning. This tendency was more pronounced in the TA muscle than in the ADM muscle. Active motor thresholds (AMT) in the TA muscle were higher in RLS patients than in controls both in the evening and in the morning. There was also a slight tendency of AMT in the ADM muscle being higher in RLS patients. Evening-morning ratios between patients and controls did not significantly differ. Central motor conduction time was similar in both groups. Mean values, standard deviations and p values are summarized in Table 1.

3.2. Silent period

The duration of the silent period in the TA muscle was much shorter in RLS patients (90.9 ± 17.7 ms) compared to controls (126.3 ± 45.1 ms) when measured in the evening ($p = 0.013$). Likewise, when measurements were performed in the morning silent period in the TA muscle was shorter in RLS patients (95.2 ± 22.5 ms) than in controls (131.7 ± 66.0 ms; $p = 0.080$). There was a difference in the duration of the SP measured in the ADM muscle between RLS patients and controls in the evening (122.7 ± 32.5 ms vs. 136.5 ± 56.1 ms, $p = 0.751$) and the morning (118.7 ± 32.4 ms vs. 138.9 ± 52.2 ms, $p = 0.383$). Without reaching statistical significance

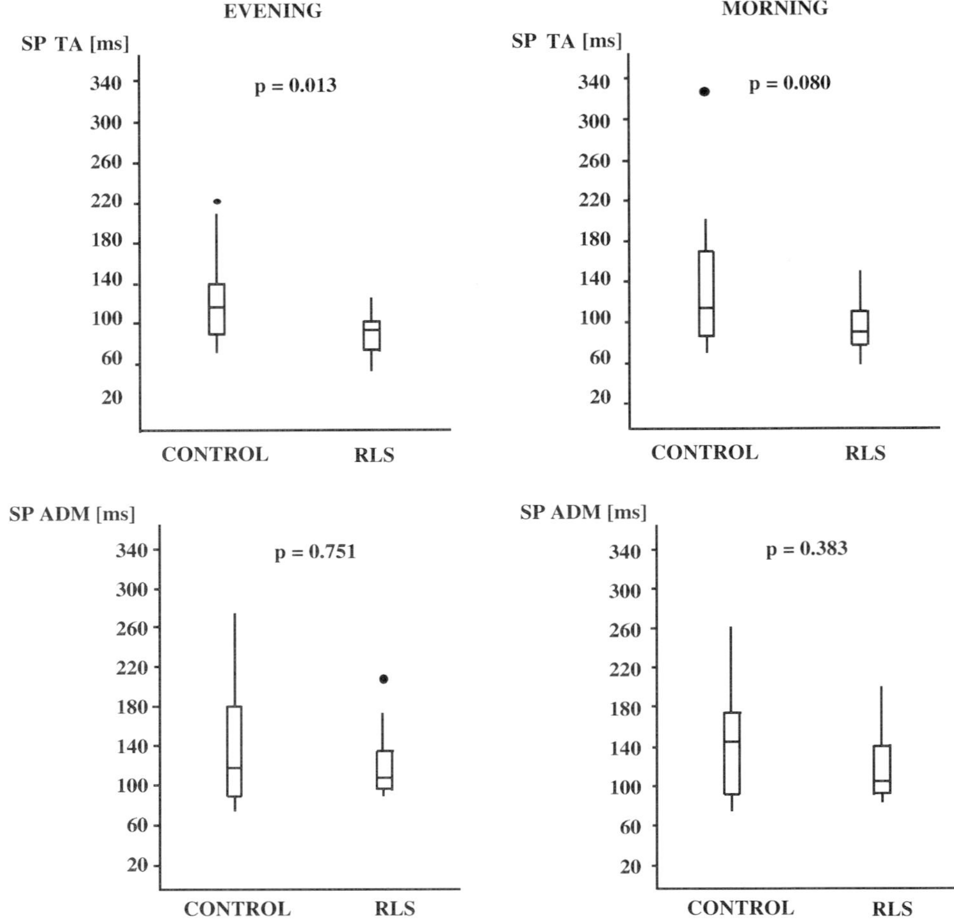

Fig. 1. Median, first and third quartile and range of silent period duration in the tibialis anterior (TA) and abductor digiti minimi (ADM) muscles).

these differences also indicate a trend of SP in the ADM to be shortened in RLS patients compared to controls. Evening-morning ratios did not significantly differ for both groups (see Table 2).

3.2. *Influence of levodopa*

An evening dose of levodopa prolonged the SP in both muscles ($n = 14$). This prolongation was mostly pronounced in the TA when measurements were performed shortly after the intake of levodopa (92.7 ± 16.9 vs. 107.6 ± 23.8; $p = 0.002$) (see Table 3). Levodopa had no influence on silent period thresholds or active motor thresholds (data not shown).

4. Discussion

This is the first study investigating the relation between the cortical silent period (SP) in leg and arm muscles and circadian rhythm in RLS symptomatology. We found that the SP in the leg muscle is considerably shortened in patients with RLS when measured in the evening with a similar shortening of the SP in the morning. The shortening of the SP in

TABLE 1

CENTRAL MOTOR CONDUCTION TIME (CMCT), SILENT PERIOD THRESHOLDS (SPT) AND ACTIVE MOTOR THRESHOLDS (AMT) OF LEG AND ARM MUSCLES IN RLS PATIENTS AND CONTROLS ($N = 15$)

	RLS patients (mean ± SD)	Controls (mean ± SD)	Wilcoxon–Mann–Whitney test
CMCT TA (ms) evening	10.7 ± 3.4	11.3 ± 1.5 (n = 14)	$p = 0.533$
CMCT TA (ms) morning	11.7 ± 2.7	13.0 ± 1.8 (n = 14)	$p = 0.186$
CMCT ADM (ms) evening	6.5 ± 1.4	6.4 ± 1.5	$p = 1.000$
CMCT ADM (ms) morning	5.8 ± 1.4	6.7 ± 1.4	$p = 0.116$
SPT TA (%) evening	55.0 ± 11.3	48.7 ± 7.2	$p = 0.064$
SPT TA (%) morning	53.0 ± 8.0	48.7 ± 5.8	$p = 0.074$
SPT TA evening/morning	1.03 ± 0.07	1.0 ± 0.1	$p = 0.297$
SPT ADM (%) evening	41.3 ± 8.8	37.0 ± 4.6	$p = 0.140$
SPT ADM (%) morning	38.7 ± 5.2	37.0 ± 4.1	$p = 0.476$
SPT ADM evening/morning	1.07 ± 0.16	1.0 ± 0.11	$p = 0.258$
AMT TA (%) evening	52.3 ± 6.2	46.7 ± 6.2	$p = 0.013$
AMT TA (%) morning	52.0 ± 7.3	46.0 ± 6.3	$p = 0.015$
AMT TA evening/morning	1.01 ± 0.1	1.02 ± 0.08	$p = 0.644$
AMT ADM (%) evening	42.7 ± 7.3	40.7 ± 7.0	$p = 0.410$
AMT ADM (%) morning	41.7 ± 6.5	38.7 ± 6.4	$p = 0.193$
AMT ADM evening/morning	1.03 ± 0.17	1.06 ± 0.12	$p = 0.717$

TA: tibialis anterior muscle; ADM: abductor digiti minimi muscle; SD: standard deviation; %: percentage of maximum stimulator output.

TABLE 2

MEANS AND STANDARD DEVIATION OF SILENT PERIOD DURATION IN LEG AND ARM MUSCLES

	RLS patients ($n = 15$)	Controls ($n = 15$)	Wilcoxon–Mann–Whitney test
SP TA (ms) evening	90.9 ± 17.7	126.3 ± 45.1	$p = 0.013$
SP TA (ms) morning	95.2 ± 22.5	131.7 ± 66.0	$p = 0.080$
SP TA evening/morning	0.97 ± 0.13	1.01 ± 0.16	$p = 0.325$
SP ADM (ms) evening	122.7 ± 32.5	136.5 ± 56.1	$p = 0.751$
SP ADM (ms) morning	118.7 ± 32.4	138.9 ± 52.2	$p = 0.383$
SP ADM evening/morning	1.06 ± 0.25	0.98 ± 0.12	$p = 0.345$
SP TA/ADM (ms) evening	0.78 ± 0.23	0.97 ± 0.26	$p = 0.061$
SP TA/ADM (ms) morning	0.83 ± 0.18	0.95 ± 0.22	$p = 0.089$

TA: tibialis anterior muscle; ADM: abductor digiti minimi muscle; SP: silent period.

TABLE 3

MEANS AND STANDARD DEVIATION OF SILENT PERIOD DURATION IN LEG AND ARM MUSCLES AFTER ADMINISTRATION OF 200/50 MG LEVODOPA/BENSERAZIDE ONE AND A HALF HOURS PRIOR TO THE EVENING MEASUREMENTS

	Untreated (n = 14)	200 mg levodopa (n = 14)	Wilcoxon signed rank test
SP TA (ms) evening	92.7 ± 16.9	107.6 ± 23.8	$p = 0.002$
SP TA (ms) morning	97.7 ± 21.1	103.0 ± 21.3	$p = 0.600$
SP ADM (ms) evening	124.0 ± 33.3	132.6 ± 42.6	$p = 0.391$
SP ADM (ms) morning	118.9 ± 33.6	124.6 ± 37.7	$p = 0.418$

TA: tibialis anterior muscle; ADM: abductor digiti minimi muscle; SP: silent period.

the arm muscle is much less pronounced compared to the legs. Comparisons of evening–morning ratios suggest that the impairment of motor-cortical inhibition does not correlate with circadian changes of symptomatology of RLS.

4.1. Silent period duration

At present there is accumulating evidence that the SP is generated at the motor cortical level resulting from intracortical inhibition and at most only the initial part is due to spinal mechanisms. Intracortical inhibition is thought to be mediated by inhibitory interneurons which are activated via recurrent collaterals from pyramidal cell axons and/or nerve fibers afferent to the motor cortex (Inghilleri et al., 1993; Roick et al., 1993; Davey et al., 1994; Schnitzler and Benecke 1994; Hallett 1995; Classen et al., 1997; Ziemann et al., 1997; Tergau et al., 1999).

In patients with lesions in the primary motor cortex the silent period is shortened (Von Giesen et al., 1994) or abolished (Schnitzler and Benecke, 1994) in muscles contralateral to the hemispheric lesions. Lesions in other motor competent cortical areas which are afferent to the primary motor cortex or thalamic lesions are associated with a prolongation of the silent period (Von Giesen et al., 1994; Faig and Busse, 1996). Shorter SP in Parkinson's disease (Haug et al., 1992; Priori et al., 1994; Nakashima et al., 1995) or Tourette syndrome (Ziemann et al., 1997) and prolonged SP in Huntington's disease (Priori et al., 1994) might reflex basal ganglia influence over the motor cortex. In RLS a significant shortening of the SP in the TA muscle with a less altered SP in ADM muscle is thus suspicious for an imbalance in the intrinsic network of the leg area of the primary motor cortex or an increased excitatory input to this area. Lesions within the primary motor cortex can almost be excluded because of the normal neurological examination, normal CMCT and the lack of structural abnormalities in MRI studies in idiopathic RLS (Bucher et al., 1996). The fact that disagreeable sensory symptoms in the legs are a major feature of RLS and that RLS may at least in some forms (Ondo and Jankovic, 1996; Rutkove et al., 1996; Gemignani et al., 1997, 1999) be more common in polyneuropathy suggests that a disorder of sensory processing may be involved in the pathogenesis of RLS. It is feasible that a hyperactivity of the afferent sensory fibers to the sensorimotor cortex may cause increased excitatory input resulting in decreased corticospinal inhibition. Previous paired pulse TMS studies in healthy subjects provided first evidence that afferent input, produced by electrical peripheral-nerve stimulation, is capable of reducing the level of intracortical inhibition by mechanisms unknown so far (Ridding and Rothwell, 1999). The hypothesis of an increased excitatory input is supported by the fact that there is a lower threshold, greater spatial spread, and prolonged duration of the

FR during sleep (Bara-Jimenez et al., 2000). These abnormalities could be explained on the basis of either abnormal sensorimotor integration at the spinal interneuronal level, the loss of supraspinal inhibitory influences or abnormal afferent input, or both (Bara-Jimenez et al., 2000). The shortened SP may also be a secondary phenomenon due to disordered dopaminergic nigrostriatal pathways like in Parkinson's disease resulting in deficient inhibition of afferents to the motor cortex (primarily the leg area). However, most receptor binding studies with positron emission tomography (PET) and single photon emission tomography (SPECT) have found normal presynaptic binding (Trenkwalder et al., 1999; Turjanski et al., 1999; Michaud et al., 2000; Eisensehr et al., 2001) which in contrast is reduced in PD. As in PD patients and also in control subjects (Priori et al., 1994) the SP was lengthened in our RLS patients by levodopa. However, about one and a half hours after levodopa intake, when levodopa plasma levels are supposed to be highest, SP was only significantly lengthened in the leg muscle. It is likely that the basal ganglia play a role at least in this modulating effect. However, it is also feasible that levodopa modulates the duration of the SP through mechanisms directly at the cortical level (Priori et al., 1994).

4.2. Silent period threshold and active motor threshold

Higher SP thresholds (SPT) in RLS patients, with differences being again more impressive in the legs, further argues for an impairment of inhibitory circuits. The duration of the SP depends to some extent on the stimulus intensity defined as 1.5 times the SPT. If the SPT is higher the stimulus for eliciting a SP also increases thus normally leading to a prolongation of the duration of the SP. Contrary we found a shortening of the silent period emphasizing the physiopathological finding. Patients not only had higher silent period thresholds but also had higher active motor thresholds (AMT) thresholds indicating a decreased neuronal excitability of the motor cortex at the membrane level (Ziemann et al., 1997). A rise of AMT seems to contradict our hypothesis of motor-cortical disinhibition, but these findings may represent compensatory mechanisms.

4.3. Circadian changes of motor-cortical disinhibition?

In the present study we recorded TMS parameters for the first time in the morning and in the evening to test the hypothesis whether cortical disinhibition correlates with the circadian pattern of RLS with aggravation of symptoms in the evening and nighttime (Trenkwalder et al., 1999). We found that the duration of the silent period did not significantly differ between morning and evening measurements and may conclude that the mechanisms responsible for shortening of the SP are not involved in the circadian periodicity. Motor disinhibition, shown by SP shortening, may be a general phenomenon in RLS and in interaction with circadian changes of other physiopathological features of RLS. This new finding may provide evidence that a permanent (possibly peripheral or basal ganglia) lesion underlie some characteristics of RLS and that at least at the beginning of the disease intact compensatory mechanisms suppress clinical RLS symptoms during the day. We know that diurnal fluctuations are less pronounced when the disease progresses and that patients may then suffer from RLS symptoms the whole day. A progression of the lesion or a decline of compensatory mechanisms may then abolish the circadian rhythm of RLS symptoms. Since our evening measurements were performed at 8 pm, however, we cannot completely exclude larger differences in the later part of the evening. Possibly correlations to the circadian pattern of RLS symptoms could have come to light if measurements were performed shortly after midnight when RLS symptoms reach a maximum (Trenkwalder et al., 1999).

Previous studies on the silent period have provided controversial findings. Tergau et al. did not find significant differences in the duration of the silent period in daytime measurements. This might be due to the fact that they investigated not the TA but a foot muscle which is probably involved in the RLS symptomatology not as much as the TA. The severity of RLS symptoms in our patients which raises the chance of detecting abnormalities may further have contributed to the different results. Nevertheless, using paired pulse inhibition they found that the whole motor cortex for upper and lower limb muscles is disinhibited in RLS. Intracortical inhibition (ICI) was significantly reduced in more severely affected patients whereas differences to control subjects were less pronounced in a subgroup of patients with milder symptoms (Tergau et al., 1999). From the findings that ICI reduction was more pronounced in the arm than in the leg muscles they concluded that impairment of motor-cortical inhibition is a general phenomenon. Since ICI is unaltered by dysfunction of corticospinal tract or spinal motoneurons (Hanajima et al., 1996) they also concluded that the reduced ICI reflects a disinhibited subcortial input to the cortex. Entezari-Taher et al. (1999) have detected a significant shortening of the silent period in RLS patients both in leg and arm muscles when TMS was performed during the day. Interestingly, the electrically elicited peripheral silent period which is known to depend on spinal inhibitory mechanisms (Shahani and Young, 1973) showed no change as compared with controls (Entezari-Taher et al., 1999). Shortening of the silent period in RLS patients may thus be due to intracortical and afferent input mechanisms and does not reflect altered inhibitory effects at the spinal level.

References

Atlas Task Force of the American Sleep Disorders Association (ASDA) B (1997) The International Classification of Sleep Disorders – Diagnostic and Coding Manual, Rochester, Minnesota.

Bara-Jimenez, W., Aksu, M., Graham, B., Sato, S. and Hallet, M. Periodic limb movements in sleep. State-dependent excitability of the spinal flexor reflex. *Neurology*, 2000, 54: 1609–1615.

Bucher, S.F., Trenkwalder, C. and Oertel, W.H. Reflex studies and MRI in the restless legs syndrome. *Acta. Neurol. Scand.*, 1996, 94: 145–150.

Classen, J., Schnitzler, A., Binkofski, F., Werhahn, K.J., Kim, Y.S., Kessler, K.R. and Benecke, R. The motor syndrome associated with exaggerated inhibition within the primary motor cortex of patients with hemiparetic stroke. *Brain*, 1997, 120: 605–619.

Davey, N.J., Romaiguere, P., Maskill, D.W. and Ellaway, P.H. Suppression of voluntary motor activity revealed using transcranial magnetic stimulation of the motor cortex in man. *J. Physiol.*, 1994, 477: 223–235.

Eisensehr, I., Wetter, T.C., Linke, R., Noachtar, S., Von Lindeiner, H., Gildehaus, F.J., Trenkwalder, C. and Tatsch, K. Normal IPT and IBZM SPECT in drug-naive and levodopa-treated idiopathic restless legs syndrome. *Neurology*, 2001, 57: 1307–1309.

Entezari-Taher, M., Singleton, J.R., Jones, C.R., Meekins, G., Petajan, J.H. and Smith, A.G. Changes in excitability of motor cortical circuitry in primary restless legs syndrome. [In Process Citation.] *Neurology*, 1999, 53: 1201–1205.

Faig, J. and Busse, O. Silent period evoked by transcranial magnetic stimulation in unilateral thalamic infarcts. *J. Neurol. Sci.*, 1996, 142: 85–92.

Gemignani, F., Marbini, A., Di Giovanni, G., Salih, S., Margarito, F.P., Pavesi, G. and Terzano, M.G. Cryoglobulinaemic neuropathy manifesting with restless legs syndrome. *J. Neurol. Sci.*, 1997, 152: 218–223.

Gemignani, F., Marbini, A., Di Giovanni, G., Salih, S. and Terzano, M.G. Charcot-Marie-Tooth disease type 2 with restless legs syndrome. *Neurology*, 1999, 52: 1064–1066.

Hallett, M. Transcranial magnetic stimulation. Negative effects. *Adv. Neurol.*, 1995, 67: 107–113.

Hanajima, R., Ugawa, Y., Terao, Y., Ogata, K. and Kanazawa, I. Ipsilateral cortico-cortical inhibition of the motor cortex in various neurological disorders. *J. Neurol. Sci.*, 1996, 140: 109–116.

Haug, B.A., Schonle, P.W., Knobloch, C. and Kohne, M. Silent period measurement revives as a valuable diagnostic tool with transcranial magnetic stimulation. *Electroencephalogr. Clin. Neurophysiol.*, 1992, 85: 158–160.

Inghilleri, M., Berardelli, A., Cruccu, G. and Manfredi, M. Silent period evoked by transcranial stimulation of the human cortex and cervicomedullary junction. *J. Physiol.* (Lond), 1993, 466: 521–534.

Martinelli, P., Coccagna, G. and Lugaresi, E. Nocturnal myoclonus, restless legs syndrome, and abnormal electrophysiological findings [letter]. *Ann. Neurol.*, 1987, 21: 515.

Michaud, M., Soucy, J.P., Chabli, A., Lavigne, G. and Montplaisir, J. Spect imaging of pre- and postsynaptic dopaminergic functions in patients with restless legs syndrome. *Sleep*, 2000, 23: A129.

Nakashima, K., Wang, Y., Shimoda, M., Sakuma, K. and Takahashi, K. Shortened silent period produced by magnetic cortical stimulation in patients with Parkinson's disease. *J. Neurol. Sci.*, 1995, 130: 209–214.

Ondo, W. and Jankovic, J. Restless legs syndrome: clinicoetiologic correlates. *Neurology*, 1996, 47: 1435–1441.

Priori, A., Berardelli, A., Inghilleri, M., Accornero, N. and Manfredi, M. Motor cortical inhibition and the dopaminergic system. Pharmacological changes in the silent period after transcranial brain stimulation in normal subjects, patients with

Parkinson's disease and drug-induced parkinsonism. *Brain*, 1994a, 117: 317–323.

Priori, A., Berardelli, A., Inghilleri, M., Polidori, L. and Manfredi, M. Electromyographic silent period after transcranial brain stimulation in Huntington's disease. *Mov. Disord.*, 1994b, 9: 178–182.

Ridding, M.C. and Rothwell, J.C. Afferent input and cortical organisation: a study with magnetic stimulation. *Exp. Brain Res.*, 1999, 126: 536–544.

Roick, H., von Giesen, H.-J. and Benecke, R. On the origin of the postexcitatory inhibition seen after transcranial magnetic brain stimulation in awake human subjects. *Exp. Brain Res.*, 1993, 94: 489–498.

Rutkove, S.B., Matheson. J.K. and Logigian, E.L. Restless legs syndrome in patients with polyneuropathy. *Muscle Nerve*, 1996, 19: 670–672.

Schnitzler, A. and Benecke, R. The silent period after transcranial magnetic stimulation is of exclusive cortical origin: evidence from isolated cortical ischemic lesions in man. *Neurosci. Lett.*, 1994, 180: 41–45.

Shahani, B.T. and Young, R.R. *Studies of the normal human silent period*. Karger, Basel, 1973.

Smith, R.C. Relationship of periodic movements in sleep (nocturnal myoclonus) and the babinski sign. *Sleep*, 1985, 8: 239–243.

Tergau, F., Wanschura, V., Canelo, M., Wischer, S., Wassermann. E.M., Ziemann, U. and Paulus, W. Complete suppression of voluntary motor drive during the silent period after transcranial magnetic stimulation. *Exp. Brain Res.*, 1999a, 124: 447–454.

Tergau, F., Wischer, S. and Paulus, W. Motor system excitability in patients with restless legs syndrome. *Neurology*, 1999b, 52: 1060–1063.

Trenkwalder, C., Hening, W.A., Walters, A.S., Campbell, S.S., Rahman, K and Chokroverty, S. Circadian rhythm of periodic limb movements and sensory symptoms of restless legs syndrome. *Mov. Disord.*, 1999a, 14: 102–110.

Trenkwalder, C., Walters, A.S., Hening, W.A., Chokroverty, S., Antonini, A., Dhawan, V. and Eidelberg, D. Positron emission tomographic studies in restless legs syndrome. *Mov. Disord.*, 1999b, 14: 141–145.

Turjanski, N., Lees, A.J. and Brooks, D.J. Striatal dopaminergic function in restless legs syndrome – 18F-dopa and 11C-raclopride PET studies. *Neurology*, 1999, 52: 932–937.

Von Giesen, H.-J., Roick, H. and Benecke, R. Inhibitory action of motor cortex following unilateral brain lesions as studied by magnetic brain stimulation. *Exp. Brain Res.*, 1994, 99: 84–96.

Walters, A.S. Toward a better definition of the restless legs syndrome. The International Restless Legs Syndrome Study Group. *Mov. Disord.*, 1995, 10: 634–642.

Wechsler, L.R., Stakes, J.W., Bhaghwan, T.S. and Busis, N.A. Periodic leg movements of sleep (nocturnal myoclonus): an electrophysiological study. *Ann. Neurol.*, 1986, 19: 168–173.

Ziemann, U., Paulus. W. and Rothenberger, A. Decreased motor inhibition in Tourette's disorder: evidence from transcranial magnetic stimulation. *Am. J. Psychiatry*, 1997, 154: 1277–1284.

Transcranial Magnetic Stimulation and Transcranial Direct Current Stimulation (Supplements to Clinical Neurophysiology, Vol. 56)
Editors: W. Paulus, F. Tergau, M.A. Nitsche, J.C. Rothwell, U. Ziemann, M. Hallett

Chapter 39

Repetitive magnetic stimulation for the treatment of chronic pain conditions

Jens D. Rollnik[a,*], Jan Däuper[a], Stefanie Wüstefeld[a], Shirin Mansouri[a], Mathias Karst[b], Matthias Fink[c], Andon Kossev[d] and Reinhard Dengler[a]

[a] *Department of Neurology and Clinical Neurophysiology,*
[b] *Department of Anesthesiology, Pain Clinic,*
[c] *Department of Physical Medicine and Rehabilitation, Medical School of Hannover, D-30623 Hannover (Germany)*
[d] *Department of Biophysics, Bulgarian Academy of Sciences, Sofia (Bulgaria)*

1. Introduction

Repetitive transcranial magnetic stimulation (rTMS) applied to the primary motor cortex (M1) may have some pain reducing effects in chronic pain conditions (Lefaucheur et al., 2001a, b). The mode of action might be comparable to electrical and invasive chronic motor cortex stimulation (MCS) (Tsubokawa et al., 1993). The pain-inhibiting mechanism of MCS is still a matter of discussion. However, it may be hypothesized that thalamic nuclei connected with motor and premotor cortices are activated by MCS (García-Larrea et al., 1999). This thalamic activation would entail a cascade of synaptic events in pain-related structures receiving afferents from these nuclei, including the medial thalamus, anterior cingulate, and upper brainstem (García-Larrea et al., 1999). While MCS is a well established neurosurgical procedure, the value of rTMS as a treatment in chronic pain conditions is still questionable (Rollnik et al., 2002).

Repetitive magnetic stimulation (rMS) administered to peripheral structures (muscle, tendon) has also been tried in chronic myofascial and musculoskeletal pain syndromes (Pujol et al., 1998; Smania et al., 2003). It has been suggested that the pain reducing mechanism of rMS is similar to that of transcutaneous electrical nerve stimulation (TENS) (Pujol et al., 1998). However, the therapeutic potential of rMS in myofascial and musculoskeletal pain conditions remains unclear, yet.

We have performed two studies in order to evaluate antalgic efficacy and safety of rTMS administered to M1 (Study 1), and peripheral rMS administered to the extensor carpi radialis muscle in chronic lateral epicondylitis patients.

* *Correspondence to*: Prof. Jens D. Rollnik, Medical School of Hannover, Department of Neurology and Clinical Neurophysiology, D-30623 Hannover, Germany.
Tel: +495115323578; Fax +495115323115;
E-mail: rollnik.jens@mh-hannover.de

2. Subjects and Methods

Primary outcome parameter in both studies was pain intensity using a conventional visual analog scale

(VAS), ranging from 0 to 100 mm (0 = “no pain at all”, 100 = “unbearable pain”). Patients were required to give three consecutive VAS ratings before and at each follow-up examination, in order to compute a mean of these three measurements. All patients in both studies gave written informed consent to participate in the study as required by local ethics committee.

2.1. *Study 1 (rTMS of M1)*

We enrolled 12 patients (6 males) with intractable chronic pain syndromes from our Pain Clinic, aged 33–67 years (mean 51.3, SD = 12.6) (Rollnik et al., 2002, Table 1). Mean duration of chronic pain was 2.7 years (SD = 2.3). Patients showed moderate depressive symptoms with a mean Beck Depression Inventory (BDI) value of 14.5 (SD = 10.2). Five of them were suffering from chronic pain at the upper, and six at the lower extremities, one patient had facial pain. The pain etiologies were brachial plexus impairment ($n = 2$), peripheral nerve lesion ($n = 1$), radiculopathy ($n = 1$), sympathetic dystrophy ($n = 2$), polyneuropathy ($n = 1$), myelopathy ($n = 2$), post herpetic neuralgia ($n = 1$), phantom limb ($n = 1$), and osteomyelitis ($n = 1$). rTMS was performed with a MagstimRapid (The Magstim Company, Whitland, Great Britain). On the initial visit the motor threshold (MT) of a muscle close to the pain region (for upper extremity: abductor digiti quinti muscle; for lower extremity: tibialis anterior muscle) was determined. Mean MT in our sample was 64.5% (± 7.8) of maximum stimulator output. Stimulation site was M1 contralateral to the pain site. A figure-8-shaped coil was used to stimulate the corresponding leg area (current in the coil was directed anteriorly) and a circular coil (current direction in the coil was anticlockwise when viewed from above) over vertex for the arm area. We performed 20 2-s, 20 Hz stimulations with 80% of motor threshold intensity over 20 min (800 pulses per session) as active treatment once. Sham stimulation occurred in the same manner as active rTMS, except that the angle of the coil, rather than being tangential to the skull was at 45° off the skull. In a sequence-controlled cross-over design, sham and active treatment were given at random order (on different days), six subjects started with placebo and six with verum rTMS.

2.2. *Study 2 (rMS in lateral epicondylitis)*

We enrolled 10 patients (two males, eight females) with therapy-resistant chronic lateral epicondylitis (tennis elbow) from the Department of Physical Medicine and Rehabilitation, Medical School of Hannover, aged 41 to 61 years (mean 44.4, SD = 6.0). All participants presented with a tender extensor carpi radialis muscle on the affected side (left elbow: $n = 4$, right elbow: $n = 6$). Duration of symptoms was 6 months at least, there was no history of surgical treatment in any of the patients. rMS was performed with a MagstimRapid (see above). On the initial visit, stimulation intensity was adjusted in each patient based on the subjectively reported pain threshold (starting at 15% of maximal stimulator output, increasing intensity by 2% steps). Stimulation site was the area of tender extensor carpi radialis muscle identified by palpation. A figure-8-shaped coil was used to enable focal stimulation. We performed 30 5-s, 20 Hz stimulations over 15 min (3000 pulses per session) as active treatment once. Sham stimulation occurred in the same manner as active rMS, except that the angle of the coil, rather than being tangential to the muscle was at 45° off the surface. In a sequence-controlled cross-over design, sham and active treatment were given at random order (on different days), five subjects started with sham and five with active rMS.

3. Results

3.1. *Study 1 (rTMS of M1)*

Under active treatment, six out of 12 patients reported an improvement of their symptoms. Mean pain reduction under verum treatment was –4.0% (SD = 14.1, range –32.6% to +16.0%). Under sham rTMS, VAS also decreased (mean –2.3, SD = 8.8, range –20.1% to +12.8%). For the whole group of patients, the difference between both conditions did not reach a level of significance ($p > 0.05$). No severe

TABLE 1

SAMPLE CHARACTERISTICS OF STUDY 1 (ROLLNIK ET AL., 2002)

Patient (initials)	Sex (m/f)	Age (years)	Pain site	Pain etiology	VAS change verum rTMS (%)	VAS change sham rTMS (%)	Motor threshold (%)
G. K.	m	51	left arm	brachial plexus injury	−2.0%	−2.3%	55%
B. M.	m	67	left arm	neuritis of the brachial plexus	−4.7%	+12.8%	67%
M. M.	f	41	right foot	radiculopathy	+4.0%	+2.8%	55%
W. N.	m	58	right hand	sympathetic dystrophy	−17.9%	–	50%
H. R.	m	64	both forearms and chest	cervical myelopathy	−25.3%	−7.4%	63%
W. R.	f	67	both feet	polyneuropathy	−32.6%	−1.1%	70%
P. R.	m	39	left foot	osteomyelitis	+0.4%	+2.3%	52%
B. K.	f	63	right leg	phantom limb	+16.1%	−3.9%	72%
D. V.	m	48	both legs	myelopathy	−15.1%	–	90%
G. K.	f	51	right foot	sympathetic dystrophy	+4.8%	–	80%
B. Z.	f	33	left hand	peripheral nerve lesion	+10.2%	−4.0%	55%
A. H.	f	34	right face	post herpetic neuralgia	+14.3%	−20.1%	65%
Mean* or sum	6/6	51.3 ± 12.6	–	–	−4.0% ± 15.6	−2.3% ± 8.8	64.5% ± 12.1

*Standard deviation is indicated (±).

adverse events could be observed. However, one patient reported the temporary occurrence of headaches at the stimulation site and did not want to participate in the study any longer.

3.2. Study 2 (rMS in lateral epicondylitis)

Immediately after active rMS, VAS was virtually unchanged (1.02, SD = 0.57) and slightly decreased to 0.90 (SD = 0.67) after 5 min, 0.92 (SD = 0.53) after 10 min, and 0.92 (SD = 0.39) 20 min after active rMS (Fig. 1). After sham treatment, the values were very similar: 0.89, SD = 0.28 (immediately after sham rMS), 0.83, SD = 0.25 (5 min post), 0.92, SD = 0.28 (10 min post), and 0.83, SD = 0.24 (20 min post). At no point of time, differences between sham and active intervention reached a level of significance.

4. Discussion

Invasive electrical motor cortex stimulation (MCS) may ameliorate symptoms in intractable chronic pain sufferers (Tsubokawa et al., 1993). Repetitive transcranial magnetic stimulation (rTMS) is a non-invasive and effective tool to stimulate and activate cortical areas. We examined whether rTMS of the motor cortex might be a useful tool in the therapy of chronic intractable pain syndromes (Rollnik et al., 2002). In a pilot study with twelve patients, we could not demonstrate significant differences between active and sham treatment, although some patients

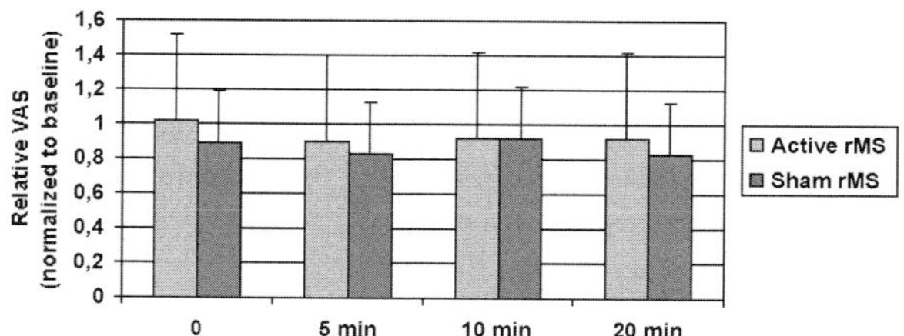

Fig. 1. Study 2: relative VAS (visual analog scale) values (normalized to baseline), 0, 5, 10, and 20 min after active or sham rMS. There were no significant differences at any point of time. Standard deviation on top of bars.

had remarkable benefit from the treatment. The findings of this study are different from previous reports (Lefaucheur et al., 2001a, b). However, it may be hypothesized that different treatment protocols have accounted for controversial results. Taken into account that MCS techniques employ a chronic stimulation, longer rTMS stimulation periods may be considered.

In another study, antalgic efficacy of rMS administered to the extensor carpi radialis muscle in chronic lateral epicondylitis patients has been examined. In contrast to previous findings (Pujol et al., 1998; Smania et al., 2003), results were negative. An explanation for different findings could be patient selection and treatment protocol. While a previous study of Pujol et al. (1998) enrolled a very heterogenous group of patients, participants of our study were suffering from chronic lateral epicondylitis, exclusively. Further, the rMS stimulation parameters of our study were slightly different from previous reports (Smania et al., 2003).

While the results of both studies defy ready summary, repetitive magnetic stimulation – both rTMS (applied to M1) and rMS (applied to the periphery) – failed to show any significant antalgic effects. Further studies are encouraged, employing larger sample sizes and using different stimulation techniques, in order to decide whether repetitive magnetic stimulation might useful in therapy-resistant chronic pain conditions.

Acknowledgements

The study was performed under the institute partnership program (Alexander-von-Humboldt foundation, Bonn, Germany).

References

García-Larrea, L., Peyron, R., Mertens. P., Gregoire. M.C., Lavenne, F., Le Bars, D., Convers, P., Mauguiere, F., Sindou, M. and Laurent, B. Electrical stimulation of the motor cortex for pain control: a combined PET-scan and electrophysiological study. *Pain*, 1999, 83: 259–273.

Lefaucheur, J.P., Drouot, X., Keravel, Y. and Nguyen, J.P. Pain relief induced by repetitive transcranial magnetic stimulation of precentral cortex. *NeuroReport*, 2001a, 12: 2963–2965.

Lefaucheur, J.P., Drouot, X. and Nguyen, J.P. Interventional neurophysiology for pain control: duration of pain relief following repetitive transcranial magnetic stimulation of the motor cortex. *Neurophysiol. Clin.*, 2001b, 31: 247–252.

Pujol, J., Pascual-Leone, A., Doltz, C., Delgado, E., Doltz, J.L. and Aldoma, J. The effect of repetitive magnetic stimulation on localized musculoskelatal pain. *NeuroReport*, 1998, 9: 1745–1748.

Rollnik, J.D., Wüstefeld, S., Däuper, J., Karst, M., Fink, M., Kossev, A. and Dengler, R. Repetitive transcranial magnetic stimulation for the treatment of pain – a pilot study. *Eur. Neurol.*, 2002, 48: 6–10.

Smania, N., Corato, E., Fiaschi, A., Pietropoli, P., Aglioti, S.M. and Tinazzi, M. Therapeutic effects of peripheral repetitive magnetic stimulation on myofascial pain syndrome. *Clin. Neurophysiol.*, 2003, 114: 350–358.

Tsubokawa, T., Katayama, Y., Yamamoto, T., Hirayama, T. and Koyama, S. Chronic motor cortex stimulation in patients with thalamic pain. *J. Neurosurg.*, 1993, 78: 393–401.

Transcranial Magnetic Stimulation and Transcranial Direct Current Stimulation (Supplements to Clinical Neurophysiology, Vol. 56)
Editors: W. Paulus, F. Tergau, M.A. Nitsche, J.C. Rothwell, U. Ziemann, M. Hallett

Chapter 40

Fluctuations of motor cortex excitability in pain syndromes

Peter Schwenkreis[a,*], Christoph Maier[b] and Martin Tegenthoff[a]

[a] *Department of Neurology, BG-Kliniken Bergmannsheil, Ruhr-University, D-44789 Bochum (Germany)*
[b] *Department of Pain Treatment, BG-Kliniken Bergmannsheil, Ruhr-University, D-44789 Bochum (Germany)*

1. Introduction

In patients with chronic pain syndromes, pain may be linked to reorganisation in the primary sensorimotor cortex. This was demonstrated for the primary somatosensory cortex (SI) in patients suffering from phantom limb pain, showing a medial shift of the lip representation (Flor et al., 1995; Birbaumer et al., 1997), as well as in patients suffering from lower back pain, showing an expansion of the cortical back representation (Flor et al., 1997). A similar reorganisation was seen in patients with phantom limb pain in the primary motor cortex (MI) (Dettmers et al., 2001; Karl et al., 2001), which is closely linked to the primary somatosensory cortex via cortical horizontal connections (Kaneko et al., 1994). Several mechanisms might contribute to cortical reorganisation: evidence of axonal sprouting as a possible long-term basis of cortical reorganisation was found in animal experiments in macaque monkeys and in cats several months after a lesion had occurred (Pons et al., 1991; Darian-Smith and Gilbert, 1994). However, other animal experiments suggest that reorganisation can occur rapidly, within minutes to hours after peripheral deafferentation (Donoghue et al., 1990), which cannot be explained by axonal sprouting. It is likely that these rapid plastic changes are based on functional synaptic changes, like changes in synaptic efficacy by NMDA mediated long-term potentiation-like mechanisms (Hess and Donoghue, 1994), and removal of local GABAergic inhibition (Jacobs and Donoghue, 1991). Additionally, an alteration of sodium channels in neuronal membranes may contribute to these rapid plastic changes (Hallett et al., 1999). These mechanisms may be linked to changes in motor cortex excitability, which can be tested by means of transcranial magnetic stimulation (TMS) using different neurophysiological parameters. Whereas motor threshold depends on the excitability of individual neurons and their density in the motor cortex, and is independent from drugs influencing synaptic transmission (Ziemann et al., 1996a), the motor evoked potential (MEP) amplitudes probably depend on postsynaptic as well as on synaptic function (Hallett et al., 1999). However, both motor threshold and MEP amplitudes are also influenced by spinal excitability changes. Exclusively cortical in origin are the phenomena of intracortical inhibition and facilitation as assessed by TMS using a paired pulses paradigm (Kujirai et al.,

* *Correspondence to*: Dr. Peter Schwenkreis, MD, BG-Kliniken Bergmannsheil, Department of Neurology, Buerkle-de-la-Camp-Platz 1, D-44789 Bochum, Germany. Tel.: ++49 234 3026819; Fax: ++49 234 3026888; E-mail: Peter.Schwenkreis@ruhr-uni-bochum.de

1993; Ziemann et al., 1996b). They are thought to reflect the activity of intracortical inhibitory and excitatory interneuronal circuits, and can be modulated by drugs influencing synaptic transmission (Ziemann et al., 1996a).

Here we review studies using TMS to detect changes in motor cortical excitability in acute experimental pain, as well as, in chronic pain syndromes, such as phantom pain or complex regional pain syndrome (CRPS).

2. Acute experimental pain and motor cortex excitability

Valeriani et al. (1999) studied the influence of painful CO_2 laser pulses, delivered on the skin of the right hand, on the MEP amplitudes recorded from the first dorsal interosseus muscle (FDI) after TMS or anodal electrical stimulation of the ipsilateral and the contralateral motor cortex in healthy humans. They found a significant bilateral reduction of the MEP amplitudes after TMS, which started about 160 ms after the laser pulse (mean N1/P1 latency of the laser evoked potentials, LEP), and lasted about 150 ms after stimulation of the contralateral and 100 ms after stimulation of the ipsilateral motor cortex. MEP amplitudes after anodal electric stimulation were not influenced by the laser pulses. Since TMS is thought to activate cortico-spinal neurons transsynaptically, whereas anodal stimulation leads to a direct activation of cortico-spinal axons (Di Lazzaro et al., 1998), it was assumed that this inhibition takes place at the motor cortex. CO_2 laser pulses are able to activate selectively nociceptive afferents (Aδ and C) (Bromm and Treede, 1984), and the N1/P1 component of the LEP is thought to be generated in the second somatosensory area (SII) (Tarkka and Treede, 1993). The authors therefore concluded that phasic nociceptive inputs, with respect to the time course presumably via Aδ afferents, lead to a bilateral inhibition of the motor cortex, which might be mediated by the SII area. In a second study, they demonstrated that CO_2 laser pulses delivered on the hand are also able to reduce the MEP amplitudes evoked by TMS of the motor cortex in proximal muscles (e.g. the biceps muscle) (Valeriani et al., 2001). MEP amplitudes after anodal stimulation of the motor cortex were not affected either. This result was interpreted as evidence for reduced excitability of the whole upper limb motor cortical area due to acute nociceptive inputs. In order to examine the influence of C fibre afferents on motor cortex excitability, Farina et al. (2001) applicated capsaicin on the skin overlying the FDI and the flexor carpi radialis (FCR) muscle. They found a significant reduction of MEP amplitudes from the FDI and FCR muscle after TMS, which started about 20 min after capsaicin application. Indices of peripheral or spinal excitability (M waves, F waves, H reflexes) were not altered. They concluded that tonic C fibre mediated skin pain induces motor cortex inhibition.

Le Pera et al. (2001) assessed the influence of tonic subcutaneous and muscle pain induced by injection of hypertonic (5%) saline on MEP amplitudes after TMS and on H reflex amplitudes, in order to detect excitability changes at a cortical and spinal level. They found an inhibition of the MEP amplitudes in the right abductor pollicis brevis muscle (ADM) after painful injection in the same as well as in a homotopic (FDI) muscle, which persisted even 20 min after the pain had disappeared. No inhibition was present after injection in the contralateral ADM, or after subcutaneous injection. H reflex amplitudes remained unchanged during an initial phase, but became reduced about 1 min after the peak-pain. Therefore these experiments demonstrated a decreased excitability of the motor cortex without spinal excitability changes during an initial phase of tonic muscle pain, whereas in a later phase both cortical and spinal excitability were reduced. With respect to positron emission tomography (PET) data (Svensson et al., 1997), the authors discussed pain-dependent inhibitory inputs on the motor cortex from the SII area.

However, in another TMS study by Romaniello et al. (2000), tonic muscle pain induced by injection of hypertonic saline in the masseter muscle did not influence MEP amplitudes recorded from this muscle. Tonic skin pain evoked by topical application of capsaicin did not alter MEP amplitudes recorded from the masseter muscle either. Therefore, this study failed to demonstrate an inhibitory influence of acute muscle or skin pain on motor cortex excitability. However, MEP in this study were recorded from the voluntary contracted masseter muscle, which might have masked an inhibitory pain effect, and which might explain the difference to the results in resting muscles reported by Le Pera et al. (2001).

3. Chronic pain syndromes and motor excitability

3.1. Phantom pain after limb amputation

A number of studies addressed the question of motor excitability changes in patients with limb amputation. Changes of motor threshold after limb amputation have been reported rather inconsistently throughout the literature. It has been reported to be lower on the amputated side of congenital (Hall et al., 1990) or traumatic upper (Cohen et al., 1991) and lower (Chen et al., 1998) limb amputees, also lower only in forearm, but not in the upper arm amputees (Röricht et al., 1999), and normal both in congenital and traumatic upper limb amputees (Kew et al., 1994; Schwenkreis et al., 2000, 2001; Irlbacher et al., 2002). These differences were attributed to a high variability in the pattern of motor threshold changes after amputation, especially in patients with a long duration since amputation (Röricht et al., 1999). However, no study could establish a relationship between changes in motor threshold and the occurrence or intensity of stump and phantom pain.

Increased MEP amplitudes (absolute or relative to CMAP after peripheral electrical stimulation) were found by different investigators when comparing proximal stump muscles of limb amputees with homologous muscles of the intact side (Cohen et al, 1991; Ridding and Rothwell, 1997; Chen et al., 1998; Karl et al., 2001; Irlbacher et al., 2002). Most of these studies did not find a relationship between increased MEP amplitudes and stump or phantom pain. However, in the study by Karl et al. (2001), only patients with phantom limb pain had larger MEP amplitudes in the biceps brachii muscle of the amputated side as compared to the intact side, whereas patients without phantom pain showed no significant side difference. Besides, MEP amplitudes on the amputated side of patients with phantom limb pain were significantly larger than in patients without. With respect to other studies (Fuhr et al., 1992; Chen et al., 1998), they argued that this MEP enlargement might be due to an increased excitability of the motor cortex, but could not exclude spinal influences on their results.

Furthermore, intracortical inhibition and facilitation were tested in different studies in lower and upper limb amputees. In lower limb amputees, Chen et al. (1998) found a significantly reduced intracortical inhibition in the hemisphere contralateral to the amputation compared to healthy subjects. Besides, there was a non-significant trend towards an enhanced intracortical facilitation in this hemisphere. Intracortical inhibition and facilitation in the hemisphere contralateral to the intact side were not significantly altered. Similar findings were obtained in upper limb amputees: upper arm amputees showed a significantly enhanced intracortical inhibition, and a non-significant trend towards a reduced intracortical inhibition, whereas forearm amputees had a significantly reduced inhibition and a trend towards an enhanced facilitation in the hemisphere contralateral to the amputation (Schwenkreis et al., 2000). Again, inhibition and facilitation in the hemisphere contralateral to the intact arm did not differ from healthy subjects. These results were interpreted in the sense of a reduction of GABA-related motor cortical inhibition, and an enhancement of NMDA-dependent excitatory mechanisms in the motor cortex of the hemisphere contralateral to limb amputation. However, neither in lower limb nor in upper limb amputees, a relationship between these cortical excitability changes and stump or phantom limb pain could be established, suggesting peripheral deafferentation rather than pain as the most important factor.

In a recent study, we again addressed the question of a possible relationship between cortical excitability changes and phantom limb pain (Schwenkreis et al.,

2003): using paired pulses TMS, we studied 16 patients who were suffering from chronic phantom limb pain (duration between 2 and 49 years) after upper limb amputation. In a randomised controlled trial, they were treated with the NMDA antagonist memantine or placebo over a period of 3 weeks, since memantine previously in healthy humans had proved to be able to enhance intracortical inhibition and to reduce intracortical facilitation (Schwenkreis et al., 1999). At baseline, intracortical inhibition was significantly reduced and intracortical facilitation was significantly enhanced in the hemisphere contralateral to the amputation compared to healthy controls. After 3 weeks of treatment with memantine, inhibition was significantly increased, and facilitation significantly decreased compared to baseline. As expected, placebo had no influence on cortical excitability. However, the reduction of cortical excitability induced by memantine was not paralleled by a reduction of phantom pain intensity, and the clinical effect of memantine did not differ significantly from placebo. We therefore concluded that chronic phantom pain is not linked to excitability changes in NMDA-dependent intracortical interneuronal circuits in the motor cortex. This could be due to the fact that cortical reorganisation in these patients is already fixed and based on axonal sprouting, with the result of new synapses. But it might be that the relationship between cortical reorganisation and phantom pain is less clear than widely believed.

3.2. Complex regional pain syndrome type I (CRPS I)

Complex regional pain syndrome type I (CRPS I) is a syndrome that develops as a consequence of trauma affecting the limbs, without obvious nerve lesion. Its main components are pain, edema, autonomic dysfunction, movement disorder, and trophic changes. An involvement of the CNS is suggested by a variety of clinical symptoms, such as hemisensory impairment or dystonia. However, the exact pathophysiolocial mechanisms of CRPS I remain unknown until now. We recently studied motor cortex excitability in a group of 25 patients suffering from CRPS I, using single and paired pulses TMS (Schwenkreis et al., 2003). Motor threshold and intracortical facilitation did not differ significantly between healthy age-matched subjects and either the patients' affected or clinically unaffected side. In contrast, intracortical inhibition was significantly reduced in both, the hemisphere contralateral to the affected and contralateral to the clinically unaffected side (Fig. 1). In the hemisphere contralateral to the affected side, the amount of disinhibition was related to the pain intensity, which was not the case in the hemisphere contralateral to the clinically unaffected side. This bilaterally reduced intracortical inhibition might be due to a reduced activity of GABA-related inhibitory mechanisms in the motor cortex, or to an enhancement of NMDA-dependent excitatory mechanisms, or both. It suggests a generalised involvement of the central motor system in the course of CRPS I, which might be at least in part related to pain. Interestingly, the finding of a bilateral motor cortex disinhibition in CRPS patients is supported by the results of a MEG study, which showed a bilaterally altered reactivity of the 20-Hz motor cortex rhythm, with a significantly

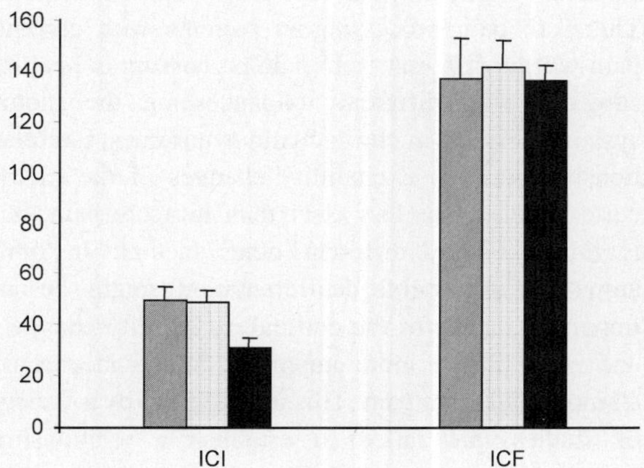

Fig. 1. Mean intracortical inhibition (ICI) and facilitation (ICF) in CRPS patients and healthy controls. Shown are the relative amplitudes (conditioned/unconditioned TMS, in %), i.e. higher bars indicate lower inhibition (ICI) and higher facilitation (ICF). The different bars refer to recordings taken from the patients' affected side (hatched), the patients' clinically unaffected side (stippled) and the dominant hand of the control group (black). Error bars are SEM.

shorter and smaller 20-Hz rebound after tactile stimuli in CRPS patients (Juottonen et al., 2002). Since the rebound of the 20-Hz rhythm is thought to reflect increased motor cortex inhibition (Salmelin and Hari, 1994), these findings also suggest a bilaterally modified inhibition of the motor cortex in CRPS.

4. Conclusions

The results of different TMS studies in experimental pain as well as in chronic pain syndromes suggest that motor cortex excitability is influenced by pain. However, there are substantial differences between acute experimental pain in healthy humans and chronic pain in patients with limb amputation or CRPS: most studies of acute pain showed a reduction of motor cortex excitability, whereas in chronic pain syndromes, an increased excitability was observed. Several reasons may be responsible for these differences: functional changes at different levels of pain processing (e.g. sensitization of peripheral afferents, central sensitization at the level of the dorsal horn, plastic changes at the level of the thalamus or cerebral cortex) are known to occur in chronic pain. Therefore pain processing in patients with chronic pain will be different from pain processing in healthy subjects, with different influences on the motor system. Besides, in chronic pain syndromes, the relationship between excitability changes of the motor cortex and pain is less clear than in acute pain, but is influenced by different other factors: In limb amputees, peripheral deafferentation might be an important factor for the cortical excitability changes, and even play a more important role than chronic stump or phantom pain. This is suggested by a variety of studies that failed to establish a relationship between cortical excitability changes and stump or phantom pain. Reduced use of a painful limb or immobilization may also contribute to cortical excitability changes. However, as seen in patients with CRPS, there is a relationship between pain and motor cortex excitability not only in acute pain, but also in patients with chronic pain syndromes.

References

Birbaumer, N., Lutzenberger, W., Montoya, P., Larbig, W., Unertl, K., Topfner, S., Grodd, W., Taub, E. and Flor, H. Effects of regional anesthesia on phantom limb pain are mirrored in changes in cortical reorganization. *J. Neurosci.*, 1997, 17: 5503–5508.

Bromm, B. and Treede, R.D. Nerve fibre discharges, cerebral potentials and sensations induced by CO_2 laser stimulation. *Hum. Neurobiol.*, 1984, 3: 33–40.

Chen, R., Corwell, B., Yaseen, Z., Hallett, M. and Cohen, L.G. Mechanisms of cortical reorganization in lower-limb amputees. *J. Neurosci.*, 1998, 18: 3443–3450.

Cohen, L.G., Bandinelli, S., Findley, T.W. and Hallett, M. Motor reorganization after upper limb amputation in man. A study with focal magnetic stimulation. *Brain*, 1991, 114: 615–627.

Darian-Smith, C. and Gilbert, C.D. Axonal sprouting accompanies functional reorganization in adult cat striate cortex. *Nature*, 1994, 368: 737–740.

Dettmers, C., Adler, T., Rzanny, R., van Schayck, R., Gaser, C., Weiss, T., Miltner, W.H., Bruckner, L. and Weiller, C. Increased excitability in the primary motor cortex and supplementary motor area in patients with phantom limb pain after upper limb amputation. *Neurosci. Lett.*, 2001, 307: 109–112.

Di Lazzaro, V., Oliviero, A., Profice, P., Saturno, E., Pilato, F., Insola, A., Mazzone, P., Tonali, P. and Rothwell, J.C. Comparison of descending volleys evoked by transcranial magnetic and electric stimulation in conscious humans. *Electroencephalogr. Clin. Neurophysiol.*, 1998, 109: 397–401.

Donoghue, J.P., Suner, S. and Sanes, J.N. Dynamic organization of primary motor cortex output to target muscles in adult rats. II. Rapid reorganization following motor nerve lesions. *Exp. Brain Res.*, 1990, 79: 492–503.

Farina, S., Valeriani, M., Rosso, T., Aglioti, S., Tamburin, S., Fiaschi, A. and Tinazzi, M. Transient inhibition of the human motor cortex by capsaicin-induced pain. A study with transcranial magnetic stimulation. *Neurosci. Lett.*, 2001, 314: 97–101.

Flor, H., Elbert, T., Knecht, S., Wienbruch, C., Pantev, C., Birbaumer, N., Larbig, W. and Taub, E. Phantom-limb pain as a perceptual correlate of cortical reorganization following arm amputation. *Nature*, 1995, 375: 482–484.

Flor, H., Braun, C., Elbert, T. and Birbaumer, N. Extensive reorganization of primary somatosensory cortex in chronic back pain patients. Neurosci. Lett., 1997, 224: 5–8.

Fuhr, P., Cohen, L.G., Dang, N., Findley, T.W., Haghighi, S., Oro, J. and Hallett, M. Physiological analysis of motor reorganization following lower limb amputation. *Electroencephalogr. Clin. Neurophysiol.*, 1992, 85: 53–60.

Hall, E.J., Flament, D., Fraser, C. and Lemon, R.N. Non-invasive brain stimulation reveals reorganized cortical outputs in amputees. *Neurosci. Lett.*, 1990, 116: 379–386.

Hallett, M., Chen, R., Ziemann, U. and Cohen, L.G. Reorganization in motor cortex in amputees an in normal volunteers after ischemic limb deafferentation. *Electroencephalogr. Clin. Neurophysiol.*, 1999 (Suppl), 51: 183–187.

Hess, G. and Donoghue, J.P. Long-term potentiation of horizontal connections provides a mechanism to reorganize cortical motor maps. *J. Neurophysiol.*, 1994, 71: 2543–2547.

Irlbacher, K., Meyer, B.U., Voss, M., Brandt, S.A. and Roricht, S. Spatial reorganization of cortical motor output maps of stump muscles in human upper-limb amputees. *Neurosci. Lett.*, 2002, 321: 129–132.

Jacobs, K.M. and Donoghue, J.P. Reshaping the cortical motor map by unmasking latent intracortical connections. *Science*, 1991, 251: 944–947.

Juottonen, K., Gockel, M., Silen, T., Hurri, H., Hari, R. and Forss, N. Altered central sensorimotor processing in patients with complex regional pain syndrome. *Pain*, 2002, 98: 315–323.

Kaneko, T., Caria, M.A. and Asanuma, H. Information processing within the motor cortex. II. Intracortical connections between neurons receiving somatosensory cortical input and motor output neurons of the cortex. *J. Comp. Neurol.*, 1994, 345: 172–184.

Karl, A., Birbaumer, N., Lutzenberger, W., Cohen, L.G. and Flor, H. Reorganization of motor and somatosensory cortex in upper extremity amputees with phantom limb pain. *J. Neurosci.*, 2001, 21: 3609–3618.

Kew, J.J., Ridding, M.C., Rothwell, J.C., Passingham, R.E., Leigh, P.N., Sooriakumaran, S., Frackowiak, R.S. and Brooks, D.J. Reorganization of cortical blood flow and transcranial magnetic stimulation maps in human subjects after upper limb amputation. *J. Neurophysiol.*, 1994, 72: 2517–2524.

Kujirai, T., Caramia, M.D., Rothwell, J.C., Day, B.L., Thompson, P.D., Ferbert, A., Wroe, S., Asselman, P. and Marsden, C.D. Corticocortical inhibition in human motor cortex. *J. Physiol.* (Lond), 1993, 471: 501–519.

Le Pera, D., Graven-Nielsen, T., Valeriani, M., Oliviero, A., Di Lazzaro, V., Tonali, P.A. and Arendt-Nielsen, L. Inhibition of motor system excitability at cortical and spinal level by tonic muscle pain. *Clin. Neurophysiol.*, 2001, 112: 1633–1641.

Pons, T.P., Garraghty, P.E., Ommaya, A.K., Kaas, J.H., Taub, E. and Mishkin, M. Massive cortical reorganisation after sensory deafferentation in adult macaques. *Science*, 1991, 252: 1857–1860.

Ridding, M.C. and Rothwell, J.C. Stimulus/response curves as a method of measuring motor cortical excitability in man. Electroencephalogr *Clin. Neurophysiol.*, 1997, 105: 340–344.

Romaniello, A., Cruccu, G., McMillan, A.S., Arendt-Nielsen, L. and Svensson, P. Effect of experimental pain from trigeminal muscle and skin on motor cortex excitability in humans. *Brain Res.*, 2000, 882: 120–127.

Röricht, S., Meyer, B.U., Niehaus, L. and Brandt, S.A. Long-term reorganization of motor cortex outputs after arm amputation. *Neurology*, 1999, 53: 106–111.

Salmelin, R. and Hari, R. Spatiotemporal characteristics of sensorimotor neuromagnetic rhythms related to thumb movement. *Neuroscience*, 1994, 60: 537–550.

Schwenkreis, P., Witscher, K., Janssen, F., Addo, A., Dertwinkel, R., Zenz, M., Malin, J.P. and Tegenthoff, M. Influence of the N-methyl-D-aspartate antagonist memantine on human motor cortex excitability. *Neurosci. Lett.*, 1999, 270: 137–140.

Schwenkreis, P., Witscher, K., Janssen, F., Dertwinkel, R., Zenz, M., Malin, J.P. and Tegenthoff, M. Changes of cortical excitability in patients with upper limb amputation. *Neurosci. Lett.*, 2000, 293: 143–146.

Schwenkreis, P., Witscher, K., Janssen, F., Pleger, B., Dertwinkel, R., Zenz, M., Malin, J.P. and Tegenthoff, M. Assessment of reorganization in the sensorimotor cortex after upper limb amputation. *Clin. Neurophysiol.*, 2001, 112: 627–635.

Schwenkreis, P., Maier, C., Pleger, B., Mansourian, N., Dertwinkel, R., Malin, J.P., Tegenthoff, M. and Zenz, M. NMDA-mediated mechanisms in cortical excitability changes after limb amputation. *Acta. Neurol. Scand.*, 2003, in press.

Schwenkreis, P., Janssen, F., Rommel, O., Pleger, B., Völker, B., Hosbach, I., Dertwinkel, R., Maier, C. and Tegenhoff, M. Bilateral motor complex disinhibition in complex regional pain syndrome (CRPS) type I of the hand. *Neurology*, 2003 (in press).

Svensson, P., Minoshima, S., Beydoun, A., Morrow, T.J. and Casey, K.L. Cerebral processing of acute skin and muscle pain in humans. *J. Neurophysiol.*, 1997, 78: 450–460.

Tarkka, I.M. and Treede, R.D. Equivalent electrical source analysis of pain-related somatosensory evoked potentials elicited by a CO_2 laser. *J. Clin. Neurophysiol.*, 1993, 10: 513–519.

Valeriani, M., Restuccia, D., Di Lazzaro, V., Oliviero, A., Profice, P., Le Pera, D., Saturno, E. and Tonali, P. Inhibition of the human primary motor area by painful heat stimulation of the skin. Clin. Neurophysiol., 1999, 110: 1475–1480.

Valeriani, M., Restuccia, D., Di Lazzaro, V., Oliviero, A., Le Pera, D., Profice, P., Saturno, E. and Tonali, P. Inhibition of biceps brachii muscle motor area by painful heat stimulation of the skin. *Exp. Brain Res.*, 2001, 139: 168–172.

Ziemann, U., Lonnecker, S., Steinhoff, B.J. and Paulus, W. Effects of antiepileptic drugs on motor cortex excitability in humans: a transcranial magnetic stimulation study. *Ann. Neurol.*, 1996a, 40: 367–378.

Ziemann, U., Rothwell, J.C. and Ridding, M.C. Interaction between intracortical inhibition and facilitation in human motor cortex. *J. Physiol.* (Lond), 1996b, 496: 873–881.

Transcranial Magnetic Stimulation and Transcranial Direct Current Stimulation (Supplements to Clinical Neurophysiology, Vol. 56)
Editors: W. Paulus, F. Tergau, M.A. Nitsche, J.C. Rothwell, U. Ziemann, M. Hallett

Chapter 41

Can epilepsies be improved by repetitive transcranial magnetic stimulation? – interim analysis of a controlled study

Frithjof Tergau[a,*], Daniela Neumann[b], Felix Rosenow[c], Michael A. Nitsche[a], Walter Paulus[a] and Bernhard Steinhoff[b]

[a] *Department of Clinical Neurophysiology, University of Göttingen, D-37075 Göttingen (Germany)*
[b] *Epilepsy Center Kork, Kehl-Kork (Germany)*
[c] *Interdisciplinary Epilepsy Center, Department of Neurology, University of Marburg, Marburg (Germany)*

1. Introduction

Since the early decades of the last century, a variety of brain stimulation techniques have been – and still are – evaluated for their therapeutical potential in the treatment of epilepsies that cannot be sufficiently improved by pharmacological and surgical strategies. Besides deep brain stimulation of various brain nuclei and other targets as well as vagal nerve stimulation (for review, see Benabid et al., 2000, 2003; Loddenkemper et al., 2001; Weinstein, 2001; Labar and Dean, 2002; Murphy and Patil, 2003), repetitive transcranial magnetic stimulation (rTMS) has gained increasing interest in the investigation of antiepileptic efficacy.

Independently of the investigation of therapeutical perspectives of rTMS as a technique to induce long-lasting modifications of the excitability of neuronal network (see below), transcrainal magnetic stimulation (TMS) with single and double pulses was introduced to explore cortical excitability. Although the studies on several epilepsy syndromes were not always easy to interpret, it is well accepted that impairment of the excitatory as well as the inhibitory properties at least in some parts of the epileptic brain can be confirmed by TMS (for review, see Ziemann et al., 1998; Macdonell et al., 2002; Tassinari, 2003). TMS can also be used to study the effect of central active drugs – most antiepileptic drugs are shown to reduce cortical excitability (Ziemann et al., 1999; Macdonell et al., 2002; Tassinari, 2003).

In the early days of transcranial magnetic stimulation (TMS) research, apprehension existed that this type of stimulation bears the risk of inducing seizures. However, from numerous studies (cf. Pascual-Leone et al., 1993; Wassermann et al., 1996; Chen et al., 1997b; Jahanshahi et al., 1997; Ziemann et al., 1998) and a consensus conference (Wassermann, 1998) it was concluded that single and double pulse TMS as well as, within certain limits, rTMS cannot be seen as pro-epileptic (for details, see also Tergau and Steinhoff, in press). Moreover, it was demonstrated that TMS series with slow repetition rates of 1 Hz or

* *Correspondence to*: Dr. Frithjof Tergau, MD, Department of Clinical Neurophysiology, University of Göttingen, Robert-Koch-Strasse 40, D-37075 Göttingen, Germany.
Tel: +49-551-39 6650; Fax: +49-551-39 8126;
E-mail: f.tergau@med.uni-goettingen.de

below (so-called low-frequency rTMS) can reduce cortical excitability (Chen et al., 1997a; Muellbacher et al., 2000). Nevertheless, rTMS with frequencies above 1 Hz (so-called high-frequency rTMS) has been shown to increase cortical excitability (Pascual-Leone et al., 1994; Berardelli et al., 1998) and with increasing frequency, stimulus intensity and/or train duration, the risk of inducing seizures increases.

Based on the findings that the effects of rTMS last beyond the period of stimulation itself, therapeutical antiepileptic potential of low-frequency rTMS was hypothesized. Here we present interim analysis of an ongoing placebo-controlled trial. The results are discussed on the bases of the existing rTMS literature regarding the treatment of epilepsies in humans.

2. Methods

A multicenter cross-over placebo-controlled three arm trial is currently performed by three German epilepsy centers. Patients with any type of medically intractable focal or generalized epilepsy with at least on average two seizures per week over a 3 month baseline period can be included. The study was approved by the local ethics committee and all patients included gave written informed consent.

By April 2003, 28 patients were enrolled, of which five patients to date have yet to complete and six patients dropped the study due to pregnancy (one), low baseline seizure frequency (one), change of residence (one), changed medication (two) or without any reason (one). The data of 17 patients, mean age 29 ± 10 years, 11 male, are presented here. Patients had the diagnosis of focal neocortical (11), focal mesial temporal (two), multifocal (two), generalized (two) epilepsy. Duration of epilepsy was 21 ± 12 years. Medication was kept constant throughout the study. The study course for each patient included three treatment periods in randomized order: two different real stimulation types were randomly intermixed with placebo stimulation. We used a MagPro Magnetic Stimulator, Dantec Medtronic, Dusseldorf, Germany with a round coil (outer diameter 9 cm) placed over the vertex. Placebo stimulation was applied by using a specially designed coil with a magnetic field intensity reduced to 10% but producing the 'click' and the cutaneous skin sensations unter the coil similar to the real coil. The three stimulation types differ in frequency: 1 Hz and 0.333 Hz for real stimulation and 0.666 Hz for placebo stimulation respectively – while all other stimulation parameters were the identical to the methods previously used (Tergau et al., 1999). Stimulation on 5 consecutive days with 1000 pulses (500 monopolar pulses with clockwise current direction followed directly by 500 pulses in anti-clockwise direction) each day, stimulus intensity for both coil orientations slightly below motor threshold, thus motor or sensory phenomena other than the acoustic and the cutaneous sensations under the coil were prevented. Treatment periods were preceded and followed by at least 4 weeks observation phases, and treatment periods were separated by at least 8 weeks. A diary record was kept by the patients, by counting all seizure or seizure-like events.

3. Results

All patients tolerated the stimulation without significant side effects, none of the patients had a major increase in seizure frequency after any of the real stimulation types.

Baseline seizure frequency during the 4 weeks prior to each of the treatment periods was relativley constant with 6.25 (median, range 2.5–320.5) seizures per week (SPW) for placebo stimulation, 5.0 (1.75– 272.25) spw for 0.333 Hz stimulation and 6.75 (1.25–350) spw for 1.0 Hz stimulation (note that one patient had frequent sensory seizures with up to 50 seizures per day, which enlarged range and standard deviation of seizure frequency of the group). For further analysis, SPW after stimulation, was individually normalized to the appropriate baseline and expressed in percent. As shown in Fig. 1, values over the 4 baseline weeks separately varied on average within the range of 80–120%. SPW during and after treatment also stayed within this range with two exceptions: (i) during 0.333 Hz stimulation seizure frequency was significantly reduced to less than 60% ($p = 0.0004$) and stayed below 80% for

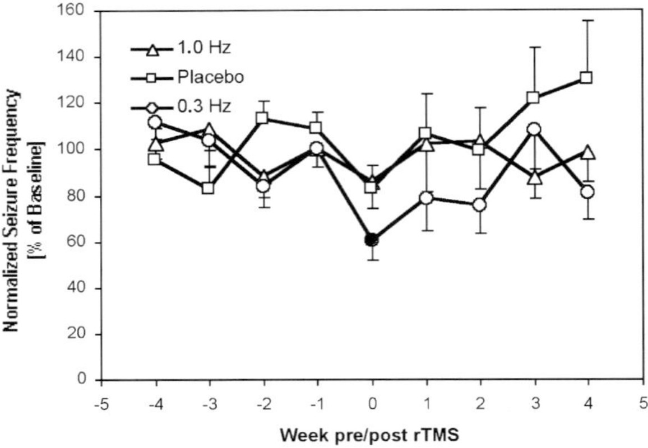

Fig. 1. The course of mean seizure frequency over a period of 9 weeks (4 weeks prior rTMS (–4 to –1), rTMS treatment week (0), 4 weeks post rTMS (1–4)) for the three stimulation modes separately. Values represent average seizure frequency for every week separately individually normalized to their mean seizure frequency during 4 weeks prior to rTMS treatment and are given in percent. Note that error bars indicate standard error of mean. Filled symbol indicates significant difference to 4-week baseline period.

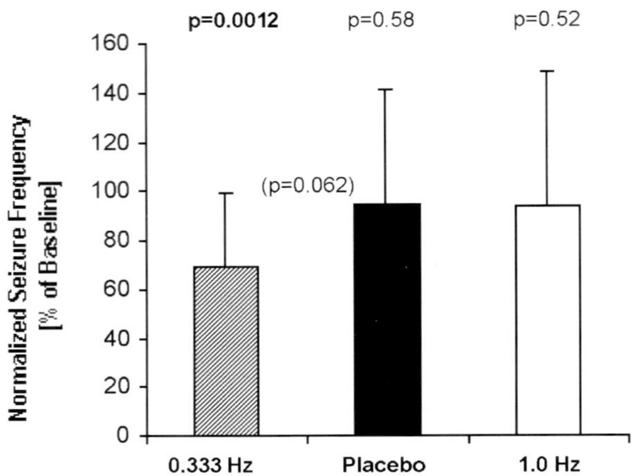

Fig. 2. Average seizure frequency is displayed for a period of 2 weeks after each of the three modes of rTMS treatment (0.333 Hz, Placebo, 1.0 Hz). Values are mean ± standard deviation of 17 subjects and are expressed as percentage of seizure frequency during 4 weeks prior to rTMS. p values of the student's t test for comparison to baseline are given at the top of the figure, bold numbers indicate statistical significance ($p < 0.05$); number in brackets indicate the p value for the comparison between 0.333 Hz and placebo stimulation which slightly failed significance.

another 2 weeks; (ii) three to four weeks after placebo stimulation, seizure frequency increased insignificantly ($p = 0.37$; $p = 0.27$) up to 120–130%. None of the weekly values of the real stimulation modes showed a statistically significant difference to placebo. For further analysis, we averaged the values of treatment and 2-weeks post-stimulation periods (cf. Theodore et al., 2002). As depicted in Fig. 2, only for 0.333 Hz stimulation was there a significant reduction in seizure frequency compared to baseline, however, the difference to placebo failed significance slightly.

4. Discussion

Antiepileptic effects of TMS pulses at first were discovered by chance when Hufnagel and Elger (1991) tried to activate the epileptic focus in 48 patients with intractable epilepsies. By using single pulse TMS they found enhancement as well as suppression of epileptiform potentials in seven patients with continuously spiking epileptic foci. Additionally, they described temporary interruption of epileptiform paroxysms for 1–3 s in nine cases and found persistent suppression of spontaneous spikes in one patient raising evidence that TMS pulses may inhibit epileptiform activity. When applying single TMS pulses repetitively every three to ten seconds (0.3 to 0.1 Hz) – before the term '*repetitive TMS*' was coined due to technical limitation of the stimulation devices – Steinhoff et al. noticed a decrease in spike frequency for at least 5 min after stimulation, most prominently bilaterally when TMS was applied contralateral to the epileptic focus in seven patients with medically intractable complex-partial seizures of mesiobasal limbic onset (Steinhoff et al., 1992; Steinhoff et al., 1993). In 1997, preliminary data on three patients with cortical action myoclonus were presented showing that 1 Hz rTMS over 30 min was able to reduce action myoclonus. Although applied over several days, the effect always vanished 2 h after rTMS (Wedegaertner et al., 1997).

The results presented here are interim analyses of the first cross-over placebo-controlled investigation on the antiepileptic efficacy of low-frequency rTMS. The data from 17 patients suggest a seizure reduction on average by 30–40% over 2 weeks after rTMS treatment with 0.333 Hz whereas, after placebo as well as after 1.0 Hz treatment there was no discernible effect on seizure frequency. Although a significant difference to placebo could not be demonstrated in this patient group, the data seems to be in line with the results of the first open pilot study on nine patients who showed reduction in seizure frequency within a similar range over a 4 week period (Tergau et al., 1999). Our results were confirmingly supplemented by a case report on a patient with focal dysplasia by another group (Menkes and Gruenthal, 2000): biweekly treatment with 100 stimuli at 0.5 Hz and 95% motor threshold intensity using an unfocal coil placed over the area of dysplasia reduced seizure frequency by 70% over a 4 weeks period of treatment.

In contrast, results of another placebo-controlled study – the first being done in this field – were not that encouraging (Theodore et al., 2002): 12 patients with focal epilepsies receiving 1 Hz stimulation on 7 days, twice daily over 15 min were compared to 12 matched patients receiving placebo stimulation. They found only 16 ± 18% seizure reduction over 2 weeks after real stimulation, while placebo stimulation yielded reduction by 1 ± 24%. This difference failed significance ($p = 0.11$).

Some methodical aspects should be discussed that may have masked better effects in the studies.

First, sample sizes were relatively small. To obtain valid information on the antiepileptic efficacy, more patients should be treated. For comparison, in the studies on vagal nerve stimulation in the tretment of epilepsy that led to FDA approval of this treatment strategy, over hundred patients were studied for significant seizure reduction, on average by 24.5% (The Vagus Nerve Stimulation Study Group, 1995).

Second, in the study by Theodore et al. (2002) a focal stimulation protocol was used, while in our studies stimulation was applied unfocally. It is known that focal stimulation at threshold intensities only activates a small area of cortex lying some 3 cm beneath the skull. It may be assumed that in some patients the epileptic focus cannot be reached properly. This could be an explanation for not being able to produce better results in the study by Theodore et al. (2002) when taken into account that 10 of the 24 patients had an temporo-mesial epileptic focus; subgroup analysis showed that neocortical epilepsies responded much better (24 ± 22% seizure reduction) than mesial epilepsies (–11 ± 28%), this difference, however, was not significant, most likely due to the small sample size. Until now, it is not known, whether the focal stimulation technique attempting to inactivate the epileptic focus is superior or whether a concept of unfocal stimulation trying to downregulate the excitability of the cortical network responsible for seizure propagation (comparable to "unfocal" effects of antiepileptic drugs or vagal nerve stimulation?) as used in our study has more advantages. Support to the latter concept can be found by neurophysiological and brain imaging studies with observations that brain areas remote from the TMS stimulation site can be modified (Paus et al., 1997; Gerschlager et al., 2001).

Third, the stimulation frequency could be of crucial importance. In our study, significant seizure reduction compared to baseline was only seen after 0.333 Hz stimulation while 1.0 Hz stimulation was quite similar to placebo. Until now, the meaning of this observation can only be speculative. 1.0 Hz is a frequency mainly inducing inhibition. This seems to be confirmed by a PET study, showing that high-frequency led to an increase of regional cerebral blood flow (rCBF) in the stimulated brain areas, whereas, under low-frequency the rCBF decreased (Post et al., 1999; Speer et al., 2000). From the existing literature we do not know where the borderline frequency between induction of facilitation and inhibition really is. Since the mechanisms behind this phenomenon are not really understood, it is, hence, not known whether the separation between those two obviously contradictory modifications of cortical excitability, facilitation and inhibition, are fixed at the same frequency for all patients. Indeed, a couple of studies demonstrated a possibly large interindividual variability in the susceptibility to inhibitory and excitatory rTMS, (Maeda et al., 2000). Moreover, it is not clear whether the results on the motor cortex (Chen et al., 1997a; Chen and Seitz, 2001) or on the visual cortex (Boroojerdi et al., 2000) can be seen as generally valid for all brain regions. Nevertheless, it is well accepted in general that activation is more likely induced when higher frequencies are used and inhibition is yielded by low frequencies. Taking this into account, it may be speculated that in some patients induced inhibition by 1.0 Hz was not strong enough. Although subgroup analysis on our data remains to be carried out, it has to be considered that interindividual differences exist in the susceptibility to inhibitory and excitatory rTMS (cf. Maeda et al., 2000).

Major criticism to the studies on rTMS in epilepsies could be that the amount of reduction in seizure frequency is not sufficient at all. However, one has to consider that techniques of brain stimulation other than rTMS failed to show superior effects so far, especially in placebo-controlled trials. This is probably due to the fact that in all studies on new treatment, the included patients suffered from very severe epilepsy syndromes and were resistant to several antiepileptic drugs. It seems unlikely that a therapeutic strategy can be developed that improves all kind of epilepsies to an extent greater than it was seen for new-developed drugs (e.g. for levetiracetam, Betts et al., 2000). As stated earlier, it should be noted that the effects of vagus nerve stimulation were at a similar range (The Vagus Nerve Stimulation Study Group, 1995). Magic effects should not be expected from rTMS.

However, many questions in this field are still to be answered. The mechanisms underlying the effects of rTMS on cortical excitability are still yet to be discovered (cf. Lisanby and Belmaker, 2000; Muller et al., 2000). The stimulation parameters such as frequency, intensity, focality, duration and repetition rate of the trains require further detailed studies. For this, rTMS has the advantages of being easy to applicate and to be non-invasive, thus, there is no risk from surgical procedures. Probably, individually optimised stimulation parameters are needed and, furthermore, it may be expected that different epilepsy syndromes may respond differently to rTMS. Also, chronic application of rTMS has to be evaluated to see whether the antiepileptic effects an be preserved over a suitable period, also possible side effects should be investigated further.

In conclusion, it will take time and numerous studies are needed before decisions can be made as to whether low-frequency rTMS may be an alternative adjunctive antiepileptic treatment in intractable epilepsy. First results are not dispiriting.

Acknowledgement

The work was supported by The Dantec/Medtronic Company, Düsseldorf, Germany

References

Benabid, A.L., Koudsie, A., Pollak, P., Kahane, P., Chabardes, S., Hirsch, E., Marescaux, C. and Benazzouz, A. Future prospects of brain stimulation. *Neurol. Res.*, 2000, 22: 237–246.

Benabid, A.L., Vercucil, L., Benazzouz, A., Koudsie, A., Chabardes, S., Minotti, L., Kahane, P., Gentil, M., Lenartz, D., Andressen, C., Krack, P. and Pollak, P. Deep brain stimulation: what does it offer? *Adv. Neurol.*, 2003, 91: 293–302.

Berardelli, A., Inghilleri, M., Rothwell, J.C., Romeo, S., Curra, A., Gilio, F., Modugno, N. and Manfredi, M. Facilitation of muscle evoked responses after repetitive cortical stimulation in man. *Exp. Brain Res.*, 1998, 122: 79–84.

Boroojerdi, B., Prager, A., Muellbacher, W. and Cohen, L.G. Reduction of human visual cortex excitability using 1-Hz transcranial magnetic stimulation. *Neurology*, 2000, 54: 1529–1531.

Chen, R. and Seitz, R.J. Changing cortical excitability with low-frequency magnetic stimulation. *Neurology*, 2001, 57: 379–380.

Chen, R., Classen, J., Gerloff, C., Celnik, P., Wassermann, E.M., Hallett, M. and Cohen, L.G. Depression of motor cortex excitability by low-frequency transcranial magnetic stimulation. *Neurology*, 1997a, 48: 1398–1403.

Chen, R., Gerloff, C., Classen, J., Wassermann, E.M., Hallett, M. and Cohen, L.G. Safety of different inter-train intervals for repetitive transcranial magnetic stimulation and recommendations for safe ranges of stimulation parameters. *Electroencephalogr. Clin. Neurophysiol.*, 1997b, 105: 415–421.

Gerschlager, W., Siebner, H.R. and Rothwell, J.C. Decreased corticospinal excitability after subthreshold 1 Hz rTMS over lateral premotor cortex. *Neurology*, 2001, 57: 449–455.

Hufnagel, A. and Elger, C.E. Responses of the epileptic focus to transcranial magnetic stimulation. *Electroencephalogr. Clin. Neurophysiol.*, 1991 (Suppl.), 43: 86–99.

Jahanshahi, M., Ridding, M.C., Limousin, P., Profice, P., Fogel, W., Dressler, D., Fuller, R., Brown, R.G., Brown, P. and Rothwell, J.C. Rapid rate transcranial magnetic stimulation – a safety study. *Electroencephalogr. Clin. Neurophysiol.*, 1997, 105: 422–429.

Labar, D. and Dean, A. Neurostimulation therapy for epilepsy. *Curr. Neurol. Neurosci. Rep.*, 2002, 2: 357–364.

Lisanby, S.H. and Belmaker, R.H. Animal models of the mechanisms of action of repetitive transcranial magnetic stimulation (RTMS): comparisons with electroconvulsive shock (ECS). *Depress Anxiety*, 2000, 12: 178–187.

Loddenkemper, T., Pan, A., Neme, S., Baker, K.B., Rezai, A.R., Dinner, D.S., Montgomery, E.B., Jr. and Luders, H.O. Deep brain stimulation in epilepsy. *J. Clin. Neurophysiol.*, 2001, 18: 514–532.

Macdonell, R.A., Curatolo, J.M. and Berkovic, S.F. Transcranial magnetic stimulation and epilepsy. *J. Clin. Neurophysiol.*, 2002, 19: 294–306.

Maeda, F., Keenan, J.P., Tormos, J.M., Topka, H. and Pascual-Leone, A. Interindividual variability of the modulatory effects of repetitive transcranial magnetic stimulation on cortical excitability. *Exp. Brain Res.*, 2000, 133: 425–430.

Menkes, D.L. and Gruenthal, M. Slow-frequency repetitive transcranial magnetic stimulation in a patient with focal cortical dysplasia. *Epilepsia*, 2000, 41: 240–242.

Muellbacher, W., Ziemann, U., Boroojerdi, B. and Hallett, M. Effects of low-frequency transcranial magnetic stimulation on motor excitability and basic motor behavior. *Clin. Neurophysiol.*, 2000, 111: 1002–1007.

Muller, M.B., Toschi, N., Kresse, A.E., Post, A. and Keck, M.E. Long-term repetitive transcranial magnetic stimulation increases the expression of brain-derived neurotrophic factor and cholecystokinin mRNA, but not neuropeptide tyrosine mRNA in specific areas of rat brain. *Neuropsychopharmacology*, 2000, 23: 205–215.

Murphy, J.V. and Patil, A. Stimulation of the nervous system for the management of seizures: current and future developments. *CNS Drugs*, 2003, 17: 101–115.

Pascual-Leone, A., Houser, C.M., Reese, K., Shotland, L.I., Grafman, J., Sato, S., Valls-Solé, J., Brasil-Neto, J.P., Wassermann, E.M., Cohen, L.G. et al. Safety of rapid-rate transcranial magnetic stimulation in normal volunteers. *Electroencephalogr. Clin. Neurophysiol.*, 1993, 89: 120–130.

Pascual-Leone, A., Valls-Solé, J., Wassermann, E.M. and Hallett, M. Responses to rapid-rate transcranial magnetic stimulation of the human motor cortex. *Brain*, 1994, 117: 847–858.

Paus, T., Jech, R., Thompson, C.J., Comeau, R., Peters, T. and Evans, A.C. Transcranial magnetic stimulation during positron emission tomography: a new method for studying connectivity of the human cerebral cortex. *J. Neurosci.*, 1997, 17: 3178–3184.

Post, R.M., Kimbrell, T.A., McCann, U.D., Dunn, R.T., Osuch, E.A., Speer, A.M. and Weiss, S.R. Repetitive transcranial magnetic stimulation as a neuropsychiatric tool: present status and future potential. *J. Ect.*, 1999, 15: 39–59.

Speer, A.M., Kimbrell, T.A., Wassermann, E.M., Repella, D., Willis, M.W., Herscovitch, P. and Post, R.M. Opposite effects of high and low frequency rTMS on regional brain activity in depressed patients. *Biol. Psychiatry.*, 2000, 48: 1133–1141.

Steinhoff, B.J., Stodieck, S.R., Paulus, W. and Witt, T.N. Transcranial stimulation. *Neurology*, 1992, 42: 1429–1430.

Steinhoff, B.J., Stodieck, S.R., Zivcec, Z., Schreiner, R., von Maffei, C., Plendl, H. and Paulus, W. Transcranial magnetic stimulation (TMS) of the brain in patients with mesiotemporal epileptic foci. *Clin. Electroencephalogr.*, 1993, 24: 1–5.

Tassinari, C.A., Cincotta, M., Zaccara, G. and Michelucci, R. Transcranial magnetic stimulation and epilepsy. *Clin. Neurophysiol.*, 2003, 114: 777–798.

Tergau, F. and Steinhoff, B.J. Therapeutic Prospects and Safety of Transcranial Magnetic Stimulation in Epilepsy. In: H. Luders (Ed.), *Deep Brain Stimulation in Epilepsy*. London: Taylor and Francis.

Tergau, F., Naumann, U., Paulus, W. and Steinhoff, B.J. Low-frequency repetitive transcranial magnetic stimulation improves intractable epilepsy. *Lancet*, 1999, 353: 2209.

Wassermann, E.M. Risk and safety of repetitive transcranial magnetic stimulation: report and suggested guidelines from the International Workshop on the Safety of Repetitive Transcranial Magnetic Stimulation, June 5–7, 1996. *Electroencephalogr. Clin. Neurophysiol.*, 1998, 108: 1–16.

Wassermann, E.M., Grafman, J., Berry, C., Hollnagel, C., Wild, K., Clark, K. and Hallett, M. Use and safety of a new repetitive transcranial magnetic stimulator. *Electroencephalogr. Clin. Neurophysiol.*, 1996, 101: 412–417.

Wedegaertner, F., Garvey, M., Cohen, L.G., Hallett, M. and Wassermann, E.M. Low frequency repetitive transcranial magnetic stimulation can reduce action myoclonus (Abstract). *Neurology*, 1997, 48: A119.

Weinstein, S. The anticonvulsant effect of electrical fields. *Curr. Neurol. Neurosci. Rep.*, 2001, 1: 155–161.

Ziemann, U., Steinhoff, B.J., Tergau, F. and Paulus, W. Transcranial magnetic stimulation: its current role in epilepsy research. *Epilepsy Res.*, 1998, 30: 11–30.

Ziemann, U., Lonnecker, S., Steinhoff, B.J. and Paulus, W. Motor excitability changes under antiepileptic drugs. *Adv. Neurol.*, 1999, 81: 291–298.

Transcranial Magnetic Stimulation and Transcranial Direct Current Stimulation (Supplements to Clinical Neurophysiology, Vol. 56)
Editors: W. Paulus, F. Tergau, M.A. Nitsche, J.C. Rothwell, U. Ziemann, M. Hallett

Chapter 42

Prefrontal cortex stimulation as antidepressant treatment: mode of action and clinical effectiveness of rTMS

Frank Padberg*, Barbara Goldstein-Müller, Peter Zwanzger and Hans-Jürgen Möller

Department of Psychiatry, Ludwig-Maximilian University, Nussbaumstr. 7, D-80336 Munich (Germany)

1. Introduction

Major goals of current research in antidepressant therapy include treating therapy resistant patients, preventing chronic depressive conditions, as well as preventing relapse of depressive episodes. This has generated tremendous interest in recent years not only in the proposal of novel principles of pharmacological treatment, e.g. substance P antagonists or CRH receptor antagonists, but also in novel non-pharmacological approaches such as sleep deprivation combined with consecutive sleep phase advance (Berger et al., 1997), transcranial magnetic stimulation (TMS) (see review by George et al., 1999; Lisanby et al., 2000; Wassermann and Lisanby, 2001), and recently vagus nerve stimulation (VNS) (Sackeim et al., 2001).

Barker et al. originally introduced TMS in 1985 as a noninvasive tool to electro-magnetically stimulate the primary motor cortex in humans (Barker et al., 1985). More recently, repetitive TMS (rTMS) has become a powerful research tool in neurophysiology and cognitive neuroscience (Hallett, 1996; George et al., 1999). Pilot studies have suggested a possible application of targeted prefrontal stimulation through rTMS as a therapeutic tool in various neurological and psychiatric disorders (George et al., 1999; Lisanby et al., 2000; Wassermann and Lisanby, 2001; Hoffman and Cavus, 2002), based on the assumption that dysfunctional prefrontal cortico-subcortical circuits are involved in the pathophysiology of these conditions. The first therapeutic application of rTMS in psychiatry was in the treatment of major depression (Höflich et al., 1993; Grisaru et al., 1994; George et al., 1995; Conca et al., 1996), and the largest panel of studies available addresses this issue. This chapter attempts to evaluate existing preclinical and clinical studies in answering the question of whether rTMS may be a useful antidepressant treatment in clinical practice.

2. Neurobiological effects of prefrontal rTMS

2.1. *Effects of rTMS in animal models*

2.1.1. *Cellular and molecular level*

Although present evidence suggests that rTMS may be considered a safe procedure, the possible effects

* *Correspondence to*: Dr. Frank Padberg, MD, Department of Psychiatry, Ludwig-Maximillian University, Nussbaumstr. 7, D-80336 Munich, Germany.
Tel: +49-89-5160-5823; Fax: +49-89-5160-5322;
E-mail: padberg@nk-i.med.uni-muenchen.de

at the structural, cellular, and molecular levels have not yet been sufficiently examined (Wassermann 1998). Early studies on adverse effects of rTMS treatment have yielded conflicting results (Sgro et al., 1991; Matsumiya et al., 1992; Counter, 1993). More recently the long-term effects of rTMS in animals have been examined under conditions analogous to those used in clinical applications (George et al., 1999). No increase in glial fibrillary acidic protein (GFAP; an indicator of reactive astrogliosis) after 11 weeks of rTMS was observed (Post et al., 1999a). These results indicate that rTMS does not result in significant structural brain alterations in rats. A profound but transient increase in GFAP mRNA throughout the molecular layer of the dentate gyrus was found after acute application of rTMS in mice (Fujiki and Steward, 1997). This increase in GFAP mRNA shows that acute rTMS can temporarily activate gene expression, which does not necessarily result in reactive astrogliosis (Steward et al., 1993). rTMS may also exhibit neuroprotective properties. Extended rTMS treatment increased the overall viability of mouse monoclonal hippocampal HT22 cells and had a neuroprotective effect against oxidative stressors such as glutamate and H_2O_2 (Post et al., 1999a). After rTMS of frontal brain regions, the intrahippocampal expression of brain-derived neurotrophic factor (BDNF) and cholecystokinin (CCK) was significantly increased (Muller et al., 2000). These results indicate that rTMS of frontal brain regions may influence the activity of hippocampal neurons. It is noteworthy that BDNF mRNA and protein expression after long-term rTMS increase in exactly the same anatomical areas as after electroconvulsive shock and antidepressant drug treatment (Nibuya et al., 1995; Zetterstrom et al., 1998, 1999). However, some differences are worth noting, e.g. rTMS has not been found to stimulate hippocampal neurogenesis as has been reported after ECT and antidepressant medication (Czéh et al., 2002).

2.1.2. *Effects on neurotransmission*

In order to address the question of the possible antidepressant effects of rTMS, several neurotransmitter systems have been examined. In theory, the stimulation of the prefrontal cortex may transsynaptically lead to an activation of dopaminergic neurons in the mesencephalon, and noradrenergic and serotonergic neurons in the brainstem.

Animal studies demonstrate effects of rTMS on dopaminergic neurotransmission. Using an in vivo microdialysis approach, a selective stimulation of dopamine release following rTMS treatment has been observed in the rat hippocampus, in the striatum, and in the nucleus accumbens septi (Keck et al., 2000b, 2002; Zangen and Hyodo, 2002). The dopamine increase was found after high frequency (20 Hz) rTMS (Keck et al., 2000b, 2002) as well as after low frequency (2 Hz) stimulation (Zangen and Hyodo, 2002). The dopamine increase within the nucleus accumbens was accompanied by an increase of extracellular glutamate in this region (Zangen and Hyodo, 2002). The effects on dopamine could be theoretically mediated both directly, via glutamatergic corticostriatal projections (Taber and Fibiger, 1995), and indirectly by an effect on mesolimbic dopaminergic neurons in the midbrain (Murase et al., 1993; Karreman et al., 1996). Simultaneous increase in dopamine and glutamate levels may indicate rTMS-induced effects of glutamate on adjacent dopaminergic nerve terminals, mediated by local ionotropic or metabotropic glutamate receptors. Cortical glutamatergic neurons originating in the prefrontal cortex and dopaminergic neurons from the ventral tegmental area (VTA) synapse in close proximity to one another on the spines of nucleus accumbens medium spiny neurons (Sesack and Pickel, 1992). A modest increase in dopamine content has also been shown in brain homogenates of striatal and hippocampal regions (Ben-Shachar et al., 1997), however, rTMS in this study was applied less focally compared to stimulation in microdialysis studies. Dopamine concentrations have also been found to increase in the striatum and the frontal cortex after ECT (McGarvey et al., 1993; Yoshida et al., 1998). In contrast, acute rTMS did not affect hippocampal noradrenaline release (Ben-Shachar et al., 1997; Keck et al., 2000b) as observed after ECT (Thomas et al., 1992) or extracellular homovanillic acid (HVA) and acetylcholine levels in the nucleus accumbens (Zangen and Hyodo, 2002).

Using in vivo microdialysis in rats, Juckel et al. was able to demonstrate that focal electrical stimulation of the medial prefrontal cortex causes a release of serotonin (5-HT) in the hippocampus and amygdala (Juckel et al., 1999). Such a 5-HT release has not been observed in a microdialysis study after high frequency rTMS (20 Hz) of frontal regions in rats (Keck et al., 2000b). In contrast, a gradual increase of the serotonin metabolite 5-hydroxy-indoleacetic acid (5-HIAA) in the nucleus accumbens occurred after frontal and caudal low frequency rTMS (2 Hz) compared to sham stimulation (Zangen and Hyodo, 2002). While the increase in dopamine was observed only during rTMS in this study, the 5-HIAA levels continued to increase > 60 min after the train. However, extracellular levels of 5-HIAA do not necessarily correlate with serotonin itself (Cumming et al., 1992). Findings showing a selective increase of 5-HT_{1A} binding sites in different frontal regions (Kole et al., 1999), a downregulation of 5-HT_{2A} receptors in the frontal cortex and striatum (Ben-Shachar et al., 1999) and rTMS-associated decrease of HT_{1A} and HT_{1B} autoreceptor sensitivity (Gur et al., 2000) offer additional evidence of rTMS action on serotonergic neurotransmission. Some of these findings coincide with changes observed after ECT and other antidepressant interventions (Zis et al., 1992; Gur et al., 1997, 2000; Post and Keck 2001).

In summary, rTMS appears to have an effect on several neurotransmitter systems which are involved in the pathophysiology of major depression. However, the comparison to prefrontal rTMS in humans is looked upon controversially (Lisanby et al., 2000) as rTMS in small rodents may be less focal due to constraints of rTMS coil sizes and differences in the functional anatomy of the prefrontal cortex between men and rodents.

2.1.3. Hypothalamic–pituitary–adrenocortical (HPA) axis

A common feature in major depression is the disinhibition of hypothalamic–pituitary–adrenocortical (HPA) system regulation. Clinical improvement after antidepressant treatment has been observed to be associated with a normalization of this system's function (Holsboer and Barden, 1996; Holsboer, 2001). The hormonal responses to stress in rats were shown to be blunted after chronic treatment with selected antidepressants (Reul et al., 1993, 1994). A hypothesis was put forward, stating that the HPA system served as a common denominator for clinically effective antidepressants (Holsboer and Barden, 1996; Holsboer, 2001). This was supported by the fact that pharmacologically different drugs similarly affected the function of the HPA system. Furthermore, recent findings on rTMS-induced changes in stress-induced corticotropin and corticosterone plasma levels suggest that rTMS of frontal brain regions attenuates the stress-induced activity of the HPA system (Keck et al., 2001). One explanation for this may be the continuous decrease in vasopressin release in the intra-paraventricular nucleus after acute frontal rTMS. It is assumed that Vasopressin plays a major role in disinhibiting HPA activity in depression (Post and Keck, 2001). This effect on stress response after a social defeat paradigm was replicated in a very recent investigation and found to overrule the effect of stress on hippocampal neurogenesis (Czéh et al., 2002).

2.1.4. Behavioral models

Various models of stress and learned helplessness in rodents, which can be regarded at least in part as behavioral models of depression, have been explored in order to investigate the antidepressant potential of rTMS. According to several research groups, it was shown that daily rTMS reduces immobility in the forced swim test (Fleischmann et al., 1995; Zyss et al., 1997; Keck et al., 2000a; Sachdev et al., 2002). Similarly, the increase in active coping strategies of animals in the Porsolt's swim test after pharmacological treatment has frequently predicted the antidepressant efficacy of the investigated drug (Borsini and Meli, 1988). Furthermore, rTMS has also been reported to increase apomorphine-induced stereotypy (Fleischmann et al., 1995). Both these findings show that in behavioral animal models rTMS may produce antidepressant effects similar to ECT (Belmaker and Grisaru, 1998).

2.2. *Effects of prefrontal rTMS in humans*

2.2.1. *Mood and emotions*

Early single pulse studies have shown individual patients and volunteers to exhibit marked emotional reactions. This has, in turn, triggered research on rTMS-induced modulation of mood and emotions in healthy volunteers. In theory, prefrontal rTMS may similarly alter measures of mood and emotions as it could transiently influence experimental parameters in neurocognitive paradigms (see review by Lisanby et al., 2000). In three pilot studies the transient effects of rTMS when applied to the dorsolateral prefrontal cortex (DLPFC) was demonstrated through mood self-rating (George et al., 1996; Pascual-Leone et al., 1996a; Dearing Martin, 1997). The so-called valence model of mood, which proposes that the left hemisphere mediates positive moods, the right hemisphere negative moods (George et al., 1997a) was supported by data provided by these studies. Observed changes in self-reported mood were nonetheless generally subtle and based solely on self-rating. More recent studies failed to replicate such clearly lateralized effects on mood (Cohrs et al., 1998; Nedjat and Folkerts, 1999; Mosimann et al., 2000; Grisaru et al., 2001; Padberg et al., 2001; Jenkins et al., 2002). The initial hypothesis of lateralized mood-effects induced by rTMS could not be substantiated.

The observed reactions varied greatly between individuals. In some cases dramatic reactions to rTMS could be seen, e.g. single subjects developed hypomanic states (Nedjat and Folkerts, 1999). Whether or not such effects are genuine functional effects of rTMS on mood or rather based on the suggestive character of these experiments remains unclear. Clarification requires further investigations in aspects of emotion and other brain regions. In contrast, a multitude of effects of prefrontal rTMS has been shown in more objective experimental models concerned with facial expression analysis, electroencephalograms (EEG) and neuroendocrine parameters, e.g. concentrations of the thyroid stimulating hormone (TSH), (George et al., 1996; Cohrs et al., 1998; Cohrs et al., 2001; Padberg et al., 2001; Schutter et al., 2001). Therefore, in addition to measures of self-reported mood, both observational and neurobiological approaches should be used to explore such hypotheses in future studies.

2.2.2. *Functional neuroimaging in healthy subjects*

Various functional imaging techniqes have been used to visualize effects of rTMS on the brain. These include functional magnet resonance imaging (fMRI), positron emission computed tomography (PET), and single photon emission computed tomography (SPECT). rTMS can serve as a probe of functional connectivity when combined with these techniques. Pioneering studies demonstrated that rTMS delivered to the frontal eye field or to the primary motor cortex produced a pattern of dose-dependent distal effects in connected brain regions (Paus et al., 1997; Fox et al., 1997). Similarly, more recent studies showed that rTMS of the prefrontal cortex modulated brain activity at both the stimulation site and in several distant regions presumably connected with the stimulated cortex, e.g. the anterior cingulate cortex (Teneback et al., 1999; Paus et al., 2001; Kimbrell et al., 2002; Shajahan et al., 2002). These findings support the hypothesis that prefrontal rTMS modulates the activity in fronto-cingulate circuits, which has been shown to be altered in major depression (Baxter et al., 1989; see also review by Drevets, 2000).

Additionally, amongst healthy volunteers rTMS of the left prefrontal cortex was shown to cause a reduction in [^{11}C]raclopride binding resulting from the release of endogenous dopamine in the left dorsal caudate nucleus (Strafella et al., 2001). It was possible to induce dopamine release by direct stimulation of corticofugal axons or by reducing GABA-mediated intracortical inhibition. This finding coincides with similar evidence from animal studies, which show a dopamine release in the rat hippocampus, striatum and nucleus accumbens septi after prefrontal rTMS (Keck et al., 2000b, 2002). Various modes of action in antidepressant pharmacotherapy are due to effects on dopamine, such as enhancement of dopaminergic neurotransmission (Post et al., 1978; Rampello et al., 1991; Kapur and Mann, 1992; Brown and Gershon, 1993) and dopamine-uptake inhibition as seen in several second-generation antidepressants (e.g. bupropione and amineptine) (Bonnet et al., 1987; Golden et al., 1988). Therefore, the observed dopamine release in mesolimbic and mesostriatal regions after rTMS may contribute to its antidepressant action. More interestingly, this may be an explanation for the clinical observation that psychotically depressed patients respond less well to rTMS treatment (Grunhaus et al., 2000), and that psychotic symptoms may occur in the course of rTMS treatment (Zwanzger et al., 2002).

2.2.3. Neuroimaging in depressed patients

Several open and controlled clinical trials have been conducted that were not primarily designed to focus on the antidepressant efficacy of rTMS but rather to test hypotheses about its mode of action. Results in numerous clinical studies of depressed patients associated improvement after rTMS with changes in prefrontal and paralimbic activity (Teneback et al., 1999; Speer et al., 2000; Catafau et al., 2001; Conca et al., 2002; Mottaghy et al., 2002). This supports the hypothesis that extended daily rTMS treatment exerts local and transsynaptically mediated effects on brain activity in depressed patients. Sham rTMS does not (Catafau et al., 2001). Speer et al. (2000) compared 20 Hz and 1 Hz rTMS over a 2-week period in a randomized cross-over design. This resulted in the main finding, that daily 20-Hz rTMS over the left prefrontal cortex at 100% MT intensity induces persistent increases in regional cortical blood flow (rCBF) in bilateral frontal, limbic, and paralimbic regions, which are involved in depression. 1-Hz rTMS produces more circumscribed decreases (including in the left amygdala). This study allows the current hypothesis of frequency-dependent, opposite effects of high and low frequency rTMS on local and distant regional brain activity to be applied to major depression. It was shown in a further study (Mottaghy et al., 2002) that significant frontal rCBF asymmetry with lower left prefrontal rCBF was no longer detectable after 2 weeks of left prefrontal 10 Hz rTMS treatment. The open nature of this study, however, limits further interpretation of these data. Placebo-induced functional changes in brain activity have recently been characterized (Mayberg et al., 2002). Such controlled designs would be optimal in neuroimaging studies in order to distinguish specific rTMS-induced from non-specific changes, and response-related from treatment-related changes.

Identifying patterns of brain activity that can be predictive of a post rTMS clinical response was an additional focus of research in neuroimaging (Kimbrell et al., 1999; Eschweiler et al., 2000; Mottaghy et al., 2002). There is evidence supporting the hypothesis of differential effects of low and high frequencies on brain activity and function (Post et al., 1997). Kimbrell et al. (1999) showed through 18-fluorodeoxyglucose positron emission tomography (FDG-PET) that patients with reduced metabolism underneath the coil responded better to 10 or 20 Hz rTMS, whereas patients with increased regional metabolism benefited more from 1 Hz rTMS. Replication studies, however, are still needed. A single-photon emission computed tomography (SPECT) study investigated perfusion using 99mTc-labeled ethylcysteinate dimer (ECD) before and after 10 sessions of 20 Hz rTMS in depressed subjects participating in a controlled trial (Teneback et al., 1999). At baseline, six of 13 patients were responders, showing a less reduced inferior frontal lobe perfusion compared to non-responders. This was further normalized after rTMS. Investigations with near infrared spectroscopy (NIRS) (Eschweiler et al., 2000) have yielded similar results. Mottaghy et al. (2002) recently observed complex patterns of correlations between clinical outcomes after rTMS and rCBF at baseline using ECD-SPECT. The rCBF in several limbic structures was negatively, and in some neocortical areas positively, correlated with the outcome (Mottaghy et al., 2002).

MRI has been useful in recently identifying another structural factor contributing to the variation of response. Several investigators found a reduction of rTMS efficacy as the distance between coil and cortex increased (Kozel et al., 2000; Mosimann et al., 2002). The distance from coil to underlying cortex determines the adjustment of the stimulation intensity to the individual motor threshold (McConnell et al., 2001). This normally corrects for skull thickness and general atrophy involving the motor cortex. Prefrontal atrophy can, however, be out of proportion in some conditions such as in long-lasting depression or in advanced age, and as the stimulation threshold is determined over the motor cortex, stimulation intensity may be too low. Prefrontal atrophy appears therefore to be a negative predictor for response and so may demand higher stimulation intensities (Padberg et al., 2002c).

2.2.4. Psychoneuroendocrine findings in depressed patients

Several groups investigated whether rTMS exerts neuroendocrine effects in depression, due to the belief that dysfunction of the hypothalamic pituitary adrenal (HPA) and the hypothalamic pituitary thyroid (HPT) axes are involved in the pathophysiology of major depression (Nemeroff and Evans, 1989; Holsboer, 2001). Normalization of the dexamethasone suppression test (DST) after rTMS treatment in medicated depressed subjects has been demonstrated by Pridmore (1999) and Reid and Pridmore (1999). This finding was additionally confirmed in drug-free patients. Normalization of the DST status was, however, associated with clinical improvement. In contrast, no effect was found on corticotropin releasing hormone-induced ACTH or cortisol increase in the combined dexamethasone suppression/CRH test (Dex/CRH) (Zwanzger et al., 2003). Szuba et al. investigated the effects of single rTMS sessions on thyroid-stimulating hormone (TSH) and mood (Szuba et al., 2001). As compared to sham conditions, TSH increased and mood improved after active rTMS conditions. However, no correlation was found between mood and TSH changes (Szuba et al., 2001). It has been suggested that neuroactive steroids that interact with the γ-aminobutyric acid type A ($GABA_A$) benzodiazepine receptor complex are involved in the pathophysiology of major depression and the action of antidepressant pharmacotherapy (Rupprecht et al., 2001). Depressed patients exhibit lowered plasma levels of 3α-reduced neuroactive steroids, which normalized following successful antidepressant pharmacotherapy (Romeo et al., 1998; Uzunova et al., 1998). In contrast, clinical improvement after rTMS was not accompanied by such changes in neuroactive steroid levels (Padberg et al., 2002a). In considering the findings, results show that effects of rTMS on various neuroendocrine axes differ in several respects from effects of antidepressant drugs. This supports the idea of a differing mode of action for rTMS.

3. Clinical efficacy in major depression

Until recently, the necessary large-scale controlled efficacy trials used to determine the efficacy of antidepressant drugs (Thase, 1999; Möller, 2001; Khan et al., 2002) have not been conducted with rTMS.

Yet most small controlled studies have demonstrated antidepressant effects superior to those shown under a sham condition. Effect sizes range from modest to substantial (Pascual-Leone et al., 1996b; George et al., 1997b; Padberg et al., 1999; Klein et al., 1999; Eschweiler et al., 2000; Berman et al., 2000; George et al., 2000; Garcia-Toro et al., 2001a; Padberg et al., 2002c; Boutros et al., 2002; Nahas et al., 2003). No significant verum-sham difference was found by only few investigators (Loo et al., 1999; Manes et al., 2001; Boutros et al., 2002; Nahas et al., 2003). Figure 1 provides an overview of the efficacy of real and sham rTMS modalities in prior controlled efficacy studies.

3.1. Methodological constraints of rTMS in clinical trials

Methodological drawbacks such as the high number of different dosing parameters, the absence of a suitable animal model to explore mechanisms of action, parameters, efficacy and side effects, and the lack of commercial development programs that are available for drug development and even VNS, have impeded a systematic development of rTMS as an antidepressant intervention. The development of rTMS as a treatment modality has not followed the usual process of antidepressant drug development running from phase I to phase III studies. Rather it has been maintained by the interest of the scientific community in a new, non-invasive, non-pharmacological approach for treating major depression, which could possibly even substitute ECT, the most effective antidepressant intervention available. Therefore, several questions will have to be answered in the future which would normally have been addressed in phase I investigations.

Several methodological constraints particular to rTMS must be considered while developing rTMS into an effective antidepressant treatment. As mentioned previously, the question of dosage and dosing schedule is a far more complex matter than in antidepressant pharmacotherapy. No systematic evaluation of stimulation parameters has yet been performed. Animal models may serve in theory to establish efficacious and safe stimulation parameters, and a few studies comparing different conditions have been published. Despite known limitations of animal models of major depression, more systematic research on dosing parameters is warranted. In a recent study using an MRI-based partial physical model, Keck et al. compared the rTMS-induced current density distribution between the rat and the human brain. Results demonstrated that stimulation parameters can be analogous by means of a similar current density distribution despite largely different brain sizes (Keck et al., 2000a).

Such partial models may enable researchers to use animal experiments in selecting promising parameters for further clinical evaluation.

There is no objective measure to determine the position of the dorsolateral prefrontal cortex (DLPFC), as is possible with the localization of the primary motor cortex by means of measuring motor evoked potentials. In clinical trials, the position of the DLPFC is commonly determined in relation to the primary motor cortex, the "standard procedure" being 5 cm anterior in a parasagittal plane. This procedure results in considerable variability (Fig. 2) in targeting the DLPFC (Herwig et al., 2001). Whether the differences in individual responses depend on anatomically different stimulation sites between individual patients remains unknown. In order to reduce the variability in rTMS localization, MRI-based neuronavigation methods may be used in clinical trials. An additional point to consider is the question of adequate placebo controls. The usual requirement to determine antidepressant efficacy is the superiority of active treatment over placebo. A placebo is not available for some interventions, however, such as sleep deprivation or ECT. Commonly sham conditions are applied as placebo comparisons in rTMS research, most often by the tilting of the coil from the skull surface. This approach poses some problems. First, some conditions, e.g. tilting the coil by 45° (Loo et al., 2000; Lisanby et al., 2001a), lead to a weak stimulation of the cortex (Fig. 1). It cannot be principally ruled out that such weak active rTMS also exerts neurobiological effects. Additionally, patients notice the differences between sham and active rTMS, because the sensation on the skull, induced twitches of scalp muscles and the acoustic artefact are absent or different under usual sham conditions. This may constitute a problem in parallel designs if patients have read about the method or communicate with other patients participating in a controlled trial. So clearly improved sham conditions need to be developed for future controlled efficacy trials.

Finally, because the person who holds the coil is normally aware of the testing condition a double-blind design in controlled rTMS studies proves to be difficult. A pseudo-double-blind approach with blind raters is therefore normally used. Several groups have tried to further restrict the possible influence of the person who conducts the rTMS by using sham coils that are inactive but otherwise not distinguishable, or by using coil holders and headrests. Such methodological constraints must be considered in future research of rTMS. Despite these limitations, the evidence for antidepressant efficacy of rTMS from previous trials has to be taken as such.

3.2. Pilot and open studies

In the 1990s Möller and coworkers as well as other groups from the U.S., Germany, Austria and Israel started independently to investigate rTMS as an antidepressant treatment (Höflich et al., 1993; Grisaru et al., 1994; George et al., 1995; Kolbinger et al., 1995; Conca et al., 1996). Single-pulse

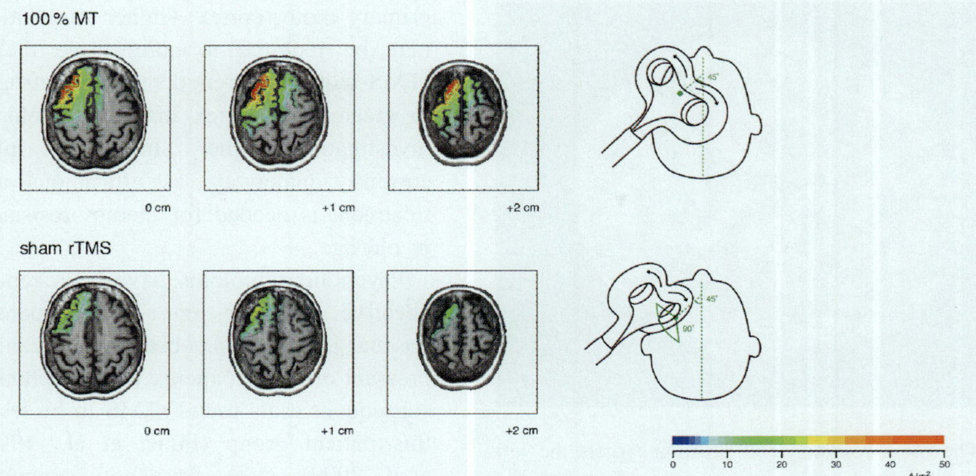

Fig. 1. MRI-based partial model of the induced current density for real and sham stimulation conditions: 100% MT intensity with normal coil position and sham coil position (also 100% MT intensity). Transversal MRI sections are shown at the level of the coil touching the skull, as well as 1 cm below and 1 cm above this level. Coil orientations are indicated. The peak current densities were related as follows: 100%: 40% (100% MT: sham). The ratios of activated volumes between sham and 100% MT were defined as function of a virtual threshold (5 to 100 A/m^2) ranging from 0.48 to 0.01.

Note: Reprinted from Neuropsychopharmacology Vol. 27; Padberg, F., Zwanzger, P., Keck, M.E., Kathmann, N., Mikhaiel, P., Ella, R., Rupprecht, P., Thoma, H., Hampel, H., Toschi, N., Möller, H.J. Repetitive transcranial magnetic stimulation (rTMS) in major depression: Relation between efficacy and stimulation intensity: 638–645, Copyright (2002), with permission from Elsevier Science.

stimulators were used in the majority of initial studies, triggered at frequencies of less than 0.3 Hz, together with large circular coils (Höflich et al., 1993; Grisaru et al., 1994; Kolbinger et al., 1995; Conca et al., 1996). Treatment was of short duration (5 days), and only one of these studies included treatment under placebo conditions comparing a supra- and subthreshold condition (Kolbinger et al., 1995). Initially, patients were only randomized to the real rTMS groups and a placebo group was added later. Antidepressant effects were postulated in most of these pilot studies, however the effect sizes were not impressive.

Data are now available from numerous open trials investigating rTMS as a putative antidepressant treatment. The average effect on depression scores was found to be modest in a recent meta analysis, with a 37.03% reduction from baseline (Burt et al., 2002). After administering rTMS in sessions on 5 consecutive days to six pharmacotherapy-resistant depressed patients, George et al. (1995) observed a reduction of the initial Hamilton Rating Scale for Depression (HRSD) (Hamilton, 1960) score by 26% with substantial improvement of depressive symptoms in two patients. Using a new stimulator with an iron core coil, Figiel et al. (1998) found a response rate of 42% after 5 rTMS sessions in the largest open trial to date, which included 56 patients. Studies (Triggs et al., 1999; Padberg et al., 2002b) continuing over a 2-week period showed a continuous clinical improvement that ranged from 30% to 41%, with response rates up to 42%.

Pridmore et al. (1999) found there to be particularly marked improvement in patients who met CORE criteria for melancholia (Parker et al., 1995). Whether observed differences in effect sizes between studies are related to the variance of stimulation parameters by means of "dose-response" relations or are

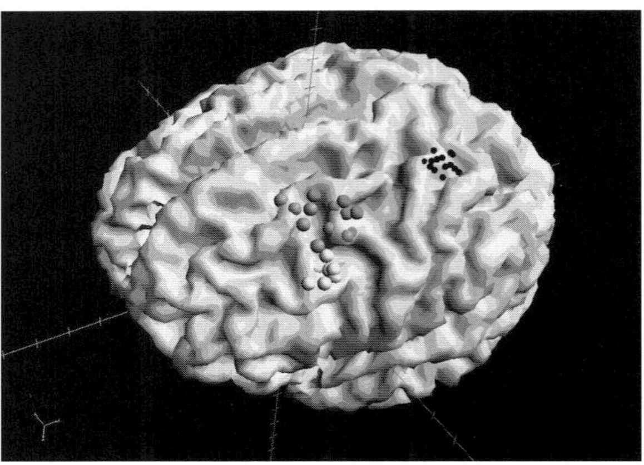

Fig. 2. The most common coil position targets the left dorsolateral prefrontal cortex by measuring 5 cm anterior (on the skull surface) to the optimal position for evoking a motor evoked potential in hand muscles. However, a considerable variability occurs with this approach, as demonstrated in a recent study applying neuronavigated rTMS (Herwig et al., 2001). The small black dots indicate the optimal sites for abductor pollicis brevis muscle stimulation over the motor cortex, i.e. the region around the lateral edge of the hand knob. The larger dots indicate the rostral coil positions over the different Brodmann areas: medium grey BA 6, dark grey BA 6/8 and 8, light grey BA 8/9 and 9. Talairach coordinates before and after "standard positioning" of the coil are visualized in an individual surface rendered MRI of the brain (white matter segmentation), which was transformed into Talairach space.

Note: Reprinted from Biological Psychiatry Vol. 50; Herwig U, Padberg F, Unger J, Spitzer M, Schonfeldt-Lecuona C. Transcranial magnetic stimulation in therapy studies: examination of the reliability of "standard" coil positioning by neuronavigation: 58–61. Copyright (2001), with permission from Elsevier Science.

due to different inclusion criteria reflecting possible predictive variables for clinical response after rTMS or both has not been determined.

Several studies have tried to identify clinical variables that enable prediction of rTMS response. Elderly patients have been found to respond poorly to rTMS in several open and controlled trials (Figiel et al., 1998; Manes et al., 2001; Mosimann et al., 2002). This has recently been explained by the increasing frontal atrophy that comes with age, which exceeds the atrophy of other cortical areas, e.g. the primary motor cortex. Higher stimulation intensities may be required to compensate the decrease of rTMS-induced current density in prefrontal areas, due to greater coil-cortex distance in old age. Studies investigating higher stimulation intensities are currently underway, as efficacious antidepressant treatment is needed for therapy-resistant depression in old age

Psychotic symptoms have been reported to be a negative predictor for rTMS response. Although Pascual-Leone et al. observed a meaningful antidepressant effect in patients with psychotic depression, subsequent trials found rTMS to be less effective in this patient group (Figiel et al., 1998; Grunhaus et al., 2000). Cases of psychotic symptoms occurring in medication-free patients for the first time ever have recently been reported (Zwanzger et al., 2002). The underlying mechanism for both the poorer response of psychotically depressed patients and newly occurring psychotic symptoms during rTMS treatment may be due to the rTMS-mediated dopamine release found in preclinical trials. Other psychopathological symptoms are less clearly associated with response after rTMS. Anxiety has been proposed as a positive predictor for rTMS outcome (Eschweiler et al., 2001), however, this has not been confirmed by others (George et al., 2000). The predictive value proposed by Pridmore et al. (1999) after finding a marked improvement in patients who met diagnostic critera for melancholia (Parker et al., 1995), has not been systematically investigated.

Theoretically, responses to other antidepressant interventions may be predictive of response to rTMS treatment, in particular if responses are based on common pathophysiology in patient subgroups. Investigation of the association between responses to different treatment modalities may therefore be useful in revealing the mode of action. As yet only non-pharmacological interventions such as partial sleep deprivation and ECT have been compared with rTMS. Non-responders to ECT have been found to be poor responders to rTMS treatment as well. Conversely, a low response rate for ECT has been reported for patients who did not previously respond to rTMS treatment (Dannon and Grunhaus, 2001).

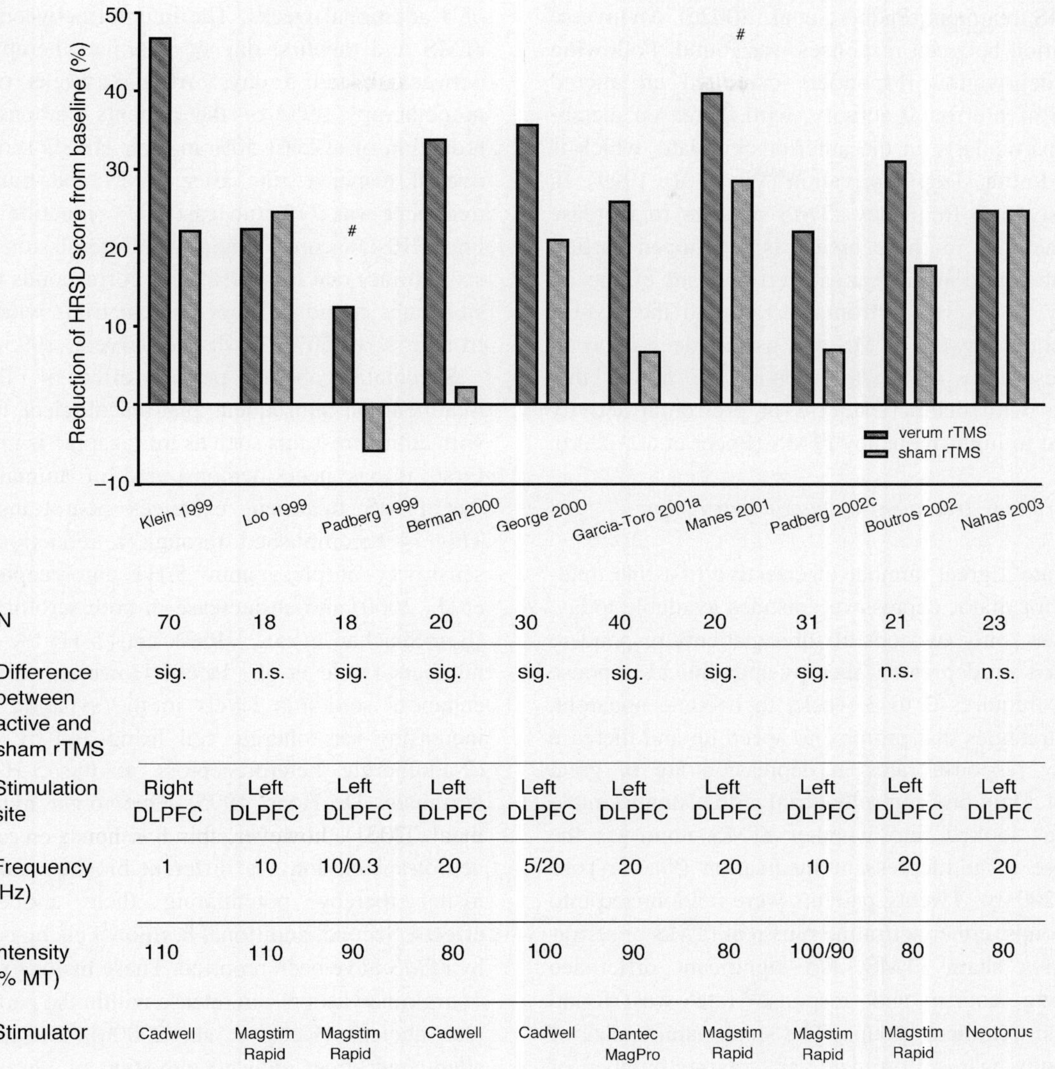

	Klein 1999	Loo 1999	Padberg 1999	Berman 2000	George 2000	Garcia-Toro 2001a	Manes 2001	Padberg 2002c	Boutros 2002	Nahas 2003
N	70	18	18	20	30	40	20	31	21	23
Difference between active and sham rTMS	sig.	n.s.	sig.	sig.	sig.	sig.	sig.	sig.	n.s.	n.s.
Stimulation site	Right DLPFC	Left DLPFC	Left DLPFC	Left DLPFC	Left DLPFC	Left DLPFC	Left DLPFC	Left DLPFC	Left DLPFC	Left DLPFC
Frequency (Hz)	1	10	10/0.3	20	5/20	20	20	10	20	20
Intensity (% MT)	110	110	90	80	100	90	80	100/90	80	80
Stimulator	Cadwell	Magstim Rapid	Magstim Rapid	Cadwell	Cadwell	Dantec MagPro	Magstim Rapid	Magstim Rapid	Magstim Rapid	Neotonus

Fig. 3. Comparison of controlled parallel design studies of rTMS as treatment in major depressive episodes. Nahas et al. (2003) investigated only bipolar type I or II patients, whereas unipolar patients or mixed groups where included in the other studies. Depicted is the reduction of baseline scores on the Hamilton Rating Scale for Depression (HRSD) for real (verum) and placebo (sham) rTMS conditions after one (#) or two weeks of rTMS. For studies with two real rTMS arms (Padberg et al., 1999; George et al., 2000; Padberg et al., 2002c) the mean HRSD reduction in both real rTMS conditions is depicted. Significant verum-sham differences and stimulation parameters are indicated below.

Note: sig. – statistically significant, n.s. – not significant, DLPFC – dorsolateral prefrontal cortex, MT – motor threshold.

Thus, there appears to be an overlap in responders to both treatments. However, non-responders to rTMS may still respond to ECT, and non-responders to ECT are more unlikely to respond to rTMS. In a recent study we investigated whether the response to partial sleep deprivation could predict the outcome of rTMS treatment (Padberg et al., 2002c). An inverse correlation between responses was found. Following sleep deprivation responders exhibited an altered pattern of prefrontal activity, with increased metabolism particularly in the anterior cingulate, which is reduced after sleep deprivation (Wu et al., 1999). In contrast, high frequency rTMS appears to increase brain activity in these areas, as mentioned earlier. Both interventions appear to exert opposite effects on activity in several prefrontal areas, and the inverse correlation between rTMS and partial sleep deprivation responses seems to support the notion that patients with distinct patterns of prefrontal activity respond to high frequency rTMS (Speer et al., 2000).

3.3. Primary treatment of major depression

There are a great number of effective first-line treatments for major depressive episodes available today. However, only two out of three patients respond to their first antidepressant therapy and clinical response usually requires 2 to 3 weeks to become apparent. New strategies that promise to speed up and increase primary response rates in depression are of great interest. Only one controlled trial with a small sample size has looked into whether rTMS improves the response to antidepressant medication (Garcia-Toro et al., 2001b). Twenty patients were randomized into two groups, either sertraline plus real rTMS or sertraline plus sham rTMS. No significant difference regarding course and response rate was found between treatment groups. The small sample size of this study was unfortunate, as a large number of patients are likely to respond quickly to sertraline treatment.

Twenty-six drug-free patients suffering from a major depressive episode according to DSM-IV criteria and who had participated in an open rTMS trial over 2 weeks receiving 10 rTMS sessions (10 Hz, left prefrontal stimulation at 100% motor threshold intensity) were recently investigated (Schüle et al., 2003). The patients were subsequently followed during standardized antidepressant pharmacotherapy with mirtazapine (monotherapy or combined with carbamazepine or lithium) for a period of 4 additional weeks. The interval between the last rTMS and the first day of pharmacotherapy varied between 1 and 5 days. After 2 weeks of rTMS monotherapy 39% of the patients demonstrated a reduction of at least 50% in their HRSD scores. The overall response rate after rTMS and mirtazapine treatment was 77% (at least 50% reduction in baseline HRSD scores), the overall remission (HRSD score (nine) rate was 39%. This corresponds to remission rates found in other clinical trials which range from 25% to 50% (Rush and Trivedi, 1995).

Speculating about a priming effect of rTMS pretreatment on subsequent pharmacological treatment with antidepressants such as mirtazapine is intriguing. First, it has been demonstrated in animal studies that rTMS treatment enhances neurotransmission. This is accomplished through a reduction of the sensitivity of presynaptic 5-HT autoreceptors (Gur et al., 2000) and an increase in both serotonin levels (Ben-Shachar et al., 1997) and 5-HT1A receptor numbers (Kole et al., 1999). However, mirtazapine enhances serotonin levels in the synaptic cleft by increasing serotonergic cell firing and by blocking (2-adrenergic heteroreceptors at the 5-HT nerve terminals (De Boer, 1995). One might hypothesize that rTMS and mirtazapine enhance serotonergic neurotransmission via different biochemical mechanisms thereby potentiating their antidepressant effects. Second, additional hormonal changes induced by rTMS have been reported. These include reduction of arginine vasopressin release within the paraventricular nucleus (Keck et al., 2000b), a significantly attenuated stress-induced elevation of plasma corticotropin and corticosterone concentrations in rats (Keck et al., 2000a, 2001; Post and Keck, 2001) and a normalization of the dexamethasone suppression test or the combined dexamethasone/suppression CRH/stimulation test in depressed patients treated with rTMS (Pridmore, 1999; Reid and Pridmore, 1999; Zwanzger et al., 2003). This attenuation of hypothalamic–pituitary–adrenocortical axis hyperactivity may favor clinical responsiveness to subsequent pharmacological treatment. Interestingly, mirtazapine is an acute inhibitor of cortisol and ACTH secretion in human subjects, presumably by blocking hypothalamic 5-$HT_{2A/C}$ and/or H_1 receptors (Schüle et al., 2002; Schüle et al., 2003). Thus, it is possible that rTMS and mirtazapine treatment work synergistically in normalizing HPA dysregulation in depressed patients.

This theoretical consideration demonstrates how rTMS might exert augmentative effects on the action of specific antidepressants and these effects may, in turn, differ depending upon the mode of action of concomitant pharmacotherapy. And so it follows that the effects of early combined treatment with other antidepressant interventions need to be systematically investigated. Eichhammer et al. showed in another small controlled study (Eichhammer et al., 2002) that the positive effects of partial sleep deprivation could successfully be maintained by subsequent 10 Hz rTMS for up to 4 days in 20 sleep deprivation responders. If this finding can be substantiated by replication, a very interesting specific therapeutic use of rTMS would arise.

3.4. Treatment of therapy-resistant depression

rTMS was originally suggested to be a potential substitute for ECT. Therefore the majority of previous trials has been conducted in rather pharmacotherapy-resistant or even refractory patients (Pascual-Leone et al., 1996b; George et al., 1997b, 2000; Padberg et al., 1999, 2002c; Berman et al., 2000; Eschweiler et al., 2000; Garcia-Toro et al., 2001a; Manes et al., 2001). Few investigators have addressed the question of efficacy in patient groups that are not explicitly treatment-resistant (Klein et al., 1999; Loo et al., 1999; George et al., 2000). Treatment-resistant patients show lower response rates, which is generally the case for antidepressant interventions including other novel, non-pharmacological approaches, e.g. VNS (Sackeim et al., 2001). It is, however, an advantage in small controlled trials that placebo response rates are also lower, and so making it easier to demonstrate placebo-verum differences with a small sample size.

Whereas in most studies investigators treated rTMS basically as an add-on treatment to a stable medication (Pascual-Leone et al., 1996b; George et al., 1997b; Klein et al., 1999; Loo et al., 1999; Padberg et al., 1999, 2002c; Eschweiler et al., 2000; Garcia-Toro et al., 2001a), several trials have included medication-free patients who received rTMS monotherapy (Berman et al., 2000; George et al., 2000; Manes et al., 2001).

Aside from differences in patient characteristics, a major confounding factor for the varying effect sizes could be the huge variation of stimulation parameters across studies. Dosing parameters of rTMS are comprised not only of a daily dosage but of a larger number of parameters including frequency, intensity, stimulation site, number of stimuli, duration of treatment, etc. All of these may have an influence on the supposed antidepressant effect. Basically all studies were conducted using different stimulation parameters (Fig. 3). Very few studies attempted to compare two conditions (Pascual-Leone et al., 1996b; Kimbrell et al., 1999; Padberg et al., 1999, 2002c; George et al., 2000; Speer et al., 2000).

A controlled study conducted by Pascual-Leone et al. used a multiple cross-over design that compared five stimulation conditions, each of which consisted of 1 week of treatment and 3 weeks follow-up (Pascual-Leone et al., 1996b). A marked improvement was seen in 11 of the 17 medication-resistant, psychotically depressed patients after only five sessions of left prefrontal 10 Hz rTMS, with the effect wearing off during the follow-up period. These findings were enthusiastically received despite the unusual design and stimulated further research on therapeutic applications of rTMS with optimistic expectations. The majority of successive studies have also shown antidepressant effects of rTMS superior to control conditions, although the effect size in the cross-over pilot study (Pascual-Leone et al., 1996b) has not to date been replicated. Results from a second cross-over study by George et al. found some clinical improvement after 2 weeks of left prefrontal 20 Hz rTMS in 12 depressed patients (George et al., 1997b). A replication study with 10 Hz rTMS and otherwise similar stimulation parameters confirmed these results, with medication-resistant patients showing modest clinical improvement (Eschweiler et al., 2000). Five of seven successive parallel studies have confirmed the superior antidepressant efficacy of rTMS over a sham condition, with effects ranging from clinically not meaningful to substantial. Padberg et al. (1999) randomized 18 patients to either 0.3 Hz, 10 Hz or sham rTMS with an equivalent number of stimuli over a 5 day period. In comparison to the other groups, patients in the 0.3 Hz group exhibited clinically marginal amelioration of depressive symptoms. Still, the duration of treatment was short and at 250/day the number of daily stimuli was much lower than in subsequent studies. In a group of 18 depressed patients, Loo et al. were unable to demonstrate an antidepressant effect of a 2-week treatment at 10 Hz rTMS compared to sham treatment, with a reduction of the HRSD score by 26% in both groups. A possible explanation for the higher sham response in this study may be the less therapy-resistant patient sample (mean number of unsuccessful antidepressant trials 1.9) as well as a potentially more active sham rTMS (Loo et al., 2000; Lisanby et al., 2001a; Padberg et al., 2002c).

A response rate of 47% was found after active rTMS compared to 17% response after sham treatment in the largest controlled trial to date ($n = 71$) which compared 1 Hz rTMS of the right DLPFC to a sham condition (Klein et al., 1999). As Pascual-Leone et al. (1996b) found no effect of 10 Hz rTMS of the right DLPFC the findings of Klein et al. appear to support the hypothesis of differential effects of slow vs fast rTMS (Post et al., 1999b). In two successive controlled studies with a parallel design only medication-free subjects were included (Berman et al., 2000; George et al., 2000). In using 20 Hz rTMS with a relatively low stimulation intensity (80% of motor threshold) in 20 patients Berman et al. (2000) found a modest antidepressant effect after real compared to sham rTMS. In a controlled trial, conducted by George et al., 30 patients were compared after treatment with 5 Hz, 20 Hz and sham rTMS (George et al., 2000). Forty-five percent of the patients were responders after active treatment (reduction of the HRSD score from baseline by at least 50%); there were no patients that responded in the sham group. There were more responders after 5 Hz rTMS than after 20 Hz rTMS, however, this difference was not statistically significant (George et al., 2000). Forty medicated patients suffering from a medication-resistant depression were studied by Garcia-Toro et al. They observed a mild antidepressant effect after 20 Hz real rTMS (Garcia-Toro et al., 2001a). The question of whether 20 Hz rTMS is effective in the treatment of depression in old age was addressed in another recent study in 20 medication-free patients (Manes et al., 2001). The results showed no significant verum-sham difference, supporting previous findings that rTMS is less effective in the elderly (Figiel et al., 1998).

We recently investigated whether stimulation intensity affects the antidepressant efficacy of rTMS in 31 patients suffering from a medication-resistant major depressive episode (Padberg et al., 2002c). We assigned patients randomly to three groups, who then underwent 10 sessions of 10 Hz rTMS over a 2-week period under various conditions: (1) stimulation of motor threshold (MT) intensity; (2) at subthreshold intensity; and (3) sham rTMS (MT intensity with the stimulation coil angled at 90°). Results indicated that antidepressant efficacy increased in a linear fashion over all the three groups, the best response being after rTMS at MT intensity (30% HRSD reduction from baseline). Thus, there is preliminary evidence that the antidepressant efficacy of rTMS depends on the applied stimulation intensity, in addition to the difference between sham and active conditions. This finding coincides firstly with evidence from a recent fMRI study (Nahas et al., 2001) that demonstrates intensity-dependent effects on brain activity in healthy volunteers and secondly, with research in elderly depressed patients where an overproportional frontal atrophy and the resulting decline of the magnetic field to the cortical surface are associated with a lower antidepressant efficacy (Kozel et al., 2000; Mosimann et al., 2002).

Boutros randomized 21 treatment-resistant patients in another very recent study (Boutros et al., 2002) to either active rTMS or to sham treatment in a double-blind design, where sub-threshold stimulation (80% MT) was delivered for 10 consecutive work days (20 Hz, 2-s trains, 20 trains). Subjects that met pre-set response criteria were entered into a follow-up phase for up to 5 months. This yielded no significant difference between groups. Six patients in the active group and one subject in the sham group met criteria for the follow-up phase. The period of time before subjects met criteria for relapse ranged greatly from two to 20 weeks.

Most previous controlled studies revealed significant verum-sham differences after short treatment periods. The studies failing to show such differences demonstrated pronounced effects of sham rTMS (Loo et al., 1999; Manes et al., 2001). Although several reasons are plausible (less-resistant patients, concomitant medication) as explanations for the differences in effect sizes, the failure of studies in showing significant placebo-verum differences is not at all unusual. More than half of adequate treatment arms in controlled trials fail to show superiority over placebo, even after the efficacy of a drug is later established (Khan et al., 2002). Results for rTMS are therefore more promising than disappointing, despite short treatment periods and inadequate sample sizes in many previous studies. More importantly, the comparably low response rates after sham rTMS may be ascribed to the rather therapy-resistant patient samples investigated as non-response to previous treatments is presumably the strongest negative predictor for all antidepressant interventions. This was recently demonstrated for VNS: response rates declined from over 50% in patients who had previously failed to respond to two or three adequate antidepressant trials to 0% in patients who had not responded to more than seven trials (Sackeim et al., 2001).

3.5. rTMS in bipolar depression

Management of depression in the context of bipolar disorders poses a major clinical problem. Although antidepressant properties have been reported, mood stabilizers such as the anticonvulsants carbamazepine and valproic acid are not particularly effective in depressed phases of the disorder. Lamotrigine, an anticonvulsant, does appear to have some antidepressant effects. The use of conventional antidepressant medication during the depressed phase may counterproductively increase a patient's cycle frequency. In several studies investigating the efficacy of rTMS in major depressive episodes also bipolar patients were included. However, separate data have not been made available from this patient group and switches to manic states have been reported in bipolar patients undergoing rTMS (Dolberg et al., 2001; Ella et al., 2002).

In a recent study (Nahas et al., 2003) rTMS was investigated in 23 depressed BPAD patients, 12 diagnosed as BPI in a depressed state, nine as BPII in a depressed state, two as BPI in mixed states. In two groups patients were randomly assigned to receive either left prefrontal rTMS (5 Hz, 110% motor threshold, 8 s on, 22 s off, over 20 min) or placebo each weekday morning for two weeks. The patients tolerated the stimulation well, exhibiting no significant events and no induction of mania. There was no statistically significant difference between the two groups in the number of antidepressant responders (> 50% decline in HRSD or HRSD < 10–4 active and 4 sham) or the mean HRSD change from baseline over 2 weeks. Compared to sham rTMS, active rTMS produced a trend but no statistically significant greater improvement in daily subjective mood ratings after treatment.

3.6. Duration of effects and maintenance

It remains to be clarified, whether subsequent antidepressant treatment is necessary to stabilize the clinical response after rTMS. A deterioration of depressive symptoms within 3 weeks after 1 week of rTMS treatment was reported by Pascual-Leone et al. (1996b) in follow-up data. However, apart from case reports, these results, as well as maintenance strategies (e.g. pharmacotherapy or maintenance rTMS) have not been confirmed nor have they been systematically studied. Dannon et al. conducted an open-label study in which they compared the medium-term outcomes of a group of patients treated with either electroconvulsive therapy or rTMS (Dannon et al., 2002). They did not find any differences in the 6-month relapse rates between both groups. However, no standardized follow-up medication was used and patients were followed up only on a monthly basis, so that a detailed assessment of the clinical course after rTMS treatment was not possible.

Schüle et al. (2003) conducted a follow-up study on drug-free patients participating in an open rTMS trial over 2 weeks. They receivied 10 rTMS sessions (10 Hz, left prefrontal stimulation at 100% motor threshold intensity) and received subsequent standardized antidepressant medication with mirtazapine (either monotherapy or combined with carbamazepine or lithium) for an additional four weeks. The interval between the last rTMS and the first day of pharmacotherapy varied between one and 5 days. A significant increase in the HRSD score of rTMS responders was observed after treatment interruption after rTMS. The length of interval without treatment coincided with the degree of the deterioration. However, under subsequent mirtazapine treatment this deterioration subsided and the further clinical course was stabilized. This corresponds with results found in the combined dexamethasone suppression/CRH test (Dex/CRH) test, in which an effect on post-dexamethasone ACTH and cortisol levels was shown, but no effect of rTMS on corticotropin releasing hormone-induced ACTH or cortisol increase resulted (Zwanzger et al., 2003). A higher risk for a relapse after remission of depressive symptoms is thus inferred (Zobel et al., 1999; Zobel et al., 2001).

Maintenance treatment with rTMS has been used successfully in single patients and case reports show favorable long-term outcomes after maintenance schedules of 0.5–2 rTMS sessions/week (Smesny et al., 2001). However, this method has its drawbacks, as it is time-consuming for patients and psychiatrists and is presumably used only in special patient populations. This treatment modality requires further systematic investigation.

3.7. Meta-analysis of efficacy in rTMS studies

Two meta analyses across controlled studies have recently been published (Burt et al., 2002; Martin et al., 2002) in spite of the huge variation of methods used in former trials. Both analyses overlap greatly in their use of selected studies, and both included unpublished data or data from manuscripts in press. After calculating effect sizes over all randomized, controlled studies without differentiating between stimulation conditions, Burt et al. (2002) concluded that the overall effect of rTMS was quite robust from the statistical angle. This supports the antidepressant action of rTMS (Burt et al., 2002). A less positive conclusion was reported in The Cochrane review (Martin et al., 2002) after analyzing different rTMS conditions (defined by stimulation side and frequency) separately. After 2 weeks of treatment, but not at other points of time a significant sham-verum difference could be established only for high frequency rTMS of the left DLPFC and low frequency rTMS of the right DLPFC. The authors reached the overall conclusion that there is not a strong case for the beneficial effects of rTMS, although the small sample sizes do not exclude the possibility of benefit (Martin et al., 2002). The explanation for the discrepancy between both analyses is the different methods applied. In theory, separate analysis for single conditions (Martin et al., 2002) is reasonable, considering the assumed specific action of rTMS. This means that each rTMS condition constitutes its own treatment modality. However, because separate analysis of each rTMS condition is based on a lower number of studies and individuals, it is more difficult to demonstrate significant differences between placebo and real rTMS conditions. Whereas Burt et al. (2002) calculated the combined effect size for 432 patients in 16 studies, the analyses of efficacy in the Cochrane review were based on fewer studies and patients (e.g. for high frequency rTMS of the left DLPFC, 11 studies with 197 individuals and for low frequency rTMS of the right DLPFC, one study with 67 patients).

3.8. Comparison with electroconvulsive therapy (ECT)

Both rTMS and ECT are means of brain stimulation. Based upon the positive findings of the first cross-over study in psychotically depressed patients (Pascual-Leone et al., 1996b), it was prematurely hypothesized that rTMS could serve as a substitute for ECT in the treatment of major depression. The basic modes of action of both treatments, however, is decidedly different. Treatment modalities for ECT have been established for decades, which is not the case for rTMS, which are, therefore, presumably less optimal. In comparison to the well-recognized strong antidepressant action of ECT (Burt et al., 2002), the results on effect sizes suggest that rTMS is less effective in therapy-resistant patients. Several groups have compared both interventions (Grunhaus et al., 2000; Pridmore et al., 2000; Janicak et al., 2002). These trials are summarized in Table 1. Pridmore et al. (2000) compared ECT and rTMS in a parallel study of 32 patients and found that patients who underwent 20 Hz rTMS improved less by means of HRSD reduction, but showed the same remission rate (69%) compared to patients who received fixed-dose, unilateral ECT. Pridmore et al. also successfully applied rTMS in place of single ECT sessions and compared this with ECT only (Pridmore, 2000). The results showed an equal improvement in both

TABLE 1

COMPARISON TRIALS OF RTMS AND ECT IN MAJOR DEPRESSIVE EPISODES (MODIFIED AFTER PADBERG AND MÖLLER, 2003): STIMULATION PARAMETERS AND THERAPEUTIC EFFECTS, MODIFIED AFTER BURT ET AL. (BURT ET AL., 2002). THE DIFFERENCES IN THE REDUCTION OF HRSD SCORES BETWEEN RTMS AND ECT GROUPS WERE STATISTICALLY NOT SIGNIFICANT

Study	Treatment groups	Design	*n*	Age (yrs)	Medication resistance	Concomitant medication	HRSD reduction
Grunhaus et al. (2000) (1–2 mg/d)	10 Hz rTMS (left DLPFC, 90% MT int.)	Parallel, randomized	20	58.4	5/15	Clonazepam	40.3%
	ECT (12 RUL, 8 RUL and BL)		20	63.6	10/10		60.6%
Pridmore et al. (2000)	20 Hz rTMS (left DLPFC, 100% MT int.)	Parallel, randomized single-masked raters	16	44.0	All	Various	55.6%
	ECT (RUL)		16	41.5	All		66.4%
Janicak et al. (2002)	10 Hz rTMS (left DLPFC, 110% MT int.)	Parallel, randomized	14	42.9	All	Minimal rescue medication	55%
	ECT (BL)		11	42.7	All		64%
Grunhaus et al. (2003)	10 Hz rTMS (left DLPFC, 90% MT int.)	Parallel, randomized single-masked raters	20	57.6	NA	Lorazepam (up to 3 mg/d)	45.5%
	ECT (13 RUL, 7 RUL and BL)		20	61.4	NA		48.2%

DLPFC – dorsolateral prefrontal cortex; MT int. – stimulation intensity related to the individual motor threshold; RUL – right unilateral; BL – bilateral; MD – major depression; BP – bipolar disorder.

treatment groups, which supports this kind of clinical application.

Grunhaus et al. (2000) studied 40 patients in an open design and reported similar findings. 10 Hz rTMS over 4 weeks proved to be less effective compared to ECT in the overall group. However, in the subgroup of non-psychotically depressed patients ($n = 20$), both interventions showed equal efficacy. In a comparison study with blind raters, Grunhaus et al. (2003) were able to replicate their findings. Forty depressed patients without psychotic symptoms were randomized to either ECT or 10 Hz rTMS groups. After ECT application 12 responders and six remitters were identified, and after rTMS application 11 responders and six remitters. In another recent controlled trial, 25 depressed patients were randomly assigned to rTMS (10–20 treatments, 10 Hz, 110% motor threshold) or a course of bitemporal ECT (4–12 treatments). Here there were no significant detectable differences in outcome variables between the two groups (e.g. HRSD reduction by 55% for the rTMS group vs. 64% for the ECT group) (Janicak et al., 2002). These results hold promise, keeping in mind, however, that blind conditions are difficult to achieve and that findings should be interpreted cautiously. The question of whether subconvulsive rTMS could be a substitute for ECT in the future requires further study.

4. Safety

The notion that rTMS is safe and well tolerated by patients within a range of parameters defined according to a consensus (Wassermann, 1998), can be substantiated by an extensive body of data. After 10 days of daily prefrontal rTMS in depressed patients there was no sign of structural changes on MR scans (Nahas et al., 2000). There was no deterioration in neuropsychologic performance, no significant mean changes in auditory threshold, and no significant EEG abnormality after 2 to 4 weeks of rTMS shown in safety studies (Padberg et al., 1999; Triggs et al., 1999; Little et al., 2000; Loo et al., 2001; Speer et al., 2001; Moser et al., 2002; Shajahan et al., 2002; Martis et al., 2003). Table 2 summarizes the neuropsychological findings in clinical studies investigating rTMS in depressed subjects. Thus, there seem to be no adverse effects on cognition as observed after ECT. On the basis that exclusion criteria are fulfilled (e.g. implanted electronical devices, previous history of seizures, etc.), the meaningful side effects are physical discomfort on the scalp during and headache after rTMS. There has been one reported case of an rTMS-associated partial seizure published since 1998 (Conca et al., 2000), whereby the risk might have been increased by both a high train duration and concomitant medication.

Particular attention, however, should be paid to the detection of psychiatric side effects and the possibility should be mentioned to the patients before obtaining their informed consent for participation in rTMS studies. Two recent case reports showed that bipolar patients treated with rTMS for depression may be at risk to switch to manic states (Dolberg et al., 2001; Ella et al., 2002). Additionally, one case has been reported in which newly developed psychotic symptoms during rTMS for depression under otherwise medication-free conditions were exhibited (Zwanzger et al., 2002).

5. Conclusions and perspectives

In addition to its powerful position as an experimental research tool in neuroscience, rTMS has established its place among possible non-pharmacological treatments for major depression. As supported by neuroimaging data, long-term rTMS modulates neuronal circuits involved in the pathophysiology of depression. Preclinical studies have shown dopaminergic and serotonergic effects, among others, as well as an attenuation of the HPA response to stress, which is hypothesized to occur at hippocampal or hypothalamic levels. The majority of clinical trials demonstrate significant antidepressant effects as compared to sham conditions, with optimal parameters yet to be identified. However, clinical efficacy has generally not been substantial, treatment periods

TABLE 2

NEUROPSYCHOLOGICAL ASSESSMENT IN CLINICAL STUDIES INVESTIGATING RTMS AS TREATMENT IN MAJOR DEPRESSIVE EPISODES

Study	*n*	Design	Medication	Stimulation site	Stimulus parameters				Measures	Findings
					Frequency (Hz)	Intensity (MT%)	Stimuli per day	Total no. of stimuli		
Padberg et al., 1999	18	Parallel, randomized, double-blind	Stable medication or drug-free	Left DLPFC	10 or 0.3 or sham	90	250	1250	Verbal learning task	Significant improvements in verbal memory after 10 Hz rTMS
Triggs et al., 1999	10	Open	Drug-free	Left DLPFC	20	80	2000	20000	MMSE, VLT, Dig. span, COWA, BWT	No significant decline in performance, significant improvement in COWA test scores post rTMS
Little et al., 2000	16	Cross-over, randomized, double-blind	Drug-free or mood stabilizers	Left DLPFC	1 or 20	80	800	8000	Buschke selective reminding test, memory cards, COWA, CPT	No adverse effects. Improvement on list recall ($p < 0.05$) one week post rTMS
Loo et al., 2001	18	Parallel, randomized, double-blind	Stable medication or drug-free	Left DLPFC	10 or sham	110	1500	15000 to 20000	MMSE, Dig. span, RAVLT, VPAL, COWA, RT, AMI	No significant mean deterioration in test scores (2 week. post rTMS) Similar results over 4 week ($n = 12$) No association between change in NP scores and clinical change. No significant differences between sham and real group

TABLE 2

CONTINUED

Study	n	Design	Medication	Stimulation site	Stimulus parameters				Measures	Findings
					Frequency (Hz)	Intensity (MT%)	Stimuli per day	Total no. of stimuli		
Speer et al., 2001	18 (14)	Cross-over, randomized, double-blind	Drug-free or valproate or carba-mazepine	Left DLPFC	1 or 20	100	1600	16000	Memory tests (see Little et al. above), CPT, COWA	No major changes in test scores (for both 1 Hz and 20 Hz group) Improvement trends on some tests No correlation with clinical improvement
Moser et al., 2002	19 (18)	Parallel, randomized, double-blind	Drug-free	Left DLPFC	20 or sham	80	800	4000	Trial Making Test A and B, WAIS-R Digit Symbol, Stroop Test, COWA, BNT, sentence repetition, Rey Auditory Verbal Learning Test, Judgement of Line Orientation	Higher digit symbol scores after real rTMS, Improvement in Trail Making Test B
Shajahan et al., 2002	15	Parallel, randomized, double-blind	Stable medication	Left DLPFC	5 or 10 or 20	80	500	5000	Stress Arousal Inventory, Auditory Verbal Learning Test, Wechsler Memory Scale, Digit Symbol Substitution Test, Traffic Light Test	No significant changes

TABLE 2. Continued.

Study	*n*	Design	Medication	Stimulation site	Stimulus parameters				Measures	Findings
					Frequency (Hz)	Intensity (MT%)	Stimuli per day	Total no. of stimuli		
Martis et al., 2003	15	Open	Drug-free	Left DLPFC	10	110	1000	10,000 to 20,000	Simple and choice reaction time, stroop COWA, WAIS-III-letter number span. Wechsler Memory Scale-Revised, Mental Alterations Test, Grooved Pegboard	No significant decline in performance. Significant improvement (baseline-post) in 3 of 4 domains: Working memory-executive function, objective memory fine motor speed, but not attention and mental speed Improvement not related to clinical change

DLPFC – left dorsolateral prefrontal cortex; MT – motor threshold.

have been relatively short, the patients mostly somewhat therapy-resistant, and follow-up not systematically included. In comparison to ECT, rTMS may be equivalent in terms of efficacy in non-psychotic, but not in psychotic patients.

On the basis of clinical data, rTMS may be beneficial as an add-on or monotherapy in the treatment of pharmacotherapy-resistant depression. Therefore rTMS has already, perhaps somewhat prematurely, been approved in Canada for this purpose. Other applications may also be feasible: (1) primary treatment as monotherapy; (2) primary treatment as an add-on to accelerate and/or increase the initial response to antidepressant medication; (3) augmentation of other non-pharmacological interventions, e.g. sleep deprivation; (4) substitution of single ECT sessions and reduction of the number of required ECT sessions; and (5) long-term maintenance treatment as in maintenance ECT.

Specific clinical applications of rTMS require further testing either in specific patient groups or through the use of specific study designs. It appears worthwhile to study these specific questions intensively when considering the possible benefit of an efficacious antidepressant treatment that is non-invasive, well-tolerated and comparably easy to conduct. In order to provide sufficient proof of antidepressant efficacy, controlled multicenter trials comparable to phase III trials in the development of antidepressant drugs are needed. Specific applications need to be investigated, particularly in its use as an early add-on treatment to facilitate response to antidepressant drugs and to maximize response rates. Follow-up data needs to be systematically evaluated to identify suitable treatment strategies for maintaining the antidepressant effect of rTMS.

Acknowledgements

This work was supported by the German Ministry for Education and Research within the promotional emphasis "German Research Network on Depression" (Subproject 6.5, F.P.) and by the Faculty of Medicine, University of Munich (Förderprogramm für Forschung und Lehre).

References

Barker, A.T., Jalinous, R. and Freeston, I.L. Noninvasive magnetic stimulation of human motor cortex. *Lancet*, 1985, ii: 1106–1107.

Baxter, L.R.J., Schwartz, J.M., Phelps, M.E., Mazziotta, J.C., Guze, B.H., Selin, C.E., Gerner, R.H. and Sumida, R.M. Reduction of prefrontal cortex glucose metabolism common to three types of depression. *Arch. Gen. Psychiatry*, 1989, 46: 243–250.

Belmaker, R.H. and Grisaru, N. Magnetic stimulation of the brain in animal depression models responsive to ECS. *J. ECT*, 1998, 14: 194–205.

Ben-Shachar, D., Belmaker, R.H., Grisaru, N. and Klein, E. Transcranial magnetic stimulation induces alterations in brain monoamines. *J. Neural. Transm.* 1997, 104: 191–197.

Ben-Shachar, D., Gazawi, H., Riboyad-Levin, J. and Klein, E. Chronic repetitive transcranial magnetic stimulation alters beta-adrenergic and 5-HT2 receptor characteristics in rat brain. *Brain Res.* 1999, 816: 78–83.

Berger, M., Vollmann, J., Hohagen, F., Konig, A., Lohner, H., Voderholzer, U. and Riemann, D. Sleep deprivation combined with consecutive sleep phase advance as a fast-acting therapy in depression: an open pilot trial in medicated and unmedicated patients. *Am. J. Psychiatry*, 1997, 154: 870–872.

Berman, R.M., Narasimhan, M., Sanacora, G., Miano, A.P., Hoffman, R.E., Hu, X.S., Charney, D.S. and Boutros, N.N. A randomized clinical trial of repetitive transcranial magnetic stimulation in the treatment of major depression. *Biol. Psychiatry*, 2000, 47: 332–337.

Bonnet, J.J., Chagraoui, A., Protais, P. and Costentin, J. Interactions of amineptine with the neuronal dopamine uptake system: neurochemical in vitro and in vivo studies. *J. Neural. Transm.*, 1987, 69: 211–220.

Borsini, F. and Meli, A. Is the forced swimming test a suitable model for revealing antidepressant activity? *Psychopharmacology* (Berl), 1988, 94: 147–160.

Boutros, N.N., Gueorguieva, R., Hoffman, R.E., Oren, D.A., Feingold, A. and Berman, R.M. Lack of a therapeutic effect of a 2-week sub-threshold transcranial magnetic stimulation course for treatment-resistant depression. *Psychiatry Res.*, 2002, 113: 245–254.

Brown, A.S. and Gershon, S. Dopamine and depression. *J. Neural. Transm. Gen. Sect* 1993, 91: 75–109.

Burt, T., Lisanby, S.H. and Sackeim, H.A. Neuropsychiatric applications of transcranial magnetic stimulation: a meta analysis. *Int. J. Neuropsychopharmacol.*, 2002, 5: 73–103.

Catafau, A.M., Perez, V., Gironell, A., Martin, J.C., Kulisevsky, J., Estorch, M., Carrio, I. and Alvarez, E. SPECT mapping of cerebral activity changes induced by repetitive transcranial magnetic stimulation in depressed patients. A pilot study. *Psychiatry Res.*, 2001, 106: 151–160.

Cohrs, S., Tergau, F., Riech, S., Kastner, S., Paulus, W., Ziemann, U., Rüther, E. and Hajak, G. High-frequency repetitive transcranial magnetic stimulation delays rapid eye movement sleep. *NeuroReport*, 1998, 9: 3439–3443.

Cohrs, S., Tergau, F., Korn, J., Becker, W. and Hajak, G. Suprathreshold repetitive transcranial magnetic stimulation elevates thyroid-stimulating hormone in healthy male subjects. *J. Nerv. Ment. Dis.* 2001, 189: 393–397.

Conca, A., Koppi, S., König, P., Swoboda, E. and Krecke, N. Transcranial magnetic stimulation: a novel antidepressive strategy? *Neuropsychobiology*, 1996, 34: 204–207.

Conca, A., Konig, P. and Hausmann, A. Transcranial magnetic stimulation induces 'pseudoabsence seizure'. *Acta Psychiatr. Scand.*, 2001, 101: 246–248.

Conca, A., Peschina, W., Konig, P., Fritzsche, H. and Hausmann, A. Effect of chronic repetitive transcranial magnetic stimulation on regional cerebral blood flow and regional cerebral glucose uptake in drug treatment-resistant depressives. A brief report. *Neuropsychobiology* 2002, 45: 27–31.

Counter, S.A. Neurobiological effects of extensive transcranial electromagnetic stimulation in an animal model. *Electroencephalogr. Clin. Neurophysiol.*, 1993, 89: 341–348.

Cumming, P., Brown, E., Damsma, G. and Fibiger, H. Formation and clearance of interstitial metabolites of dopamine and serotonin in the rat striatum: an in vivo microdialysis study. *J. Neurochem.*, 1992, 59: 1905–1914.

Czéh, B., Welt, T., Fischer, A.K., Erhardt, A., Schmitt, W., Müller, M.B., Toschi, N., Fuchs, E. and Keck, M.E. Chronic psychosocial stress and concomitant repetitive transcranial magnetic stimulation: Effects on stress hormone levels and adult hippocampal neurogenesis. *Biol. Psychiatry*, 2002, 52: 1057–1065.

Dannon, P.N. and Grunhaus, L. Effect of electroconvulsive therapy in repetitive transcranial magnetic stimulation non-responder MDD patients: a preliminary study. *Int. J. Neuropsycho-pharmacol.* 2001, 4: 265–268.

Dannon, P.N., Dolberg, O.T., Schreiber, S. and Grunhaus, L. Three and six-month outcome following courses of either ECT or rTMS in a population of severely depressed individuals – preliminary report. *Biol. Psychiatry*, 2002, 51: 687–690.

De Boer, T. and Ruigt, G.S.F. The selective alpha–2-adrenoceptor antagonist mirtazapine (Org 3770) enhances noradrenergic and 5-HT1A-mediated serotonergic neurotransmission. *CNS Drugs*, 1995, 4 (Suppl.): 29–38.

Dearing, M.J. Mood effects of prefrontal repetitive high-frequency TMS in healthy volunteers. *CNS Spectrums*, 1992, 2: 53 and 68.

Dolberg, O.T., Schreiber, S. and Grunhaus, L. Transcranial magnetic stimulation-induced switch into mania: a report of two cases. *Biol. Psychiatry*, 2001, 49: 468–470.

Drevets, W.C. Functional anatomical abnormalities in limbic and prefrontal cortical structures in major depression. *Prog. Brain. Res.*, 2000, 126: 413–431.

Eichhammer, P., Kharraz, A., Wiegand, R., Langguth, B., Frick, U., Aigner, J.M. and Hajak, G. Sleep deprivation in depression stabilizing antidepressant effects by repetitive transcranial magnetic stimulation. *Life Sci.*, 2002, 70: 1741–1749.

Ella, R., Zwanzger, P., Stampfer, R., Preuss, U., Müller-Siecheneder, F., Möller, H.-J. and Padberg, F. Switch to mania after slow rTMS of the right prefrontal cortex. *J. Clin. Psychiatry* 2002, 63: 249.

Eschweiler, G.W., Wegerer, C., Schlotter, W., Spandl, C., Stevens, A., Bartels, M. and Buchkremer, G. Left prefrontal activation predicts therapeutic effects of repetitive transcranial magnetic stimulation (rTMS) in major depression. *Psychiatry Res.*, 2000, 99: 161–172.

Eschweiler, G.W., Plewnia, C. and Bartels, M. Welche depressiven Patienten profitieren von präfrontaler transkranieller Magnetstimulation (rTMS)? Which patients with major depression benefit from prefrontal repetitive magnetic stimulation? [article in German]. *Fortschr. Neurol. Psychiatr.*, 2001, 69: 402–409.

Figiel, G., Epstein, C., McDonald, W., Amazon-Leece, J., Figiel, L., Saldivia, A. and Glover, S. The use of rapid-rate transcranial magnetic stimulation (rTMS) in refractory depressed patients. *J. Neuropsychiatry Clin. Neurosci.*, 1998, 10: 20–25.

Fleischmann, A., Prolov, K., Abarbanel, J. and Belmaker, R.H. The effect of transcranial magnetic stimulation of rat brain on behavioral models of depression. *Brain Res.*, 1995, 699: 130–132.

Fox, P., Ingham, R., George, M.S., Mayberg, H., Ingham, J., Roby, J., Martin, C. and Jerabek, P. Imaging human intra-cerebral connectivity by PET during TMS. *NeuroReport* 1997, 8: 2787–2791.

Fujiki, M. and Steward, O. High frequency transcranial magnetic stimulation mimics the effects of ECS in upregulating astroglial gene expression in the murine CNS. *Brain Res. Mol. Brain. Res.*, 1997, 44: 301–308.

Garcia-Toro, M., Mayol, A., Arnillas, H., Capllonch, I., Ibarra, O., Crespi, M., Mico, J., Lafau, O., Lafuente, L. Modest adjunctive benefit with transcranial magnetic stimulation in medication-resistant depression. *J. Affect. Disord.*, 2001a, 64: 271–275.

Garcia-Toro, M., Pascual-Leone, A., Romera, M., Gonzalez, A., Mico, J., Ibarra, O., Arnillas, H., Capllonch, I., Mayol, A. and Tormos, J.M. Prefrontal repetitive transcranial magnetic stimulation as add on treatment in depression. *J. Neurol. Neurosurg. Psychiatry*, 2001b, 71: 546–548.

George, M.S., Wassermann, E.M., Williams, W.A., Callahan, A., Ketter, T.A., Basser, P., Hallett, M. and Post, R.M. Daily left prefrontal repetitive transcranial magnetic stimulation (rTMS) improves mood in depression. *NeuroReport*, 1995, 6: 1–6.

George, M.S., Wassermann, E.M., Williams, W.A., Steppel, J., Pascual-Leone, A., Basser, P., Hallett, M. and Post, R.M. Changes in mood and hormone levels after rapid-rate transcranial magnetic stimulation (rTMS) of the prefrontal cortex. *J. Neuropsychiatry Clin. Neurosci.*, 1996, 8: 172–180.

George, M.S., Speer, A.M., Wassermann, E.M., Kimbrell, T.A., William, W.A., Kellner, C.H., Risch, S.C., Stallings, L. and Post, R.M. Repetitive TMS as a probe of mood in health and disease. *CNS Spectrums*, 1997a, 2: 39–44.

George, M.S., Wassermann, E.M., Kimbrell, T.A., Little, J.T., Williams, W.E., Danielson, A.L., Greenberg, B.D., Hallett, M. and Post, R.M. Mood improvement following daily left prefrontal repetitive transcranial magnetic stimulation in patients with depression: A placebo-controlled crossover trial. *Am. J. Psychiatry*, 1997b, 154: 1752–1756.

George, M.S., Lisanby, S.H. and Sackeim, H.A. Transcranial magnetic stimulation. *Arch. Gen. Psychiatry*, 1999, 56: 300–311.

George, M.S., Nahas, Z., Molloy, M., Speer, A.M., Oliver, N.C., Li, X.B., Arana, G.W., Risch, S.C. and Ballenger, J.C. A controlled trial of daily left prefrontal cortex TMS for treating depression. *Biol. Psychiatry*, 2000, 48: 962–970.

Golden, R.N., Rudorfer, M.V., Sherer, M.A., Linnoila, M. and Potter, W.Z. Bupropion in depression. I. Biochemical effects and clinical response. *Arch. Gen. Psychiatry*, 1988, 45: 139–143.

Grisaru, N., Yarovslavsky, U., Abarbanel, J., Lamberg, T. and Belmaker, R.H. Transcranial magnetic stimulation in depression and schizophrenia. *European Neuropsychopharmacology*, 1994, 4: 287–288.

Grisaru, N., Bruno, R. and Pridmore, S. Effect on the emotions of healthy individuals of slow repetitive transcranial magnetic stimulation applied to the prefrontal cortex. *J. ECT* 2001, 17: 184–189.

Grunhaus, L., Dannon, P.N., Schreiber, S., Dolberg, O.H., Amiaz, R., Ziv, R. and Lefkifker, E. Repetitive transcranial magnetic stimulation is as effective as electroconvulsive therapy in the treatment of nondelusional major depressive disorder: an open study. *Biol. Psychiatry*, 2000, 47: 314–324.

Grunhaus, L., Schreiber, S., Dolberg, O.T., Polak, D. and Dannon, P.N. A randomized controlled comparison of electroconvulsive therapy and repetitive transcranial magnetic stimulation in severe and resistant nonpsychotic major depression. *Biol. Psychiatry*, 2003, 53: 324–331.

Gur, E., Lerer, B. and Newman, M.E. Chronic electroconvulsive shock and 5-HT autoreceptor activity in rat brain: an in vivo microdialysis study. *J. Neural. Transm.*, 1997, 104: 795–804.

Gur, E., Lerer, B., Dremencov, E. and Newman, M.E. Chronic repetitive transcranial magnetic stimulation induces subsensitivity of presynaptic serotonergic autoreceptor activity in rat brain. *Neuroreport* 2000, 11: 2925–2929.

Hallett, M. Transcranial magnetic stimulation: a tool for mapping the central nervous system. *Electroencephalogr. Clin. Neurophysiol.*, 1996, (Suppl.) 46: 43–51.

Hamilton, M. A rating scale for depression. *J. Neurol. Neurosurg. Psychiatry*, 1960, 23: 56–62.

Herwig, U., Padberg, F., Unger, J., Spitzer, M. and Schonfeldt-Lecuona, C. Transcranial magnetic stimulation in therapy studies: examination of the reliability of "standard" coil positioning by neuronavigation. *Biol. Psychiatry*, 2001, 50: 58–61.

Hoffman, R.E. and Cavus, I. Slow transcranial magnetic stimulation, long-term depotentiation, and brain hyperexcitability disorders. *Am. J. Psychiatry*, 2002, 159: 1093–1102.

Höflich, G., Kasper, S., Hufnagel, A., Ruhrmann, S. and Möller, H.-J. Application of transcranial magnetic stimulation in treatment of drug-resistant major depression. *Human Psychopharmacology*, 1993, 8: 361–365.

Holsboer, F. Stress, hypercortism and corticosteroid receptors in depression: implications for therapy. *J. Affect. Disord.*, 2001, 62: 77–91.

Holsboer, F. and Barden, N. Antidepressants and hypothalamic-pituitary-adrenocortical regulation. *Endocr. Rev.*, 1996, 17: 187–205.

Janicak, P.G., Dowd, S.M., Martis, B., Alam, D., Beedle, D., Krasuski, J., Strong, M.J., Sharma, R., Rosen, C. and Viana, M. Repetitive transcranial magnetic stimulation vs. electroconvulsive therapy for major depression: Preliminary results of a randomized trial. *Biol. Psychiatry*, 2002, 51: 659–667.

Jenkins, J., Shajahan, P.M., Lappin, J.M. and Ebmeier, K.P. Right and left prefrontal transcranial magnetic stimulation at 1 Hz does not affect mood in healthy volunteers. *BMC Psychiatry*, 2002, 2: 1

Juckel, G., Mendlin, A. and Jacobs, B.L. Electrical stimulation of rat medial prefrontal cortex enhances forebrain serotonin output: implications for electroconvulsive therapy and transcranial magnetic stimulation in depression. *Neuropsychopharmacology*, 1999, 21: 391–398.

Kapur, S. and Mann, J.J. Role of the dopaminergic system in depression. *Biol. Psychiatry*, 1992, 32: 1–17.

Karreman, M., Westerink, B.H. and Moghaddam, B. Excitatory amino acid receptors in the ventral tegmental area regulate dopamine release in the ventral striatum. *J. Neurochem.*, 1996, 67: 601–607.

Keck, M.E., Engelmann, M., Müller, M.B., Henniger, M.S.H., Hermann, B., Rupprecht, R., Neumann, I.D., Toschi, N., Landgraf, R. and Post, A. Repetitive transcranial magnetic stimulation induces active coping strategies and attenuates the neuroendocrine stress response in rats. *J. Psychiatr. Res.*, 2000a, 34: 265–276.

Keck, M.E., Sillaber, I., Ebner, K., Welt, T., Toschi, N., Kaehler, S.T., Singewald, N., Philippu, A., Elbel, G.K., Wotjak, C.T., Holsboer, F., Landgraf, R. and Engelmann, M. Acute transcranial magnetic stimulation of frontal brain regions selectively modulates the release of vasopressin, biogenic amines and amino acids in the rat brain. *Eur. J. Neurosci.*, 2000b, 12: 3713–3720.

Keck, M.E., Welt, T., Post, A., Müller, M.B., Toschi, N., Wigger, A., Landgraf, R., Holsboer, F. and Engelmann, M. Neuroendocrine and behavioral effects of repetitive transcranial magnetic stimulation in a psychopathological animal model are suggestive of antidepressant-like effects. *Neuropsycho-pharmacology*, 2001, 24: 337–349.

Keck, M.E., Welt, T., Müller, M.B., Erhardt, A., Ohl, F., Toschi, N., Holsboer, F. and Sillaber, I. Repetitive transcranial magnetic stimulation increases the release of dopamine in the mesolimbic and mesostriatal system. *Neuropharmacology*, 2002, 43: 101–109.

Khan, A., Khan, S. and Brown, W.A. Are placebo controls necessary to test new antidepressants and anxiolytics? *Int. J. Neuropsychopharm.*, 2002, 5: 193–197.

Kimbrell, T.A., Little, J.T., Dunn, R.T., Frye, M.A., Greenberg, B.D., Wassermann, E.M., Repella, J.D., Danielson, A.L., Willis, M.W., Benson, B.E., Speer, A.M., Osuch, E., George, M.S. and Post, R.M. Frequency dependence of antidepressant response to left prefrontal repetitive transcranial magnetic stimulation (rTMS) as a function of baseline cerebral glucose metabolism. *Biol. Psychiatry*, 1999, 46: 1603–1613.

Kimbrell, T.A., Dunn, R.T., George, M.S., Danielson, A.L., Willis, M.W., Repella, J.D., Benson, B.E., Herscovitch, P., Post, R.M. and Wassermann, E.M. Left prefrontal-repetitive transcranial magnetic stimulation (rTMS) and regional cerebral glucose metabolism in normal volunteers. *Psychiatry Res.*, 2002, 115: 101–113.

Klein, E., Kreinin, I., Chistyakov, A., Koren, D., Mecz, L., Marmur, S., Ben-Shachar, D. and Feinsod, M. Therapeutic efficacy of right prefrontal slow repetitive transcranial magnetic stimulation in major depression. *Arch. Gen. Psychiatry*, 1999, 56: 315–320.

Kolbinger, H.M., Höflich, G., Hufnagel, A., Möller, H.-J. and Kasper, S. Transcranial magnetic stimulation (TMS) in the treatment of major depression – a pilot study. *Human Psychopharmacology*, 1995, 10: 305–310.

Kole, M.H., Fuchs, E., Ziemann, U., Paulus, W. and Ebert, U. Changes in 5-HT1A and NMDA binding sites by a single rapid transcranial magnetic stimulation procedure in rats. *Brain Res.*, 1999, 826: 309–312.

Kozel, F.A., Nahas, Z., deBrux, C., Molloy, M., Lorberbaum, J.P., Bohning, D., Risch, S.C. and George, M.S. How coil-cortex distance relates to age, motor threshold, and antidepressant response to repetitive transcranial magnetic stimulation. *J. Neuropsychiatry Clin. Neurosci.*, 2000, 12: 376–384.

Lisanby, S.H., Luber, B., Perera, T. and Sackeim, H.A. Transcranial magnetic stimulation: Applications in basic neuroscience and neuropsychopharmacology. *Int. J. Neuropsychopharm.*, 2000, 3: 259–273.

Lisanby, S.H., Gutman, D., Luber, B., Schroeder, C. and Sackeim, H.A. Sham TMS: intracerebral measurement of the induced electrical field and the induction of motor-evoked potentials. *Biol. Psychiatry*, 2001, 49: 460–463.

Little, J.T., Kimbrell, T.A. and Wassermann, E.M. Cognitive effects of 1- and 20-hertz repetitive transcranial magnetic stimulation in depression: preliminary report. *Neuropsychiatry Neuropsychol. Behav. Neurol.*, 2000, 13: 119–124

Loo, C., Mitchell, P., Sachdev, P., McDarmont, B., Parker, G. and Gandevia, S. Double-blind controlled investigation of transcranial magnetic stimulation for the treatment of resistant major depression. *Am. J. Psychiatry*, 1999, 156: 946–948.

Loo, C.K., Taylor, J.L., Gandevia, S.C., McDarmont, B.N., Mitchell, P.B. and Sachdev, P.S. Transcranial magnetic stimulation (TMS) in controlled treatment studies: are some "sham" forms active? *Biol. Psychiatry*, 2000, 47: 325–331.

Loo, C.K., Sachdev, P.S., Elsayed, H., McDarmont, B.N., Mitchell, P.B., Wilkinson, M., Parker, G. and Gandevia, S.C. Effects of a 2- to 4-week course of repetitive transcranial magnetic stimulation (rTMS) on neuropsychological functioning, electroencephalogram and auditory threshold in depressed patients. *Biol. Psychiatry*, 2001, 49, 615–623.

Manes, F., Jorge, R., Morcuende, M., Yamada, T., Paradiso, S. and Robinson, R.G. A controlled study of repetitive transcranial magnetic stimulation as a treatment of depression in the elderly. *Int. Psychogeriatr.*, 2001, 13: 225–231.

Martin, J.L., Barbanoj, M.J., Schlaepfer, T.E., Clos, S., Perez, V., Kulisevsky, J. and Gironell, A. Transcranial magnetic stimulation for treating depression. *Cochrane Database Syst. Rev.*, 2002 (2), CD003493.

Martis, B., Alam, D., Dowd, S.M., Hill, S.K., Sharma, R.P., Rosen, C., Pliskin, N., Martin, E., Carson, V. and Janicak, P.G. Neurocognitive effects of repetitive transcranial magnetic stimulation in severe major depression. *Clin. Neurophysiol.*, 2003, 114: 1125–1132.

Matsumiya, Y., Yamamoto, T., Yarita, M., Miyauchi, S. and Kling, J.W. Physical and physiological specification of magnetic pulse stimuli that produce cortical damage in rats. *J. Clin. Neurophysiol.*, 1992, 9: 278–287.

Mayberg, H.S., Silva, J.A., Brannan, S.K., Tekell, J.L., Mahurin, R.K., McGinnis, S. and Jerabek, P.A. The functional neuroanatomy of the placebo effect. *Am. J. Psychiatry*, 2002, 159: 728–737.

McConnell, K.A., Nahas, Z., Shastri, A., Lorberbaum, J.P., Kozel, F.A., Bohning, D.E. and George, M.S. The transcranial magnetic stimulation motor threshold depends on the distance from coil to underlying cortex: a replication in healthy adults comparing two methods of assessing the distance to cortex. *Biol. Psychiatry*, 2001, 49: 454–459.

McGarvey, K.A., Zis, A.P., Brown, E.E., Nomikos, G.G. and Fibiger, H.C. ECS-induced dopamine release: effects of electrode placement, anticonvulsant treatment, and stimulus intensity. *Biol. Psychiatry*, 1993, 34: 152–157.

Möller, H.-J. Methodological aspects in the assessment of severity of depression by the Hamilton Depression Scale. *Eur. Arch. Psychiatry Clin. Neurosci.*, 2001, 251 (Suppl.) 2, II: 13–20.

Moser, D.J., Jorge, R.E., Manes, F., Paradiso, S., Benjamin, M.L. and Robinson, R.G. Improved executive functioning following repetitive transcranial magnetic stimulation. *Neurology*, 2002, 58: 1288–1290.

Mosimann, U.P., Rihs, T.A., Engeler, J., Fisch, H. and Schlaepfer, T.E. Mood effects of repetitive transcranial magnetic stimulation of left prefrontal cortex in healthy volunteers. *Psychiatry Res.*, 2000, 94: 251–256.

Mosimann, U., Marré, S.C., Werlen, S., Schmitt, W., Hess, C.W., Fisch, H.U. and Schlaepfer, T.E. Antidepressant effects of repetitive transcranial magnetic stimulation in the elderly – Correlation between effect size and coil-cortex distance. *Arch. Gen. Psychiatry*, 2002, 59: 560–561.

Mottaghy, F., Keller, C., Gangitano, M., Ly, J., Thall, M., Parker, J. and Pascual-Leone, A. Correlation of cerebral blood flow and treatment effects of repetitive transcranial magnetic stimulation in depressed patients. *Psychiatry Res.*, 2002, 115: 1–14.

Muller, M.B., Toschi, N., Kresse, A.E., Post, A., Keck, M.E. Long-term repetitive transcranial magnetic stimulation increases the expression of brain-derived neurotrophic factor and cholecystokinin mRNA, but not neuropeptide tyrosine mRNA in specific areas of rat brain. *Neuropsychopharmacology*, 2000, 23: 205–215.

Murase, S., Grenhoff, J., Chouvet, G., Gonon, F.G. and Svensson, T.H. Prefrontal cortex regulates burst firing and transmitter release in rat mesolimbic dopamine neurons studied in vivo. *Neurosci. Lett.*, 1993, 157: 53–56.

Nahas, Z., DeBrux, C., Chandler, V., Lorberbaum, J.P., Speer, A.M., Molloy, M.A., Liberatos, C., Risch S.C. and George, M.S. Lack of significant changes on magnetic resonance scans before and after 2 weeks of daily left prefrontal repetitive transcranial magnetic stimulation for depression. *J. ECT*, 2000, 16: 380–390.

Nahas, Z., Lomarev, M., Roberts, D.R., Shastri, A., Lorberbaum, J.P., Teneback, C., McConnell, K., Vincent, D.J., Li, X., George, M.S. and Bohning, D.E. Unilateral left prefrontal transcranial magnetic stimulation (TMS) produces intensity-dependent bilateral effects as measured by interleaved BOLD fMRI. *Biol. Psychiatry*, 2001, 50: 712–720.

Nahas, Z., Kozel, F.A., Li, X., Anderson, B. and George, M.S. Left prefrontal transcranial magnetic stimulation (TMS) treatment of depression in bipolar affective disorder: a pilot study of acute safety and efficacy. *Bipolar Disord.*, 2003, 5: 40–47.

Nedjat, S. and Folkerts, H.W. Induction of a reversible state of hypomania by rapid-rate transcranial magnetic stimulation over the left prefrontal cortex. *J. ECT*, 1999, 15: 166–168.

Nemeroff, C.B. and Evans, D.L. Thyrotropin releasing hormone (TRgH), the thyroid axisand affective disorders. *Ann. NY Acad. Sci.*, 1989, 533: 304–310.

Nibuya, M., Morinobu, S. and Duman, R.S. Regulation of BDNF and trkB mRNA in rat brain by chronic electroconvulsive seizure and antidepressant drug treatments. *J. Neurosci.*, 1995, 15: 7539–7547.

Padberg, F. and Möller, H.J. Repetitive transcranial magnetic stimulation: does it have potential in the treatment of depression? *CNS Drugs*, 2003, 17: 383–403.

Padberg, F., Zwanzger, P., Thoma, H., Kathmann, N., Haag, C., Greenberg, B.D., Hampel, H. and Möller H.-J. Repetitive transcranial magnetic stimulation (rTMS) in pharmacotherapy-refractory major depression: comparative study of fast, slow and sham rTMS. *Psychiatry Res.*, 1999, 88: 163–171.

Padberg, F., Juckel, G., Präßl, A., Zwanzger, P., Mavrogiorgou, P., Hegerl, U., Hampel, H. and Möller, H.-J. Facial expressions and mood after transcranial magnetic stimulation of the prefrontal cortex. *J. Neuropsychiatry Clin. Neurosci.*, 2001, 13: 206–212.

Padberg, F., di Michele, F., Zwanzger, P., Romeo, E., Bernardi, G., Schüle, C., Baghai, T.C., Ella, R., Pasini, A. and Rupprecht, R. Plasma concentrations of neuroactive steroids before and after repetitive transcranial magnetic stimulation (rTMS) in major depression. *Neuropsychopharmacology*, 2002a, 27: 874–878, corrigendum in *Neuropsychopharmacology*, 2003, 28: 610–611.

Padberg, F., Schüle, C., Zwanzger, P., Baghai, T., Ella, R., Mikhaiel, P., Hampel, H., Möller, H.-J. and Rupprecht, R. Relation between responses to repetitive transcranial magnetic stimulation and partial sleep deprivation in major depression. *J. Psychiatr. Res.*, 2002b, 36: 131–135.

Padberg, F., Zwanzger, P., Keck, M. E., Kathmann, N., Mikhaiel, P., Ella, R., Rupprecht, P., Thoma, H., Hampel, H., Toschi, N. and Möller, H.-J. Repetitive transcranial magnetic stimulation (rTMS) in major depression: Relation between efficacy and stimulation intensity. *Neuropsychopharmacology*, 2002c, 27: 638–645.

Parker, G., Hadzi-Pavlovic, D., Brodaty, H., Austin, M. P., Mitchell, P., Wilhelm, K. and Hickie, I. Sub-typing depression, II. Clinical distinction of psychotic depression and non-psychotic melancholia. *Psychol. Med.*, 1995, 25: 825–832.

Pascual-Leone, A., Catalá, M.D. and Pascual-Leone, A. Lateralized effect of rapid-rate transcranial magnetic stimulation of the prefrontal cortex on mood. *Neurology*, 1996a, 46: 499–502.

Pascual-Leone, A., Rubio, B., Pallardó, F. and Catalá, M.D. Rapid-rate transcranial magnetic stimulation of left dorsolateral prefrontal cortex in drug-resistant depression. *Lancet*, 1996b, 348: 233–237.

Paus, T., Jech, R., Thompson, C.J., Comeau, R., Peters, T. and Evans, A.C. Transcranial magnetic stimulation during positron emission tomography: a new method for studying connectivity of the human cerebral cortex. *J. Neurosci.*, 1997, 17: 3178–3184.

Paus, T., Castro-Alamancos, M.A. and Petrides, M. Cortico-cortical connectivity of the human mid-dorsolateral frontal cortex and its modulation by repetitive transcranial magnetic stimulation. *Eur. J. Neurosci.*, 2001, 14: 1405–1411.

Post, A. and Keck, M.E. Transcranial magnetic stimulation as a therapeutic tool in psychiatry: what do we know about the neurobiological mechanisms? *J. Psychiatr. Res.*, 2001, 35: 193–215.

Post, A., Müller, M.B., Engelmann, M. and Keck, M.E. Repetitive transcranial magnetic stimulation in rats – evidence for a neuro-protective effect in vitro and in vivo. *Eur. J. Neurosci.*, 1999, 11: 3247–3254.

Post, R.M., Gerner, R.H., Carman, J.S., Gillin, J.C., Jimerson, D.C., Goodwin, F.K. and Bunney, W.E.J. Effects of a dopamine agonist piribedil in depressed patients: relationship of pretreatment homovanillic acid to antidepressant response. *Arch. Gen. Psychiatry*, 1978, 35: 609–615.

Post, R.M., Kimbrell, T., Frye, M., George, M., McCann, U., Little, J., Dunn, R., Li, H. and Weiss, S.R.B. Implications of kindling and quenching for the possible frequency dependence of rTMS. *CNS Spectrums*, 1997, 2: 54–60.

Post, R.M., Kimbrell, T.A., McCann, U.D., Dunn, R.T., Osuch, E.A., Speer, A.M. and Weiss, S.R.B. Repetitive transcranial magnetic stimulation as a neuropsychiatric tool: present status and future potential. *J. ECT*, 1999, 15: 39–59.

Pridmore, S. Rapid transcranial magnetic stimulation (rTMS) and normalisation of the dexamethasone suppression test (DST). *Psychiatry Clin. Neurosci.*, 1999, 53: 33–37.

Pridmore, S. Substitution of rapid transcranial magnetic stimulation treatments for electroconvulsive therapy treatments in a course of electroconvulsive therapy. Depress. *Anxiety*, 2000, 12: 118–123.

Pridmore, S., Rybak, M., Turnier-Shea, Y., Reid, P., Bruno, R., Couper, D. A naturalistic study of response in melancholia to transcranial magnetic stimulation (TMS). *German J. Psychiatry*, 1999, 2: 13–21.

Pridmore, S., Bruno, R., Turnier-Shea, Y., Reid, P., Rybak, M. Comparison of unlimited numbers of rapid transcranial magnetic stimulation (rTMS) and ECT treatment sessions in major depressive episode. *Int. J. Neuropsychopharmacol.*, 2000, 3: 129–134.

Rampello, L., Nicoletti, G. and Raffaele, R. Dopaminergic hypothesis for retarded depression: a symptom profile for predicting therapeutical responses. *Acta Psychiatr. Scand.*, 1991, 84: 552–554.

Reid, P.D. and Pridmore, S. Dexamethasone suppression test reversal in rapid transcranial magnetic stimulation-treated depression. Australian and New Zealand *J. Psychiatry*, 1999, 33: 274–277.

Reul, J.M., Stec, I., Soder, M. and Holsboer, F. Chronic treatment of rats with the antidepressant amitriptyline attenuates the activity of the hypothalamic-pituitary-adrenocortical system. *Endocrinology*, 1993, 133: 312–320.

Reul, J.M., Labeur, M.S., Grigoriadis, D.E., De Souza E.B. and Holsboer, F. Hypothalamic-pituitary-adrenocortical axis changes in the rat after long-term treatment with the reversible monoamine oxidase-A inhibitor moclobemide. *Neuroendocrinology*, 1994, 60: 509–519.

Romeo, E., Strohle, A., Spalletta, G., Di Michele, F., Hermann, B., Holsboer, F., Pasini, A. and Rupprecht, R. Effects of antidepressant treatment on neuroactive steroids in major depression. *Am. J. Psychiatry*, 1998, 155: 910–913.

Rupprecht, R., Di Michele, F., Hermann, B., Strohle, A., Lancel, M., Romeo, E. and Holsboer, F. Neuroactive steroids: molecular mechanisms of action and implications for neuropsychopharmacology. *Brain Res.*, 2001, 37: 59–67.

Rush, A.J. and Trivedi, M.H. Treating depression to remission. *Psychiatric Annals*, 1995, 25: 704–705.

Sachdev, P.S., McBride, R., Loo, C.K., Mitchell, P.M., Malhi, G.S. and Croker, V. Effects of Different Frequencies of Transcranial Magnetic Stimulation (TMS) on the Forced Swim Test Model of Depression in Rats. *Biol. Psychiatry*, 2002, 51: 474–479.

Sackeim, H.A., Rush, A.J., George, M.S., Marangell, L.B., Husain, M.M., Nahas, Z., Johnson, C.R., Seidman, S., Giller, C., Haines, S., Simpson, R.K.J. and Goodman, R.R. Vagus nerve stimulation (VNS) for treatment-resistant depression: efficacy, side effects, and predictors of outcome. *Neuropsychopharmacology*, 2001, 25: 713–728.

Schüle, C., Baghai, T., Bidlingmaier, M., Strasburger, C. and Laakmann, G. Endocrinological effects of mirtazapine in healthy volunteers. *Prog. Neuropsychopharmacol. Biol. Psychiatry*, 2002, 26: 1253–1261.

Schüle, C., Baghai, T., Zwanzger, P., Ella, R., Eser, D., Padberg, F., Möller, H.-J. and Rupprecht, R. Attenuation of hypothalamic-pituitary-adrenocortical hyperactivity in depressed patients by mirtazapine. *Psychopharmacology* (Berl), 2003a, 166: 271–275.

Schüle, C., Zwanzger, P., Baghai, T., Mikhaiel, P., Thoma, H., Möller, H.-J., Rupprecht, R. and Padberg, F. Effects of antidepressant pharmacotherapy after repetitive transcranial magnetic stimulation in major depression: an open follow-up study. *J. Psychiatr. Res.*, 2003b, 37: 145–153.

Schutter, D., van Honk, J., d'Alfonso, A., Postma, A. and de Haan, E. Effects of slow rTMS at the right dorsolateral prefrontal cortex on EEG asymmetry and mood. *Neuroreport* 2001, 12: 445–447.

Sesack, S.R. and Pickel, V.M. Prefrontal cortical efferents in the rat synapse on unlabeled neuronal targets of catecholamine terminals in the nucleus accumbens septi and on dopamine neurons in the ventral tegmental area. *J. Comp. Neurol.* 1992, 320: 145–160.

Sgro, J.A., Ghatak, N.R., Stanton, P.C., Emerson, R.G. and Blair, R. Repetitive high magnetic field stimulation: the effect upon rat brain. In W.J. Levy, R.Q. Cracco, A.T. Barker and J. Rothwell (Eds), *Magnetic Motor Stimulation: Basic Principles and Clinical Experience* (EEG Suppl. 43). Amsterdam: Elsevier, 1991, 180–185.

Shajahan, P.M., Glabus, M.F., Steele, J.D., Doris, A.B., Anderson, K., Jenkins, J.A., Gooding, P.A. and Ebmeier, K.P. Left dorsolateral repetitive transcranial magnetic stimulation affects cortical excitability and functional connectivity, but does not impair cognition in major depression. *Neuro-Psychopharmacology and Biological Psychiatry* 2002, 26: 945–954.

Smesny, S., Volz, H.P., Liepert, J., Tauber, R., Hochstetter, A. and Sauer, H. [Repetitive transcranial magnetic stimulation (rTMS) in the acute and long-term therapy of refractory depression – a case report] (Article in German). *Nervenarzt*, 2001, 72: 734–738.

Speer, A.M., Kimbrell, T.A., Wassermann, E.M., D Repella, J., Willis, M.W., Herscovitch, P. and Post, R.M. Opposite effects of high and low frequency rTMS on regional brain activity in depressed patients. *Biol Psychiatry*, 2000, 48: 1133–1141.

Speer, A.M., Repella, J.D., Figueras, S., Deminan, N.K., Kimbrell, T.A., Wasserman, E.M. and Post, R.M. Lack of adverse cognitive effects on 1 Hz and 20 Hz repetitive transcranial magnetic stimulation at 100% of motor threshold over left prefrontal cortex in depression. *J. ECT*, 2001, 17: 259–263.

Steward, O., Kelley, M.S. and Torre, E.R. The process of reinnervation in the dentate gyrus of adult rats: temporal relationship between changes in the levels of glial fibrillary acidic protein (GFAP) and GFAP mRNA in reactive astrocytes. *Exp. Neurol.*, 1993, 124: 167–183.

Strafella, A.P., Paus, T., Barrett, J. and Dagher, A. Repetitive transcranial magnetic stimulation of the human prefrontal cortex induces dopamine release in the caudate nucleus. *J. Neurosci.*, 2001, 21: RC157.

Szuba, M., O'Reardon, J.P., Rai, A.S., Snyder-Kastenberg, J., Amsterdam, J.D., Gettes, D.R., Wassermann, E.M. and Evans, D.L. Acute mood and TSH effects of transcranial magnetic stimulation in major depression. *Biol. Psychiatry*, 2001, 50: 22–27.

Taber, M.T. and Fibiger, H.C. Electrical stimulation of the prefrontal cortex increases dopamine release in the nucleus accumbens of the rat: modulation by metabotropic glutamate receptors. *J. Neurosci.*, 1995, 15: 3896–3904.

Teneback, C.C., Nahas, Z., Speer, A.M., Molloy, M., Stallings, L.E., Spicer, K.M., Risch, S.C. and George, M.S. Changes in prefrontal cortex and paralimbic activity in depression following two weeks of daily left prefrontal TMS. *J. Neuropsychiatry Clin. Neurosci.*, 1999, 11: 426–435.

Thase, M.E. How should efficacy be evaluated in randomized clinical trials of treatments for depression? *J. Clin. Psychiatry*, 1999, 60 (Suppl. 4): 23–31.

Thomas, D.N., Nutt, D.J. and Holman, R.B. Effects of acute and chronic electroconvulsive shock on noradrenaline release in the rat hippocampus and frontal cortex. *Br. J. Pharmacol.*, 1992, 106: 430–434.

Triggs, W.J., McCoy, K.J.M., Greer, R., Rossi, F., Bowers, D., Kortenkamp, S., Nadeau, S.E., Heilman, K.M. and Goodman, W.K. Effects of left frontal transcranial magnetic stimulation on depressed mood, cognition, and corticomotor threshold. *Biol. Psychiatry*, 1999, 45: 1440–1446.

Uzunova, V., Sheline, Y., Davis, J.M., Rasmusson, A., Uzunov, D.P., Costa, E. and Guidotti, A. Increase in the cerebrospinal fluid content of neurosteroids in patients with unipolar major depression who are receiving fluoxetine or fluvoxamine. *Proc. Natl. Acad. Sci. USA*, 1998, 95: 3239–3244.

Wassermann, E.M. Risk and safety of repetitive transcranial magnetic stimulation: report and suggested guidelines from the International Workshop on the Safety of Repetitive Transcranial Magnetic Stimulation, June 5–7, 1996. *Electroenceph. Clin. Neurophysiol.*, 1998: 1–16.

Wassermann, E.M. and Lisanby, S.H. Therapeutic application of repetitive transcranial magnetic stimulation: a review. *Clin. Neurophysiol.*, 2001, 112: 1367–1377.

Wu, J., Buchsbaum, M.S., Gillin, J.C., Tang, C., Cadwell, S., Wiegand, M., Najafi, A., Klein, E., Hazen, K., Bunney, W.E.J., Fallon, J.H., Keator, D. Prediction of antidepressant effects of sleep deprivation by metabolic rates in the ventral anterior cingulate and medial prefrontal cortex. *Am. J. Psychiatry*, 1999, 156: 1149–1158.

Yoshida, K., Higuchi, H., Kamata, M., Yoshimoto, M., Shimizu, T. and Hishikawa, Y. Single and repeated electroconvulsive shocks activate dopaminergic and 5-hydroxytryptaminergic neurotransmission in the frontal cortex of rats. *Prog. Neuropsychopharmacol. Biol. Psychiatry*, 1998, 22: 435–444.

Zangen, A. and Hyodo, K. Transcranial magnetic stimulation induces increases in extracellular levels of dopamine and glutamate in the nucleus accumbens. *NeuroReport*, 2002, 13: 2401–2405.

Zetterstrom, T.S., Pei, Q. and Grahame-Smith, D.G. Repeated electroconvulsive shock extends the duration of enhanced gene expression for BDNF in rat brain compared with a single administration. *Brain Res. Mol. Brain Res.*, 1998, 57: 106–110.

Zetterstrom, T.S., Pei, Q., Madhav, T.R., Coppell, A.L., Lewis, L. and Grahame-Smith, D.G. Manipulations of brain 5-HT levels affect gene expression for BDNF in rat brain. *Neuropharmacology*, 1999, 38: 1063–1073.

Zis, A.P., Nomikos, G.G., Brown, E.E., Damsma, G. and Fibiger, H.C. Neurochemical effects of electrically and chemically induced seizures: an in vivo microdialysis study in the rat hippocampus. *Neuropsychopharmacology*, 1992, 7: 189–195.

Zobel, A.W., Yassouridis, A., Frieboes, R.M. and Holsboer, F. Prediction of medium-term outcome by cortisol response to the combined dexamethasone-CRH test in patients with remitted depression. *Am. J. Psychiatry*, 1999, 156: 949–951.

Zobel, A.W., Nickel, T., Sonntag, A., Uhr, M., Holsboer, F. and Ising, M. Cortisol response in the combined dexamethasone/CRH test as predictor of relapse in patients with remitted depression. a prospective study. *J. Psychiatr. Res.*, 2001, 35: 83–94.

Zwanzger, P., Ella, R., Keck, M.E., Rupprecht, R. and Padberg, F. Occurrence of delusions during repetitive transcranial magnetic stimulation (rTMS) in major depression. *Biol. Psychiatry*, 2002, 51: 602–603.

Zwanzger, P., Baghai, T.C., Padberg, F., Ella, R., Minov, C., Mikhaiel, P., Schüle, C., Thoma, H. and Rupprecht, R. The combined dexamethasone-corticotropin-releasing-hormone test (DEX/CRH test) before and after treatment with repetitive - transcranial magnetic stimulation in major depression. *Psychoneuroendocrinology*, 2003, 28: 376–385.

Zyss, T., Gorka, Z., Kowalska, M. and Vetulani, J. Preliminary comparison of behavioral and biochemical effects of chronic transcranial magnetic stimulation and electroconvulsive shock in the rat. *Biol. Psychiatry*, 1997, 42: 920–924.

Transcranial Magnetic Stimulation and Transcranial Direct Current Stimulation (Supplements to Clinical Neurophysiology, Vol. 56)
Editors: W. Paulus, F. Tergau, M.A. Nitsche, J.C. Rothwell, U. Ziemann, M. Hallett

Chapter 43

Motorcortical excitability after electroconvulsive therapy in patients with major depressive disorder

Malek Bajbouj[a], Jürgen Gallinat[a], Undine E. Lang[a], Peter Neu[a] and Ludwig Niehaus[b]

[a] *Department of Psychiatry, Charité – University Medicine Berlin, Campus Benjamin Franklin, Berlin (Germany)*

[b] *Department of Neurology, Charité – University Medicine Berlin, Campus Virchow, Berlin (Germany)*

1. Introduction

Induction of seizures by electroconvulsive therapy (ECT) has been used for the treatment of psychiatric disorders for more than 60 years. Particularly in the treatment of severe major depression, evidence for the effectiveness and superiority of ECT over other antidepressant treatments is convincing (Janicak and Martis, 1999). The exact mode of action remains unclear. One of the main hypotheses is a compensatory increase in the activity of the inhibitory neurotransmitter gamma-aminobutyric acid (GABA) (Sackeim, 1999).

Therefore, it has been suggested that the GABA neurotransmitter system may contribute to the mechanism of action in the treatment of major depressive disorders (Sanacora et al., 2000). Reports demonstrating increased GABA receptor binding in rodent brains after chronic administration of different classes of clinically effective antidepressants and electroshock (Lloyd et al., 1989) initially led to a GABAergic hypothesis of antidepressant mechanism of action. In accordance with these findings recent studies using proton magnetic resonance spectroscopy showed an increase in cortical GABA concentrations following electroconvulsive therapy (ECT) in patients with major depression (Sanacora et al., 2003). Although later studies have yielded inconsistent results regarding antidepressant effects on GABA receptor binding (Cross and Horton, 1988), the recent use of several anticonvulsant agents (Bowden, 2001; Schmidt do Prado-Lima and Bacaltchuck, 2002) and neuroactive steroids (Rupprecht, 2003) with GABA-enhancing properties in the treatment of mood disorders has renewed interest in the role of GABA in the treatment of major depression.

In the past few years transcranial magnetic stimulation (TMS) has been introduced as a powerful tool to explore the integrity and excitability of the corticospinal system in patients with neurological and psychiatric diseases (Puri and Lewis, 1996; Fitzgerald et al., 2002).

* *Correspondence to*: Dr. Malek Bajbouj, Department of Psychiatry, Charité – University Medicine Berlin, Campus Benjamin Franklin, Eschenallee 3, 14050 Berlin, Germany.
Tel: +49-30 8445 8622; Fax: +49-30 8445 8233;
E-mail: malek.bajbouj@medzin.fu-berlin.de

Recent studies in patients with major depression showed abnormalities of motorcortical excitability (Maeda et al., 2000; Steele et al., 2000) and changes of motorcortex excitability in the ECT course in a single patient (Sommer et al., 2002).

TMS has been used to demonstrate at least two different cortical inhibitory processes (Sanger et al., 2001). First, the postexcitatory inhibition (PI) succeeds the contralateral MEP and refers to a silence in the EMG following the MEP in a contralateral target muscle. Second, one can monitor intracortical inhibition (ICI) and intracortical facilitation (ICF) in humans with the use of TMS in the paired-pulse-paradigm (Rothwell, 1991; Kujirai et al., 1993).

In the context of our study, it is of interest that there are hints for a modulation of the cortical excitability by central GABAergic activity, e.g. GABA agonists like tiagabine and lorazepam alter intracortical inhibition (Ziemann et al., 1996; Werhahn et al., 1999; Di Lazzaro et al., 2000). Therefore, measuring the duration of the PI and parameters of intracortical inhibition and facilitation seemed to be reasonable to monitor acute ECT effects in depressive patients.

The aim of the present study was to clarify the effect of electroconvulsive therapy in patients with major depressive disorder on TMS parameters associated with central GABAergic neurotransmission.

2. Patients and methods

2.1. Patients

The study was approved by the Ethics Committee of the Benjamin-Franklin-University Hospital of the Free University of Berlin. All subjects gave written informed consent. Hospitalized patients meeting the DSM-IV criteria for major depression were studied. Diagnosis was made in consensus between the attending physician and a senior house officer. Exclusion criteria for patients were mental retardation, significant other psychiatric or neurological illness such as epilepsy, organic mental disorder, alcohol or substance abuse within 1 year before the study. We studied 12 right-handed patients with major depressive episode (7 women, 5 men). Patients received the following antidepressant medication, which was kept constantly in the 4 weeks prior to investigation: venlafaxine (5 patients, dose range 150 to 225 mg/day), tranylcypromine (3 patients, dose range from 20 to 40 mg/day), mirtazapine (1 patient, 30 mg/day), sulpiride (1 patient, 150 mg/day), no psychopharmacological treatment (2 patients). No patient received anticonvulsants, benzodiazepines or mood stabilizers.

Clinical symptoms were assessed using the Hamilton Depression Scale (HAMD) (Hamilton, 1967) before electrophysiological examination (further clinical data: see Table 1).

2.2. Magnetic stimulation and recording

2.2.1. General procedure

Focal TMS with monophasic pulses was performed with a figure-of-eight-shaped coil (MC-B70) of the Maglite stimulator with the Twin Top option (Dantec Medtronic, Skovlunde, Denmark), with the coils center (contact point of both half-coils) placed over the hand-associated motor cortex. For each subject, the stimulation point for eliciting maximal hand motor responses was determined individually and lay, on average, 6 cm lateral to the vertex and 1 cm anterior to the interaural line. For optimal stimulation, the induced currents were directed posteroanteriorly. The elicited surface compound muscle action potential (electrode area 28 mm^2) was recorded bilaterally from the first dorsal interosseus (ID) muscle. Data were amplified, bandpass filtered (20 Hz to 2 kHz), digitized (sampling rate 5 kHz) and stored on a personal computer for offline-analysis.

TMS was performed 1 day before and six hours after first session of ECT.

2.2.2. Response parameters

The *threshold* (percentage of maximum stimulator output) for eliciting contralateral hand motor responses was determined for the relaxed hand muscles and defined as the stimulus intensity at which responses of at least 0.05 mV occurred in about half of ten trials.

TABLE 1

CLINICAL DATA OF 12 PATIENTS WITH MAJOR DEPRESSION AND PARAMETERS OF ELECTRO-CONVULSIVE THERAPY

HAMD (24)	32.2 ± 7.1
Age (in years)	51.1 ± 15.5
Duration of episode (in week)	26.8 ± 17.3
Number of episodes	4.7 ± 3.9
Thiopental dose (in mg)	304.2 ± 33.1
Seizure duration (EEG, in s)	38.8 ± 22.2
Seizure duration (EMG, in s)	29.2 ± 19.0

Cortex stimulation was then performed during maximal tonic hand muscle contraction. The stimuli were applied over each hemisphere at an intensity of 80% of the maximum stimulator output. The duration of postexcitatory inhibition was measured from the onset of the corticospinally mediated EMG response to the end of the silent period, which was set at a point where the averaged tonic EMG activity again reached the amplitude of the mean EMG activity before the cortex stimulus. To assess inhibitory effects 20 consecutive EMG signals elicited by stimulation over each hemisphere were rectified. The duration of each trial was then measured and then averaged. Amplitudes of the contralateral EMG responses were determined baseline-to-peak.

Intracortical inhibition (ICI) and intracortical facilitation (ICF) were investigated with the previously described paired-pulse technique (Kujirai et al., 1993). Since it was known from previous studies that short interstimulus intervals (ISI 2 and 3 ms) have an inhibitory and long ISIs (10 and 15 ms) have a facilitatory effect, intracortical inhibition and facilitation were calculated across these intervals, respectively. The intensity of the conditioning stimulus was adjusted to 80% of the resting motor threshold, and the intensity of the test stimulus was set so that the test stimulus alone produced a response of about 1 mV peak-to-peak amplitude. Ten trials of the unconditioned control single test stimuli and 10 paired pulse stimuli of each ISI were recorded, delivered 10 s apart in random order. The peak-to-peak amplitudes of the conditioned response were averaged and expressed as a percentage of the average of the test response amplitudes.

2.3. Electroconvulsive therapy (ECT)

ECT was administered with a square-wave, constant-current, brief-pulse device (Thymatron DG, Somatics Inc, Lake Bluff, Ill, USA). Anaesthesia was performed in a standard manner with succinylcholine and thiopental. Patients were treated with the standard right unilateral electrode placement, with stimulus intensity two times the initial seizure threshold. Seizure duration was monitored with electromyography and electroencephalography (see Table 1).

2.4. Statistical methods

The Wilcoxon two-sample test was used for statistical analysis of the neurophysiological data comparing parameters before, and six hours after, electroconvulsive therapy. Analysis of variance (Spearman correlation coefficient) was used to assess the effects of anaesthesia and seizure duration on the measured neurophysiological parameters. Level of significance was set at 5%.

3. Results

3.1. Single pulse TMS

Duration of postexcitatory inhibition was significantly prolonged after the first session of ECT compared to baseline, while motor threshold and response amplitude remained unchanged (Table 2). No side differences were observed. Single recordings from one patient with exemplary findings are shown in Fig. 1.

3.2. Paired-pulse TMS

In all patients inhibition of test motor responses occurred at ISIs of 2 and 3 ms (values < 100%), whereas facilitation occurred at ISIs of 10 and 15 ms (values > 100%). ICI was significantly increased and ICF was significantly decreased after ECT in

TABLE 2

RESPONSE AMPLITUDE (AMP), MOTOR THRESHOLD (MT), DURATION OF POSTEXCITATORY INHIBITION (PI; MS), INTRACORTICAL INHIBITION (ICI) AND INTRACORTICAL FACILITATION (ICF) IN 12 PATIENTS WITH MAJOR DEPRESSION BEFORE AND AFTER ELECTROCONVULSIVE THERAPY (ID: INTEROSSEUS DORSALIS MUSCLE)

	Baseline	6 h post ECT	*p*
Amp left ID (mV)	4.4 ± 0.6	4.5 ± 0.8	0.33
Amp right ID (mV)	4.7 ± 0.4	4.9 ± 0.9	0.36
MT left ID (%)	43.8 ± 7.4	46.1 ± 8.9	0.19
MT right ID (%)	42.8 ± 7.9	43.9 ± 10.6	0.39
PI left ID (ms)	236.0 ± 46.4	269.7 ± 37.0	0.01
PI right ID(ms)	224.0 ± 57.3	269.6 ± 51.8	0.01
ICI left ID (%)	44.2 ± 33.4	23.7 ± 19.2	0.01
ICI right ID (%)	42.5 ± 25.9	25.1 ± 11.6	0.01
ICF left ID (%)	196.7 ± 119.1	118.9 ± 58.3	0.01
ICF right ID (%)	226.7 ± 166.6	119.9 ± 41.6	0.01

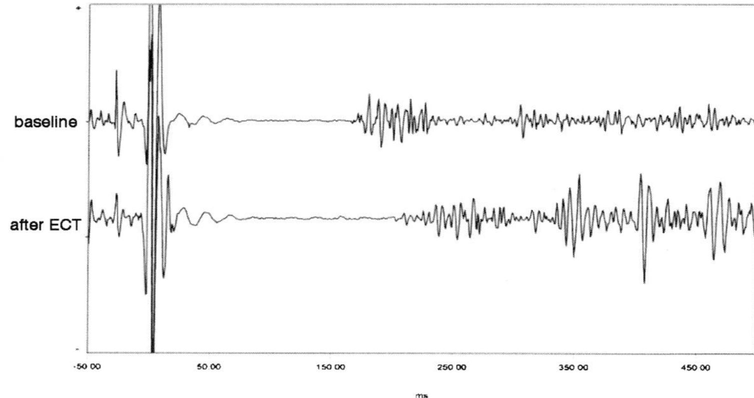

Fig. 1. Postexcitatory inhibition of ongoing EMG activity in the left interosseus dorsalis muscle in a patient with major depression before (upper trace) and six hours after single electroconvulsive therapy (lower trace).

comparison to baseline (Table 2). No side differences were observed.

3.3. Parameters of electroconvulsive therapy and clinical data

Parameters of the single session of electroconvulsive therapy are summarized in Table 1. There was no significant correlation between a dose of thiopental and the duration of postexcitatory inhibition (left ID: $p = 0.32$, right ID: $p = 0.28$), ICI (left ID: $p = 0.37$, right ID: $p = 0.44$) and ICF (left ID: $p = 0.31$, right ID: $p = 0.29$). Using the Spearman's correlation coefficient a correlation between seizure duration and duration of postexcitatory inhibition ($r = 0.44$; $p = 0.04$) respectively intracortical inhibition ($r = 0.54$; $p = 0.03$) was observed (Fig. 2). No correlation was observed between ICF and seizure parameters. No correlations

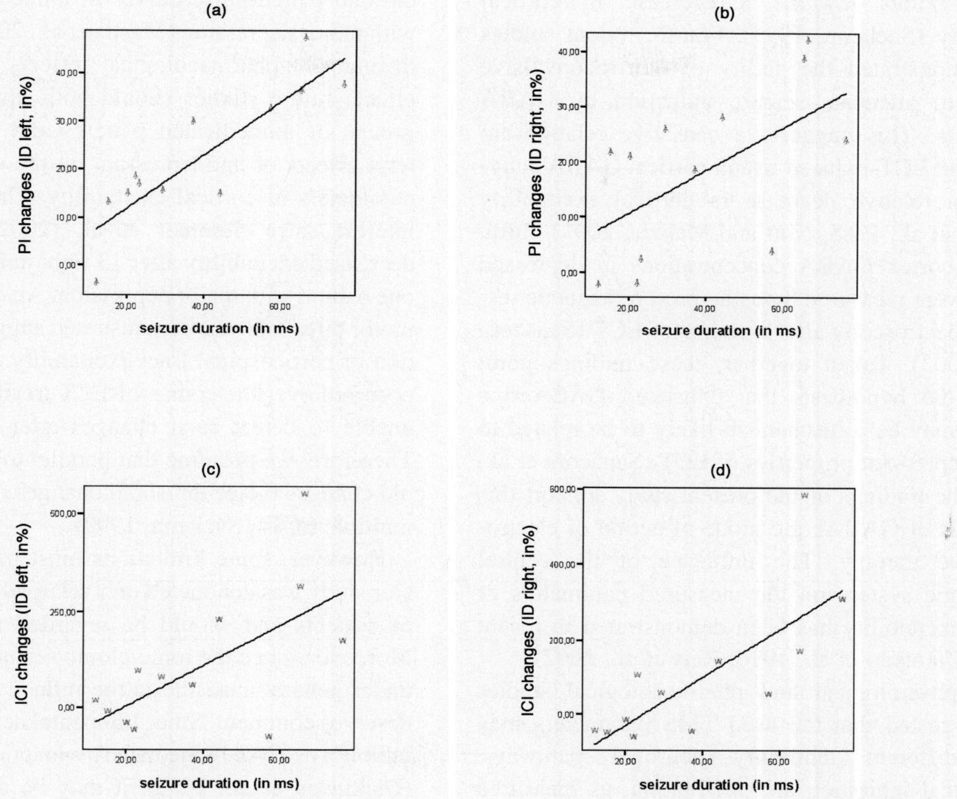

Fig. 2. Correlation between seizure duration and changes of the duration of the postexcitatory inhibition (PI) of the left (a) and right (b) interisseus dorsalis muscle (ID) and correlation between the seizure duration and ICI changes of the left (c) and right (d) interosseus dorsalis muscle.

were observed between HAMD score and motor threshold (left ID: $r = 0.23, p = 0.47$; right ID: $r = 0.27, p = 0.39$), duration of postexcitatory inhibition (left ID: $r = 0.30, p = 0.92$; right ID: $r = 0.30, p = 0.30$), intracortical inhibition (left ID: $r = 0.01, p = 0.99$; right ID: $r = 0.19, p = 0.54$) and intracortical facilitation (left ID: $r = 0.09, p = 0.76$; right ID: $r = 0.21, p = 0.51$).

4. Discussion

Using transcranial magnetic stimulation we investigated excitatory and inhibitory cortical functions after a single tonic-clonic seizure induced by electroconvulsive therapy in patients with major depressive disorder. The main findings of the present study were that after ECT the duration of PI increased, the ICI increased and the ICF decreased. These findings indicate an enhanced activity of inhibitory circuits in human motor cortex following a single ECT.

Several lines of evidence suggest that an enhanced activity of inhibitory circuits is involved in the mechanism of action of electroconvulsive therapy. First, animal studies demonstrate elevated GABA concentrations in several brain regions following repeated electroconvulsive seizures (Green, 1986; Lipcsey et al., 1986; Nutt and Malizia, 2001; Sanacora et al., 2003). Second, an elevation of GABA concentration in the cerebrospinal fluid in patients receiving a course of ECT was observed (Lipcsey et al., 1986). Third, in the course of ECT a decrease in seizure duration points towards a decrease in cortical excitability (Sackeim, 1999). Fourth, rodent studies have demonstrated the ability of electroconvulsive seizures to attenuate seizure induction by GABA antagonists. This suggests a causative relationship between an ECT-induced rise in cortical GABA activity and a relative decrease in cortical excitability (Wielosz et al., 1985; Nutt and Malizia, 2001). Fifth, elevated cortex GABA concentrations in depressed patients were measured by using proton magnetic resonance spectroscopy after a course of ECT (Sanacora et al., 2003). Taken together, these findings point towards the hypothesis that enhanced GABAergic function may be a mechanism likely to be related to the antidepressant properties of ECT (Sanacora et al., 2003). The findings of the present study support this hypothesis of GABAergic mode of action of electroconvulsive therapy. The influence of the central GABAergic system on the measured parameters of cortical excitability has been demonstrated in recent studies (Ziemann et al., 1996; Reis et al., 2002).

Both physiological and pharmacological studies have suggested that the used TMS parameters may reflect different inhibitory neuronal pathways. Intracortical inhibition and facilitation, as measured by the paired pulse technique, may be mediated by the $GABA_A$ interneurones (Hanajima et al., 1998). Conversely, the PI may mainly be mediated by the $GABA_B$ interneurones (Roick et al., 1993; Siebner et al., 1998; Werhahn et al., 1999; Sanger et al., 2001).

The potential influence of antidepressant medication with noradrenergic properties on two aspects of the present study should be kept in mind. First, Herwig et al. (2002) were able to show an increased intracortical excitability after ingestion of the norepinephrin-reuptake-inhibitor reboxetine. Therefore, it seems reasonable that antidepressant medication may also be responsible for the noticeable high ICF values at baseline. Due to the longitudinal design of our study it was not possible to answer the question whether this phenomena was a consequence of inner tension or of pharmacological treatment. Second, it is conceivable that antidepressant medication masks possible interhemispheric differences which we were unable to detect and which had been described for motor threshold and paired-pulse curves in unmedicated patients with major depression (Maeda et al., 2000). To clearly distinguish pharmacological effects from disease effects future studies should both investigate larger groups of unmedicated patients and estimate long-term effects of antidepressant on the course of these parameters of cortical excitability. This is of special interest since Sommer et al. (2002) described a decreased excitability after 13 right unilateral ECTs in one patient with major depression. An elevated resting motor threshold was demonstrated suggesting a reduction of corticospinal tract excitability. These changes occurred over the course of ECT treatment. We were unable to detect such changes after a single ECT. Therefore, we presume that parallel to seizure threshold changes motor threshold changes only occur after multiple ECTs (Sackeim, 1999).

However, some limitations must be kept in mind. Our study was conducted on a relatively small number of patients and should be regarded as preliminary. Moreover, since the tonic-clonic seizure was artificial under general anaesthesia the influence of thiopental deserves comment. Since thiopental acts by enhancing inhibitory GABA-mediated synaptic transmission (Dickinson et al., 2002), it may be argued that this substance would explain the reduced cortical excitability. There are at least three arguments contrary to this point. First, Inghilleri et al. (1996) were unable to find an influence of thiopental on cortical excitability. Second, it is unlikely that an ultra short-acting barbiturate like thiopental with duration of action of 6–8 min still influences parameters of cortical excitability six hours after termination of anaesthesia (Dickinson et al., 2002). Third, we were unable to find a correlation between the amount of thiopental and the parameters of cortical excitability, while seizure duration correlated significantly with PI and ICI. Therefore, it seems more likely that enhanced cortical inhibition is rather influenced by seizure duration than by thiopental dosage.

In conclusion, our findings indicate that inhibitory circuits play a role after a single electroconvulsive therapy. Future studies should address the question of the time course of changes after a single ECT at different time points and the effect of repetitive ECT on the mentioned parameters of cortical excitability. Furthermore the predictive value of the measured TMS parameters on antidepressant potential of ECT.

Acknowledgements

This work was supported in part by Sonnenfeldstiftung Berlin. The authors are grateful to Florence Hellen, Christina Schindowski and Agnieszka Slezak for technical assistance.

References

Bowden, C.L. Introduction: the role of anticonvulsants as mood stabilizers. *J. Clin. Psychiatry*, 2001, 62 (Suppl. 14): 3–4.

Cross, J.A. and Horton, R.W. Effects of chronic oral administration of the antidepressants, desmethylimipramine and zimelidine on rat cortical GABA-B binding sites: a comparison with 5-HT2 binding site changes. *Br. J. Pharmacol.*, 1988, 93: 331–336.

Di Lazzaro, V., Oliviero, A., Meglio, M., Cioni, B., Tamburrini, G., Tonali, P. and Rothwell, J.C. Direct demonstration of the effect of lorazepam on the excitability of the human motor cortex. *Clin. Neurophysiol.*, 2000, 111: 794–799.

Dickinson, R., De Sousa, S.L., Lieb, W.R. and Franks, N.P. Selective synaptic actions of thiopental and its enantiomers. *Anesthesiology*, 2002, 96: 884–892.

Fitzgerald, P.B., Brown, T.L. and Daskalakis, Z.J. The application of transcranial magnetic stimulation in psychiatry and neurosciences research. *Acta. Psychiatr. Scand.*, 2002, 105: 324–340.

Green, A.R. Changes in gamma-aminobutyric acid biochemistry and seizure threshold. *Ann. NY Acad. Sci.*, 1986, 462: 105–119.

Hamilton, M. Development of a rating scale for primary depressive illness. *Br. J. Soc. Clin. Psychol.*, 1967, 6: 278–296.

Hanajima, R., Ugawa, Y., Terao, Y., Sakai, K., Furubayashi, T., Machii, K. and Kanazawa, I. Paired-pulse magnetic stimulation of the human motor cortex: differences among I waves. *J. Physiol.*, I 1998, 509 (Pt. 2): 607–618.

Herwig, U., Brauer, K., Connemann, B., Spitzer, M. and Schonfeldt-Lecuona, C. Intracortical excitability is modulated by a norepinephrine-reuptake inhibitor as measured with paired-pulse transcranial magnetic stimulation. *Psychopharmacology* (Berl), 2002, 164: 228–232.

Inghilleri, M., Berardelli, A., Marchetti, P. and Manfredi, M. Effects of diazepam, baclofen and thiopental on the silent period evoked by transcranial magnetic stimulation in humans. *Exp. Brain Res.*, 1996, 109: 467–472.

Janicak, P.G. and Martis, B. Strategies for treatment-resistant depression. *Clin. Cornerstone*, 1999, 1: 58–71.

Kujirai, T., Caramia, M.D., Rothwell, J.C., Day, B.L., Thompson, P.D., Ferbert, A., Wroe, S., Asselman, P. and Marsden, C.D. Corticocortical inhibition in human motor cortex. *J. Physiol.* 1993, 471: 501–519.

Lipcsey, A., Kardos, J., Prinz, G. and Simonyi, M. Effect of electroconvulsive therapy on the GABA level in the cerebrospinal fluid. *Psychiatr. Neurol. Med. Psychol.* (*Leipz*), 1986, 38: 554–555.

Lloyd, K.G., Zivkovic, B., Scatton, B., Morselli, P.L. and Bartholini, G. The gabaergic hypothesis of depression. *Prog. Neuropsychopharmacol. Biol. Psychiatry*, 1989, 13: 341–351.

Maeda, F., Keenan, J.P. and Pascual-Leone, A. Interhemispheric asymmetry of motor cortical excitability in major depression as measured by transcranial magnetic stimulation. *Br. J. Psychiatry*, 2000, 177: 169–173.

Nutt, D.J. and Malizia, A.L. New insights into the role of the GABA(A)-benzodiazepine receptor in psychiatric disorder. *Br. J. Psychiatry*, 2001, 179: 390–396.

Puri, B.K. and Lewis, S.W. Transcranial magnetic stimulation in psychiatric research. *Br. J. Psychiatry*, 1996, 169: 675–677.

Reis, J., Tergau, F., Hamer, H.M., Muller, H.H., Knake, S., Fritsch, B., Oertel, W.H. and Rosenow, F. Topiramate selectively decreases intracortical excitability in human motor cortex. *Epilepsia*, 2002, 43: 1149–1156.

Roick, H., von Giesen, H.J. and Benecke, R. On the origin of the postexcitatory inhibition seen after transcranial magnetic brain stimulation in awake human subjects. *Exp. Brain Res.*, 1993, 94: 489–498.

Rothwell, J.C. Physiological studies of electric and magnetic stimulation of the human brain. *Electroencephalogr. Clin. Neurophysiol.*, 1991, 43: 29–35.

Rupprecht, R. Neuroactive steroids: mechanisms of action and neuropsychopharmacological properties. *Psychoneuroendocrinology*, 2003, 28: 139–168.

Sackeim, H.A. The anticonvulsant hypothesis of the mechanisms of action of ECT: current status. *J. ECT.* 1999, 15: 5–26.

Sanacora, G., Mason, G.F. and Krystal, J.H. Impairment of GABAergic transmission in depression: new insights from neuroimaging studies. *Crit. Rev. Neurobiol.*, 2000, 14: 23–45.

Sanacora, G., Mason, G.F., Rothman, D.L., Hyder, F., Ciarcia, J.J., Ostroff, R.B., Berman, R.M. and Krystal, J.H. Increased Cortical GABA Concentrations in Depressed Patients Receiving ECT. *Am. J. Psychiatry*, 2003, 160: 577–579.

Sanger, T.D., Garg, R.R. and Chen, R. Interactions between two different inhibitory systems in the human motor cortex. *J. Physiol.*, 2001, 530: 307–317.

Schmidt do Prado-Lima, P.A. and Bacaltchuck, J. Topiramate in treatment-resistant depression and binge-eating disorder. *Bipolar Disord.*, 2002, 4: 271–273.

Siebner, H.R., Dressnandt, J., Auer, C. and Conrad, B. Continuous intrathecal baclofen infusions induced a marked increase of the transcranially evoked silent period in a patient with generalized dystonia. *Muscle Nerve* 1998, 21: 1209–1212.

Sommer, M., Dieterich, A., Ruther, E., Paulus, W. and Wiltfang, J. Increased transcranial magnetic motor threshold after ECT A case report. Eur Arch Psychiatry *Clin. Neurosci.*, 2002, 252: 250–252.

Steele, J.D., Glabus, M.F., Shajahan, P.M. and Ebmeier, K.P. Increased cortical inhibition in depression: a prolonged silent period with transcranial magnetic stimulation (TMS). *Psychol. Med.* 2000, 30: 565–570.

Werhahn, K.J., Kunesch, E., Noachtar, S., Benecke, R. and Classen, J. Differential effects on motorcortical inhibition induced by blockade of GABA uptake in humans. *J. Physiol.*, 1999, 517 (Pt. 2): 591–597.

Wielosz, M., Stelmasiak, M., Ossowska, G. and Kleinrok, Z. Effects of electroconvulsive shock on central GABA-ergic mechanisms. *Pol. J. Pharmacol. Pharm.*, 1985, 37: 113–122.

Ziemann, U., Lonnecker, S., Steinhoff, B.J. and Paulus, W. The effect of lorazepam on the motor cortical excitability in man. *Exp. Brain Res.*, 1996, 109: 127–135.

Transcranial Magnetic Stimulation and Transcranial Direct Current Stimulation (Supplements to Clinical Neurophysiology, Vol. 56)
Editors: W. Paulus, F. Tergau, M.A. Nitsche, J.C. Rothwell, U. Ziemann, M. Hallett

Chapter 44

Transcranial magnetic brain stimulation and the cerebellum

K. Wessel

Department of Neurology, Municipal Hospital, and Cognitive Neurology, Institute at the Technical University, Salzdahlumer Strasse 90, D-38126 Braunschweig (Germany)

In general, there are three types of studies dealing with TMS and the cerebellum. First, studies focussing on the question whether the excitatory state of the primary motor cortex (M1) is changed either physiologically in relation to cerebellar stimulation or clinically in relation to cerebellar dysfunction in cerebellar diseases (question 1). Second, TMS-studies dealing with the influence of the cerebellum on the integration of different (e.g. cutaneous) afferences to M1 (question 2). And third, studies undertaken under the purpose to differentiate different degenerative (e.g. polyglutamine) diseases according to TMS findings, for example examinations comparing central motor conduction times (CMCT) in patients with spino-cerebellar atrophy type 1 (SCA 1) and other SCA-types; as well as possible therapeutic effects of TMS over the cerebellum (question 3).

1. Studies in relation to question 1

By transcranial electrical stimulation over the lateral occiput, a reduction of motor cortex excitabilty could be produced (Ugawa et al., 1991). In patients with cerebellar dysfunction this effect was absent (Ugawa et al., 1994a, b). It was concluded that stimulation activates cerebellar structures that suppress motor cortex excitability through cerebello-thalamo-cortical pathways. In contrast, Meyer et al. (1994) found that the anatomic structure, activated by stimulation over the lateral occiput, remains unclear, but probably activation of brain stem structures rather than the cerebellum plays the major role. Furthermore, this group described increased thresholds for the excitation of the motor cortex contralateral to cerebellar lesions. Further single-pulse TMS over the cerebellum affects corticospinal excitability by a cerebellar and a peripheral mechanism. Gerschlager et al. (2002) found with repetitive TMS (rTMS) that stimulation over either the right cerebellum or the right posterior neck (peripheral stimulation) facilitated MEPs in right hand an forearm muscles up to 30 min after the end of the train. Much of the persisting effects of rTMS over the cerebellum on corticospinal excitability appear to be mediated through stimulation of peripheral rather than central structures.

We found significantly increased motor thresholds in patients with severe (not with mild to moderate) ataxia (Wessel et al., 1996). This may suggest facilitory influences of the cerebellum on the corticospinal system, which are lacking in patients with cerebellar lesions. Presumably, the cerebellum exerts a tonic

* *Correspondence to*: Dr. Karl Wessel,
Tel: +49 531 5952300; Fax: +49 531 5952659;
E-mail: k.wessel@klinikum-braunschweig.de

facilitory effect on the motor cortex via the cerebellar nuclei, that is restrained to a certain extent by the Purkinje cells.

A recent study (Okabe et al., 2003) demonstrated the connectivity between the cerebellum and M1 the other way around. rTMS over the left M1 evoked an increase of regional cerebral blood flow in the contralateral (right) cerebellar hemisphere.

Excitatory and inhibitory effects of TMS on the motor system are mediated by distinct cortical elements. Inhibitory actions can be elicited by TMS which appear directly after MEP (postexcitatory inhibition; pI-S) and can be measured by blockade of tonic EMG activity. It is suggested that pI-S is generated in the primary motor cortex and that intracortical inhibitory interneurones may play the major role (van Giesen et al., 1994). We found a prolonged pI-S in most patients with cerebellar degeneration, indicating enhanced inhibitory mechanisms in the motor cortex (Wessel et al., 1996). Additionally, patients with cerebellar degeneration had an abnormal excitability build-up in M1 prior to movement onset as tested with TMS (Liepert et al., 1996) or with recordings of movement related cortical potentials (Wessel et al., 1994; Gerloff et al., 1996). This is supported by TMS experiments on pre-movement facilitation. In normal subjects TMS before voluntary movements (between the "go" signal and the onset of voluntary EMG activity) produces a facilitation of the MEP (pre-movement facilitation). This premovement facilitation is significantly decreased in patients with cerebellar disease (Nomura et al., 2001).

Intracortical inhibition and intracortical facilitation can be studied by using the technique of paired transcranial magnetic pulses (Kujirai et al., 1993; Liepert et al., 1998). In this technique the intensity of the first, conditioning stimulus is below the motor threshold, the intensity of the second test stimulus is suprathreshold and produces a MEP. Short interstimulus intervals of 1–4 ms suppress the ampitude of the test stimulus, longer interstimulus intervals of 8–20 ms induce a facilitation of the test stimulus response. Both, inhibitory as well as facilitory phenomena, are thought to be of cortical origin (Ziemann et al., 1996). Using this technique we performed a study with the aim to find out whether, by the use of cerebro-cerebellar interconnections, the excitatory state of M1 is changed in patients with cerebellar degeneration as compared to normal controls (Liepert et al., 1998; Wessel et al., 1999). The main finding was a significant impairment of facilitation in M1 in patients with cerebellar degeneration. Motor thresholds and intracortical inhibition phenomena in cerebellar patients were normal. The fact that in patients with cerebellar degeneration intracortical inhibition was normal, and intracortical facilitation was abnormal, indicates again that these phenomena are mediated independently by different neurons.

Pinto and Chen (2001) investigated conditioning magnetic stimulation of the cerebellum which in normal subjects reduces MEP amplitudes after motor cortex stimulation (test MEP) 5–8 ms later. Small test MEPs of about 0.5 mV were markedly inhibited at interstimulus intervals of 5–8 ms, but there was much less inhibition for test MEPs of about 2 mV. There was no significant MEP suppression during voluntary activation of the target muscle (first dorsal interosseus muscle) or during arm extension on the same side. Findings indicate that cerebellar stimulation has a much stronger effect on motor cortex neurons activated near threshold intensities than those activated at higher intensities. Activation of contralateral (to the stimulated hand area) but not ipsilateral arm muscles reduces the excitability of the cerebellothalamocortical projections to the motor cortex.

The deep cerebellar nuclei exert a tonic excitatory influence on the motor cortex. Inactivation of these neurons by stimulation of inhibitory Purkinje cells may suppress this effect. Cooling or a lesion of the dentate nucleus results in ataxia. Thus, a predominant dysfunction of the cerebellar nuclei could be assumed in patients with cerebellar degeneration. A reduction of the excitatory drive of cerebellar nuclei to the motor cortex might be the reason for the impairment of facilitation in patients with cerebellar degeneration. This may, in part, also explain some of the clinical symptoms in cerebellar disease such as delayed onset of movement and slowing of the velocity of motion. But, as pathological abnormalities in cerebellar degeneration are not restricted to cerebellar neurons, even if clinical signs of an extracerebellar involvement of the disease are lacking, it cannot completely be ruled out that other structures could contribute to the reduced facilitation. Although the transcranial magnetic double stimulation is supposed to reflect intracortical phenomena, additional effects from subcortical areas cannot be completely excluded.

If facilitory influences on the motor cortex are reduced, the equilibrium of inhibition and excitation may also be disturbed, resulting in a predominance of inhibitory phenomena. Such a dysbalance between inhibitory and excitatory phenomena could explain the prolongation of pI-S, which has been ascribed to enhanced inhibitory mechanisms in the motor cortex in the presence of cerebellar dysfunction (Wessel et al., 1996). pI-S in general is a complex phenomenon; the early portion is supposed to be due to spinal mechanisms and the late portion is mediated by supraspinal, presumably cortical mechanisms (Roick et al., 1993; Triggs et al., 1993). A relative disinhibition of inhibitory cortical interneurons could be the reason for a prolongation of pI-S in our patients.

2. Studies in relation to question 2

Recent investigations have demonstrated the cerebellar involvement in higher order tasks such as sensorimotor learning (Deuschl et al., 1996), classic conditioning (Topka et al., 1993) and cognitive functions (Schmahmann and Sherman, 1998). Most of these tasks involve the integration of sensory afferences in complex motor activities. The cerebellum has been regarded as an instrument for analysing somatosensory information in order to optimise movements, suggesting that it plays a role in the mechanisms of sensorimotor integration (Fellows et al., 2001). Using rTMS Théoret et al. (2001) studied the effect of transient disruption of the lateral or medial cerebellum on a paced-finger-tapping (PFT) task. The results show greater variability on the PFT task following a 5 min train of 1 Hz rTMS to the medial cerebellum. Magnetic stimulation of the lateral cerebellum or motor cortex, and sham stimulation, had no effect. These data show the causal link between activity in the medial cerebellum and the production of timed movements.

TMS has been shown to be a sensitive tool in studying sensorimotor integration. MEP facilitation and inhibition also depend upon proprioceptive (Komori et al., 1992) and cutaneous afferences (Tamburin et al., 2001). Stimulation of cutaneous afferences has an inhibitory effect on M1 excitability in TMS experiments in normal subjects (Tamburin et al., 2001). The effect of peripheral nerve stimulation on TMS has been investigated in patients with movement disorders, such as Parkinson's disease (Yokota et al., 1995), corticobasal degeneration (Strafella et al., 1997) and dystonia (Abbruzzese et al., 2001). Up to now there is no study on the conditioning effect of such peripheral nerve stimulation on M1 excitability in patients with cerebellar disease. Functional neuroimaging studies have shown multiple tactile projections to the cerebellum (Nitschke et al., 1998; Bushara et al., 2001), but failed to demonstrate cerebellar activation in response to proprioceptive stimulation (Fox et al., 1985; Mima et al., 1999). Therefore, in patients with cerebellar disease, it might in particular be interesting to study the effect of stimulating cutaneous afferences on M1 excitability in TMS experiments.

3. Studies in relation to question 3

Studies on TMS findings in patients with spinocerebellar ataxias have reported different and in part contradictory results (Wessel et al., 1993; Perretti et al., 1996; Abele et al., 1997; Schöls et al., 1997a, b; Yokota et al., 1998; Revisto et al., 2000). This is in part explained by the examination of different and also inhomogenous patient groups. Since many of the cerebellar diseases now can be classified on the basis of molecular genetic findings the question arises whether the different types of diseases can also be differentiated phenotypically on the basis of e.g. electrophysiological/neurophysiological, and in this context, TMS findings. Regarding this type of studies a special interest arose, whether the spino-cerebelar atrophy type 1 (SCA 1) can be differentiated from other SCA types (SCA 2, 3, 6) on the basis of TMS findings. Perretti et al. (1996) and Abele et al. (1997) found a prolonged CMCT or a lacking MEP in all patients with SCA 1 (10 years mean duration of the disease). The CMCT was prolonged in only few patients with SCA 2, 3, or 6. Schöls et al. (1997a, b) and Yokota et al. (1998) also found significantly increased CMCT times in SCA 1 patients without much overlap to the other SCA types. Revisto et al. (2000) on the other hand described prolonged CMCT times also in SCA 2 patients with a long duration of the disease (mean 17 years). Thus, CMCT findings in patients with SCA not only depend on the moleculargenetic classification of the disease, but in part also on the severity and duration of the disease.

Two recent studies examined the possible therapeutic effect of TMS over the cerebellum. There is some evidence that an overactivity of the cerebellum plays a role in the pathophysiology of essential tremor. Gironell et al. (2002) performed low-frequency rTMS over the cerebellum in patients with essential tremor and found a notable tremor improvement within 5 min after rTMS. And in patients with degenerative ataxic disorders Shiga et al. (2002) found that a session of several single pulse TMSs over the cerebellum on 21 consecutive days improved truncal ataxia.

References

Abbruzzese, G., Marchese, R., Buccolieri, A., Gasparetto, B. and Trompetto, C. Abnormalities of sensorimotor integration in focal dystonia. A transcranial magnetic stimulation study. *Brain*, 2001, 124: 537–545.

Abele, M., Burk, K., Andres, F., Topka, H., Laccone, F., Bosch, S., Brice, A., Cancel, G. and Dichgans, J. Autosomal dominant cerebellar ataxia type I. Nerve conduction and evoked potential studies in families with SCA1, SCA2, and SCA3. *Brain*, 1997, 120: 2141–2148.

Bushara, K.O., Wheat, J.M., Khan, A., Mock, B.J., Turski, P.A. and Sorenson, J. et al. Multiple tactile maps in the human cerebellum. *NeuroReport*, 2001, 12: 2483–2486.

Deuschl, G., Toro, G., Zeffiro, T., Massaquoi, S. and Hallett, M. Adaptation motor learning of arm movements in patients with cerebellar disease. *J. Neurol. Neurosurg. Psychiat.*, 1996, 60: 515–519.

Fellows, S.J., Ernst, J., Schwarz, M., Topper, R. and Noth, J. Precision grip deficits in cerebellar disorders in man. *Clin. Neurophysiol.*, 2001, 112: 1793–1802.

Fox, P.T., Raichle, M.E. and Thach, W.T. Functional mapping of the human cerebellum with positron emission tomography. *Proc. Natl. Acad. Sci. USA*, 1985, 82: 7462–7466.

Gerloff, C., Altenmüller, E. and Dichgans, J. Disintegration and reorganization of cortical motor processing in two patients with cerebellar stroke. *Electroenceph. Clin. Neurophysiol.*, 1996, 98: 59–68.

Gerschlager, W., Christensen, L.O., Bestmann, S. and Rothwell, J.C. rTMS over the cerebellum can increase corticospinal excitability through a spinal mechanism involving activation of peripheral nerve fibres. *Clin. Neurophysiol.*, 2002, 113: 1435–1440.

Gironell, A., Kulisevski, J., Lorenzo, J., Barbanoj, M., Pascual-Sedano, B. and Otermin, P. Transcranial magnetic stimulation of the cerebellum in essential tremor: a controlled study. *Arch. Neurol.*, 2002, 59: 413–417.

Komori, T., Watson, B. and Brown, W. Influence of peripheral afference on cortical and spinal motoneuron excitability. *Muscle Nerve*, 1992, 15: 48–51.

Kujirai, T., Caramia, M.D. and Rothwell, J.C. Corticocortical inhibition in human motor cortex. *J. Physiol.*, 1993, 471: 501–519

Liepert, J., Wassermann, E.M., Cohen, L.G., Samii, A. and Hallett, M. Motor cortex excitability and reaction time in cerebellar degeneration. *Electroenceph. Clin. Neurophysiol.*, 1996, 99: 392.

Liepert, J., Classen, J., Cohen, L.G., Hallett, M. Task-dependent changes of intracortical inhibition. *Exp. Brain Res.*, 1998, 118: 421–426

Mally, J., and Stone, T.W. Transcranial magnetic stimulation alleviates truncal ataxia in spinocerebellar degeneration. *J. Neurol. Neurosurg. Psychiat.*, 2002, 72: 124–126.

Matsuda, H., Yagishita, A. and Tsuji, S. Transcranial magnetic stimulation alleviates truncal ataxia in spinocerebellar degeneration. *J. Neurol. Neurosurg. Psychiat.*, 2002, 72: 124–126.

Meyer, B.U., Röricht, S. and Machetanz, J. Reduction of corticospinal excitability by magnetic stimulation over the cerebellum in patients with large defects of one cerebellar hemisphere. *Electroenceph. Clin. Neurophysiol.*, 1994, 93: 372–379.

Mima, T., Sadato, N., Yazawa, S., Hanakawa, T., Fukuyama, H., Yonekura, Y. et al. Brain structures related to active and passive finger movements in man. *Brain*, 1999, 122: 1989–1997.

Nitschke, M.F., Hahn, C., Melchert, U.H., Handels, H. and Wessel, K. Activation of the cerebellum by sensory finger stimulation and by finger opposition movements. A functional magnetic resonance imaging study. *J. Neuroimaging.*, 1998, 8: 127–131.

Nomura, T., Takeshima, T. and Nakashima, K. Reduced pre-movement facilitation of motor evoked potentials in spinocerebellar degeneration. *J. Neurol. Sci.*, 2001, 187: 41–47.

Okabe, S., Hanajima, R., Ohnishi, T., Nishikawa, M., Imabayashi, E., Takano, H., Kawachi, T., Matsuda, H., Shiio, Y., Iwata, N.K., Furubayashi, T., Terao, Y. and Ugawa, Y. Funktional connectivity revealed by single-photon emission computed tomography (SPECT) during repetitive transcranial magnetic stimulation (rTMS) of the motor cortex. *Clin. Neurophysiol.*, 2003, 114: 450–457.

Pascual-Leone, A., Rubio, B. and Pallardo, F. Transcranial magnetic stimulation alleviates truncal ataxia in spinocerebellar degeneration. *J. Neurol. Neurosurg. Psychiat.*, 2002, 72: 124–126.

Perretti, A., Santoro, L., Lanzillo, B., Filla, A., De Michele, G., Barbieri, F., Martino, G., Ragno, M., Cocozza, S. and Caruso, G. Autosomal dominant cerebellar ataxia type I: multimodal electrophysiological study and comparison between SCA1 and SCA2 patients. *J. Neurol. Sci.*, 1996, 142: 45–53.

Pinto, A.D. and Chen, R. Suppression of the motor cortex by magnetic stimulation of the cerebellum. *Exp. Brain Res.*, 2001, 140: 505–510.

Restivo, D.A., Giuffrida, S., Rapisarda, G., Antonuzuo, A., Saponara, R., Reggio, A., Trovato, S., Raffaele, R., Domina, E., Trovato, A., Condorelli, D.F. and Pennisi, G. Central motor conduction to lower limb after transcranial magnetic stimulation in spinocerebellar ataxia type 2 (SCA2). *Clin. Neurophysiol.*, 2000, 111: 630–635.

Roick, H., Von Giessen, H.J. and Benecke, R. On the origin of the post-excitatory inhibition seen after transcranial magnetic brain stimulation in awake human subjects. *Exp. Brain Res.*, 1993, 94: 489–498.

Schmahmann, J.D. and Sherman, J.C. The cerebellar cognitive affective syndrome. *Brain*, 1998, 121: 561–579.

Schöls, L., Amoiridis, G., Büttner, T., Przuntek, H., Epplen, J.T. and Riess, O. Autosomal dominant cerebellar ataxia: phenotypic differences in genetically defined subtypes? *Ann. Neurol.*, 1997a, 42: 924–932.

Schöls, L., Amoiridis, G., Langkafel, M., Schöls, S. and Przuntek, H. Motor evoked potentials in the spinocerebellar ataxias type 1 and type 3. *Muscle Nerve*, 1997b, 20: 226–228.

Shiga, Y., Tsuda, T., Itoyama, Y., Shimizu, H., Miyazawa, K.I., Jin, K. and Yamazaki, T. Transcranial magnetic stimulation alleviates truncal ataxia in spinocerebellar degeneration. *J. Neurol. Neurosurg. Psychiat.*, 2002, 72: 124–126.

Strafella, A., Ashby, P. and Lang, A.E. Reflex myoclonus in corticobasal ganglionic degeneration involves a transcortical pathway. *Mov. Discord.*, 1997, 12: 360–369.

Tamburin, S., Manganotti, P., Zanette, G. and Fiaschi, A. Cutaneomotor integration in human hand motor areas: somatotopic effect and interaction of afferents. *Exp. Brain Res.*, 2001, 141: 232–241.

Théoret, H., Haque, J. and Pascual-Leone, A. Increased variability of paced finger tapping accuracy following repetitive magnetic stimulation of the cerebellum in humans. *Neurosci. Lett.*, 2001, 306: 29–32.

Topka, H., Valls-Sole, J., Massaquoi, S.G. and Hallett, M. Deficit in classical conditioning in patients with cerebellar degeneration. *Brain*, 1993, 116: 961–969.

Triggs, W.J., Cros, D., Macdonell, R.A.L., Chiappa, K.H., Fang, J. and Day, B.J. Cortical and spinal motor excitability during the transcranial magnetic stimulation silent period in humans. *Brain Res.*, 1993, 628: 39–48.

Ugawa, Y., Day, B.L., Rothwell, J.C., Thompson, P.D., Merton, P.A. and Marsden, C.D. Modulation of motor cortex excitability by electrical stimulation over the cerebellum in man. *J. Physiol.*, 1991, 93: 225–229.

Ugawa, Y., Genba-Shimizu, K., Rothwell, J.C., Iwata, M. and Kanazawa, I. Supression of motor cortical excitability by electrical stimulation over the cerebellum in ataxie. *Ann. Neurol.*, 1994a, 36: 225–229.

Ugawa, Y., Hanajima, R. and Kanazawa, I. Motor cortex inhibition in patients with ataxia. *Electroenceph. Clin. Neurophysiol.* 1994b, 93: 225–229.

Van Giesen, H.J., Roick, H. and Benecke, R. Inhibitory actions of motor cortex following unilateral brain lesions as studied by magnetic brain stimulation. Exp *Brain Res.*, 1994, 99: 84–96.

Wessel, K., Huss, G.P., Brückmann, H. and Kömpf, D. Follow-up of neurophysiological tests and CT in late-onset cerebellar ataxia and multiple system atrophy. *J. Neurol.*, 1993, 240: 168–176.

Wessel, K., Verleger, R., Nazarenus, D., Vieregge, P. and Kömpf, D. Movement-related cortical potentials preceding sequential and goaldirected arm and finger movements in patients with cerebellar atrophy. *Electroenceph. Clin. Neurophysiol.*, 1994, 92: 331–341.

Wessel, K., Tegenthoff, M., Vorgerd, M., Otto, V., Nitschke, M. F. and Malin, J.-P. Enhancement of inhibitory mechanisms in the motor cortex of patients with cerebellar degeneration: a study with transcranial magnetic brain stimulation. *Electroenceph Clin Neurophysiol.*, 1996, 101: 273–280.

Yokota, T., Saito, Y. and Shimizu, Y. Increased corticomotoneural excitability after peripheral nerve stimulation in DOPA non responsive hemiparkinsonism. *J. Neurol. Sci.*, 1995, 129: 34–39.

Yokota, T., Sasaki, H., Iwabuchi, K., Schiojiri, T., Yoshino, A., Otagiri, A., Inaba, A. and Yuasa, T. Electrophysiological features of central motor conduction in spinocerebellar atrophy type 1, type 2, and Machado-Joseph desease. *J. Neurol. Neurosurg. Psychiat.* 1998, 65: 530–534.

Ziemann, U., Rothwell, J.C. and Ridding, M.C. Interaction between intracortical inhibition and facilitation in human motor cortex. *J. Physiol.*, 1996, 496: 873–881.

Subject Index